Lung Cancer Rehabilitation

Lung Cancer Rehabilitation

Edited by

ADRIAN CRISTIAN, MD MHCM FAAPMR
Chief
Cancer Rehabilitation
Miami Cancer Institute
Miami, Florida

ELSEVIER

Lung Cancer Rehabilitation   ISBN: 978-0-323-83404-9

Notices

Publisher: Sarah E. Barth
Acquisitions Editor: Humayra R. Khan
Editorial Project Manager: Barbara L. Makinster
Project Manager: Kiruthika Govindaraju
Cover Designer: Christian Bilbow

3251 Riverport Lane
St. Louis, Missouri 63043

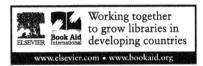

Working together to grow libraries in developing countries

www.elsevier.com • www.bookaid.org

This book is dedicated to

My wife Eliane, children Alexander and Chloe for their constant support, inspiration, and love, Steluta and Cali Cristian and Rasela Cru for their exceptional strength, grace, and wisdom, Randi Lynn Zuller for her extraordinary encouragement and unwavering support, Daniela Spector and Vivian Brash for their optimism and dedication to family, Drs. Mark Hupart and Alexis Renta Torres for their life-long friendship, my patients, teachers, and students who have enriched my professional journey in medicine.

List of Contributors

Elisa Alpert, MD
Department of Physical Medicine and Rehabilitation
Northwell Health
Manhasset, NY, United States

Haley R. Appel, PA-C, MMS
Miami Cancer Institute
Miami, FL, United States

Jennifer Baima, MD
Associate Professor
University of Massachusetts Medical school
Worcester, MA, United States

Kimberly Bancroft, PhD
Clinical Psychologist
Mary Free Bed Rehabilitation Hospital
Holland, MI, United States

Betty Chernack, MD
Perelman School of Medicine
University of Pennsylvania
Philadelphia, PA, United States

Ady M. Correa-Mendoza, MD
Cancer Rehabilitation Fellow, PGY-5
Physical Medicine & Rehabilitation
University of Miami/Jackson Memorial Hospital
Miami, FL, United States

Adrian Cristian, MD, MHCM
Chief
Cancer Rehabilitation
Miami Cancer Institute
Miami, FL, United States

Christian M. Custodio, MD
Attending Physiatrist
Memorial Sloan Kettering Cancer Center
Associate Clinical Professor
Weill Cornell Medicine

Chanel Davidoff, DO
Resident Physician
Department of Physical Medicine & Rehabilitation
Donald and Barbara Zucker School of Medicine at
    Hofstra/Northwell Health
Manhasset, NY, United States

Monica Diaz, RD/LDN, CPT
Miami Cancer Institute
Miami, FL, United States

J. Anthony Garcia, DO
PGY-2 Resident
Department of Physical Medicine and Rehabilitation
Donald and Barbara Zucker School of Medicine at
    Hofstra/Northwell Health
Manhasset, NY, United States

Alexandra I. Gundersen, MD
Harvard Medical School
Boston, MA, United States

Spaulding Rehabilitation Hospital
Department of Physical Medicine and Rehabilitation
Boston, MA, United States;

Massachusetts General Hospital
Boston, MA, United States

Sherry Hite, MOT, OTR/L
Manager of Occupational Therapy
Department of Rehabilitation
City of Hope Medical Center
Duarte, CA, United States

Naomi M. Kaplan, MBBS
Attending Physician
Mary Free Bed Rehabilitation Hospital
Grand Rapids, MI, United States

Clinical Assistant Professor
Michigan State University College of Human Medicine
Grand Rapids, MI, United States

Ben Kestenbaum, DO
Resident Physician
Larkin Community Hospital
Miami, FL, United States

Vinita Khanna, LCSW, MPH, ACHP-SW, OSW-C
Manager of Clinical Social Work
Department of Clinical Social Work
Keck Hospital of USC/USC Norris Comprehensive
    Cancer Center
Los Angeles, CA, United States

Lynn Kim, OTD, OTR/L
Lead Occupational Therapist
Department of Rehabilitation
City of Hope Medical Center
Duarte, CA, United States

Sasha E. Knowlton, MD
Harvard Medical School
Boston, MA, United States

Spaulding Rehabilitation Hospital
Department of Physical Medicine and Rehabilitation
Boston, MA, United States

Massachusetts General Hospital
Boston, MA, United States

Franchesca König, MD
Assistant Attending
Neurology - Division of Rehabilitation Medicine
Memorial Sloan Kettering Cancer Center
New York, NY, United States

Assistant Attending
Physical Medicine & Rehabilitation
Weill Cornell Medical Center
New York, NY, United States

Rupesh Kotecha, MD
Chief of Radiosurgery
Department of Radiation Oncology
Miami Cancer Institute
Baptist Health South Florida
Miami, FL, United States

Department of Radiation Oncology
Herbert Wertheim College of Medicine
Florida International University
Miami, FL, United States

Department of Translational Medicine
Herbert Wertheim College of Medicine
Florida International University
Miami, FL, United States

Susan Maltser, DO
Vice-Chair and Associate Professor
Department of Physical Medicine and Rehabilitation
Zucker School of Medicine at Hofstra/Northwell
Hempstead, NY, United States

Chair and Medical Director
Department of Physical Medicine and Rehabilitation
Glen Cove Hospital
Glen Cove, NY, United States

Director, Cancer Rehabilitation
Rehabilitation Service Line
Northwell Health
New York, NY, United States

Genevieve Marshall, DO
Resident Physician
Physical Medicine & Rehabilitation
Northwell Health
Manhasset, NY, United States

Patrick Martone, DO
Assistant Professor
Department of Physical Medicine and Rehabilitation
Donald and Barbara Zucker School of Medicine at
    Hofstra/Northwell Health
Bay Shore, NY, United States

Suleyki Medina, MD
Palliative Medicine Attending
Symptom Management and Palliative Medicine
Miami Cancer Institute
Baptist Health South Florida
Miami, FL, United States

Assistant Professor
Florida International University
Herbert Wertheim College of Medicine
    (FIU-HWCOM)
Miami, FL, United States

Diana Molinares, MD
Assistant Professor
Physical Medicine and Rehabilitation
University of Miami Miller School of Medicine
Miami, FL, United States

Cancer Rehabilitation Medicine Director
Physical Medicine and Rehabilitation
Sylvester Comprehensive Cancer Center
Miami, FL, United States

Lindsay M. Niccolai, PhD
Department of Supportive Care Medicine
Moffitt Cancer Center
Tampa, FL, United States

Hanna Oh, MD
Assistant Professor
Department of Rehabilitation
University of Washington
School of Medicine
Seattle, WA, United States

Medical Director of Cancer Rehabilitation
Rehabilitation Medicine
Seattle Cancer Care Alliance
Seattle, WA, United States

Romer B. Orada, DO
Miami Cancer Institute
Baptist Health South Florida
Miami, FL, United States

Jesuel Padro-Guzman, MD
Assistant Attending
Neurology, Memorial Sloan Kettering
New York, NY, United States

Assistant Professor
Rehabilitation Medicine
Weill Cornell Medical College
New York, NY, United States

Amy K. Park, DO
Resident Physician
Department of Physical Medicine & Rehabilitation
Zucker School of Medicine at Hofstra/Northwell
Manhasset, NY, United States

Christina Paul, MD
Fellow
Memorial Sloan Kettering Cancer Center

Jennie L. Rexer, PhD
Department of Neuro-Oncology
Section of Neuropsychology
The University of Texas MD Anderson
    Cancer Center
Houston, TX, United States

Muni Rubens, MD, PhD
Miami Cancer Institute
Miami, FL, United States

Lisa Marie Ruppert, MD
Associate Attending
Rehabilitation Medicine Service-Department of
    Neurology
Memorial Sloan Kettering Cancer Center
New York, NY, United States

Assistant Professor
Department of Rehabilitation Medicine
Weill Cornell Medical College
New York, NY, United States

Eileen R. Slavin, DO, MPH
Physical Medicine and Rehabilitation Fellow
Larkin Community Hospital
Miami, FL, United States

Jordan Stumph, MD
Resident Physician
New York Presbytarian/Weill Cornell Medical Center
New York, NY, United States

Dominique Symonette, MS, RD/LDN, CNSC
Miami Cancer Institute
Miami, FL, United States

Suzanne Gutiérrez Teissonniere, MD
Assistant Attending
Rehabilitation Medicine
Department of Neurology
Memorial Sloan Kettering Cancer Center
New York, NY, United States

Assistant Professor
Rehabilitation Medicine
Weill Cornell Medicine
New York, NY, United States

Martin C. Tom, MD
Radiation Oncologist
Department of Radiation Oncology
Miami Cancer Institute
Baptist Health South Florida
Miami, FL, United States

Department of Radiation Oncology
Herbert Wertheim College of Medicine
Florida International University
Miami, FL, United States

Raees Tonse, MD
Research Fellow
Department of Radiation Oncology
Miami Cancer Institute
Baptist Health South Florida
Miami, FL, United States

Alexander G. Watson, MD, MBA
Department of Physical Medicine and Rehabilitation
University of Pittsburgh Medical Center
Pittsburgh, PA, United States

Vanessa Monique Yanez, MSOT, OTR/L
Contributing Faculty
University of St. Augustine
Health Sciences
Austin, TX, United States

Jasmine Zheng, MD
Perelman School of Medicine
University of Pennsylvania
Philadelphia, PA, United States

Preface

According to the American Cancer Society, lung cancer is the second most common cancer in both men and women. The lifetime risk of developing lung cancer is about 1:15 for men and 1:17 for women and 541,000 people in the United States have at some point in their lives been diagnosed with lung cancer. Lung cancer is most often diagnosed in more advanced stages of disease, and in adults over the age of 65.[1] In this older population, age-related changes as well as the presence of other medical diagnoses such heart disease, diabetes mellitus, and emphysema make it more challenging for those affected to tolerate lung cancer treatments. Lung cancer treatment often consists of chemotherapy, radiation therapy, surgery and immunotherapy, and each of these can be associated with a range of adverse effects that can contribute to the development of physical impairments. These impairments can adversely affect physical function and quality of life. It is important to identify those individuals at risk for development of cancer and cancer-related physical and psychological impairments as well as those whom have already developed them, and initiate treatments as early as possible.

The rehabilitation of the person with lung cancer often requires a multidisciplinary team approach by clinicians whose goal is to improve quality of life and minimize loss of function in individuals with lung cancer. Ideally, this team works closely with the oncology treatment team in a variety of settings such as inpatient, outpatient, and the patient's home using a proactive approach to identify and treat physical and psychological impairments.

This book is meant to provide the reader with a holistic and integrative approach to the care of the person with lung cancer. It contains information on the epidemiology, staging, and treatment of lung cancer as well as the evaluation and treatment of common cancer and cancer treatment–related physical and psychological impairments.

I want to thank the authors for their important contributions to this book. My hope is that readers of this text will use this knowledge to provide compassionate and effective care that will enhance the quality of life of those affected by lung cancer.

Adrian Cristian MD MHCM FAAPMR
Miami Cancer Institute
Miami, Florida, USA

REFERENCE

1. American Cancer Society. *Cancer Facts and Figures 21021*. Atlanta: American Cancer Society; 2020.

Contents

An Overview of the Epidemiology, Types of Lung Cancer, Staging, and Rehabilitation Continuum of Care

ALEXANDER G. WATSON, MD, MBA • ROMER B. ORADA, DO

EPIDEMIOLOGY

Lung cancer incidence and prevalence trends have evolved due to changes in screening and primary prevention, while early detection and improved treatments increase survivorship. Data from 2012[1] report that providers are annually diagnosing approximately 1.8 million new cases of lung cancer with 1.6 million related deaths. In developed countries, the age standardized risk (ASR) of incidence and mortality was 1.4−1.5-fold higher and 1.5−1.8 fold higher, respectively, than in less developed countries. ASR is used for comparing rates between populations in diseases for which age contributes significantly to risk.[2]

Within the United States, most cases of lung cancer are attributable to exposures like tobacco smoke, asbestos, and radon. Although incidence declined in the United States from 2007 to 2016, there are still approximately 150,000 annual lung cancer deaths.[3] The rate of incidence decline varies based on age, sex, and geographic status. For individuals 55 years and older, rates were highest in men from nonmetropolitan counties. In individuals 35−54 years old, there were no sex differences in incidence, but the same nonmetropolitan geographic predominance persisted. This difference appears to be growing as rates decline in both men and women from metropolitan areas faster than nonmetropolitan areas.

RACIAL/ETHNIC DIFFERENCES

When not adjusting for smoking status, African American and Native Hawaiian men had the highest incidence of lung cancer of 252.1 per 100,000 individuals.[4] For women, incidence was similar among African Americans, Native Hawaiians, and whites, with 146.8, 167.4, and 135.1 individuals per 100,000,

respectively. For all lung cancer types, Japanese American and Latino individuals had significantly lower risk than African Americans, with relative risks ranging from 0.36 (95% CI = 0.33 to 0.45) for Latino women to 0.59 (95% CI = 0.52 to 0.65) for Japanese-American men. Native Hawaiians had a much higher rate of developing small cell lung cancer (SCLC) than any other group, and African Americans had the highest incidence of nonsmall cell lung cancer (NSCLC).

Smoking dramatically increases excess relative risk (ERR) relative to nonsmokers in a dose-dependent relationship when stratified by 25 pack-years versus 50 pack-years.[4] ERR for all types of lung cancer in the 25 pack-years subgroup increases to 21.9 (Native Hawaiian), 19.1 (African American), 11.9 (White), 10.1 (Japanese American), and 8 (Latino) with the highest proportion being SCLC and squamous cell carcinomas (SCCs). In the 50 pack-years group, ERR for all lung cancer subtypes increased to 35.3 (Native Hawaiian), 31.7 (AA), 24.0 (White), 21.4 (Japanese American), and 20.0 (Latino). Similarly, the greatest increases in risk were for developing SCLC and squamous cell.

SCREENING

Researchers have attempted to identify the best method and frequency of lung cancer screening. The National Lung Screening Trial (NLST)[5] aimed to determine if low-dose helical computed tomography (LDCT) could screen for lung cancer and reduce mortality. Patients with substantial (30+ pack-years) and recent/current smoking histories were included; former smokers must have quit within the previous 15 years. Study participants underwent three screenings using either radiography or LDCT (T0, T1, and T2) at 1-year intervals, with the first screening (T0) soon after the time of randomization. All-cause mortality in the LDCT group was reduced by 6.7% (95% CI, 1.2 to 13.6; $P = .02$) relative to the radiography group; however, 96.4% of the positive screening results in the low-dose CT group and 94.5% in the radiography group were false positives.

After a median of 6.5 years of follow-up, the LDCT participants sustained a significant reduction in lung cancer mortality,[6] replicating and demonstrating the durability of the initial NLST findings. Therefore, the 3.3% absolute risk reduction (ARR) did not suggest a length time bias of distant cases caught earlier but instead suggested screening with LDCT likely prevented additional deaths.

SUBTYPES OF LUNG CANCER

"Lung cancer" comprises malignancies in the trachea, bronchus, and lung. Certain subtypes have greater associations with smoking than others, and evolving trends in subtype incidence may be the result of changes in tobacco consumption amount or delivery.[7] Classification designations have changed over time, as previously, lung cancer was mainly divided into two major histologic groups based on World Health Organization (WHO) guidelines. Cancers were designated either SCLC or NSCLC, which includes SCC, large cell carcinoma, and adenocarcinoma.[8]

In 2015, the WHO modified these classifications.[9] Improvement in genetic testing of tumor cells provided a strong foundation for reclassification of SCC, adenocarcinoma, and large cell carcinoma, and targeted medicines make these classifications more clinically relevant. New concepts in adenocarcinoma classification including lepidic versus invasive pattern designations impact the approach to tumor size measurement for Tumor, Node, Metastasis (TNM) staging of small tumors $\leq$3 cm, which determines the surgical management of patients. Now, pathology includes histologic pattern descriptions such as lepidic, acinar, papillary, micropapillary, and solid.

With SCC, descriptions include morphologic details such as unequivocal keratinization and well-formed classical bridges. For both adenocarcinoma and SCC, when pathologists cannot clearly differentiate by simple microscopy, at least one immunohistochemical stain is used to classify the tumor and, for adenocarcinoma, rule out the potential for it being a metastasis from different site. Tumors that do not resemble squamous cell or adenocarcinoma under microscopy or staining are designated non-small cell carcinoma (NSCC) since metastasis cannot be ruled out. If the tumor expresses pneumocyte markers, the designation is "NSCC favor adenocarcinoma," and should be specified as "NSCC

favor squamous cell carcinoma" when expressing SCC markers. Additionally, other IHC stains such as hormonal staining could add specificity beyond NSCC not otherwise specified (NOS).

Beyond the IHC descriptions, adenocarcinoma is designated in situ[9] versus minimally invasive if:

ADENOCARCINOMA

In situ:	Minimally Invasive:
3 cm or smaller	Predominantly lepidic growth with invasive component measuring at most 0.5 cm in greatest dimension within any one focus.
Solitary tumor	Cell type of tumor is mostly nonmucinous, but rarely can be mucinous.
Demonstrates pure lepidic growth with no invasion of stroma/vascular/pleural structures or air spaces, and no pattern of invasive adenocarcinoma subtypes such as acinar, papillary, micropapillary, solid, colloid, enteric, fetal, or invasive mucinous adenocarcinoma Cells are mostly nonmucinous Nuclear atypia is absent/inconspicuous nuclear atypia Common septal widening with sclerosis/elastosis	The invasive component is any histologic subtype other than lepidic pattern and cells infiltrating myofibroblastic stroma cannot invade lymphatics, blood vessels, air spaces*, or pleura, and cannot contain tumor necrosis or spread through air spaces.

* May spread through air spaces if micropapillary clusters, solid nests, or single cells beyond the tumor edge into air spaces in lung parenchyma.

The updated recommendations discontinued the use of the "small cell" subtype of SCC due to the confusion with SCLC. "Clear cell" is now recognized as a cytologic feature that may occur in other subtypes. The remaining recognized subtypes include keratinizing, nonkeratinizing, and basaloid.

In neuroendocrine tumors, many unique features of carcinoid (nonlarge cell neuroendocrine) tumors differentiate them from higher-grade small cell carcinoma and large cell neuroendocrine carcinomas. These typically carry better prognoses, are less associated with smoking, occur in younger populations, and, unlike SCLC and LCNEC, have fewer genetic abnormalities.[10] The most important criterion for differentiating carcinoid subtypes from high-grade SCLC or LCNEC is the mitotic rate, and the presence of necrosis is important to consider as SCLC/LCNEC has higher mitotic rates with greater necrosis.[11]

Small Cell Lung Cancer

The prototypical patient with SCLC is a male current/past heavy smoker over 70 years old with other cardiopulmonary comorbidities,[12] although literature has documented rare cases in never smokers.[13] Symptom onset is rapid either due to intrathoracic growth, distant spread, or paraneoplastic syndromes.[12]

Likely, given the association with smoking and due to the decline in smoking rates in industrialized nations,[14] annual incidence of SCLC has been declining over the past 30 years. SCLC is often clinically suspected from presenting signs and symptoms, but pathology/cytology is required to confirm. Using bronchoscopy or fine-needle aspiration, providers retrieve a sample from the primary tumor, lymph nodes, or other metastatic sites. A bronchial biopsy, cytologic brushing, or sputum samples may result in a false negative, because the tumor grows under the mucosal surface.[12] Chest radiography will demonstrate predominantly central and bulky tumors. SCLC metastasizes early to the brain, liver, adrenals, and bone[15,16] but also has a high response rates to chemotherapy.[12]

The most typical symptoms associated with SCLC are cough/wheeze, dyspnea, and hemoptysis caused by local intrapulmonary tumor growth as well as effects of intrathoracic spread to the superior vena cava (SVC), chest wall, or esophagus causing recurrent laryngeal nerve palsy, and pain, fatigue, or anorexia.[16] Additionally, remote symptoms due to distant spread and paraneoplastic syndromes are more common with SCLC than NSCLC.[15] With local invasion of the SVC, tumors may elicit an SVC syndrome, which most commonly occurs with SCLC.[17] Symptoms will be swelling of the face, neck, and upper extremity with dyspnea/cough, although these may be confounded by other effects of the tumor. Due to obstruction of flow into the SVC, approximately one third of cases may have visibly dilated vasculature on the chest.[17]

Pancoast syndrome/tumors or superior pulmonary sulcus tumors occur due to local invasion of the lower trunk of the brachial plexus and typically present with pain in the arm that radiates proximally/superiorly to the head and neck or inferiorly/distally to the medial scapula, the axilla and anterior chest, or the ipsilateral arm favoring the distribution of the ulnar nerve.[18] With invasion of the adjacent stellate ganglion, the patient may demonstrate Horner's Syndrome with ipsilateral myosis, ptosis, anhidrosis, and enophthalmos. These tumors are typically adenocarcinoma or SCC; very rarely these tumors will be SCLC.[19]

NEUROLOGIC SYNDROMES

The variety of paraneoplastic neurologic syndromes (PNSs) is too extensive to cover thoroughly considering that fewer than 1% of patients with cancer will develop any of the potential manifestations,[20] although rates are higher in SCLC at approximately 3%−5%.[21] Typically, PNSs are progressive and debilitating within weeks to months.[22] The higher incidence in SCLC is due to tumors' expression of various antigens and patients' development of targeted antibodies. For example, approximately 20% of patients with SCLC have detectable levels of circulating antibodies targeting the Hu protein, which is also a normal component of neurons.[23] Some cases suggest a favorable prognosis with anti-Hu antibody-related PNS, as the targeted immune response has even resulted in spontaneous regression of the tumor.[24−26] Often, treating the underlying malignancy improves symptoms of PNS.[27] Immunosuppressives may also temporarily improve symptoms,[28] but without lasting effect.

These unique paraneoplastic syndromes and local structural impacts are relevant to rehabilitation specialists as they may result in impairments that therapies should target or restrictions around which therapies must be designed. Moreover, understanding the etiology of progressive weakness, worsening pain, or a new-onset movement disorder may provide an accurate diagnosis when imaging may be negative. This would allow for targeted workup instead of wasting resources and delaying rehabilitation.

Encephalomyelitis is a classical PNS which includes subacute cerebellar degeneration (SCD), myelitis, brainstem encephalitis, and limbic encephalitis.[29,30] Cases of SCD have been documented in SCC and SCLC,[31−33] and the same antibodies associated with Lambert−Eaton Myasthenic Syndrome (antibodies to voltage gated calcium channels) are present in a significant percentage of SCD cases.[34] Lambert−Eaton Myasthenic Syndrome, almost always associated with SCLC and rarely with NSCLC,[35,36] is a neuromuscular junction disorder in which antibodies impair calcium release in the presynaptic neuron with hallmark proximal muscle weakness that improves with activity and autonomic changes such as dry mouth or constipation.[37,38]

Opsoclonus-myoclonus, like LEMS, is predominantly associated with SCLC but has been reported in patients with NSCLC.[39] This disorder is characterized by rapid, randomly directed conjugate eye movements (opsoclonus) with myoclonus occurring in muscles of the head/neck, trunk, and limbs.[40] Subacute sensory neuropathy is often characterized by subacute/asymmetric numbness and/or a stocking-glove distribution of pain29,41,42. Chronic gastrointestinal pseudoobstruction is autonomic dysfunction with symptoms of nausea/vomiting, gastroparesis, and constipation without mechanical obstruction often seen in SCLC but has been documented in NSCLC.[43,44]

In cases of polymyositis and dermatomyositis associated with lung cancer,[45] SCLC (29%) and SCC (21%) were the most common types[46]; both are myopathic disorders, and dermatomyositis also features distinct cutaneous findings. Some patients that have recovered from cancer and dermatomyositis may have reactivation of the dermatomyositis without cancer recurrence.[47] "Stiff-man syndrome" (SMS) (with many variants) is characterized by skeletal muscle stiffness and spasms seen in patients with SCLC. SMS is associated with antiglutamic acid decarboxylase antibodies in cerebrospinal fluid or serum, symptoms of continuous muscle activity in trunk, and proximal limb muscles, and heightened reflexes.[48] Patients with lung cancer (often SCLC[49]) may develop movement disorders such as classic symmetric choreoathetosis involving the muscles of the neck, trunk, and limbs, although some patients may have unilateral presentation of chorea, dystonia, or orobuccal dyskinesia.[48]

Additional PNSs include the following:
- Acute necrotizing myopathy
- Syndromes of the peripheral nervous system
- Syndromes of the neuromuscular junction and muscle (including myasthenia gravis)
- Guillain–Barre syndrome
- Acute pandysautonomia
- Acquired neuromyotonia
- Acute sensorimotor neuropathy
- Brachial neuritis
- Subacute/chronic sensorimotor neuropathies
- Neuropathy and paraproteinaemia
- Neuropathy with vasculitis
- Autonomic neuropathies
- Optic neuritis
- Cancer-associated retinopathy
- Melanoma-associated retinopathy
- Necrotizing myelopathy
- Motor neuron diseases

RHEUMATOLOGIC CONDITIONS

Hypertrophic pulmonary osteoarthropathy (HPO) is a constellation of symptoms including symmetric polyarthritis, periostitis of long tubular bones, and clubbing of fingers that is associated with pulmonary disorders—not exclusively lung cancer[50]). At least 70% of HPO cases are associated with lung cancer, typically NSCLC[51]; alternatively, cases of HPO are rare in lung cancer. The hallmark symptom of HPO is periostitis, often the tibia or fibula, but may include any tubular bone.[50] Possibly related to the noninflammatory etiology, NSAIDs have only modest effect on pain. Like other paraneoplastic syndromes, one of the most effective treatments for HPO is to treat the underlying malignancy,[52,53] and other treatments include bisphosphonates,[54–56] octreotide,[57,58] and gefitinib.[59]

DETERMINING PROGNOSIS

Although the oncologist will likely be primary in providing prognostic information to the patient, rehabilitation practitioners benefit in being able to determine general prognosis to aid in goal setting and discharge planning. The first consideration of establishing prognosis is designating the patient's malignancy SCLC or NSCLC.

In NSCLC, prognostic information is predominantly based off initial staging using the TNM classification.[60] TNM staging categorizes tumors based on primary tumor characteristics (T), regional lymph node involvement (N), and metastases (M). Presently, molecular features of lung cancer tumors are not included in the TNM system. The ultimate stage (I through IV) is determined by the combination of T, N, and M descriptors. Metastatic sites such as skin, liver, and four or more sites carry particularly worse prognostic weight.[61] Previous racial associations between worse outcomes with NSCLC and African descent have been discounted after rigorous multivariate analysis[62] demonstrated the association was the result of socioeconomic and performance status. Important survival factors include performance status (baseline functional status), which is the greatest nonstaging factor,[63,64] smoking status,[65] and anorexia/weight loss.[63] Presently, studies attempting to add prognostic value from specific types of NSCLC have shown inconsistent results.

With SCLC, initial prognostication had traditionally used a two-stage system between designations of limited versus extensive disease (ED). "Limited" disease is restricted to the ipsilateral hemithorax/regional lymph nodes and can be encompassed in a safe radiotherapy field. This is significant, because SCLC is highly responsive to radiation due to its rapid growth. However, the designation now differentiates timing of treatment modalities as treatment for extensive stage SCLC also includes radiotherapy.[66] Recent data have shown benefits of using the full TNM staging system to qualify SCLC stage,[67] and overall, prognostic factors for SCLC and NSCLC are similar[68]: extent of disease, ECOG performance status, and presence of weight loss. Other considerations include presence of anemia, leukocytosis, and elevations in serum erythrocyte sedimentation rate, lactate dehydrogenase (LDH), and neuron-specific enolase (NSE). Data suggest prognostic value of these in univariate analysis in both limited and ED although the difference in median survival within subgroups was less substantial for these factors in ED.

IMPORTANCE OF PREHABILITATION IN PATIENTS WITH LUNG CANCER

Comprehensive cancer rehabilitation begins with prehabilitation. Surgeons are integrating prehabilitation into preoperative planning, given that this represents an investment in functional and physiological capacity with hopes of improving their tolerance to stressful interventions that benefit recovery.[69] In one study of cardiothoracic surgeons, an overwhelming majority of respondents were willing to delay surgical resection beyond the current average 20-day waiting period to allow patients to participate in prehabilitation.[70]

The Enhanced Recovery after Surgery (ERAS) gradually refers to patient-centered, evidence-based, multidisciplinary pathways to reduce patients' stress response to surgery, facilitate recovery, and optimize physiologic function.[71] This team updates recommendations on best practices for different surgical procedures. In a recent update for lung surgical procedures,[69] ERAS and the European Society of Thoracic Surgeons (ESTS) included key recommendations of prehabilitation for high-risk patients as well as other components of a multimodal program such as nutritional screening and smoking cessation.

Maximizing Adherence

Given the number of medical appointments required after initial diagnosis, the new psychological burden, and the onset of symptoms, preoperative programs should prioritize patient convenience and medical team buy-in. In the PROLUCA study,[72] patients designated to the preoperative home-based exercise program were mostly unable to adhere to the schedule due to the number of appointments required within the average preoperative 8-day window. Another prospective study recruited patients newly diagnosed with NSCLC and high-performance status (PS = 0 or 1) to assess the

feasibility of adhering to a structured exercise program prior to- and during treatment initiation.[73] Of all consented patients (n = 25), 20% were unable to complete the initial baseline evaluation. The completion rate for the 16-session program was 44%; the most commonly cited reasons for nonadherence were physical deterioration and/or feeling unwell.

Given the likelihood of posttreatment rehabilitation intolerance due to symptoms and decline in health status,[73–75] clinicians should stress the benefits of prehabilitation both as a means of maintaining current function and protecting against future decline. In terms of *initiating* a prehabilitation program, one study[70] reported access to professionals, comorbidities, and transportation as the top three barriers. Cancer diagnosis and treatment is an interdisciplinary process that requires specialists to coordinate for patients to meet with each team member in succession. Therefore, one means of addressing transportation limitations is to coordinate further by including prehabilitation into a day's visit with the treatment team.

Exercise Intervention

One primary prehabilitation objective is to improve baseline cardiopulmonary function, given the effects of treatment on lung function and association of lung cancer with pulmonary comorbidities. Initial treatments including resection of cancer and surrounding parenchyma, chemotherapy, and radiation negatively impact exercise tolerance and endurance.[76,77] Maintaining or building lean mass has additional utility as a target for exercise, since the presence of lung cancer and treatment significantly impacts strength and muscle mass. One prospective study found nearly 70% of patients with advanced lung cancer experience cachexia and nearly 50% experienced sarcopenia.[78]

Examples of Regimens

Prehabilitation exercise regimens vary in the existing literature. Table 1.1 below demonstrates common components of exercise and respiratory training when included (Table 1.2).

Lifestyle Intervention

Undoubtedly, smoking cessation is the highest yield lifestyle intervention for patients who smoke at the time of diagnosis. Analyzing data from the prospective Cancer Prevention Study (CPS)-II Nutrition cohort, researchers determined the rates of smoking cessation were significantly higher in those respondents who were diagnosed with cancer than those who were

TABLE 1.1
Adopted With Permission From Avancini and Colleagues.[79]

Training	Description	Intensity
Aerobic	Endurance is usually proposed with activities involving dynamical work with large muscle mass, e.g., walking, cycling, running. It can be divided into two methodologies: • continuous, i.e., characterized by long-duration sessions performed continuously without rest. • With interval, i.e., composed by short bouts (e.g., 4 min) of high intensity interspersed by active recovery (e.g., 3 min), usually at low intensity, repeated 3–4 times/session.	Moderate and vigorous, i.e., at 40%–89% of heart rate recovery. This intensity can be linear, i.e., the same for each session or can progressively increase during the training session. Moderate and vigorous, i.e., at 40%–89% of heart rate recovery.
Strength	Strength training applies the use of resistance to muscular contraction to build strength, anaerobic endurance, and size of skeletal muscles. It involves use of different tools: elastic bands, free-weights, machines, or bodyweight exercises	60%–70% of one repetition maximum
Respiratory	Involves a range of training methodologies: • Respiratory muscle training, with or without a device to increase strength of respiratory muscles • Inspiratory muscle training, with or without a device to increase strength of inspiratory muscles • Expiratory muscle training, with or without a device to increase strength of expiratory muscles.	80% of maximal vital capacity 20%–60% of maximal inspiratory pressure N/A

not.[80] Given the possibility of worsening respiratory function for 1–2 weeks immediately following smoking cessation,[81] patients should quit immediately and receive resources such as nicotine replacement therapy to allow for adequate symptom resolution prior to possible surgery. One study[82] used a 4-week cessation time period prior to initiation of chemotherapy without related adverse effects. Moreover, smokers' decreased cough sensitivity can return to baseline as early as 2 weeks from cessation.[83]

Other potential lifestyle interventions include nutritional supplementation. Prior to initiating supplements, clinicians should screen patients for malnutrition and directly replete deficiencies through dietary counseling, oral supplementation, or parenteral nutrition when warranted and in accordance with the patient's wishes.[84] If a patient does not screen positive for malnutrition at baseline, it is critical to monitor for weight loss, poor enteral intake, and serologic markers of malnutrition as patients with lung cancer have increased risk of developing malnutrition, with higher rates in metastatic disease. Further, there is a high risk of significant weight loss within 90 days of radiotherapy due to the incidence of esophagitis and secondary food aversion.[85]

Psychiatric Intervention-Addressing Stigma
Patients with lung cancer possess the greatest levels of psychological distress of all cancers, largely the result of health-related stigma[86] suggesting the patient's behavior caused their illness. This shame is associated with anxiety and depression[87] leading to worse survival and quality of life in patients with cancer, regardless of whether they actually smoked.[88,89] One aspect of mitigating stigma lies in health care professionals using positive, clear, and open communication. This nonjudgmental tone is crucial to providing the highest level of care, as patients with lung cancer may be reluctant to discuss behaviors they perceive as contributing to their diagnosis.

Multimodal Perioperative Programs
The existing literature demonstrates the necessity of a multimodal intervention to maximize benefits, target multiple deficits, and reach objectives in a shorter timeframe. A

TABLE 1.2
Example of a High-Intensity Interval Training (HIIT) Program Adapted With Permission From Avancini and Colleagues.[79]

Frequency	Warm-up	HIGH-INTENSITY PHASE				RECOVERY PHASE				Cool-down	Total Duration (min)
		Intensity (% HR max)	Duration (min)	No. of intervals	Sum of high-intensity duration (min)	Intensity (% HR max)	Duration (min)	No. of intervals	Sum of recovery duration (min)		
3 times per week	5 min at 40%–50% HRmax	75%–85%	4	4	16	50%–60%	3	4	12	5 min at 40%–50% HRmax	38

multimodal RCT[90] randomized patients before NSCLC resection to either a 4-week prehabilitation program followed by an 8-week rehabilitation program versus an 8-week rehabilitation program alone. The program included home-based moderate-intensity exercise of aerobic training 3 days per week, resistance training 3 days per week, personalized nutritional counseling with whey protein supplementation, and anxiety reducing strategies via guided relaxation 2–3 times per week. Functional capacity was not significantly different between the groups at 4 weeks postoperatively; however, the prehabilitation group had significantly better measures of physical health and total health at 4 weeks as measured by the SF-36 Physical Summary and SF-36 Total, respectively.

Limitations to Prehabilitation

Arguably the most significant potential limitations to prehabilitation are patient/surgeon buy-in, the potential for comorbidities or neoplastic/paraneoplastic symptoms to limit participation, and grief/psychological limitations associated with the new diagnosis. A new cancer diagnosis involves a grieving process like any other life-changing negative event,[91] and adjustment disorders are not uncommon in this population.[92] The mood impact may dramatically diminish motivation during a crucial window where every day

screen, the patient will require confirmation testing and appropriate staging, including a biopsy for histologic diagnosis. This should be completed as timely as possible to both minimize potential progression[93] and afford the patient maximum time for prehabilitation and medical management before surgery/chemoradiation. If the patient is presenting with symptoms, their prognosis carries higher mortality risks.[63] Additional workup at that time will likely be symptom-directed such as radiographs for bone pain and a standard battery of serum laboratory tests, screening for electrolyte and hematologic abnormalities.

As part of coordinated interdisciplinary care, rehabilitation specialists will establish timelines for rehabilitation care while accounting for oncologic treatment. Consultation with a physical medicine and rehabilitation physician will establish a patient's suitability for rehabilitation and set initial goals. The treatment team will consider delaying surgery/chemoradiation and likely factor in the type/stage of cancer, baseline health status, goals of treatment, prognosis, and deficits at presentation. At this time, one may perform screening tests for undiagnosed comorbidities such as spirometry to assess for COPD, fasting glucose/hemoglobin A1C for diabetes, polysomnography for obstructive sleep apnea, etc.

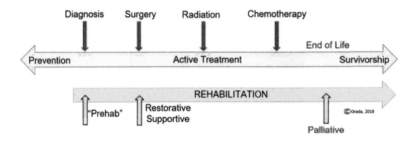

of therapeutic interventions could tangibly reduce surgical risk and foster resilience for withstanding treatment. Persuading stakeholders to delay surgical resection and allow time for prehabilitation may be a difficult but necessary conversation. Ultimately, concessions may require compromise and accelerating timeframes as patient preference and risk/benefit considerations dictate.

THE CONTINUUM OF CARE FOR LUNG CANCER REHABILITATION

From Diagnosis

After presenting with signs/symptoms concerning for lower respiratory malignancy or following a positive

Risk Considerations During the Continuum of Care

One important consideration is the safety of rehabilitation for patients with boney metastases and the risk of pathologic fracture while weight-bearing. For some patients, prophylactic repair may be beneficial, and orthopedic referral at diagnosis of bone metastases may be warranted. One retrospective study compared rates of pathologic fracture across cancer types, finding patients with multiple myeloma had the highest rate of fracture (43%) and lung cancer had the lowest rate (17%).[94] Physicians can quantify the risk using measures such as the Mirels' Classification,[64] which considers details of lesion size, site, appearance, and associated pain.

Due to poor healing of long bone fractures in patients with metastatic disease,[65] clinicians may consider prophylactic fixation for Mirels' scores of at least 9. Some lesions with scores up to eight can be managed with local radiotherapy and medications[95] such as denosumab[96,97] or bisphosphonates.[98] Alternatively, the appropriate use of orthoses can stabilize and effectively "reinforce" vulnerable bones.[99]

Multiple reviews evaluating the safety of rehabilitation with bone metastases suggest refraining from manual muscle testing, resistance training, and any activities that generate sheer forces in limbs affected by metastases.[95,100] A study of patients with vertebral metastases demonstrated the safety and efficacy with isometric exercises of paravertebral muscles, effectively preventing atrophy that would occur with standard bedrest absent pathologic fractures.[101] Other research advocates the use of neuromuscular electrical stimulation and biofeedback-assisted exercises as means of passive and (guarded) active muscle contractions,[102,103] although practitioners should not place heat/current directly over metastatic lesions.

During treatment, patients are also at risk of medication side effects and interactions. Beyond the well-known side effects of chemotherapy and radiation such as anorexia, nausea/diarrhea, neuropathic symptoms, and anemia, other common medications like steroids may cause myopathy, further immunosuppression, and poor wound healing which may be relevant to the rehabilitation specialist.

Logistical safety concerns mirror those in other areas of medical care. With large care teams spanning multiple medical specialties, case workers, prosthetists/orthotists, and other vendors, each transition of care requires a handoff that provides the opportunity for communication errors. Providers may minimize risks by thoroughly documenting visits and providing a verbal handoff that highlight any changes to care plans. In this patient population, documentation such as a physician order for life sustaining treatment becomes vitally important for respecting patient wishes if one provider revisits goals of care with the patient and family.

General Prehabilitation Program Recommendations

Initiation date for the first cancer therapy will determine the length of prehabilitation. From this date, clinicians can discuss goals of prehabilitation with the patient and build a multimodal prehabilitation schedule. The following sample program represents a four-pillared framework based on the present literature that

clinicians should tailor to the patient's exercise tolerance and preintervention timeline.

Exercise pillar: The literature currently supports high-intensity interval training at least 3 days per week[104] for 4 weeks if able. If possible, increasing the frequency may yield greater benefit or offset shorter durations; patients may participate up to 5 days/week likely without increased risk.[105] Progressive resistance exercise training[106] 3 days per week on nonconsecutive days may complement the aerobic benefits of HIIT and build/maintain lean mass. Practitioners can determine starting resistance and repetition ranges from either a direct assessment of 1 repetition max[107] or using a calculation based on $7-10$[108] or $4-6$ repetitions.[109]

Respiratory pillar: Pulmonary training is an integral component of a multimodal prehabilitation program, as exercise alone has limited efficacy in improving spirometry values,[110–113] and research supports the tangible benefits with improvements in FVC and FEV1.[114–117] Therefore, integrating the techniques utilized in the literature offers patients the opportunity to perform beneficial therapies at home. Much of the literature features the use of inspiratory muscle training,[105,118] with devices that provide objective targets for resistance. During the first screen, therapists should determine the patient's maximum inspiratory pressure (MIP) as this will be the benchmark on which future device settings will be based. Then, the patient should perform slow inspiration/expiration with starting resistance of 20%–30% of MIP and increase the resistance 5%–10% if he or she is able to perform the exercise for at least 10 min without rest. The patient should perform this exercise at least 20 min per day. Additionally, the objective feedback of increasing resistance as the patient tolerates greater load may provide positive reinforcement and facilitate further participation.

Lifestyle pillar: The first lifestyle recommendation in a multimodal prehabilitation program is to begin the process of smoking cessation, particularly given the recommended lead-time of quitting smoking prior to surgical interventions or chemotherapy. Research suggests that early conversations regarding smoking cessation may be most effective as patients are more receptive to significant lifestyle changes at the time of a cancer diagnosis,[119] and patients who welcome assistance are 40% more likely to quit smoking.[120] There are limited studies of smoking cessation in the specific context of patients with cancer; however, one trial found bupropion to be minimally effective and only if the patient has symptoms of depression.[121] Of note, with the potential association between bupropion and lowered seizure threshold,[122] clinicians should exercise caution in patients with metastatic disease or those with electrolyte abnormalities; however, at present dosage schedules and formulations, bupropion may carry a *lower* seizure risk than other antidepressants.[123]

The psychological pillar of the program includes previously discussed aspects such as smoking cessation therapy or as needed treatments for sleep disorders such as cognitive behavioral therapy for insomnia.[124] Beyond these, patients would likely benefit from peer support programs and other techniques for stress management. Participants in one study remarked that the group exercise component of their intervention had positive benefits on their mood by providing a sense of community with others in similar situations.[125] This aspect would include palliative care specialists to comanage care of patient comfort, optimize quality of life, and help facilitate discussions about goals of care and end of life planning.[126]

ACUTE HOSPITALIZATION

A patient may require acute hospitalization following a diagnosis of lung cancer for several reasons. Patients may have a planned admission for resection of cancer and will ideally have completed a prehabilitation program to medically optimize them. Postoperative impairments from surgery will typically be related to pain and fatigue and the method of resection dictates the severity and duration. Pulmonary resections are increasingly being performed by minimally invasive approaches such as video-assisted thoracoscopic surgery or robot-assisted thoracoscopic surgery due to technological improvements, better outcomes, and shorter recovery periods.[127] Length of stay is shortened by the trend toward minimally invasive techniques, and patients report less pain and require less opioid pain medications postoperatively.

Common complications following lung resection include atelectasis, respiratory failure, (prolonged) air leak, and bronchopleural fistula formation. Air leak is common following lobectomy and 10%−15% of patients exhibit a prolonged leak[128] lasting longer than 7 days.[129] These are managed conservatively with maintaining chest tubes[129] which have implications for therapy participation. Recent literature suggests approximately 10% of pneumonectomies develop a fistula between bronchi and the pleural space (bronchopleural fistula),[130] with lower rates following lobectomy. Unlike air leaks, these are managed surgically with closure of the bronchus, drainage of the pleural space, and subsequent sterilization.[131] Arrhythmia is a common nonpulmonary complication, with some studies reporting atrial fibrillation (AF) in

>5% of cases.[132] Premorbid history of paroxysmal AF or intraoperative lymph node dissections and transfusions increased the likelihood of postoperative AF.

Following surgery, patients will almost immediately begin participating in physical therapy, occupational therapy, and respiratory therapies to minimize complications. The extent and intensity of these therapies are related to the type of resection, as thoracotomy is associated with higher rates of pulmonary complications, pain, and longer recover periods than less invasive methods of resection.[133] Physical therapy within hours of emergence from general anesthesia is encouraged, largely to mitigate the potentially significant postoperative pain and effects of reduced inspiratory volumes/cough. Some patients limit upper extremity range of motion due to pain, which may predispose them to secondary pathology. In addition to traditional multimodal analgesics such as acetaminophen and opioid medications, clinicians can employ transcutaneous electrical nerve stimulation and topical medications like lidocaine or diclofenac. Oral NSAIDs are relatively contraindicated due to their effect on bone healing postoperatively[134,135] and efficacy of pleurodesis[136] but may be warranted in short durations for certain procedures.

Simple interventions after surgery can help reduce pulmonary complications. Upright positioning both in and out of bed improves ventilatory volumes and gas exchange ([133,137]); however, the patient may be placed in a side-lying position for comfort when in bed. In these situations, the patient should lay with the nonoperated side down unless they have had a full pneumonectomy, in which case they should be carefully placed with the operated side down to minimize complications.[133] Previous guidelines recommended early patient mobilization on postoperative day 1 (POD 1); research indicates that edge of bed mobilization with sustained upright sitting followed by ambulation as tolerated improves outcomes.[138] Considerations for mobilization/ambulation include generally stable vital signs—heart rate (HR) 40−140/min, respiration rate (RR) 8−36, oxygen saturation >85%, and mean arterial pressure >65/systolic blood pressure (SBP) 80−200/diastolic BP (DBP) < 110—as well as monitoring chest and feeding tubes to ensure they do not migrate, and controlling pain prior to initiation of activity (particularly if the patient has drains in place).[139]

In most cases, patients should participate in therapies with graduated intensity[140] with the clinician monitoring the patients' tolerance and any signs/symptoms of overexertion. Patients should begin with short sessions, multiple times per day to ensure tolerance and safety with mild/moderate perceived exertion reaching heart rates up to 60% of the calculated maximum heart rate.[141] As able, the patient graduates to increasing walking distances and then ambulating up/down stairs approximately on POD 3–5, based on their overall risk level, perceived exertion, and exercise/pain tolerance.

This program is contraindicated in patients with unstable vital signs, altered mental status, untreated thromboembolism, significant ventilatory requirements, uncontrolled arrhythmia/heart failure, acute renal failure, or weight-bearing limitations to ambulation[141]; alternatively, patients unable to participate in physical therapy can prioritize respiratory training interventions. These pulmonary interventions mirror those employed during prehabilitation. Clinicians may utilize multiple deep-breathing techniques that vary by position and goals. Generally, upright deep breathing helps to prevent atelectasis/reverse mild atelectasis[142,143] and improve oxygenation; patients may perform 5 breaths each with a 3 s hold hourly[144] to support equal lung filling. The pelvis should have a posterior tilt to maximize the mechanical advantage of the diaphragm.

In nonsurgical cases, patients may require acute hospitalization for conditions indirectly related to their lung cancer diagnosis such as electrolyte disturbances, COPD exacerbations, common infections, and pain. Cancer-related pain differs from postoperative pain in the severity, variability of its character, and prognosis for resolution.[145] Some patients may require short inpatient visits for pain control including optimizing medications and, when applicable, XRT to malignant lesions that are sources of pain.

Patients that have received chemotherapy, are malnourished, or have advanced disease may be at higher risk for hospital-acquired.[146] In one multiyear study of over 2000 patients with any type of cancer in a community hospital setting, nearly 9% of patients required at least one hospitalization in association with their chemotherapy regimen. The two primary reasons were gastrointestinal side effects and infection; risk increased with greater comorbidity burden, increased age, and creatinine elevation. Unsurprisingly, patients admitted for symptom management had longer LOS and were more likely to die during the hospitalization than patients admitted for diagnostic or therapeutic procedures.[147]

Postacute Care

The first of several factors that dictates disposition from acute hospitalizations is patient need. To qualify for inpatient rehabilitation, the patient must have treatable impairments such as diffuse muscular weakness, focal deficits due to local pathology such as pathologic fracture or tumor invasion into peripheral nerves, or decreased cardiopulmonary function from comorbidities. Moreover, the patient must be able to participate at least 3 hours a day, 5 days per week unless a waiver is available. If a patient is functionally *too* close to baseline or, alternatively, too ill for intense therapy, he or she may instead benefit from a skilled nursing facility for lower intensity therapies. Other excluding factors reflect the intent for inpatient rehabilitation to bridge a patient for discharge home, and therefore the patient should be medically well enough to participate, have pain controlled without intravenous (IV) opioid medications, nor require IV antihypertensives—the latter typically requires the patient to be on a heart monitor to ensure hemodynamic stability, implying the patient should remain on an acute medical service.

A typical inpatient therapy regimen includes physical therapy, occupational therapy, and as needed speech/cognitive therapy. If resources allow, the patient may work with neuropsychologists or respiratory therapists as needed. Physical therapists may implement different modalities of resistance and aerobic training to promote greater exercise tolerance, endurance, and measures of global function. In one prospective study, aerobic exercise training alone[148] promoted a significant increase in overall performance as quantified by power generation (bicycle ergometry from 68 ± 3 to 86 ± 4 W, $P < .001$) and 6-minute walk test (from 322 ± 11 to 385 ± 13 m, $P < .001$). Fatigue was significantly improved and quality of life, typically associated with cancer-related fatigue, improved as well.

Resistance training is necessary to foster lasting gains in skeletal muscle mass[149] and strength[150] and is associated with resilience to physical trauma such as falls and improvements in global measures such as HRQoL. While high-intensity resistance training will have near-term improvements in fatigue, HRQoL, and cardiopulmonary efficiency, muscle strength gains remain durable and significantly greater than control at 68 weeks follow-up.[150]

Cancer Cachexia

Cancer cachexia is a component of both the pathophysiology of malignancy[151] and the anorexic effects of treatment. Cancer cachexia is a syndrome of inflammation, skeletal muscle breakdown, (often) lipolysis, and decreased appetite.[79] Since it is not reversible simply with increased caloric intake, appetite stimulants alone may not be adequate. Treatment modalities span multiple nutritional, behavioral, and pharmacologic mechanisms.

Generally, begin by optimizing apparent nutritional deficits. Some amino acids are conditionally essential in oncology such as glutamine,[152] and others are more traditionally anabolic in individuals without cancer such as leucine.[153] Omega 3 fatty acids may mitigate the inflammatory aspect of cachexia and, similarly, nonsteroidal antiinflammatory drugs have been shown to be beneficial, particularly in combination with L-carnitine[154] in some trials.

Some medications are used as appetite stimulants with only modest efficacy such as megestrol acetate,[155] which may increase appetite but with poor overall effect on lean mass. Practitioners utilize mirtazapine, a tetracyclic antidepressant, for its common side effect of appetite stimulation. Dronabinol, a constituent of cannabis, is also often prescribed, but some studies suggest poor efficacy in meaningfully improving appetite and lean mass in patients with cancer.[156] Research is also investigating ghrelin, the "hunger hormone" and related analogues such as anamorelin as a means of targeting appetite while minimizing side effects. Two RCTs—ROMANA 1 and 2—found improvements in weight and lean mass with anamorelin157. Although these studies did not demonstrate benefit for survival or strength, an additional trial showed benefit for QoL.[158] Also of note, if a patient's cancer is responsive to chemotherapy, they may begin to regain weight as treatment progresses.[151]

Pain and Fatigue Management

One of the primary distressing and activity-limiting effects of treatment for lung can cancer is fatigue that ensues from treatment. Research shows that in surgical resection for NSCLC (stages IA and IB), 57% of patients reported fatigue of any severity (mild—severe)[159]; patients treated with chemotherapy reported fatigue at a rate of 88%.[160] This is relevant since fatigue impacts HRQoL[161] more than depression and anxiety.[162] Studies report mixed efficacy of physical activity interventions on improving fatigue symptoms in patients with lung cancer. One randomized controlled trial found a 6 month intervention with weekly supervised physical activity sessions was not effective in significantly improving symptoms of fatigue.[163] This may be the result of the advanced stage of the population's disease, inadequate intensity of the intervention, or other mitigating factors that could have been better addressed with a multimodal intervention.

Another RCT[164] compared rehabilitation within 2 weeks of resection(early) versus greater than 2 weeks (late) in reducing fatigue. The early rehabilitation group (ERG) initially appeared to be protected from the worsening fatigue symptoms in the first 14 weeks that the late rehabilitation group (LRG) demonstrated. By 26 weeks, this fatigue significantly improved in the LRG, and there were no significant differences between the two groups. This study did not include a nonintervention control, and therefore, conclusions cannot be drawn regarding expected fatigue symptoms from resection alone. Objectively, the ERG demonstrated a smaller decrease in VO2 peak at 14 weeks relative to the LRG, and by the next time point (14 weeks postop to 26 weeks), the LRG had a significant increase in VO2 peak such that both groups were no longer significantly different in their VO2 peak values. The improvement seen in both groups from 14 to 26 weeks resulted in no significant difference in VO2 peak from baseline-26 weeks or baseline-52 weeks. Essentially, the VO2 peak recovered from the initial decline in both groups.

Even with the mixed efficacy in these trials, a systematic review and metaanalysis demonstrated that, in comparison with psychological, pharmacologic, and exercise + psychological interventions, exercise alone had the greatest weighted effect size (0.30, $P < 0.001$) in reducing cancer-related fatigue.[165] Psychological (0.27, $P < 0.001$) and psychological + exercise (0.26, $P < 0.001$) were only modestly less effective, whereas pharmacologic treatment had a low impact (0.09, $P = 0.05$). The pharmacologic interventions assessed were SSRIs, modafinil/armodafinil, methylphenidate/dexmethylphenidate, dexamphetamine, and methylprednisolone.

Myriad reasons may explain the mixed results of exercise efficacy in reducing fatigue. One aspect may be exercise modalities are not all created equal. In one RCT of patients with any stage of NSCLC and SCLC comparing performance of a tai chi program versus "low impact exercise," the tai chi intervention group reported greater improvement in CRF after both 6 and 12 weeks. One important critique of the study is the control group; "low impact exercise" participants performed "arm, neck, and leg circles, followed by stretches for upper and lower body muscle groups along with deep abdominal breathing." Based on this description and without any objective measures of exertion, one may presume these exercises may mitigate performance bias for a control group but likely do not afford the same benefits of more effortful exercise. At the least, however, exercise program participation does not *exacerbate* CRF.[166]

Emerging/Nontraditional Treatments

The legality of agents such as cannabis, psilocybin, and methylenedioxymethamphetamine (MDMA) continues to evolve with changing public perception and research demonstrating efficacy with treating pain and psychiatric disease. Cannabis contains dozens of cannabinoid compounds and terpenes that stimulate appetite and can improve pain, anxiety, and insomnia.[167–169] MDMA may be highly effective in coordination with extended therapy sessions in treating conditions such as posttraumatic stress disorder (PTSD) so much, that (at the time of this publication) the FDA is reviewing applications to approve it for breakthrough status.[170] Psilocybin, the primary active constituent of psychedelic mushrooms, has also been approved as a breakthrough medication due to its efficacy in treatment-resistant depression. Other research demonstrates benefits in depression for patients with terminal diseases.[171,172]

Continuation of Chemotherapy/Radiation During Inpatient Rehabilitation

Often, patients will begin in IPR between treatments for cancer. For instance, they would recover from the acute surgical/initial chemotherapeutic treatment, be admitted to IPR for 2–3 weeks, and discharged with the intention of resuming chemoradiation. The goals of IPR during this window include optimizing pain management, fostering resilience, and maximizing function prior to the subsequent side effects of continued therapeutic or palliative treatments.[173]

Postacute Skilled Nursing Facilities and Long-Term Care Facilities

Some situations require patients to be discharged to SNFs or LTACs following hospitalization. SNFs offer varying levels of rehabilitation and care based on location and patient need. For patients unable to participate in the intensity required by IPR, SNFs allow for fewer therapy sessions during the daytime ("subacute" rehabilitation) but provide closer medical oversight than outpatient rehabilitation. Alternatively, patients may also benefit who have significant deficits that preclude them from safe discharge home but not substantial enough to warrant IPR. For some, gains made during IPR are insufficient for a safe discharge home, or the patient may lack suitable support from existing caregivers. In these situations, patients may be safest with discharge to an SNF. LTAC facilities, alternatively, allow for select features of acute-level care such as ventilation management/weaning in patients whose condition does not otherwise warrant inpatient acute medical care. Rehabilitation therapies in LTAC facilities are site dependent but are typically less frequent/rigorous than in SNFs and limited by physical constraints such as being physically tethered to a ventilator.

Home Rehabilitation

After discharge from acute medical care (for higher-functioning patients) or inpatient rehabilitation, patients often transition to home-based rehabilitation therapies. These programs are ideal for deficits that may be addressed with less equipment and/or for whom travel limitations make participation in outpatient rehabilitation difficult. Therapies maximize safety and functioning in the home environment and may have less efficacy than other settings in improving global strength and functioning but offer improvements in measures of HRQoL and perceived symptom severity.[174] These are guided by home physical, occupational, and speech therapists. For higher-functioning patients without significant cognitive impacts, other research supports patient-facilitated home exercise programs (HEPs) as a means of personal involvement and maintaining motivation in treatment, stress management, and even preventing boredom.[175] For these patients, the conclusion of therapist-directed treatment in the home or outpatient setting culminates in a transition to an HEP for maintaining functional gains and mitigating subsequent decline.

After achieving a level of independence, simple interventions may yield positive results, particularly in global measures of function and self-perceptions of health. In one longitudinal study of patients with lung cancer, researchers found a dose-dependent relationship between walking time and QoL measures. For each additional minute of walking per week, patients averaged an increase of 0.03 in objective measures of QoL.[176] This study also drew conclusions regarding therapy adherence. After transition to home rehabilitation, adherence to therapies typically decreases,[177] especially with regards to self-directed HEPs. Factors that improve the likelihood of walking adherence were treatment status—those who had completed treatment were more likely to walk—as well as social support and self-efficacy/confidence in continuing exercise.[176] In the PROLUCA study, adherence to postoperative group exercise interventions was not related to timing of program initiation; participants who began "early" (after 2 weeks) and "late" (after 6 weeks) had equal rates of adherence.[72] Like the study's findings on preoperative exercise programs, patients attributed nonadherence to lack of time, too many hospital appointments/hospitalization, and lack of motivation.

Even one program designed to foster adherence that screened for motivation at inclusion suffered from high rates of nonadherence.[178] The most common reasons cited were fatigue and performance status declines despite similar baseline characteristics between patients that completed the program and those that dropped out. Although this study may be limited by sample size, practitioners may draw conclusions from it, corroborating data,[74] and those mentioned previously regarding nonadherence with prehabilitation/perioperative rehabilitation plans.

Given the high rate of dropout due to symptoms and performance status declines, the ideal time for therapy may be in the prehabilitation phase (prior to treatment initiation), although this may conflict with patients' wishes. Within one study[75] of patients at least "possibly interested in receiving exercise counseling," the majority prefer counseling to occur during (28.1% of respondents) or after treatment (28.1%). This may be modifiable with counseling regarding benefits of prehabilitation from rehabilitation practitioners, palliative care, and oncology teams.

Outpatient Rehabilitation

Patients will transition to outpatient rehabilitation following discharge from their acute hospitalization. Typically, the regimen will be a continuation of the therapies from which they were benefitting at the end of inpatient rehabilitation but prioritize activities that require observation or specialized equipment. Therapies will continue to target impairments from tumors/metastases, treatment side effects, or general deconditioning. Symptoms such as cancer-related fatigue benefit greatly from exercise yet can limit motivation for initiating exercise[179]; therefore, a set schedule of outpatient rehabilitation may help maintain participation until symptoms improve. As some higher-functioning patients may not have membership to local fitness centers or have safety concerns due to balance impairment or weight-bearing status, outpatient rehabilitation affords them the opportunity to resistance and aerobically train under licensed supervision.

Outpatient therapy often occurs 2–3 visits per week for 6–8 weeks with a transition to an HEP. Goals often include increasing proficiency with therapies such that the patient can safely continue written therapy instructions with minimal guidance. Exercise prescriptions written by the patient's physiatrist will include the intended frequency, duration, restrictions/precautions, and further recommendations based on the patient's current functional status and goals. Factoring in patients' preferred exercise modalities is an easy way to boost adherence.

Cancer Survivorship and Surveillance

Cancer survivors often have residual deficits that may benefit from therapeutic intervention such as fatigue, peripheral neuropathy, musculoskeletal pain, lower bone density, contractures, or decreased pulmonary function. Moreover, these predispose survivors to serious secondary injury from events such as falls.[179] Ongoing treatment for nutritional deficits and exercise programs to foster physical resilience may improve these symptoms and reduce future risk. Also, although only a minority of patients develop PTSD from cancer diagnosis/treatment,[180] those affected may benefit from early recognition. PTSD rates in patients treated for any cancer increases with invasive treatment(s); this trend suggests the prevalence of PTSD after lobectomy/pneumonectomy in patients with lung cancer may be higher than in oncology overall.

When in remission, patients undergo regular surveillance to monitor for recurrence. Given the high rate of advanced disease at recurrence (~2/3 of patients), current recommendations include 6-month follow-up for the first 2 years following intent-to-cure treatment[181] including CT of the chest through adrenal glands, preferably with contrast. In subsequent years, patients are screened using noncontrast, low-dose chest CT. These imaging modalities should only be utilized in patients who would be able to undergo further treatment should cancer recur. Patients treated for SCLC who did not undergo prophylactic cranial irradiation should be monitored with brain MRI every 3 months during the first year and every 6 months during the second year following treatment; this does not apply to patients treated for NSCLC.

Advanced Stages/End of Life

Timing the transition from aggressive treatment to hospice care is not always intuitive and requires clinicians to recognize the appropriate time and emotionally prepare the patient and family. Merely proposing this transition to hospice requires emotional awareness given the implication treatment has reached a point of futility. The appropriateness of the timing of the suggestion requires the clinician to understand treatment goals, which typically relies on conversations that began much earlier.

When the patient and treatment team agree to prioritize comfort and quality of life over aggressive life-extending treatment, rehabilitation therapies may retain a role for patients in end of life care. One study assessed patients' willingness to participate in rehabilitation in the setting of late-stage lung cancer diagnoses.[182] Nearly one third of patients were interested in continuing rehabilitation, and rates were highest if patients had specific musculoskeletal complaints. Reasons for disinterest were lack of perceived benefit and available time, often relative to other more pressing demands.

Therefore, treatment strategies begin with revised goal setting—is the patient's priority to attend specific upcoming life events, prevent hospital admissions, maintain independence, or minimize pain and anxiety? One study of patients in hospice with any terminal malignancy demonstrated a 6% rate of hospital admission. Of these, over one third of patients received aggressive care and over one third of patients died during the hospitalization, likely in lieu of their preferred setting.[183]

One multimodal study of patients with advanced lung cancer utilized group exercise, individualized home-exercise plan, and nutrition and palliative care consults.[184] The study achieved 44% enrollment with respondents stating the program improved their confidence in physical abilities and gave them a sense of a "return to normal." Group exercise provided social engagement with others who can relate to their diagnosis and sessions had immediate benefits on pain, tiredness/drowsiness, shortness of breath, depression/anxiety, fatigue, energy, and well-being. Tiredness benefits were durable and lasted beyond a pre/postexercise class improvement. Qualitative data highlight the need for exercise variability and enthusiastic instructors. Respondents suggested extending the palliative consults to one-on-one counseling.[184]

In end-of-life care, clinicians will target symptoms of pain, delirium/restlessness, secretions, dyspnea, and cough[185] as these are distressing to both patients and family. Oral medications may need to be administered transdermally, intravenously, or subcutaneously as the patient loses the ability to safely swallow. Care transitions to a supportive role and mere physical presence can be therapeutic. Educating the patient and family on what the patient's final moments may entail can alleviate fear and instill/maintain trust; this education includes how to recognize the "dying phase" so everyone may adequately prepare. Patients may qualify for hospice care in their home or inpatient setting, depending on the complexity of their medical comorbidities and if they are in the active dying phase.

Although controversial, physician-assisted dying (PAD) has increasingly gained acceptance to maintain control and dignity in patients' final moments. For others, religious or ethical conflicts may prohibit them from considering the practice. Patients that ultimately participate in PAD often cite their "inability to engage in enjoyable activities," or their loss of dignity and autonomy.[186] Ultimately, utilizing PAD is a personal decision during a patient's end of life care.

CONCLUSION

Lung cancer incidence is declining in the developed world largely due to decreased smoking rates, while survivorship is increasing due to improved screening and treatments. With emerging immunotherapies and genomic-targeted treatments, survivorship is likely to increase further. This growing population of survivors requires clinicians to anticipate and address likely impairments early in the continuum of care, which spans prehabilitation, inpatient rehabilitation, home/outpatient therapies, and end of life care.

Rehabilitation in the setting of lung cancer includes exercise modalities, pulmonary training, optimizing nutrition, managing pain and fatigue, and facilitating psychiatric support when warranted as stigma is significant in this population, regardless of prior smoking status. Therapies at all stages can increase participation adherence by increasing group/peer involvement and minimizing time expenditure, as these are highly preferred by patients. Compassionate care demands recognition of the appropriate time to transition to end-of-life care, prioritize quality of life, and recognize rehabilitation's role in this setting. With these patient goals and physicians' roles, lung cancer rehabilitation is a highly interdisciplinary practice.

REFERENCES

1. Wong MCS, Lao X, Ho K-F, Goggins W, Tse SLA. Incidence and mortality of lung cancer: global trends and association with socioeconomic status. *Sci Rep.* 2017;7(1):14300.
2. Ahmad OB, Boschi-Pinto C, Lopez AD, Murray CJL, Lozano R, Inoue M. *Age Standardization of Rates: A New WHO Standard.* Vol. 9(10). Geneva: World Health Organization; 2001.
3. O'Neil ME, Henley SJ, Rohan EA, Ellington TD, Gallaway MS. Lung cancer incidence in nonmetropolitan and metropolitan counties - United States, 2007–2016. *MMWR.* 2019;68(44):993–998.
4. Stram DO, Park SL, Haiman CA, et al. Racial/ethnic differences in lung cancer incidence in the multiethnic cohort study: an update. *J Natl Cancer Inst.* 2019;111(8):811–819.
5. Aberle DR, Adams AM, Berg CD, et al. Reduced lung-cancer mortality with low-dose computed tomographic screening. *N Engl J Med.* 2011;365(5):395–409.
6. National Lung Screening Trial Research Trail. Lung cancer incidence and mortality with extended follow-up in the national lung screening trial. *J Thorac Oncol.* 2019; 14(10):1732–1742.
7. Cheng T-YD, Cramb SM, Baade PD, Youlden DR, Nwogu C, Reid ME. The international Epidemiology of lung cancer: latest trends, disparities, and tumor characteristics. *J Thorac Oncol.* 2016;11(10):1653–1671.

8. Gosney J. *Pathology and Genetics of Tumours of the Lung, Pleura, Thymus and Heart.* World Health Organization classification of tumors; 2004:76−77.

9. Travis WD, Brambilla E, Nicholson AG, et al. The 2015 World Health Organization classification of lung tumors: impact of genetic, clinical and radiologic advances since the 2004 classification. *J Thorac Oncol.* 2015;10(9): 1243−1260.

10. A genomics-based classification of human lung tumors. *Sci Transl Med.* 2013;5(209):209ra153.

11. Caplin ME, Baudin E, Ferolla P, et al. Pulmonary neuroendocrine (carcinoid) tumors: European Neuroendocrine Tumor Society expert consensus and recommendations for best practice for typical and atypical pulmonary carcinoids. *Ann Oncol.* 2015;26(8):1604−1620.

12. van Meerbeeck JP, Fennell DA, De Ruysscher DK. Small-cell lung cancer. *Lancet.* 2011;378(9804):1741−1755.

13. Torres-Durán M, Ruano-Ravina A, Kelsey KT, et al. Small cell lung cancer in never-smokers. *Eur Respir J.* 2016; 47(3):947−953.

14. Islami F, Torre LA, Jemal A. Global trends of lung cancer mortality and smoking prevalence. *Transl Lung Cancer Res.* 2015;4(4):327−338.

15. Masters GA. Clinical presentation of small cell lung cancer. In: *Principles and Practice of Lung Cancer.* Philadelphia, PA: Lippincott Williams & Wilkins; 2010:341−351.

16. Wilson LD, Detterbeck FC, Yahalom J. Superior vena cava syndrome with malignant causes. *N Engl J Med.* 2007; 356(18):1862−1869.

17. Rice TW, Rodriguez RM, Light RW. The superior vena cava syndrome: clinical characteristics and evolving etiology. *Medicine.* 2006;85(1):37−42.

18. Arcasoy SM, Jett JR. Superior pulmonary sulcus tumors and Pancoast's syndrome. *N Engl J Med.* 1997;337(19): 1370−1376.

19. Foroulis CN, Zarogoulidis P, Darwiche K, et al. Superior sulcus (Pancoast) tumors: current evidence on diagnosis and radical treatment. *J Thorac Dis.* 2013;5(Suppl 4): S342−S358.

20. Dalmau J, Rosenfeld MR. Paraneoplastic syndromes of the CNS. *Lancet Neurol.* 2008;7(4):327−340.

21. Elrington GM, Murray NM, Spiro SG, Newsom-Davis J. Neurological paraneoplastic syndromes in patients with small cell lung cancer. A prospective survey of 150 patients. *J Neurol Neurosurg Psychiatry.* 1991;54(9):764−767.

22. Honnorat J, Antoine J-C. Paraneoplastic neurological syndromes. *Orphanet J Rare Dis.* 2007;2:22.

23. Spiro SG, Gould MK, Colice GL. Initial evaluation of the patient with lung cancer: symptoms, signs, laboratory tests, and paraneoplastic syndromes: ACCP evidenced-based clinical practice guidelines. *Chest.* 2007;132(3 Suppl):149s−160s.

24. Gill S, Murray N, Dalmau J, Thiessen B. Paraneoplastic sensory neuronopathy and spontaneous regression of small cell lung cancer. *Can J Neurol Sci.* 2003;30(3): 269−271.

25. Hirano S, Yoshifumi N, Morinoa E, et al. A case of spontaneous regression of small cell lung cancer with progression of paraneoplastic sensory neuropathy. *Lung Cancer.* 2007;58(2):291−295.

26. Mawhinney E, Gray OM, McVerry F, McDonnell GV. Paraneoplastic sensorimotor neuropathy associated with regression of small cell lung carcinoma. *BMJ Case Rep.* 2010;2010. bcr0120091486.

27. Suzuki M, Kimura H, Tachibana I, et al. Improvement of anti-Hu-associated paraneoplastic sensory neuropathy after chemoradiotherapy in a small cell lung cancer patient. *Intern Med.* 2001;40(11):1140−1143.

28. Keime-Guibert F, Grausd F, Fleurya A, et al. Treatment of paraneoplastic neurological syndromes with antineuronal antibodies (Anti-Hu, anti-Yo) with a combination of immunoglobulins, cyclophosphamide, and methylprednisolone. *J Neurol Neurosurg Psychiatry.* 2000; 68(4):479−482.

29. Graus F, Delattre JY, Antoine JC, et al. Recommended diagnostic criteria for paraneoplastic neurological syndromes. *J Neurol Neurosurg Psychiatry.* 2004;75(8): 1135−1140.

30. Gultekin SH, Rosenfeld MR, Voltz R, Eichen J, Posner JB, Dalmau J. Paraneoplastic limbic encephalitis: neurological symptoms, immunological findings and tumour association in 50 patients. *Brain.* 2000;123(Pt 7): 1481−1494.

31. Bruylant K, Crols R, Humbel RL, Appel B, De Deyn PP. Probably anti-Tr associated paraneoplastic cerebellar degeneration as initial presentation of a squamous cell carcinoma of the lung. *Clin Neurol Neurosurg.* 2006; 108(4):415−417.

32. Konishi J, Yamazaki K, Chikai K, et al. Paraneoplastic cerebellar degeneration (PCD) associated with squamous cell carcinoma of the lung. *Intern Med.* 2004;43(7):602−606.

33. Sabater L, Bataller L, Carpentier AF, et al. Protein kinase Cgamma autoimmunity in paraneoplastic cerebellar degeneration and non-small-cell lung cancer. *J Neurol Neurosurg Psychiatry.* 2006;77(12):1359−1362.

34. Sabater L, Höftberger R, Boronat A, Saiz A, Dalmau J, Graus F. Antibody repertoire in paraneoplastic cerebellar degeneration and small cell lung cancer. *PLoS One.* 2013; 8(3):e60438.

35. O'Neill JH, Murray NM, Newsom-Davis J. The Lambert-Eaton myasthenic syndrome. A review of 50 cases. *Brain.* 1988;111(Pt 3):577−596.

36. Nair SG, Kumar BS, Rajan B. Poorly differentiated carcinoma of the lung presenting with Lambert−Eaton myasthenic syndrome. *Am J Clin Oncol.* 2000;23(1):58−59.

37. Keogh M, Sedehizadeh S, Maddison P. Treatment for Lambert-Eaton myasthenic syndrome. *Cochrane Database Syst Rev.* 2011;2011(2):Cd003279.

38. Titulaer MJ, Lang B, Verschuuren JJ. Lambert-Eaton myasthenic syndrome: from clinical characteristics to therapeutic strategies. *Lancet Neurol.* 2011;10(12): 1098−1107.

39. Bataller L, Graus F, Saiz A, Vilchez JJ. Clinical outcome in adult onset idiopathic or paraneoplastic opsoclonus-myoclonus. *Brain*. 2001;124(Pt 2):437–443.

40. Ohara S, Iijima N, Hayashida K, Oide T, Katai S. Autopsy case of opsoclonus-myoclonus-ataxia and cerebellar cognitive affective syndrome associated with small cell carcinoma of the lung. *Mov Disord*. 2007;22(9): 1320–1324.

41. Chalk CH, Windebank AJ, Kimmel DW, McManis PG. The distinctive clinical features of paraneoplastic sensory neuronopathy. *Can J Neurol Sci*. 1992;19(3):346–351.

42. de Beukelaar JW, Sillevis Smitt PA. Managing paraneoplastic neurological disorders. *Oncol*. 2006;11(3): 292–305.

43. Lucchinetti CF, Kimmel DW, Lennon VA. Paraneoplastic and oncologic profiles of patients seropositive for type 1 antineuronal nuclear autoantibodies. *Neurology*. 1998; 50(3):652–657.

44. Lee HR, Lennon VA, Camilleri M, Prather CM. Paraneoplastic gastrointestinal motor dysfunction: clinical and laboratory characteristics. *Am J Gastroenterol*. 2001; 96(2):373–379.

45. Zahr ZA, Baer AN. Malignancy in myositis. *Curr Rheumatol Rep*. 2011;13(3):208–215.

46. Fujita J, Tokuda M, Bandoh S, et al. Primary lung cancer associated with polymyositis/dermatomyositis, with a review of the literature. *Rheumatol Int*. 2001;20(2):81–84.

47. Mori H, Habe K, Hakamada A, Isoda K-I, Mizutani H. Relapse of dermatomyositis after 10 years in remission following curative surgical treatment of lung cancer. *J Dermatol*. 2005;32(4):290–294.

48. Bentea G, Sculier C, Grigoriu B, et al. Autoimmune paraneoplastic syndromes associated to lung cancer: a systematic review of the literature: part 3: neurological paraneoplastic syndromes, involving the central nervous system. *Lung Cancer*. 2017;106:83–92.

49. Vigliani MC, Honnorat J, Antoine J-C, et al. Chorea and related movement disorders of paraneoplastic origin: the PNS EuroNetwork experience. *J Neurol*. 2011; 258(11):2058–2068.

50. Davis MC, Sherry V. Hypertrophic osteoarthropathy as a clinical manifestation of lung cancer. *Clin J Oncol Nurs*. 2011;15(5):561–563.

51. Ito T, Goto K, Yoh K, et al. Hypertrophic pulmonary osteoarthropathy as a paraneoplastic manifestation of lung cancer. *J Thorac Oncol*. 2010;5(7):976–980.

52. Shih WJ. Pulmonary hypertrophic osteoarthropathy and its resolution. *Semin Nucl Med*. 2004;34(2):159–163.

53. Albrecht S, Keller A. Postchemotherapeutic reversibility of hypertrophic osteoarthropathy in a patient with bronchogenic adenocarcinoma. *Clin Nucl Med*. 2003;28(6): 463–466.

54. King MM, Nelson DA. Hypertrophic osteoarthropathy effectively treated with zoledronic acid. *Clin Lung Cancer*. 2008;9(3):179–182.

55. Bernardo SG, Emer J, Burnett M, Gordon M. Hypertrophic osteoarthropathy presenting as unilateral cellulitis

with successful treatment using pamidronate disodium. *J Clin Aesthet Dermatol*. 2012;5(9):37–46.

56. Amital H, Applbaum YH, Vasiliev L, Rubinow A. Hypertrophic pulmonary osteoarthropathy: control of pain and symptoms with pamidronate. *Clin Rheumatol*. 2004; 23(4):330–332.

57. Angel-Moreno Maroto A, Martinez-Quintana E, Suarez-Castellano L, Perez-Arellano J-L. Painful hypertrophic osteoarthropathy successfully treated with octreotide. The pathogenetic role of vascular endothelial growth factor (VEGF). *Rheumatology*. 2005;44(10):1326–1327.

58. Johnson SA, Spiller PA, Faull CM. Treatment of resistant pain in hypertrophic pulmonary osteoarthropathy with subcutaneous octreotide. *Thorax*. 1997;52(3):298–299.

59. Hayashi M, Sekikawa A, Saijo A, Takada W, Yamawaki I, Ohkawa S-I. Successful treatment of hypertrophic osteoarthropathy by gefitinib in a case with lung adenocarcinoma. *Anticancer Res*. 2005;25(3c): 2435–2438.

60. Goldstraw P, Chansky K, Crowley J, et al. The IASLC lung cancer staging project: proposals for revision of the TNM stage groupings in the forthcoming (eighth) edition of the TNM classification for lung cancer. *J Thorac Oncol*. 2016;11(1):39–51.

61. Hoang T, Xu R, Schiller JH, Bonomi P, Johnson DH. Clinical model to predict survival in chemonaive patients with advanced non–small-cell lung cancer treated with third-generation chemotherapy regimens based on eastern cooperative oncology group data. *J Clin Oncol*. 2005;23(1):175–183.

62. Blackstock AW, Herndon, JE, Paskett ED, et al. Outcomes among African-American/non-African-American patients with advanced non-small-cell lung carcinoma: report from the Cancer and Leukemia Group B. *J Natl Cancer Inst*. 2002;94(4):284–290.

63. Athey VL, Walters SJ, Rogers TK. Symptoms at lung cancer diagnosis are associated with major differences in prognosis. *Thorax*. 2018;73(12):1177–1181.

64. Jawad MU, Scully SP. In brief: classifications in brief: Mirels' classification: metastatic disease in long bones and impending pathologic fracture. *Clin Orthop Relat Res*. 2010;468(10):2825–2827.

65. Gainor BJ, Buchert P. Fracture healing in metastatic bone disease. *Clin Orthop Relat Res*. 1983;(178):297–302.

66. Palma DA, Warner A, Louie AV, Senan S, Slotman B, Rodrigues GB. Thoracic radiotherapy for extensive stage small-cell lung cancer: a meta-analysis. *Clin Lung Cancer*. 2016;17(4):239–244.

67. Shirasawa M, Fukui T, Kusuhara S, et al. Prognostic significance of the 8th edition of the TNM classification for patients with extensive disease small cell lung cancer. *Cancer Manag Res*. 2018;10:6039–6047.

68. Bremnes RM, Sundstrom S, Aasebø U, Kaasa S, Hatlevoll R, Aamdal S. The value of prognostic factors in small cell lung cancer: results from a randomised multicenter study with minimum 5 year follow-up. *Lung Cancer*. 2003;39(3):303–313.

69. Batchelor TJP, Rashburn NJ, Abdelnour-Berchtold E, et al. Guidelines for enhanced recovery after lung surgery: recommendations of the enhanced recovery after surgery (ERAS®) Society and the European Society of Thoracic Surgeons (ESTS). *Eur J Cardio Thorac Surg.* 2019;55(1): 91−115.

70. Shukla A, Granger CL, Wright GM, Edbrooke L, Denehy L. Attitudes and perceptions to prehabilitation in lung cancer. *Integr Cancer Ther.* 2020;19. p. 1534735420924466.

71. Ljungqvist O, Scott M, Fearon KC. Enhanced recovery after surgery: a review. *JAMA Surg.* 2017;152(3):292−298.

72. Sommer MS, Trier K, Vibe-Peterson J, et al. Perioperative rehabilitation in operable lung cancer patients (PRO-LUCA): a feasibility study. *Integr Cancer Ther.* 2016; 15(4):455−466.

73. Temel JS, Greer JA, Goldberg S, et al. A structured exercise program for patients with advanced non-small cell lung cancer. *J Thorac Oncol.* 2009;4(5):595−601.

74. Missel M, Pedersen JH, Hendriksen C, Tewes M, Adamsen L. Exercise intervention for patients diagnosed with operable non-small cell lung cancer: a qualitative longitudinal feasibility study. *Support Care Cancer.* 2015;23(8):2311−2318.

75. Leach H, Devonish JA, Bebb DG, Krenz KA, Culos-Reed SN. Exercise preferences, levels and quality of life in lung cancer survivors. *Support Care Cancer.* 2015; 23(11):3239−3247.

76. Bobbio A, Chetta A, Carbognani P, et al. Changes in pulmonary function test and cardio-pulmonary exercise capacity in COPD patients after lobar pulmonary resection. *Eur J Cardio Thorac Surg.* 2005;28(5):754−758.

77. Nowicki A, Piekarska J, Farbicka E. The assessment of cancer-related fatigue syndrome in patients with lung cancer during palliative chemotherapy. *Adv Respir Med.* 2017;85(2):69−76.

78. Srdic D, Plestina S, Sverko-Peternac A, Nikolac N, Simundic A- M, Samarzija M. Cancer cachexia, sarcopenia and biochemical markers in patients with advanced non-small cell lung cancer-chemotherapy toxicity and prognostic value. *Support Care Cancer.* 2016;24(11): 4495−4502.

79. Avancini A, Cavallo A, Trestini I, et al. Exercise prehabilitation in lung cancer: getting stronger to recover faster. *Eur J Surg Oncol.* 2021;47(8):1847−1855.

80. Westmaas JL, Newton CC, Stevens VL, Flanders WD, Gapstur SM, Jacobs EJ. Does a recent cancer diagnosis predict smoking cessation? An analysis from a prospective US cohort. *J Clin Oncol.* 2015;33(15):1647−1652.

81. Ussher M, West R, Steptoe A, McEwen A. Increase in common cold symptoms and mouth ulcers following smoking cessation. *Tobac Control.* 2003;12(1):86−88.

82. Tarumi S, Yokomise H, Gotoh M, et al. Pulmonary rehabilitation during induction chemoradiotherapy for lung cancer improves pulmonary function. *J Thorac Cardiovasc Surg.* 2015;149(2):569−573.

83. Dicpinigaitis PV, Sitkauskiene B, Stravinskaite K, Appel DW, Negassa A, Sakalauskas R. Effect of smoking cessation on cough reflex sensitivity. *Eur Respir J.* 2006; 28(4):786−790.

84. Arends J, Bachmann P, Baracos V, et al. ESPEN guidelines on nutrition in cancer patients. *Clin Nutr.* 2017;36(1): 11−48.

85. Kiss N. Nutrition support and dietary interventions for patients with lung cancer: current insights. *Lung Cancer.* 2016;7:1−9.

86. Cataldo JK, Slaughter R, Jahan T, Pongquan VL, Hwang WJ. Measuring stigma in people with lung cancer: psychometric testing of the cataldo lung cancer stigma scale. *Oncol Nurs Forum.* 2011;38(1):E46−E54.

87. Brown Johnson CG, Brodsky JL, Cataldo JK. Lung cancer stigma, anxiety, depression, and quality of life. *J Psychosoc Oncol.* 2014;32(1):59−73.

88. Chapple A, Ziebland S, McPherson A. Stigma, shame, and blame experienced by patients with lung cancer: qualitative study. *BMJ.* 2004;328(7454):1470.

89. Shen MJ, Hamann HA, Thomas AJ, Ostroff JS. Association between patient-provider communication and lung cancer stigma. *Support Care Cancer.* 2016;24(5): 2093−2099.

90. Ferreira V, Minnella EM, Awasthi R, et al. Multimodal prehabilitation for lung cancer surgery: a randomized controlled trial. *Ann Thorac Surg.* 2020;112(5): 1600−1608.

91. Gökler-Danışman I, Yalçınay-İnan M, Yiğit İ. Experience of grief by patients with cancer in relation to perceptions of illness: the mediating roles of identity centrality, stigma-induced discrimination, and hopefulness. *J Psychosoc Oncol.* 2017;35(6):776−796.

92. Zhu J, Fang F, Sjölander A, Fall K, Adami HO, Valdimarsdóttir U. First-onset mental disorders after cancer diagnosis and cancer-specific mortality: a nationwide cohort study. *Ann Oncol.* 2017;28(8):1964−1969.

93. Mohammed N, Kestin LL, Grills IS, et al. Rapid disease progression with delay in treatment of non−small-cell lung cancer. *Int J Radiat Oncol Biol Phys.* 2011;79(2): 466−472.

94. Saad F, Lipton A, Cook R, Chen Y-M, Smith M, Coleman R. Pathologic fractures correlate with reduced survival in patients with malignant bone disease. *Cancer.* 2007;110(8):1860−1867.

95. Sheill G, Guinan EM, Peat N, Hussey J. Considerations for exercise prescription in patients with bone metastases: a comprehensive narrative review. *PM R.* 2018;10(8): 843−864.

96. Scagliotti GV, Hirsh V, Siena S, et al. Overall survival improvement in patients with lung cancer and bone metastases treated with denosumab versus zoledronic acid: subgroup analysis from a randomized phase 3 study. *J Thorac Oncol.* 2012;7(12):1823−1829.

97. De Castro J, Garcia R, Garrido P, et al. Therapeutic potential of denosumab in patients with lung cancer: beyond prevention of skeletal complications. *Clin Lung Cancer.* 2015;16(6):431−446.

98. Lopez-Olivo MA, Shah N, Pratt G, Risser J, Symanski E, Suarez-Almazor ME. Bisphosphonates in the treatment

of patients with lung cancer and metastatic bone disease: a systematic review and meta-analysis. *Support Care Cancer.* 2012;20(11):2985–2998.

99. Cheville A. 29 - Cancer rehabilitation. In: Cifu DX, ed. *Braddom's Physical Medicine and Rehabilitation.* 6th ed. Philadelphia: Elsevier; 2021:568–593.e7.

100. Bunting RW, Shea B. Bone metastasis and rehabilitation. *Cancer.* 2001;92(S4):1020–1028.

101. Rief H, Omlor G, Akbar M, et al. Feasibility of isometric spinal muscle training in patients with bone metastases under radiation therapy - first results of a randomized pilot trial. *BMC Cancer.* 2014;14(1):67.

102. Crevenna R. From neuromuscular electrical stimulation and biofeedback-assisted exercise up to triathlon competitions—regular physical activity for cancer patients in Austria. *Eur Rev Aging Phys Act.* 2013;10(1):53–55.

103. Crevenna R, Kainberger F, Wiltschke C, et al. Cancer rehabilitation: current trends and practices within an Austrian University Hospital Center. *Disabil Rehabil.* 2020;42(1):2–7.

104. Rispoli M, Salvi R, Cennamo A, et al. Effectiveness of home-based preoperative pulmonary rehabilitation in COPD patients undergoing lung cancer resection. *Tumori J.* 2020;106(3):203–211.

105. Morano MT, Araujo AS, Nascimento FB, et al. Preoperative pulmonary rehabilitation versus chest physical therapy in patients undergoing lung cancer resection: a pilot randomized controlled trial. *Arch Phys Med Rehabil.* 2013;94(1):53–58.

106. Peddle-McIntyre CJ, Bell G, Fenton D, McCargar L, Courneya KS. Feasibility and preliminary efficacy of progressive resistance exercise training in lung cancer survivors. *Lung Cancer.* 2012;75(1):126–132.

107. Phillips WT, Batterham AM, Valenzuela JE, Burkett LN. Reliability of maximal strength testing in older adults. *Arch Phys Med Rehabil.* 2004;85(2):329–334.

108. Knutzen KM, Brilla LR, Caine D. Validity of 1RM prediction equations for older adults. *J Strength Condit Res.* 1999;13(3):242–246.

109. Dohoney P, Chromiak JA, Lemiere D, Abadie BR, Kovacs C. Prediction of one repetition maximum (1-RM) strength from a 4-6 RM and a 7-10 RM submaximal strength test in healthy young adult males. *J Exerc Physiol.* 2002;5(3):54–59.

110. Bobbio A, Chetta A, Ampollini L, et al. Preoperative pulmonary rehabilitation in patients undergoing lung resection for non-small cell lung cancer. *Eur J Cardio Thorac Surg.* 2008;33(1):95–98.

111. Jones LW, Peddle C, Eves N, et al. Effects of presurgical exercise training on cardiorespiratory fitness among patients undergoing thoracic surgery for malignant lung lesions. *Cancer.* 2007;110(3):590–598.

112. Perrotta F, Cennamo A, Cerqua FS, et al. Effects of a high-intensity pulmonary rehabilitation program on the minute ventilation/carbon dioxide output slope during exercise in a cohort of patients with COPD undergoing lung resection for non-small cell lung cancer. *J Bras Pneumol.* 2019;45(6).

113. Coats V, Maltais F, Simard S, et al. Feasibility and effectiveness of a home-based exercise training program before lung resection surgery. *Can Respir J J Can Thorac Soc.* 2013;20(2):e10–e16.

114. Liptay MJ, Basu S, Hoaglin M, et al. Diffusion lung capacity for carbon monoxide (DLCO) is an independent prognostic factor for long-term survival after curative lung resection for cancer. *J Surg Oncol.* 2009;100(8):703–707.

115. Dales RE, Dionne G, Leech JA, Lunau M, Schweitzer I. Preoperative prediction of pulmonary complications following thoracic surgery. *Chest.* 1993;104(1):155–159.

116. Sekine Y, Chiyo M, Iwata T, et al. Perioperative rehabilitation and physiotherapy for lung cancer patients with chronic obstructive pulmonary disease. *Jpn J Thorac Cardiovasc Surg.* 2005;53(5):237–243.

117. Licker M, Karenovics W, Diaper J, et al. Short-term preoperative high-intensity interval training in patients awaiting lung cancer surgery: a randomized controlled trial. *J Thorac Oncol.* 2017;12(2):323–333.

118. Benzo R, Wigle D, Novotny P, et al. Preoperative pulmonary rehabilitation before lung cancer resection: results from two randomized studies. *Lung Cancer.* 2011;74(3):441–445.

119. Bluethmann SM, Basen-Engquist K, Vernon SW, et al. Grasping the "teachable moment": time since diagnosis, symptom burden and health behaviors in breast, colorectal and prostate cancer survivors. *Psycho Oncol.* 2015;24(10):1250–1257.

120. Park ER, Gareen IF, Japuntich S, et al. Primary care provider-delivered smoking cessation interventions and smoking cessation among participants in the national lung screening trial. *JAMA Intern Med.* 2015;175(9):1509–1516.

121. Schnoll RA, Martinez E, Tatum K, et al. A bupropion smoking cessation clinical trial for cancer patients. *Cancer Causes Control.* 2010;21(6):811–820.

122. Pesola GR, Avasarala J. Bupropion seizure proportion among new-onset generalized seizures and drug related seizures presenting to an emergency department. *J Emerg Med.* 2002;22(3):235–239.

123. Finkelstein Y, Macdonald EM, Li P, Mamdani MM, Gomes T, Juurlink DN. Second-generation antidepressants and risk of new-onset seizures in the elderly. *Clin Toxicol.* 2018;56(12):1179–1184.

124. Garland SN, Johnson JA, Savard J, et al. Sleeping well with cancer: a systematic review of cognitive behavioral therapy for insomnia in cancer patients. *Neuropsychiatric Dis Treat.* 2014;10.

125. Wiskemann J, Hummler S, Diepold C, et al. POSITIVE study: physical exercise program in non-operable lung cancer patients undergoing palliative treatment. *BMC Cancer.* 2016;16(1):499.

126. Santiago-Palma J, Payne R. Palliative care and rehabilitation. *Cancer.* 2001;92(S4):1049–1052.

127. Klapper J, D'Amico TA. VATS versus open surgery for lung cancer resection: moving toward a minimally invasive approach. *J Natl Compr Cancer Netw.* 2015;13(2): 162–164.

128. Okereke I, Murthy SC, Alster JM, Blackstone EH, Rice TW. Characterization and importance of air leak after lobectomy. *Ann Thorac Surg.* 2005;79(4):1167–1173.

129. Rivera C, Bernard A, Falcoz P-E, et al. Characterization and prediction of prolonged air leak after pulmonary resection: a nationwide study setting up the index of prolonged air leak. *Ann Thorac Surg.* 2011;92(3): 1062–1068.

130. Gursoy S, Yazgan S, Ucvet A, et al. Postpneumonectomy bronchopleural fistula in non-small cell lung cancer patients: incidence, survival, mortality, and treatment analysis. *Surg Today.* 2018;48(7):695–702.

131. Sirbu H, Busch T, Aleksic I, Schreiner W, Oster O, Dalichau H. Bronchopleural fistula in the surgery of non-small cell lung cancer: incidence, risk factors, and management. *Ann Thorac Cardiovasc Surg.* 2001;7(6): 330–336.

132. Muranishi Y, Sonobe M, Menju T, et al. Atrial fibrillation after lung cancer surgery: incidence, severity, and risk factors. *Surg Today.* 2017;47(2):252–258.

133. Ahmad AM. Essentials of physiotherapy after thoracic surgery: what physiotherapists need to know. A narrative review. *Kor J Thoracic Cardiovasc Surg.* 2018;51(5):293.

134. Dahners LE, Mullis BH. Effects of nonsteroidal anti-inflammatory drugs on bone formation and soft-tissue healing. *J Am Acad Orthopaedic Surgeon.* 2004;12(3): 139–143.

135. Chen MR, Dragoo JL. The effect of nonsteroidal anti-inflammatory drugs on tissue healing. *Knee Surg Sports Traumatol Arthrosc.* 2013;21(3):540–549.

136. Lardinois D, Vogt P, Yang L, Hegyi I, Baslam M, Weder W. Non-steroidal anti-inflammatory drugs decrease the quality of pleurodesis after mechanical pleural abrasion. *Eur J Cardio Thorac Surg.* 2004;25(5):865–871.

137. Nielsen KG, Holte K, Kehlet H. Effects of posture on postoperative pulmonary function. *Acta Anaesthesiol Scand.* 2003;47(10):1270–1275.

138. Kaneda H, Saito Y, Okamoto M, Maniwa T, Minami K, Imamura H. Early postoperative mobilization with walking at 4 hours after lobectomy in lung cancer patients. *Gen Thoracic Cardiovasc Surg.* 2007;55(12):493–498.

139. Yousef K, Pinsky MR, DeVita MA, Sereika S, Hravnak M. Characteristics of patients with cardiorespiratory instability in a step-down unit. *Am J Crit Care.* 2012;21(5): 344–350.

140. Pryor JA, Prasad AS. *Physiotherapy for Respiratory and Cardiac Problems: Adults and Paediatrics.* Elsevier Health Sciences; 2008.

141. Hillegass E. *Essentials of Cardiopulmonary Physical Therapy-E-Book.* Elsevier Health Sciences; 2016.

142. Hess D, MacIntyre NR, Mishoe SC, Galvin WF, Adams AB. *Respiratory Care: Principles and Practice.* Jones & Bartlett Learning; 2011.

143. Duggan M, Kavanagh BP, Warltier DC. Pulmonary atelectasis: a pathogenic perioperative entity. *J Am Soc Anesthesiol.* 2005;102(4):838–854.

144. Platell C, Hall JC. Atelectasis after abdominal surgery. *J Am Coll Surg.* 1997;185(6):584–592.

145. Caraceni A, Portenoy RK. An international survey of cancer pain characteristics and syndromes. *Pain.* 1999;82(3): 263–274.

146. Hassett MJ, Rao SR, Brozovic S, et al. Chemotherapy-related hospitalization among community cancer center patients. *Oncologist.* 2011;16(3):378–387.

147. Numico G, Cristofano A, Mozzicafreddo A, et al. Hospital admission of cancer patients: avoidable practice or necessary care? *PLoS One.* 2015;10(3):e0120827.

148. Riesenberg H, Lübbe AS. In-patient rehabilitation of lung cancer patients—a prospective study. *Support Care Cancer.* 2010;18(7):877–882.

149. Codima A, das Neves Silva W, de Souza Borges AP, de Castro Jr G. Exercise prescription for symptoms and quality of life improvements in lung cancer patients: a systematic review. *Support Care Cancer.* 2020:1–13.

150. De Backer IC, Vreugdenhil G, Nijziel MR, Kester AD, van Breda E, Schep G. Long-term follow-up after cancer rehabilitation using high-intensity resistance training: persistent improvement of physical performance and quality of life. *Br J Cancer.* 2008;99(1):30–36.

151. Dev R, Wong A, Hui D, Bruera E. The evolving approach to management of cancer cachexia. *Oncology.* 2017;31(1): 23–32.

152. Topkan E, Yavuz MN, Onal C, Yavuz AA. Prevention of acute radiation-induced esophagitis with glutamine in non-small cell lung cancer patients treated with radiotherapy: evaluation of clinical and dosimetric parameters. *Lung Cancer.* 2009;63(3):393–399.

153. Engelen M, Safar AM, Bartter T, Koeman F, Deutz NEP. High anabolic potential of essential amino acid mixtures in advanced nonsmall cell lung cancer. *Ann Oncol.* 2015; 26(9):1960–1966.

154. Madeddu C, Dessi M, Panzone F, et al. Randomized phase III clinical trial of a combined treatment with carnitine+ celecoxib±megestrol acetate for patients with cancer-related anorexia/cachexia syndrome. *Clin Nutr.* 2012;31(2):176–182.

155. Garcia VR, Ortiz Z. Megestrol acetate for treatment of anorexia-cachexia syndrome. *Cochrane Database Syst Rev.* 2013;3.

156. Jatoi A, Windschitl HE, Loprinzi CL, et al. Dronabinol versus megestrol acetate versus combination therapy for cancer-associated anorexia: a North Central Cancer Treatment Group study. *J Clin Oncol.* 2002;20(2):567–573.

157. Temel JS, Abernethy AP, Currow DC, et al. Anamorelin in patients with non-small-cell lung cancer and cachexia (ROMANA 1 and ROMANA 2): results from two randomised, double-blind, phase 3 trials. *Lancet Oncol.* 2016; 17(4):519–531.

158. Katakami N, Uchino J, Yokoyama T, et al. Anamorelin (ONO-7643) for the treatment of patients with non–small

cell lung cancer and cachexia: results from a randomized, double-blind, placebo-controlled, multicenter study of Japanese patients (ONO-7643-04). *Cancer.* 2018;124(3):606–616.

159. Hung R, Krebs P, Coups EJ, et al. Fatigue and functional impairment in early-stage non-small cell lung cancer survivors. *J Pain Symptom Manag.* 2011;41(2):426–435.

160. Sha F, Zhuang S, Zhou L, et al. Biomarkers for cancer-related fatigue and adverse reactions to chemotherapy in lung cancer patients. *Mol Clin Oncol.* 2015;3(1):163–166.

161. Bower JE. Cancer-related fatigue—mechanisms, risk factors, and treatments. *Nat Rev Clin Oncol.* 2014;11(10):597–609.

162. Jung JY, Lee JM, Kim MS, Shim YM, Zo JI, Yun YH. Comparison of fatigue, depression, and anxiety as factors affecting posttreatment health-related quality of life in lung cancer survivors. *Psycho Oncol.* 2018;27(2):465–470.

163. Dhillon HM, Bell ML, van der Ploeg HP, et al. Impact of physical activity on fatigue and quality of life in people with advanced lung cancer: a randomized controlled trial. *Ann Oncol.* 2017;28(8):1889–1897.

164. Quist M, Sommer MS, Vibe-Petersen J, et al. Early initiated postoperative rehabilitation reduces fatigue in patients with operable lung cancer: a randomized trial. *Lung Cancer.* 2018;126:125–132.

165. Mustian KM, Alfano CM, Heckler C, et al. Comparison of pharmaceutical, psychological, and exercise treatments for cancer-related fatigue: a meta-analysis. *JAMA Oncol.* 2017;3(7):961–968.

166. Avancini A, Sartori G, Gkountakos A, et al. Physical activity and exercise in lung cancer care: Will promises be fulfilled? *Oncologist.* 2020;25(3):e555–e569. https://doi.org/10.1634/theoncologist.2019-0463.

167. Ebbert JO, Scharf EL, Hurt RT. Medical cannabis. *Mayo Clin Proc.* 2018;93(12):1842–1847.

168. Babson KA, Sottile J, Morabito D. Cannabis, cannabinoids, and sleep: a review of the literature. *Curr Psychiatr Rep.* 2017;19(4):23.

169. Piper BJ, DeKeuster RM, Beals ML, et al. Substitution of medical cannabis for pharmaceutical agents for pain, anxiety, and sleep. *J Psychopharmacol.* 2017;31(5):569–575.

170. Kargbo RB. Psilocybin therapeutic research: the present and future paradigm. *ACS Med Chem Lett.* 2020;11(4):399–402.

171. Ross S, Bossis A, Guss J, et al. Rapid and sustained symptom reduction following psilocybin treatment for anxiety and depression in patients with life-threatening cancer: a randomized controlled trial. *J Psychopharmacol.* 2016;30(12):1165–1180.

172. Grob CS, Bossis AP, Griffiths RR. *Use of the Classic Hallucinogen Psilocybin for Treatment of Existential Distress Associated with Cancer. Psychological Aspects of Cancer.* 2013:291–308.

173. Chasen MR, Feldstain A, Gravelle D, MacDonald N, Pereira J. An interprofessional palliative care oncology rehabilitation program: effects on function and predictors of program completion. *Curr Oncol.* 2013;20(6):301–309.

174. Edbrooke L, Aranda S, Granger CL, et al. Multidisciplinary home-based rehabilitation in inoperable lung cancer: a randomised controlled trial. *Thorax.* 2019;74(8):787–796.

175. Edbrooke L, Denehy L, Granger CL, Kapp S, Aranda S. Home-based rehabilitation in inoperable non-small cell lung cancer—the patient experience. *Support Care Cancer.* 2020;28(1):99–112.

176. Lin YY, Liu MF, Tzeng J-I, Lin C-C. Effects of walking on quality of life among lung cancer patients: a longitudinal study. *Cancer Nurs.* 2015;38(4):253–259.

177. Medina-Mirapeix F, Escolar-Reina P, Gascón-Cánovas JJ, Montilla-Herrador J, Jimeno-Serrano FJ, Collins SM. Predictive factors of adherence to frequency and duration components in home exercise programs for neck and low back pain: an observational study. *BMC Muscoskel Disord.* 2009;10(1):155.

178. Andersen AH, Vinther A, Poulsen L-L, Mellemgaard A. A modified exercise protocol may promote continuance of exercise after the intervention in lung cancer patients–a pragmatic uncontrolled trial. *Support Care Cancer.* 2013;21(8):2247–2253.

179. Silver JK, Gilchrist LS. Cancer rehabilitation with a focus on evidence-based outpatient physical and occupational therapy interventions. *Am J Phys Med Rehabil.* 2011;90(5).

180. Cordova MJ, Riba MB, Spiegel D. Post-traumatic stress disorder and cancer. *Lancet Psychiatr.* 2017;4(4):330–338.

181. Schneider BJ, Ismaila N, Aerts J, et al. Lung cancer surveillance after definitive curative-intent therapy: ASCO guideline. *J Clin Oncol.* 2020;38(7):753–766.

182. Cheville AL, Rhudy L, Basford JR, Griffin JM, Flores AM. How receptive are patients with late stage cancer to rehabilitation services and what are the sources of their resistance? *Arch Phys Med Rehabil.* 2017;98(2):203–210.

183. Cintron A, Hamel MB, Davis RB, Burns RB, Phillips RS, McCarthy EP. Hospitalization of hospice patients with cancer. *J Palliat Med.* 2003;6(5):757–768.

184. Ester M, Culos-Reed SN, Abdul-Razzak A, et al. Feasibility of a multimodal exercise, nutrition, and palliative care intervention in advanced lung cancer. *BMC Cancer.* 2021;21(1):1–13.

185. Lim RBL. End-of-life care in patients with advanced lung cancer. *Ther Adv Respir Dis.* 2016;10(5):455–467.

186. Loggers ET, Starks H, Shannon-Dudley M, Back AL, Appelbaum FR, Stewart FM. Implementing a death with dignity program at a comprehensive cancer center. *N Engl J Med.* 2013;368(15):1417–1424.

Systemic Therapy and Radiation Therapy in Lung Cancer

RAEES TONSE, MD • MARTIN C. TOM, MD • RUPESH KOTECHA, MD

INTRODUCTION

Lung cancer is the most common cause of cancer-related death in both men and women around the world.[1] Given that lung cancer can remain asymptomatic when it presents with a low disease burden in its early stages, it is usually discovered only after it has progressed to an advanced stage. Nonsmall cell lung cancer (NSCLC) accounts for about 85% of lung cancer cases.[2] Screening with low-dose computed tomography (CT) has recently been shown to have a mortality benefit in high-risk patients (i.e., 50 years and older, 20 or more pack-year smoking history, exposure to radon and asbestos, family history of lung cancer), and its use is increasing given its incorporation into national guidelines.[3] However, the majority of patients come in for diagnostic evaluation of specific symptoms or because of an unexpected finding on chest imaging (not performed during screening assessment). The goal of the initial examination is to gather enough clinical and radiologic information to guide diagnostic tissue biopsy, complete staging, and determine a treatment plan. Treatment is governed by the cancer's subtype and stage, and there are now several personalized treatments that were previously unavailable based on the molecular profile of the disease.[4] In general, the role of multidisciplinary teams to optimize treatment is crucial, especially as patients receive multimodal therapies.

EPIDEMIOLOGY OF LUNG CANCER

Lung cancer caused an estimated 1.8 million deaths in 2020 worldwide.[5] In the United States, it causes about 230,000 new cases and 130,000 deaths per year.[1,5] Due to advancements in systemic therapies, such as the development of newer targeted agents against specific actionable molecular alterations, as well as the introduction of immunotherapeutics into the treatment space, improvements in survival have been observed in recent population-based analyses.[6,7] Before the fifth decade of life, lung cancer is quite uncommon; after that, the risk increases with age. Men are generally more affected than women. Lung cancer deaths are slowly declining, largely due to cessation in smoking as it reduces lung cancer risk.[8] Even reducing the number of cigarettes smoked daily has shown to be beneficial.[3] In general, any form of smoking, including secondhand smoke, cigars, and pipes, raises the risk of lung cancer. Due to inconsistent results, the link between marijuana and e-cigarettes is less apparent with lung cancer that traditional tobacco exposures.[9] Radon exposure and select types of interstitial lung disease are other risk factors. Lung cancer is also linked to chronic obstructive pulmonary disease and prior family history.

The most common presenting manifestations in lung cancer include cough, hemoptysis, dyspnea, and chest pain.[10] Patients with these symptoms often undergo a chest radiograph at initial presentation due to the low radiation exposure and ease of testing. An enlarged hilar or paratracheal node, an endobronchial lesion, postobstructive pneumonia, or segmental or lobar atelectasis can all be seen on a chest radiograph.[11] Additional testing with a contrast-enhanced chest CT can be performed based on suspicious radiograph findings. A solitary lung nodule, uneven or spiculated margins, and thick-walled cavitation on CT are potential indicators of malignancy. On the other hand, lung cancer is highly unlikely to be represented by solid-appearing lesions on chest CTs that have remained consistent in size for at least 2 years. Asymptomatic patients may have incidental findings during routine screening.

STAGING FOR LUNG CANCER

Whether lung cancer is localized in the lungs or has extended to regional lymph nodes or other organs determines the stage. Tumors can grow in the lungs for a long period before being discovered. As a result, it is difficult to diagnose lung cancer in its early stages

Lung Cancer Rehabilitation. https://doi.org/10.1016/B978-0-323-83404-9.00011-6

(stages I and II). A positron emission tomography (PET/CT) is recommended for extracranial systemic staging and magnetic resonance imaging (MRI) of the brain for those with Stage II–IV NSCLC and any patient diagnosed with small cell lung cancer (SCLC).

The Tumor, Node, Metastasis (TNM) stage at presentation is the most important factor in determining the prognosis in individuals with NSCLC. Currently, the American Joint Committee on Cancer (AJCC) eighth edition is in use for staging of NSCLC (see Table 2.1).[13] The various stages for NSCLC are as follows:

TABLE 2.1
TNM Staging of Lung Cancer.[12]

T: PRIMARY TUMOR

Tx	Primary tumor cannot be assessed or tumor proven by presence of malignant cells in sputum or bronchial washings but not visualized by imaging or bronchoscopy
T0	No evidence of primary tumor
Tis	Carcinoma in situ
T1	Tumor ≤3 cm in greatest dimension surrounded by lung or visceral pleura without bronchoscopic evidence of invasion more proximal than the lobar bronchus
T1a(mi)	Minimally invasive adenocarcinoma
T1a	Tumor ≤1 cm in greatest dimension
T1b	Tumor >1 cm but ≤2 cm in greatest dimension
T1c	Tumor >2 cm but ≤3 cm in greatest dimension
T2	Tumor >3 cm but ≤5 cm or tumor with any of the following features: - Involves main bronchus regardless of distance from the carina but without involvement of the carina - Invades visceral pleura - Associated with atelectasis or obstructive pneumonitis that extends to the hilar region, Involving part or all of the lung
T2a	Tumor >3 cm but ≤4 cm in greatest dimension

TABLE 2.1
TNM Staging of Lung Cancer.[12]—cont'd

T2b	Tumor >4 cm but ≤5 cm in greatest dimension
T3	Tumor >5 cm but ≤7 cm in greatest dimension or associated with separate tumor nodule(s) in the same lobe as the primary tumor or directly invades any of the following structures: Chest wall (including the parietal pleura and superior sulcus tumors), phrenic nerve, parietal pericardium
T4	Tumor >7 cm in greatest dimension or associated with separate tumor nodule(s) in a different ipsilateral lobe than that of the primary tumor or invades any of the following structures: diaphragm, mediastinum, heart, great vessels, trachea, recurrent laryngeal nerve, esophagus, vertebral body, and carina

N: REGIONAL LYMPH NODE INVOLVEMENT

Nx	Regional lymph nodes cannot be assessed
N0	No regional lymph node metastasis
N1	Metastasis in ipsilateral peribronchial and/or ipsilateral hilar lymph nodes and intrapulmonary nodes, including involvement by direct extension
N2	Metastasis in ipsilateral mediastinal and/or subcarinal lymph node(s)
N3	Metastasis in contralateral mediastinal, contralateral hilar, ipsilateral or contralateral scalene, or supraclavicular lymph node(s)

M: DISTANT METASTASIS

M0	No distant metastasis
M1	Distant metastasis present
M1a	Separate tumor nodule(s) in a contralateral lobe; tumor with pleural or pericardial nodule(s) or malignant pleural or pericardial effusion
M1b	Single extrathoracic metastasis
M1c	Multiple extrathoracic metastases in one or more organs

- Stage I - A tumor that has not spread to any lymph nodes. Stage I is further divided into subcategories based on the tumor's size: Stage IA cancers are 3 cm or less in size, and are further split into IA1, IA2, and IA3 (depending on size). Tumors in stage IB are greater than 3 cm but less than 4 cm in diameter.
- Stage II - It is subdivided into two stages: Stage IIA lung cancer is defined as a tumor that is larger than 4 cm but smaller than 5 cm and has not spread to adjacent lymph nodes. Stage IIB lung cancer is defined as a tumor that is smaller than 5 cm in diameter and has progressed to the lymph nodes.
- Stage III - They are further classified as stage IIIA, IIIB, or IIIC and is determined by the size of the tumor and the number of lymph nodes to which the malignancy has spread.
- Stage IV - It indicates that the cancer has spread to other parts of the body, such as the other lung, pleural effusion, pericardial effusion, or distant areas of the body, via the bloodstream. Based on the extent of the disease, stage IV NSCLC is further classified into stage IVA, IVB, or IVC.

TREATMENT OPTIONS

Basics of Surgery

For stage I and II NSCLC, surgery is the treatment of choice.[14,15] The different types of surgery for NSCLC include the following:

- **Pneumonectomy:** The entire lung, as well as its lymph nodes, is removed during this procedure and it is usually indicated for tumors that are centrally located.[16]
- **Lobectomy:** During this treatment, an entire lung lobe is removed along with the regional lymph nodes.[17]
- **Segmentectomy:** Only a portion of the lung is removed, not the complete lobe. Usually indicated if the patient's normal lung function is insufficient to sustain the removal of the entire lobe. This procedure may be performed via a video-assisted thoracoscopic surgery (VATS) or robotic-assisted thoracoscopic surgery (RATS).[18]
- **Wedge resection:** This procedure involves removal of a small nonanatomic wedge of the affected lung. This is typically performed with VATS or RATS techniques. These strategies have been shown to reduce surgical morbidity, including perioperative discomfort, and appear to be especially beneficial for patients with comorbidities.[18]

Despite the fact that surgical decisions are made based on provider and institution preferences, recent studies support the use of VATS procedures. For example, in a randomized study of VATS versus open thoracotomy, VATS procedures were linked to a reduction in operation time, blood loss, and hospital stays, as well as less postoperative pain and better quality of life.[19]

Radiation Therapy

In general, radiation therapy (RT) is often used either in a curative sense or for those needing palliation for metastatic disease. Patients who are unable to have surgery due to comorbidities or who refuse resection may be treated with definitive RT.[20–22] It may be utilized depending on the stage of NSCLC and other factors: for patients with early-stage disease, as a first-line treatment, occasionally in combination with chemotherapy, especially if the lung tumor cannot be removed, or if the patient refuses surgery in those with locally advanced disease. RT can also be used after surgery (along with chemotherapy) for patients who have resected tumors with positive margins. RT can also be used before surgery (usually along with chemotherapy) to make it easier to operate on a lung tumor by reducing the size and extent of disease. RT is also often used to treat areas of metastatic disease to the brain or bones and can also be used to relieve pain, bleeding, and cough associated with growth of the primary disease.

The various types of RT techniques used are as follows:

- **Three-dimensional conformal radiation therapy (3D-CRT):** RT beams are shaped and focused from a variety of angles on the tumor, reducing the risk of injury to healthy tissues.[23]
- **Intensity-modulated radiation therapy (IMRT):** Sophisticated inverse planning and computational algorithms are used to maximize RT delivery to the treatment volume while minimizing RT to normal tissue outside of the target.[24] When tumors are in close proximity to critical structures, such as the spinal cord, this approach is useful.
- **Stereotactic body radiation therapy (SBRT):** It employs concentrated high-dose RT beams that are delivered in five or fewer treatments.[21] Several beams are targeted at the tumor from various angles. SBRT is usually recommended for lesions less than 5 cm in diameter.
- **Particle therapy:** Patients with stage I NSCLC have received proton beam and carbon ion therapy, with similar outcomes to SBRT.[25] Particle therapy's unique depth-dose characteristics allow for dose escalation to tumors while sparing normal tissues and enhancing quality of life.

- **Brachytherapy:** Radioactive material (typically in the form of small pellets/seeds) is placed directly into the tumor or the airway next to it via a bronchoscope or surgery.[26] The radiation only travels a short distance from the source, minimizing the impact on healthy tissues in the area.

Chemotherapy/Systemic Therapy

Chemotherapy may be suggested in a variety of settings for patients with NSCLC, depending on the tumor stage.[27] Neoadjuvant chemotherapy is used to try to reduce a tumor so that it can be removed with less extensive surgery. Adjuvant chemotherapy is used to try to destroy any residual cancer cells or any subclinical microscopic clinical disease not visible on imaging studies. For locally advanced lung disease, chemotherapy coupled with RT is the preferred treatment. Chemotherapy is used to treat lung cancer that has progressed to other organs such as the bones, liver, or brain.[28] Cisplatin, carboplatin, paclitaxel, docetaxel, gemcitabine, vinorelbine, etoposide, and pemetrexed are the most often utilized chemotherapeutic drugs for NSCLC.

Targeted therapies differ from conventional chemotherapy drugs in their administration, side effect profile, and disease response. Patients who have certain molecular characteristics are frequently treated with specific targeted therapies:

- Patients with activating mutations in the epidermal growth factor receptor (EGFR) gene are more likely to be never smokers, women, and Asian in origin.[29] Patients that have EGFR mutations have a much better prognosis and respond to EGFR tyrosine kinase inhibitors such as erlotinib, osimertinib, gefitinib, and afatinib.[30]
- Other NSCLC subtypes are identified by the presence of ROS1 or EML4-ALK fusion oncogenes, which are more common in former smokers and appear earlier in life.[31] Anaplastic lymphoma kinase (ALK) inhibitors [i.e., crizotinib, ceritinib, alectinib, brigatinib, and lorlatinib] have high response rates in these select patients.[32]
- Less common driver mutations and corresponding targeted drugs include BRAF [dabrafenib, trametinib], Kirsten rat sarcoma viral oncogene homolog [sotorasib], ROS1 [crizotinib, ceritinib, lorlatinib], neurotrophic receptor tyrosine kinase [larotrectinib, entrectinib], MET [capmatinib, tepotinib], and RET [selpercatinib, pralsetinib].[33] Whole-genome testing is needed to discover the presence of these rare potential targets.

- Programmed death-ligand 1 (PD-L1) tumor expression can help guide treatment decisions in both first-line and second-line settings by predicting response to various immunotherapies.[13,34] Various checkpoint inhibitors used in the treatment of NSCLC are anticytotoxic T-lymphocyte antigen 4 (CTLA-4) [ipilimumab], antiprogrammed cell death protein-1 (PD1) [pembrolizumab, nivolumab], and anti-PD-L1 [durvalumab, atezolizumab].

STAGE BY STAGE TREATMENTS

Different treatment options may be recommended for each stage of NSCLC.

Stage I and II NSCLC

Patients with stage I or II NSCLC should be treated with complete surgical resection whenever possible. Several criteria, such as the presence of lymphovascular space invasion, tumor size, and the presence of lymph nodes, should be addressed when determining whether individuals might benefit from adjuvant chemotherapy treatment for postexcision.[35] Patients who are medically inoperable should be considered for definitive treatment with SBRT.[36] Several fractionation schedules have been developed for this patient population ranging from treatment in a single fraction,[37] three fractions,[36] four fractions,[38] or five fractions,[39] depending on tumor size, location, proximity to nearby organs-at-risk, and institutional practice. The SPACE study investigated two RT delivery modalities for patients with Stage I peripheral NSCLC: SBRT (66 Gy in 3 fractions) and 3D-CRT (70 Gy in 35 fractions).[40] There was an improvement in local control with SBRT compared to 3DCRT as well as improved toxicity profile and quality of life. Similarly, the CHISEL trial was a phase III trial for peripheral T1-T2a NSCLC with a 2:1 randomization to SBRT versus conventional RT, which also demonstrated the superiority of SBRT with regards to local control.[41]

The promising outcomes with SBRT compared to surgery have led to multiple attempts to directly compare to the two treatment techniques for patients with early-stage NSCLC. Despite the failure of multiple comparative studies to start or enroll patients, the STARS/ROSEL combined analysis of two trials randomly assigning patients to SBRT or surgery found that patients treated with SBRT had comparable rates of recurrence-free survival and higher rates of overall survival (OS).[42] Further trials are currently ongoing to better compare these treatment approaches.

Stage III NSCLC

About one-third of NSCLC patients are diagnosed with Stage III disease and as this stage grouping represents not only a large proportion of patients but also encompasses those with a variety of tumor sizes and differing extents of lymph node involvement, treatment is typically multimodal. Patients who are medically operable can be treated with neoadjuvant chemotherapy and resection[43] or neoadjuvant chemoradiotherapy and resection.[44] For resected patients who are found unexpectedly to have Stage III disease after final pathology review, adjuvant chemotherapy is usually recommended.[45,46] For select patients with N2 disease, sequential RT was initially considered[46,47]; however, the results of recent studies have failed to show any benefit in disease-free survival.[48] Chemotherapy and RT may be given together (concurrent chemoradiotherapy) or may be given one after the other (sequential chemoradiotherapy) in select patients.[49] The addition of consolidative chemotherapy to patients receiving concurrent chemotherapy has not improved survival outcomes[50] nor has increasing radiation dose.[51] However, the addition of durvalumab in the adjuvant setting has led to significant improvements in survival for nonoperable patients.[52]

Stage IV NSCLC

Systemic therapy or a palliative strategy based on symptoms is typically used to treat patients with advanced disease. Chemotherapy, molecularly targeted therapy, and/or immunotherapy may all help to extend life expectancy in appropriately selected patients without significantly adversely affecting quality of life. Whenever possible, the tumor's mutation status should be used to guide treatment decisions in these situations. Moreover, although the definition of oligometastatic disease is evolving, the role of local therapies—such as SBRT, surgery, or other ablative approaches—is increasing in this patient population. In a randomized phase II study, local consolidative treatment was found to improve OS in patients with oligometastatic NSCLC when compared to maintenance therapy.[53] Furthermore, the phase II randomized SABR-COMET study found that local treatment, in conjunction with systemic therapy, enhanced survival in patients with synchronous or metachronous metastatic disease.[54] Current studies are ongoing to further define the role of these local therapies in patients with metastatic disease to determine which patients should be selected for local therapy, the optimal time point for intervention, and the potential interactions and toxicities among different treatment choices.

Limited Stage SCLC

Approximately one-third of patients with SCLC will be diagnosed with limited-stage disease. Although this term traditionally referred to patients being eligible for treatment in a single RT port, there are evolving controversies regarding the inclusion of patients with supraclavicular and contralateral mediastinal/hilar lymphadenopathy. However, this usually applies to patients in Stages I–III of the disease. Patients with stage I SCLC who are incidentally detected, undergo complete surgical resection, and have no evidence of mediastinal lymph node involvement should receive adjuvant chemotherapy. Similarly, SBRT followed by adjuvant chemotherapy can be explored for medically inoperable patients with early-stage disease.[55] For patients with limited-stage disease, four cycles of doublet chemotherapy with early initiation of RT, during the first or second cycle, is recommended. Twice-daily RT (45 Gy in 30 fractions) was initially demonstrated to be superior to once-daily low-dose RT (45 Gy in 25 fractions).[56] More recently, the CONVERT trial compared the same twice-daily RT schedule to high-dose daily RT (66 Gy in 30 fractions) and failed to show superiority with the high-dose daily fractionation schedule.[57]

Extensive Stage SCLC

Approximately two-thirds of patients with SCLC are diagnosed with extensive-stage disease. Recent studies have shown that triple therapy, which includes doublet chemotherapy plus atezolizumab, improves progression-free survival and OS when compared to traditional doublet chemotherapy alone.[58] Consolidative chest RT with a dose of 30 Gy in 10 fractions is indicated for patients who have had a partial response to therapy and have residual disease in the chest.[59] In RTOG 0937, adding consolidative RT to intrathoracic disease and extracranial metastases failed to improve OS.[60]

Prophylactic Cranial Irradiation

Prophylactic cranial irradiation (PCI) has been found to reduce the risk of intracranial relapse and increase OS in patients with limited-stage disease who respond well to upfront chemoradiotherapy.[61] For patients who have extensive-stage disease, however, the role of PCI is now controversial. Initially, a European study found that individuals who got PCI had a lower probability of intracranial relapse and better OS compared to standard surveillance.[62,63] However, a recent Japanese study demonstrated no survival benefit compared to modern MRI screening during the initial treatment and RT at the time of disease relapse.[64] Surveillance, stereotactic radiosurgery, and hippocampal-avoidance PCI are all being investigated in this patient population currently.

TOXICITIES

During and shortly after surgery, anesthesia reactions, bleeding, pulmonary embolism, and wound infections are all potential complications.[65] RT can result in fatigue, lack of appetite, weight loss, as well as skin changes in the treated area.[66] RT, along with chemo-

fractions (radiation treatment plan, middle). She tolerated radiation treatment without acute or late toxicity. Follow-up CT chest showed mild consolidation and peripheral ground glass opacities at the treatment site, typical of post-RT changes, without evidence of recurrent or metastatic disease (right).

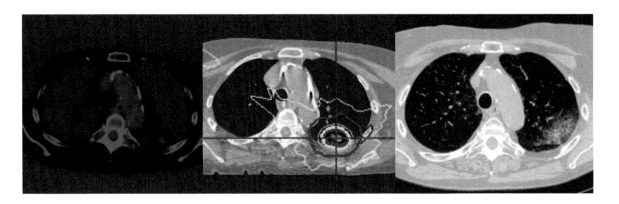

therapy, targeted therapies, and immunotherapies, can result in pneumonitis and pulmonary fibrosis, which presents as cough, respiratory difficulties, and shortness of breath. Most chemotherapy regimens induce nausea and vomiting of varying intensities, but these side effects can be treated efficiently with aggressive treatments and prophylactic measures.[67] Hematologic toxicity, which includes anemia and neutropenia, as well as an increased risk of infection. Common side effects related to targeted therapy include acne-like rash on face and upper body, dry and itchy skin, and enhanced sensitivity to sunlight.[33] Immune checkpoint inhibitors function by eliminating the body's immune system defenses leading to autoimmune reactions. Dermatologic, diarrhea/colitis, hepatotoxicity, pneumonitis, and endocrinopathies represent some of the common adverse effects.[68]

CASE STUDIES

Case 1: Stage I NSCLC Treated With SBRT

An 87-year-old female, former smoker, presented with an incidentally discovered left upper lobe nodule initially measuring 1.6×1.5 cm. She was lost to follow-up, but 2 years later repeat CT chest showed that the nodule had increased to 2.3×1.6 cm. PET/CT demonstrated an SUV max of 2.0 without evidence of regional or metastatic disease (left). She was deemed to be a high risk for biopsy and was not a surgical candidate. She was treated with curative RT using SBRT to a dose of 60 Gy in five

Case 2: Stage III NSCLC Treated With Trimodality Therapy

A 57-year-old male, active smoker, presented with hoarse voice. CT chest demonstrated a lung mass and PET/CT revealed left hilar lymphadenopathy measuring 3.2×3.0 cm with an SUV of 10.81, as well as a $9.0 \times 7.1 \times 4.9$ cm mass of the left upper lobe with an SUV of 18.88 with direct invasion into the mediastinum (top left). MRI brain was negative and biopsy of the left level 4 lymph node revealed lung adenocarcinoma. He was staged as cT4N2M0, stage IIIB by AJCC eighth edition, and recommended to undergo trimodality therapy. He received preoperative RT using IMRT to a dose of 60 Gy in 30 fractions (radiation treatment plan, top right) with concurrent carboplatin and paclitaxel. Postchemoradiotherapy CT chest showed interval reduction in the size of the mass and lymph nodes (bottom left). He underwent a left pneumonectomy (postpneumonectomy CT chest, bottom right) with pathology revealing a pathologic complete response to neoadjuvant therapy, ypT0N0M0.

Case 3: Stage III NSCLC Treated With Concurrent Chemoradiotherapy Followed by Immunotherapy

A 63-year-old male, active smoker, presented with blood-tinged sputum. CT chest showed a right lung mass and PET/CT revealed a 4.7 cm right upper lobe mass with an SUV max of 5.2 (left), a 1.4 cm FDG avid lung nodule in the right upper lobe concerning

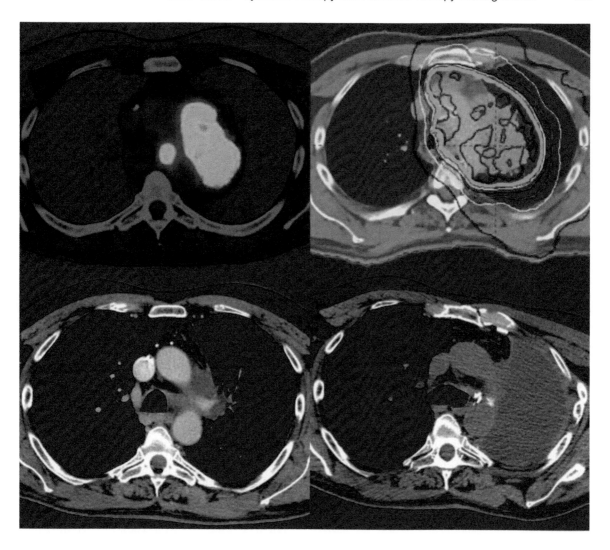

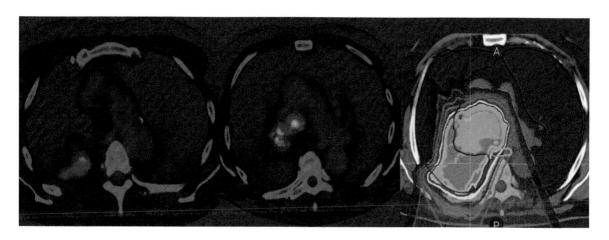

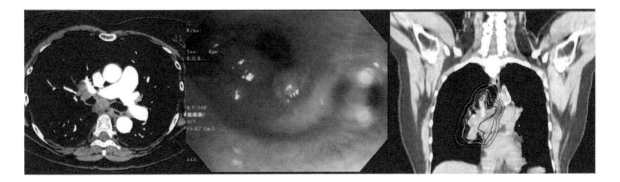

for a satellite lesion, as well as mediastinal and hilar lymphadenopathy (middle). Bronchoscopic biopsy was consistent with lung adenocarcinoma. MRI brain was negative and the patient was staged T3N2M0, stage IIIB by AJCC eighth edition. He was treated with proton RT to a dose of 70 Gy in 35 fractions (proton radiation treatment plan, right) with concurrent carboplatin and paclitaxel on clinical trial RTOG 1308, followed by consolidation durvalumab.

Case 4: Stage IV NSCLC Treated With Palliative RT for Hemoptysis

A 69-year-old female, former smoker, presented with cough and blood-tinged sputum. CT chest showed a right perihilar mass causing bronchial compression (left), as well as extensive mediastinal lymphadenopathy and bilateral metastatic pulmonary nodules and bone metastases. Bronchoscopy revealed extensive endobronchial lesions obstruction partially the right main stem and right upper lobe bronchus (middle). Biopsy returned lung adenocarcinoma. She was staged T4N3M1c, stage IVB by AJCC eighth edition. Her cough

and hemoptysis worsened, and she was treated with palliative RT using 3D-CRT, 30 Gy in 10 fractions, to the right hilar/mediastinal disease (radiation treatment plan, right). Her symptoms resolved during the course of treatment and she went on to receive palliative systemic therapy.

Case 5: LS-SCLC Treated With Chemoradiotherapy and PCI

A 57-year-old female, active smoker, presented with cough. CT chest showed a right hilar mass and bulky mediastinal lymphadenopathy, which were demonstrated on PET/CT without evidence of metastatic disease (left). MRI brain was negative, and bronchoscopic biopsy returned small cell lung carcinoma. She was staged T1bN2M0, stage IIIA (limited stage). She was treated with RT using IMRT to 45 Gy in 30 fractions delivered twice daily (radiation treatment plan, middle) with concurrent and adjuvant carboplatin and etoposide. Posttreatment CT chest showed a partial response. She subsequently received PCI using 3D-CRT to a dose of 25 Gy in 10 fractions (radiation treatment plan, right).

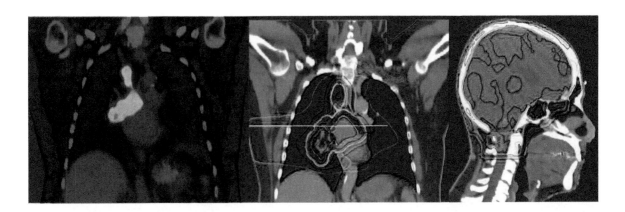

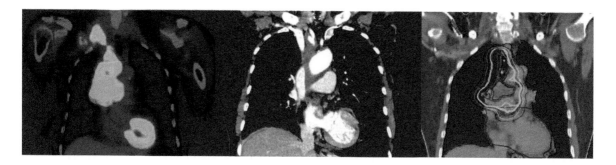

Case 6: ES-SCLC Treated With Consolidative Chest RT

A 72-year-old female, active smoker, presented with cough and back pain. CT chest showed bulky right hilar, mediastinal, and supraclavicular lymphadenopathy. PET/CT redemonstrated the thoracic lymphadenopathy (left) and revealed extensive bony metastatic disease. MRI brain was negative for metastasis, and biopsy of the right supraclavicular lymphadenopathy returned SCLC. She was staged T4N3M1c, stage IVB (extensive stage). She completed four cycles of carboplatin, etoposide, and atezolizumab. Postchemotherapy CT chest demonstrated significant reduction in the size of her thoracic disease (middle). She underwent consolidation RT to the residual mediastinal disease using IMRT, 30 Gy in 10 fractions (RT plan, right). Rather than undergoing PCI, she opted for surveillance MRI imaging of the brain every 3 months.

CONCLUSION

Lung cancer remains one of the most lethal cancers, with a high mortality rate. Screening for lung cancer holds promise to aid in the diagnosis of patients with earlier stage disease and allow for the opportunity to provide curative treatments. Various minimally invasive diagnostic and staging modalities are now available, and our understanding of lung cancer biology has advanced dramatically, resulting in a plethora of new therapeutic options. This biologically driven understanding of the disease process coupled with novel minimally invasive surgical approaches and advanced RT modalities will pave the way for improved lung cancer outcomes. Finally, immunotherapy holds great promise in the treatment of lung cancer and additional research is currently underway in order to further define its use.

REFERENCES

1. Sung H, Ferlay J, Siegel RL, et al. Global cancer statistics 2020: GLOBOCAN estimates of incidence and mortality worldwide for 36 cancers in 185 countries. *CA Cancer J Clin.* 2021;71(3):209–249.
2. Rodriguez-Canales J, Parra-Cuentas E, Wistuba II. Diagnosis and molecular classification of lung cancer. *Cancer Treat Res.* 2016;170:25–46.
3. Bade BC, Dela Cruz CS. Lung cancer 2020: epidemiology, etiology, and prevention. *Clin Chest Med.* 2020;41(1):1–24.
4. Sholl LM. Biomarkers in lung adenocarcinoma: a decade of progress. *Arch Pathol Lab Med.* 2015;139(4):469–480.
5. Siegel RL, Miller KD, Fuchs HE, Jemal A. Cancer statistics, 2021. *CA Cancer J Clin.* 2021;71(1):7–33.
6. Kalia M. Biomarkers for personalized oncology: recent advances and future challenges. *Metabolism.* 2015;64(3 Suppl 1):S16–S21.
7. Bernicker E. Biomarker testing in non-small cell lung cancer: a clinician's perspective. *Arch Pathol Lab Med.* 2015;139(4):448–450.
8. Nasim F, Sabath BF, Eapen GA. Lung cancer. *Med Clin N Am.* 2019;103(3):463–473.
9. Thrul J, Vijayaraghavan M, Kalkhoran S, Satterfield JM. Patterns of cigarette, e-cigarette, and cannabis use among adult smokers in primary care 2014–2015. *Addict Behav.* 2020;100:106109.
10. Collins LG, Haines C, Perkel R, Enck RE. Lung cancer: diagnosis and management. *Am Fam Physician.* 2007;75(1):56–63.
11. Neal RD, Sun F, Emery JD, Callister ME. Lung cancer. *BMJ.* 2019;365:l1725.
12. Amin MB, Stephen BE, Frederick LG, et al. *AJCC Cancer Staging Manual.* 8 ed. Springer International Publishing; 2018. XVII, 1032.
13. Hirsch FR, Scagliotti GV, Mulshine JL, et al. Lung cancer: current therapies and new targeted treatments. *Lancet.* 2017;389(10066):299–311.
14. Lackey A, Donington JS. Surgical management of lung cancer. *Semin Intervent Radiol.* 2013;30(2):133–140.

15. Abbas AE. Surgical management of lung cancer: history, evolution, and modern advances. *Curr Oncol Rep.* 2018; 20(12):98.

16. Manerikar A, Querrey M, Cerier E, et al. Comparative effectiveness of surgical approaches for lung cancer. *J Surg Res.* 2021;263:274–284.

17. Howington JA, Blum MG, Chang AC, Balekian AA, Murthy SC. Treatment of stage I and II non-small cell lung cancer: diagnosis and management of lung cancer, 3rd ed: American College of Chest Physicians evidence-based clinical practice guidelines. *Chest.* 2013;143(5 Suppl):e278S–e313S.

18. Hoy H, Lynch T, Beck M. Surgical treatment of lung cancer. *Crit Care Nurs Clin N Am.* 2019;31(3):303–313.

19. Bendixen M, Jørgensen OD, Kronborg C, Andersen C, Licht PB. Postoperative pain and quality of life after lobectomy via video-assisted thoracoscopic surgery or anterolateral thoracotomy for early stage lung cancer: a randomised controlled trial. *Lancet Oncol.* 2016;17(6):836–844.

20. Parashar B, Arora S, Wernicke AG. Radiation therapy for early stage lung cancer. *Semin Intervent Radiol.* 2013; 30(2):185–190.

21. Crabtree TD, Denlinger CE, Meyers BF, et al. Stereotactic body radiation therapy versus surgical resection for stage I non-small cell lung cancer. *J Thorac Cardiovasc Surg.* 2010;140(2):377–386.

22. Brown S, Banfill K, Aznar MC, Whitehurst P, Faivre FC. The evolving role of radiotherapy in non-small cell lung cancer. *Br J Radiol.* 2019;92(1104):20190524.

23. Badellino S, Muzio JD, Schivazappa G, et al. No differences in radiological changes after 3D conformal vs VMAT-based stereotactic radiotherapy for early stage non-small cell lung cancer. *Br J Radiol.* 2017;90(1078):20170143.

24. Chun SG, Hu C, Komaki RU, et al. Impact of intensity-modulated radiation therapy technique for locally advanced non-small-cell lung cancer: a secondary analysis of the NRG oncology RTOG 0617 randomized clinical trial. *J Clin Oncol.* 2017;35(1):56–62.

25. Gjyshi O, Liao Z. Proton therapy for locally advanced non-small cell lung cancer. *Br J Radiol.* 2020;93(1107): 20190378.

26. Stewart A, Parashar B, Patel M, et al. American Brachytherapy Society consensus guidelines for thoracic brachytherapy for lung cancer. *Brachytherapy.* 2016;15(1):1–11.

27. Nagasaka M, Gadgeel SM. Role of chemotherapy and targeted therapy in early-stage non-small cell lung cancer. *Expert Rev Anticancer Ther.* 2018;18(1):63–70.

28. Gadgeel SM. Role of chemotherapy and targeted therapy in early-stage non-small cell lung cancer. *Am Soc Clin Oncol Educ Book.* 2017;37:630–639.

29. Lim SM, Syn NL, Cho BC, Soo RA. Acquired resistance to EGFR targeted therapy in non-small cell lung cancer: mechanisms and therapeutic strategies. *Cancer Treat Rev.* 2018;65:1–10.

30. Gelatti ACZ, Drilon A, Santini FC. Optimizing the sequencing of tyrosine kinase inhibitors (TKIs) in epidermal growth factor receptor (EGFR) mutation-positive non-small cell lung cancer (NSCLC). *Lung Cancer.* 2019;137:113–122.

31. Sgambato A, Casaluce F, Maione P, Gridelli C. Targeted therapies in non-small cell lung cancer: a focus on ALK/ ROS1 tyrosine kinase inhibitors. *Expert Rev Anticancer Ther.* 2018;18(1):71–80.

32. Skoulidis F, Heymach JV. Co-occurring genomic alterations in non-small-cell lung cancer biology and therapy. *Nat Rev Cancer.* 2019;19(9):495–509.

33. Ruiz-Cordero R, Devine WP. Targeted therapy and checkpoint immunotherapy in lung cancer. *Surg Pathol Clin.* 2020;13(1):17–33.

34. Dafni U, Tsourti Z, Vervita K, Peters S. Immune checkpoint inhibitors, alone or in combination with chemotherapy, as first-line treatment for advanced non-small cell lung cancer. A systematic review and network meta-analysis. *Lung Cancer.* 2019;134:127–140.

35. Artal Cortes A, Calera Urquizu L, Hernando Cubero J. Adjuvant chemotherapy in non-small cell lung cancer: state-of-the-art. *Transl Lung Cancer Res.* 2015;4(2):191–197.

36. Timmerman RD, Hu C, Michalski JM, et al. Long-term results of stereotactic body radiation therapy in medically inoperable stage I non-small cell lung cancer. *JAMA Oncol.* 2018;4(9):1287–1288.

37. Ma SJ, Serra LM, Syed YA, Hermann GM, Gomez-Suescun JA, Singh AK. Comparison of single- and three-fraction schedules of stereotactic body radiation therapy for peripheral early-stage non-small-cell lung cancer. *Clin Lung Cancer.* 2018;19(2):e235–e240.

38. Videtic GM, Paulus R, Singh AK, et al. Long-term follow-up on NRG oncology RTOG 0915 (NCCTG N0927): a randomized phase 2 study comparing 2 stereotactic body radiation therapy schedules for medically inoperable patients with stage I peripheral non-small cell lung cancer. *Int J Radiat Oncol Biol Phys.* 2019;103(5):1077–1084.

39. Bezjak A, Paulus R, Gaspar LE, et al. Safety and efficacy of a five-fraction stereotactic body radiotherapy schedule for centrally located non-small-cell lung cancer: NRG oncology/ RTOG 0813 trial. *J Clin Oncol.* 2019;37(15):1316–1325.

40. Nyman J, Hallqvist A, Lund JÅ, et al. SPACE - a randomized study of SBRT vs conventional fractionated radiotherapy in medically inoperable stage I NSCLC. *Radiother Oncol.* 2016;121(1):1–8.

41. Ball D, Mai GT, Vinod S, et al. Stereotactic ablative radiotherapy versus standard radiotherapy in stage 1 non-small-cell lung cancer (TROG 09.02 CHISEL): a phase 3, open-label, randomised controlled trial. *Lancet Oncol.* 2019;20(4):494–503.

42. Chang JY, Senan S, Paul MA, et al. Stereotactic ablative radiotherapy versus lobectomy for operable stage I non-small-cell lung cancer: a pooled analysis of two randomised trials. *Lancet Oncol.* 2015;16(6):630–637.

43. Betticher DC, Depierre A. Pre-operative chemotherapy in non-small cell lung cancer. *Rev Mal Respir.* 2005;22(6 Pt 2):8S112–8S117.

44. Rusch VW, Albain KS, Crowley JJ, et al. Surgical resection of stage IIIA and stage IIIB non-small-cell lung cancer after concurrent induction chemoradiotherapy. A Southwest Oncology Group Trial. *J Thorac Cardiovasc Surg.* 1993; 105(1):97–104. discussion 104-6.

45. Douillard JY, Rosell R, De Lena M, et al. Adjuvant vinorelbine plus cisplatin versus observation in patients with completely resected stage IB-IIIA non-small-cell lung cancer (Adjuvant Navelbine International Trialist Association [ANITA]): a randomised controlled trial. *Lancet Oncol.* 2006;7(9):719−727.

46. Douillard JY, Rosell R, De Lena M, et al. Impact of postoperative radiation therapy on survival in patients with complete resection and stage I, II, or IIIA non-small-cell lung cancer treated with adjuvant chemotherapy: the adjuvant Navelbine International Trialist Association (ANITA) Randomized Trial. *Int J Radiat Oncol Biol Phys.* 2008;72(3):695−701.

47. Robinson CG, Patel AP, Bradley JD, et al. Postoperative radiotherapy for pathologic N2 non-small-cell lung cancer treated with adjuvant chemotherapy: a review of the National Cancer Data Base. *J Clin Oncol.* 2015;33(8):870−876.

48. Hui Z, Men Y, Hu C, et al. Effect of postoperative radiotherapy for patients with pIIIA-N2 non-small cell lung cancer after complete resection and adjuvant chemotherapy: the phase 3 PORT-C randomized clinical trial. *JAMA Oncol.* 2021;7(8):1178−1185.

49. Auperin A, Le Péchoux C, Rolland E, et al. Meta-analysis of concomitant versus sequential radiochemotherapy in locally advanced non-small-cell lung cancer. *J Clin Oncol.* 2010;28(13):2181−2190.

50. Tsujino K, Kurata T, Yamamoto S, et al. Is consolidation chemotherapy after concurrent chemo-radiotherapy beneficial for patients with locally advanced non-small-cell lung cancer? A pooled analysis of the literature. *J Thorac Oncol.* 2013;8(9):1181−1189.

51. Bradley JD, Paulus R, Komaki R, et al. Standard-dose versus high-dose conformal radiotherapy with concurrent and consolidation carboplatin plus paclitaxel with or without cetuximab for patients with stage IIIA or IIIB non-small-cell lung cancer (RTOG 0617): a randomised, two-by-two factorial phase 3 study. *Lancet Oncol.* 2015;16(2):187−199.

52. Antonia SJ, Villegas A, Daniel D, et al. Overall survival with durvalumab after chemoradiotherapy in stage III NSCLC. *N Engl J Med.* 2018;379(24):2342−2350.

53. Gomez DR, Blumenschein GR, Lee JJ, et al. Local consolidative therapy versus maintenance therapy or observation for patients with oligometastatic non-small-cell lung cancer without progression after first-line systemic therapy: a multicentre, randomised, controlled, phase 2 study. *Lancet Oncol.* 2016;17(12):1672−1682.

54. Palma DA, Olson R, Harrow S, et al. Stereotactic ablative radiotherapy for the comprehensive treatment of oligometastatic cancers: long-term results of the SABR-COMET phase II randomized trial. *J Clin Oncol.* 2020;38(25):2830−2838.

55. Verma V, Simone CB, Allen PK, et al. Multi-institutional experience of stereotactic ablative radiation therapy for stage I small cell lung cancer. *Int J Radiat Oncol Biol Phys.* 2017;97(2):362−371.

56. Turrisi 3rd AT, Kim K, Blum R, et al. Twice-daily compared with once-daily thoracic radiotherapy in limited small-cell lung cancer treated concurrently with cisplatin and etoposide. *N Engl J Med.* 1999;340(4):265−271.

57. Faivre-Finn C, Snee M, Ashcroft L, et al. Concurrent once-daily versus twice-daily chemoradiotherapy in patients with limited-stage small-cell lung cancer (CONVERT): an open-label, phase 3, randomised, superiority trial. *Lancet Oncol.* 2017;18(8):1116−1125.

58. Horn L, Mansfield AS, Szczesna A, et al. First-line atezolizumab plus chemotherapy in extensive-stage small-cell lung cancer. *N Engl J Med.* 2018;379(23):2220−2229.

59. Slotman BJ, Njo KH, De Jonge A, Meyer OW, Karim AB. Consolidative thoracic radiotherapy and prophylactic cranial irradiation in limited disease small cell lung cancer. *Lung Cancer.* 1993;10(3−4):199−208.

60. Gore EM, Hu C, Sun AY, et al. Randomized phase II study comparing prophylactic cranial irradiation alone to prophylactic cranial irradiation and consolidative extracranial irradiation for extensive-disease small cell lung cancer (ED SCLC): NRG oncology RTOG 0937. *J Thorac Oncol.* 2017;12(10):1561−1570.

61. Auperin A, Arriagada R, Pignon JP, et al. Prophylactic cranial irradiation for patients with small-cell lung cancer in complete remission. Prophylactic Cranial Irradiation Overview Collaborative Group. *N Engl J Med.* 1999;341(7):476−484.

62. Slotman BJ. Should all patients with SCLC receive prophylactic cranial irradiation if they have responded to treatment? PCI should be offered in nearly all cases. *Clin Adv Hematol Oncol.* 2015;13(11):729−731.

63. Slotman BJ, Mauer ME, Bottomley A, et al. Prophylactic cranial irradiation in extensive disease small-cell lung cancer: short-term health-related quality of life and patient reported symptoms: results of an international Phase III randomized controlled trial by the EORTC Radiation Oncology and Lung Cancer Groups. *J Clin Oncol.* 2009;27(1):78−84.

64. Takahashi T, Yamanaka T, Seto T, et al. Prophylactic cranial irradiation versus observation in patients with extensive-disease small-cell lung cancer: a multicentre, randomised, open-label, phase 3 trial. *Lancet Oncol.* 2017;18(5):663−671.

65. Templeton R, Greenhalgh D. Preoperative rehabilitation for thoracic surgery. *Curr Opin Anaesthesiol.* 2019;32(1):23−28.

66. Fang P, Swanick CW, Pezzi TA, et al. Outcomes and toxicity following high-dose radiation therapy in 15 fractions for non-small cell lung cancer. *Pract Radiat Oncol.* 2017;7(6):433−441.

67. Rossi A, Di Maio M. Platinum-based chemotherapy in advanced non-small-cell lung cancer: optimal number of treatment cycles. *Expert Rev Anticancer Ther.* 2016;16(6):653−660.

68. Patel SA, Weiss J. Advances in the treatment of non-small cell lung cancer: immunotherapy. *Clin Chest Med.* 2020;41(2):237−247.

The Assessment of the Person With Lung Cancer and Implications for the Rehabilitation Clinician

ADRIAN CRISTIAN, MD, MHCM • BEN KESTENBAUM, DO • MUNI RUBENS, MD, PHD

INTRODUCTION

Lung cancer patients are often diagnosed later in life and at advanced stages of the disease. The treatment of lung cancer often consists of a combination of systemic therapy (chemotherapy, immunotherapy), radiation therapy, and surgery. These treatments as well as age-related changes, comorbid conditions such as emphysema and heart disease can have adverse effects on physical function. Cancer and cancer treatment—related physical impairments can develop and can lead to a decreased quality of life. This chapter provides an overview of the anatomy and physiology of lung cancer, toxicities associated with common lung cancer treatments, and then provides a framework for the assessment of lung cancer patient from a holistic perspective.

EPIDEMIOLOGY OF LUNG CANCER

Lung cancer is the most common cause of cancer mortality in the United States.[1] The age of its occurrence is 50–70 years, with the mean age of presentation being 60 years. The risk of developing lung cancer is higher among men in all age groups over 40, and is more common in men than in women. In the United States, Northern Europe, and Western Europe, the prevalence of lung cancer has been decreasing in men; however, the incidence of lung cancer has been increasing in Eastern and Southern Europe. Western countries are seeing an increase in prevalence of lung cancer in women, as well as in younger individuals. Women have a higher incidence of localized disease at presentation, higher incidence of adenocarcinoma, and are typically younger when they present with symptoms. Over the past 20 years, the incidence of lung cancer has generally decreased in both men and women 30–54 years of age in all races and ethnic groups, with the incidence declining more steeply in men. Rates of incidence in women, ages 30–39 years, have increased when compared to those in men of the same age group.[2]

The predominant risk factors for lung cancer are cigarette smoke, asbestos, and radon exposure.[1] Radioactive decay of uranium results in the production of radon.[1] Asbestos and arsenic are carcinogens and are risk factors associated with occupational exposure.[2] Pack-years, or the amount smoked × duration of smoking, are directly related to risk of lung cancer.[2]

It has been estimated that 10%–15% of all lung cancers occur in those who have never smoked, resulting in the mortality of 16,000–24,000 people.[3] Those who do not smoke still have the potential to be exposed to secondhand smoke, radon, and indoor air pollutants such as cooking fumes.[3] The risk of developing lung cancer in those who have never smoked increases by 20%–30% when exposed to secondhand smoke at home or at work.[4] The likelihood of developing lung cancer due to secondhand smoke increases in the same manner it does for those who smoke, with greater duration and levels of exposure leading to increased risk.

TYPES OF LUNG CANCER

Small cell carcinoma represents approximately 15% of lung cancer cases and is treated with chemotherapy and radiation, and does not involve surgical resection.[1] On histology, poorly differentiated small cells are observed that are derived from neuroendocrine cells. This type of cancer has a primary tumor located centrally within the lung and is common among male smokers.

Nonsmall cell carcinomas compose the other 85% of all lung cancers, with 40% being adenocarcinoma, 30%

Lung Cancer Rehabilitation. https://doi.org/10.1016/B978-0-323-83404-9.00005-0

squamous cell carcinoma, 10% large cell carcinoma, and 5% carcinoid tumor.[1] Squamous cell carcinoma has keratin pearls or intracellular bridges on histology and is the most common tumor in male smokers. The primary tumor in squamous cell carcinoma is centrally located within the lung and may produce PTHrP which is associated with hypercalcemia.[1] Treatment of squamous cell carcinoma is through surgical resection, chemotherapy, and radiation.

Adenocarcinoma is the most common tumor in nonsmokers as well as female smokers, with a peripherally located primary tumor.[1] A peripheral mass along with pleural plaques can cause the pleura to "pucker." This can also be seen as a result of asbestosis. Adenocarcinoma in situ exhibits columnar cells growing along bronchioles and alveoli which can present on imaging as a consolidation that can resemble a pneumonia.[1] Treatment of adenocarcinoma is chemotherapy, radiation, and resection/surgery.

Large cell carcinoma is identified by poorly differentiated large cells. This type of carcinoma has an association with smoking and has a primary tumor that can be located either centrally or peripherally in the lung. When a primary tumor's location is described as central, this pertains to the trachea, bronchi, or segmental bronchi, while a peripherally located primary tumor will be at the subsegmental bronchi and distal structures within the lung.

Carcinoid tumors appear as well-differentiated neuroendocrine cells on histology and have no significant association with smoking. The primary tumor can be located centrally or peripherally within the lung; however, when located centrally, it forms a poly-like mass in the bronchus.[1]

STAGING OF LUNG CANCER

Staging of lung cancer is vital in order to provide the most appropriate treatment. Staging via PET-CT occurs before treatment and is performed utilizing the TNM staging system.[1] T is indicative of the primary tumor size and local extension. N represents spread to regional lymph nodes. In the case of lung cancer, this refers to hilar as well as mediastinal lymph nodes.[1] N0 represents no regional lymph node metastasis, N1 is ipsilateral peri-bronchial and/or ipsilateral hilar nodes and intra-pulmonary nodes, N2 is ipsilateral mediastinal and/or subcarinal nodes, and N3 is contralateral node involvement or ipsilateral scalene node involvement or supra-clavicular node involvement. M indicates the presence of metastasis with M0 representing no metastasis and M1 representing distant metastasis.[1]

LUNG ANATOMY AND PHYSIOLOGY

It is important to understand basic principles of lung anatomy and physiology to grasp the changes that take place to the pulmonary system when affected by cancer. As air enters through the pharynx, the first structures encountered are the trachea and bronchial tree. The tracheal mucosa is composed of ciliated pseudostratified columnar epithelium and numerous mucus-secreting goblet cells on a basement membrane with a thin collagenous lamina propria. The submucosa contains sero-mucous glands and the adventitia contains cartilaginous rings interconnected by connective tissue. The hyaline cartilage rings are opened posteriorly with the open ends connected by fibro elastic tissue and a band of smooth muscle.[5]

The trachea bifurcates at the carina into the left and right main bronchi. Each bronchus then has lobar branches extending into each respective lung. In order to pass more horizontally over the heart, the left main bronchus diverges from the bifurcation at a sharper angle. The right main bronchus separates into superior, middle, and inferior lobar bronchi, each corresponding to the lobes of the right lung. The left main bronchus separates into superior and inferior lobar bronchi, each corresponding to the lobes of the left lung. The conducting portion of bronchial tree is from the carina to the terminal bronchiole, with the responsibility of moving gas into and out of the lungs. This includes the segmental bronchus, which is covered by cartilaginous plates, the large subsegmental bronchus, and the small subsegmental bronchus. The epithelium of the bronchus is comprised of pseudostratified columnar ciliated epithelium with goblet cells, which transitions first into a simple columnar ciliated epithelium and then into a cuboidal epithelium as it moves distally, branching into smaller bronchioles. The cartilaginous support is lost at the bronchiolar level and the muscle layer becomes the dominant structure, which is made of smooth muscle and elastic fibers.[5]

The terminal bronchiole is a part of the bronchiole that does not possess the cartilage plates of the more proximal portions of the bronchus and demarcates the end of the conducting portion of the airway and the beginning of the respiratory portion of the airway. Distal to the conducting portion of the airway, the respiratory portion of the airway is responsible for the transfer of oxygen and carbon dioxide and contains the respiratory bronchiole, alveolar ducts, alveolar sacs, and alveoli. Respiratory bronchioles are composed of pulmonary alveoli, smooth muscle, and elastic fibers. The epithelium of the respiratory bronchiole is primary cuboidal, may be ciliated, does not contain goblet cells, and has a supporting layer formed by collagen and smooth muscle. Alveoli interrupt the main wall and are the smallest and most numerous subdivisions of the respiratory system. The interalveolar septum contains openings between alveoli to promote equalization of air pressures among them.[5]

Alveoli have an epithelial lining and lumen which contains alveolar macrophages, surfactant, type I and type II pneumocytes, elastic fibers, capillary endothelial cells, capillary lumens, and erythrocytes. Gas exchange occurs between alveolar and capillary lumens in the alveoli, during which oxygen is transferred to erythrocytes and carbon dioxide is transferred to the alveolar airway. Basement membranes of capillary endothelial cells are fused with the basement membrane of type I alveolar epithelial cells, which decreases distance for gas exchange at the air–blood barrier where gas exchange occurs. Type I pneumocytes are thin and squamous, joined by tight junctions to limit fluid infiltration into alveoli, and are responsible for gas exchange, maintenance of ion and fluid balance, and communication with type II pneumocytes. Type II pneumocytes are large and cuboidal, produce and secrete surfactant, express immuno-modulatory proteins required for host defense, and are responsible for the regeneration of alveolar epithelium following injury. Surfactant decreases surface tension of the alveoli, enabling easier lung expansion. (4).

As can be seen from staging of lung cancer, the lymphatic system is very important to the spread of lung cancer. Pulmonary lymph nodes along the bronchial tree drain from lungs into hilar (bronchopulmonary) lymph nodes. From there, lymph moves through inferior and superior bronchial nodes, paratracheal lymph nodes, the broncho–mediastinal trunk, and then to the right lymphatic or thoracic duct. (5).

The collection of alveolar sacs makes up an acinus. A combination of multiple acini, pulmonary arteries, pulmonary veins, and lymphatics make up the normal secondary pulmonary lobule, which is the functional unit of the lung.

Respiratory mechanics relates directly to the physiology of the lungs and is characterized by inspiratory and expiratory phases. In inspiration, the diaphragm contracts and lowers, thus increasing volume of the pleural cavity. The external intercostal scalene and posterior serratus muscles contract to elevate ribs and expand pleural cavity further. Expansion of pleural cavity generates negative intrapleural pressure and results in inspiration. Due to surface tension, increases in volume of pleural cavity coincide with increase in lung volume.

When the muscles previously described relax and diaphragm returns to superior expiratory position, this is referred to as passive expiration. Lung contraction increases pulmonary pressure and results in expiration. Contrast this with forced expiration, where internal intercostal muscles actively lower rib cage more than passive elastic recoil and more rapidly.[6]

The entire bronchial tree moves within the lung as the volume of the lung changes throughout the inspiratory and expiratory process of respiration. As you move more distally along the bronchial tree, movements are more pronounced.

ANATOMY, PHYSIOLOGY, AND PATHOPHYSIOLOGY OF LUNG CANCER

Now that the normal structure and function of the respiratory system has been described, the effects of cancer on anatomy and physiology, along with the pathophysiology of cancer itself, can be described. Carcinogens damage DNA, resulting in mutations that disrupt regulatory systems and enable growth and spread of cancer. Polycyclic hydrocarbons of cigarette smoke are known to be particularly carcinogenic. Uncontrolled cell growth in the lungs involves the structures and tissues of the lung itself, as well as the surrounding structures and their respective tissues. Cancer cells develop resistance to oxidative stress, which enables them to withstand and exacerbate inflammatory conditions that inhibit the activity of the immune system against the tumor.[7]

Anatomic changes seen in lung carcinoma cause pathophysiologic variation that is similar to that which is observed in a myriad of other lung diseases. Imaging will show a solitary nodule, also known as a coin lesion. Coin lesions are also seen in granulomatous conditions, as well as in individuals with bronchial hamartoma.[1] Nonspecific presenting symptoms such as cough, dyspnea, hemoptysis, obstructive pneumonia, and weight loss are seen in patients with lung carcinoma.[1] As the disease progresses, increased invasion occurs that can affect several of the anatomical structures described above. An example of this is T2 in the staging of the lung cancer. This involves the main bronchus, invades visceral pleura, and or shows atelectasis/obstructive pneumonitis into the hilum.[8] Invasion and expansion by the primary tumor can cause damage to structures typically used for defense of infection, resulting in pneumonia.[1] Examples of defenses against pneumonia are cough reflex, muco-ciliary escalator, and mucus plugging (2). Inflammation that incorporates bronchioles and damages cells can perpetuate bronchoconstriction and promote respiratory compromise.

The location of the cancer/tumor determines the signs/symptoms observed. An endobronchial location can present with cough, hemoptysis, bronchial obstruction, as well as pneumonitis, pneumonia, and/or pleural effusion. Mediastinal location can cause dyspnea, postprandial cough, wheezing, stridor, hoarseness, chylothorax, and dysphagia. Hoarseness typically occurs in this case due to irritation of recurrent laryngeal nerve. Upper airway obstruction is the cause of stridor and/or wheezing. Chylothorax relates to obstruction of lymph at the thoracic duct. A postprandial cough as well as dysphagia can be the result of enlargement of subcarinal lymph nodes and thus compression of the middle third of the esophagus.[9] Bronchial and tracheal stenosis as result of cancer results in obstruction and thus changes in airflow and decreased oxygenation.[5] Superior vena cava syndrome occurs when the tumor obstructs the superior vena cava, which results in distended head and neck veins, as well as blue discoloration of arms and face.[1] Diaphragmatic paralysis can occur if the tumor is pressing on the phrenic nerve.[1] Paralysis or weakness of the diaphragm impacts the respiratory mechanism and will lead to respiratory compromise. Horner syndrome presents with ptosis, anhidrosis, and miosis when the sympathetic chain is involved. Shoulder pain and hand weakness can be seen with brachial plexus involvement of apical tumors that involve the superior sulcus, also known as Pancoast tumors.[1]

In adenocarcinoma, when the lung is biopsied, the histological analysis shows a tumor arising from the bronchial glands as well as substantial mucus production. Adenocarcinomas arise from acinar, papillary, broncho-alveolar, and mucus-secreting cells. Adenocarcinoma may spread directly to pleura, diaphragm, pericardium, or bronchi with advanced disease spreading to the mediastinum, great vessels, trachea, esophagus, vertebral column, or adjacent lobe. Spread can result in superior vena cava obstruction, phrenic nerve dysfunction, Horner syndrome, brachial plexus compression, and/or pericardial effusion (12).

Airway obstruction at any level interferes with one's oxygenation and ventilation ability. Any pathology that limits the flow of air into and out of the body will limit ventilation. Malignant airway obstruction can occur due to obstruction within central airways, which includes the trachea, main-stem bronchi, and right bronchus intermedius. Complications related to central airway obstruction include but are not limited to dyspnea, atelectasis, hypoxemia, hemoptysis, postobstructive pneumonia or respiratory distress.[10]

Accumulation of inflammatory mucus and loss of elastic recoil due to lung tissue destruction and/or increased resistance within the airway causes pathology that is also seen in COPD. Patients with this condition will have permanent enlargement of air spaces beyond the terminal bronchioles, increasing diffusion distance, and thus worsening ventilation perfusion mismatch.[5] Changes in pulmonary function tests (PFTs) observed due to this pathology are decreased functional vital capacity (FVC), decreased forced expiratory volume during first second of expiration (FEV1), decreased FEV1:FVC ratio, and increased total lung capacity (TLC) due to air trapping.

Inflammation in lung that exceeds ability of antiproteases to balance protease activity will lead to destruction of alveolar air sacs.[1] Destruction of alveoli results in a decrease of surface area for gas exchange, which can cause necrotizing inflammation with damage to airway walls resulting in air trapping due to sustained dilation of bronchioles and bronchi, as well as loss of airway tone.[1] Air trapping can result in hypoxemia, which can then lead to secondary pulmonary hypertension and progress to right-sided heart failure and further dyspnea on exertion.

Pleural effusion with inflammation, leaky capillaries, and increased oncotic pressure can result in decreased lung volume and restrictive lung disease. Restrictive lung disease reduces the total volume of air that the lungs can hold. Pathophysiology that is seen in these instances is poor lung compliance, as well as poor chest wall compliance, depending on if the restriction is intrinsic or extrinsic. PFT changes observed due to these changes are decreased TLC, residual volume (RV), FEV1, and normal or increased functional vital capacity (VC) ratio of FEV1:FVC. Lung cancer is an exudative process which leads to decrease in exchange of oxygen and thus ventilation mismatch. Decrease in ventilation can result in atelectasis and respiratory compromise.

Development of pneumonia or pneumonitis can cause alveoli to be filled with exudate, inflammatory cells, and fibrin. This process worsens ventilation mismatch and can cause changes in lung parenchyma which will decrease lung volume and cause further ventilation perfusion mismatch.[5] Both diffusion defects and ventilation perfusion mismatch could lead to hypoxemia, which will cause hypoxia and eventual further cellular injury.

METASTASIS

The metastasis of lung cancer requires a transition from epithelial to mesenchymal cell types. This may occur through the activation of signaling pathways such as Akt/GSK3Beta, MEK-ERK, Fas, and Par6.[11] Lymphatic spread is the usual route of metastasis with initial spread to lymph nodes that drain regionally. In adeno-carcinoma, for example, lymph node metastasis occurs in peri-bronchial lymph nodes before moving to mediastinal or subcarinal nodes and then the contralateral lung. Distant metastasis includes extension to a contra-lateral lobe, pleural nodules, malignant pleural or peri-cardial effusion, or any distant site such as the brain, bones, or liver.

Different types of metastasis are seen in different types of lung cancer, with varied effects on the individual and specific organ systems within the body. Small cell carcinoma has early metastasis producing endocrine or nervous system paraneoplastic syndromes. SIADH is seen in small cell carcinoma, resulting in hyponatremia. ACTH overproduction can also be observed in small cell carcinoma resulting in Cushing's syndrome. Bone pain and spinal cord impingement can be seen. Neurologic problems may develop, such as headache, weakness or numbness of limbs, dizziness, and seizures. Lambert–Eaton syndrome occurs in some instances with nonsmall cell lung cancer (NSCLC). This is a paraneoplastic autoimmune disorder in which antibodies are formed against presynaptic calcium channels at the neuromuscular junction producing proximal muscle weakness that is gradual in onset. Metastatic spread of lung cancer to the liver is most common, which can result in nausea, vomiting, and abdominal pain/discomfort.

CHANGES TO LUNG FUNCTION IN TREATMENT OF LUNG CANCER

Surgical resection, systemic therapy, and radiotherapy are commonly used to treat lung cancer; however, each of them can have major effects on the physiology of the lungs and respiratory system as a whole.

SURGERY

Surgical resection is a valuable treatment method for lung cancer, because substantial number of patients can be cured by this intervention and long-term survival rates increase significantly. Lobectomy, pneumonectomy, and video-assisted thorascopic surgery are surgeries that are utilized in treatment of NSCLC stages I–IIIA. Most patients with a preoperative forced expiratory volume in one second (FEV_1) of greater than 2.5 L are able to tolerate pneumonectomy. With an FEV_1 of 1.1–2.4 L, a lobectomy is possible; however, patients with an FEV_1 of less than 1 L are not considered candidates for surgery.[9]

Compared with preoperation data, arterial pressure of oxygen divided by inspired oxygen concentration (P/F) and arterial oxygen partial pressure divided by alveolar oxygen partial pressure (a/A) decreased significantly in 3 days($P < .01$) and PaCO2 P50O2 increased significantly on the day after operation ($P < .01$), especially in the group of pneumonectomy and abnormal ventilation, hypoxemia measured presurgery.[12] P50O2 represents the affinity of hemoglobin–oxygen and is the tension of oxygen when hemoglobin saturation is 50%. When hemoglobin–oxygen affinity increases, a left shift is seen in the oxyhemoglobin dissociation curve and the P50O2 value decreases. An increase in P50O2, as described in the study, means an increase in venous oxygen tension and increased delivery of oxygen to tissues. A study that measured health-related quality of life in patients who underwent lung cancer surgery found that survivors exhibited worsening dyspnea, coughing, and chest pain.[13]

The loss of pulmonary function subsequent to surgical resection depends upon the extent of lung tissue removed as well as baseline derangements in pulmonary function. The volume of lung tissue extracted is important because adult lung cannot regenerate new alveolar septal tissues, thereby leading to some persistent residual loss of pulmonary function.[14] Surgical resection adversely affects the VC and FEV1 acutely as well as chronically. Within 1 month after surgical resection, VC recovers to the maximum possible extent, whereas FEV1 recovers gradually and may take up to 3 months due to the time taken for the surgical pain and injury to disappear completely.[14] Several years after surgical resection, VC and FEV1 further decrease due to weakening respiratory muscle strength, loss of elastic recoil of the lung tissue, increasing chest wall stiffness, altered surfactant composition, and increasing ventilation perfusion mismatch. Both American College of Chest Physicians and the British Thoracic Society recommend that FEV1 and DLCO should be measured preoperatively in order to estimate postoperative levels of FEV1 and DLCO, which could help in appropriate patient selection for surgical resection.[15] The functional loss after surgical resection can be estimated using quantitative radionuclide pulmonary perfusion scintigraphy for split lung function.[16]

Postoperative complications in surgical resections occur and have serious impacts on length of stay and mortality. For pneumonectomies' in particular, examples of these complications include arrhythmias, vocal cord paralysis, pneumonia, pulmonary embolism, and pulmonary edema.[17] In a separate study, pneumonia.

pulmonary embolism, and arrhythmia were listed as major morbidities and resulted in more than doubling the patient's length of stay compared to those patients who did not have one of them.[18] In addition to the effect on length of stay, complications following pneumonectomy also resulted in a high mortality rate.[19]

SYSTEMIC THERAPY

Approximately 80% of all patients with lung cancer are considered for chemotherapy at some point during the course of their illness[9] Systemic treatment for lung cancer has evolved significantly in the recent years and has been focusing on individually tailored treatment approaches. Combination chemotherapy with cisplatin or carboplatin and additional drugs such as paclitaxel, docetaxel, gemcitabine, vinorelbine, etoposide, and pemetrexed, remain the mainstay of adjuvant chemotherapy for NSCLCs. In addition, recent developments in cancer treatment have introduced targeted agents such as epidermal growth factor receptor tyrosine kinase inhibitors such as erlotinib, gefitinib, afatinib, and osimertinib, and anaplastic lymphoma kinase inhibitors such as crizotinib, ceritinib, alectinib, and brigatinib. Various immunotherapeutic agents such as ipilimumab, pembrolizumab, nivolumab, and durvalumab have been used as first- and second-line agents. Chemotherapeutic drugs such as pemetrexed, gemcitabine, and paclitaxel are associated with pneumonitis, while carboplatin, paclitaxel, cisplatin and gemcitabine are associated with impaired DLCO.[20] Vinorelbine is associated with adverse effects such as bronchospasm, dyspnea, diffuse interstitial infiltration, alveolar infiltration, and acute respiratory distress syndrome.[21] Oxaliplatin is associated with interstitial lung disease and diffuse alveolar damage. Targeted therapies such as gefitinib and erlotinib are associated with interstitial lung disease. Erlotinib is additionally associated with interstitial pneumonia, pneumonitis, acute respiratory distress syndrome, pulmonary fibrosis, and alveolitis. The pulmonary side effects of immunotherapeutic agents are primarily due to immune-related reactions, and hence present with nonspecific symptoms such as cough, fever, chest discomfort, and dyspnea. Pulmonary toxicities due to immunotherapeutic agents commonly present with a restrictive pattern in PFT and show decreased diffusion capacity. Specifically, ipilimumab is associated with pulmonary sarcoid-like granulomatosis.[22]

Although not directly related to lung function, platinum-based chemotherapeutic agents have been shown to cause significant peripheral neuropathy. Peripheral neuropathy can limit a person's ability to be active, and this decrease in activity can further compromise respiratory mechanics.

RADIOTHERAPY

Radiotherapy-Induced Lung Injury (RILI) includes any lung damage associated with ionizing radiation used for treating cancers. RILI consists of two stages: an early-stage known as radiation pneumonitis (RP) and a late stage known as radiation fibrosis (RF). RP is characterized by acute inflammation of the lung tissue and subsequent to exposure to the radiation. RF is a clinical sequela that results from chronic damage and fibrosis of the lung tissue and constitutes a long-term side effect of radiotherapy. Though the exact mechanism for RILI is not completely understood, it has been imputed to be radiation-induced destruction of alveolar epithelium and pulmonary capillary endothelium, thereby compromising the alveolar barrier functions. This acutely triggers cytokine release and initiates an inflammatory response leading to RP.[23] Subsequently, these initial cytokines attract macrophages and other chronic inflammatory cells. Macrophage accumulation stimulates the production of reactive oxygen and nitrogen species, which in turn unleash a cascade of proinflammatory, proangiogenic, and profibrinogenic cytokines. These changes in the milieu sustain a continuous and progressive inflammatory and fibrotic response, which could lead to long-term adverse effects such as RF.[24] Both clinical assessment and radiological findings are used for diagnosing RILI. The incidence of RILI and other lung toxicities have significantly decreased in the recent years due to introduction of newer forms of radiotherapy such as Stereotactic Body Radiation Therapy and Intensity-modulated radiotherapy, which significantly decrease both dosage as well as the area treated by radiotherapy.

Pulmonary function can be estimated through a number of methods such as spirometry, diffusion capacity for carbon monoxide (DLCO), and body plethysmography. These tests are commonly indicated in patients before beginning thoracic radiotherapy in order to assess the fitness of the patient, as well as to obtain baseline estimates of pulmonary function so that comparisons could be done after treatment. Since the structure of lung is not uniform, radiotherapy to the lung produces differential responses.[25] Ventilation parameters such as VC could increase or decrease corresponding to improvements resulting from radiotherapy or deterioration due to treatment side effects.[26] Improvements could be due to reopening of the obstructed airways after destruction of the cancer cells due to radiotherapy, whereas deterioration could be due to fibrotic narrowing and new onset obstruction due to the side effects. However, unlike VC, diffusion, which is a measure of conductance of gas across alveolocapillary lining, measured using DLCO, is commonly reported to decrease after radiotherapy and does not recuperate several months after treatment.[26] Decrease in FEV1 after radiotherapy could be due to acute bronchial obstruction resulting from swelling of the tissues. Changes in lung compliance following radiotherapy are indicated by decrease in FVC and TLC. If greater volumes of the lung are exposed to radiotherapy, a significant decrease in lung compliance occurs as reflected by lowered FVC, TLC, and FEV1. The 6-min walking test (6-MWT) could be used as an instrument to predict RP among patients receiving radiotherapy for lung cancers. 6-MWT/FVC values < 4 ft/L are indicative of chronic RP.[27]

EFFECT OF CANCER TREATMENT ON MUSCLES AND NERVES

A number of peripheral nervous system lesions such as plexopathies, peripheral neuropathies, and mononeuropathies could be precipitated by direct or indirect damages to the nervous system due to cancer treatments such as chemotherapy, radiotherapy, and surgery. In addition, the damage can also involve muscles, especially in radiotherapy due to RF. As much as 38% of patients who have undergone multiple schedules of chemotherapy report symptoms of chemotherapy-induced neuropathy. The incidence of neuropathy is significantly higher for platinum-based agents, vinca alkaloids, taxanes, and proteasome inhibitors.[28] In addition, corticosteroids which are used for cancer treatment and antiinflammatory effects can lead to myopathies due to catabolic and antianabolic effects. Chemotherapies primarily involve either complete or irreversible damage to dorsal root ganglia, or partial injuries to distal axons resulting in neurological symptoms. Similarly, radiotherapy can lead to either direct destruction of neuromuscular tissue or secondary destruction due to fibrosis and compression leading to neurological symptoms.[29] The mechanism of action of radiation-induced fibrosis of neuromuscular tissues is similar to RILI. Though poorly understood, it is generally accepted that RF occurs due to gradual physiological response of the radiated tissues which progressively undergo sclerosis and eventually fibrosis. Initially, there is an acute inflammatory response that kills rapidly proliferating cell types through apoptosis and free radical–mediated DNA damage. This leads to the healing steps such as fibroblastic proliferation, extracellular matrix deposition, and copious release of proinflammatory cytokines and reactive oxygen species. This leads to further cell damage and death due to microvascular ischemia and hypoxia, thus potentiating further fibroblast proliferation and the repeat cycles of subsequent release of proinflammatory cytokine and reactive oxygen species. Eventually, over a period of many years, the tissues become poorly vascularized, friable, and fragile and eventually fibrosis sets in. A number of tissues such a skin, nerve, muscle, tendon, ligament, and fascia could undergo fibrosis and potentiate nerve impingement and associated neuromuscular sequalae. In corticosteroid-induced myopathy, it is believed that corticosteroid-mediated upregulation of proteolytic enzyme systems such as calpains, cathepsins, and ubiquitin–proteasome system increases lysis of myofibrillar proteins through dissociation of actin and myosin.[30] In addition, corticosteroids inhibit protein synthesis and muscle building by blocking the incorporation of amino acid by the myocytes and downregulation of transcription factor called myogenin. Corticosteroids also lower serum potassium and phosphate, precipitating muscle weakness and atrophy.

THE ASSESSMENT OF THE PATIENT WITH LUNG CANCER—AN OVERVIEW

Clinicians practicing rehabilitation medicine will often encounter patients with a history of lung cancer in a variety of clinical settings such as during acute hospitalizations for cancer treatment or other medical conditions, acute inpatient rehabilitation units, sub-acute rehabilitation and skilled nursing facilities, outpatient rehabilitation clinics, and the patient's home. Given the complexity of challenges facing lung cancer patients and survivors, it is important for rehabilitation clinicians to have a strategy to assess the individual with lung cancer that encompasses all of the complexities and that can be used to establish a treatment plan to address these challenges. In this section, such an assessment will be explored.

Lung cancer often affects older adults and it is not unusual that the initial presentation of the lung cancer is at a more advanced stage. It is important to obtain an accurate chronological history of the lung cancer and its treatment. This includes collecting information about the date of diagnosis, stage of cancer at time of diagnosis, location of metastatic disease such as to the brain, liver, and skeletal system as well as treatments. Common treatments for lung cancer include systemic therapy, radiation therapy, and surgery as mentioned above, each with its own side effects that can in turn contribute to the development of physical impairments that affect quality of life. At times, it may be a combination of factors contributing to the development of these impairments. For example, the combination of prior lung surgery, chemotherapy, and radiation therapy to the lung can significantly limit pulmonary function. A pathological fracture treated surgically or brain metastasis treated with radiotherapy and surgery can lead to additional impairments that can adversely affect quality of life.

The individual affected by lung cancer, may also have one of more precancer medical conditions such as emphysema, heart disease, and diabetes as well as age-related physical changes that may have adversely impacted their level of function even before the cancer diagnosis and now may further reduce the person's margin of good health and contribute to the development of frailty. Fig. 3.1 depicts various factors, that when combined can contribute to the development of physical impairments, loss of physical function, and decline in quality of life.

It is useful to follow a checklist when assessing the lung cancer patient to ensure that all possible factors affecting that person's quality of life are addressed. Table 3.1 provides an example of this checklist.

To begin with, it is important to determine the chief complaint since there may be several different factors contributing to the person's functional decline. In the acute hospitalization setting, it may be an inability to tolerate systemic therapy for the cancer that contributes to dehydration and poor nutritional intake. Alternatively, it may be a pneumonia, new pathological fracture of the femur, or pain from metastatic disease to the spine from a vertebral compression fracture. In the outpatient setting, it may be a painful neuropathy affecting hands and feet associated with a decreased ability to use the hands or difficulty walking due to impaired balance or a postthoracotomy pain that brings the patient to seek medical attention. It is important to note that several factors may be linked together contributing to the reason that the person is now seeking care from rehabilitation clinicians. The combination of poor appetite and weight loss, shortness of breath due to decreased pulmonary function, fatigue, and limited endurance for walking can all limit the ability to perform daily activities. If the individual lives alone or has limited social support system and income, it may also contribute to the development of frailty. This in turn may affect their ability to receive and tolerate further lung cancer treatments.

MEDICAL INTERVIEW

In the medical interview, it is important to ask about the presence of fatigue to perform activities of daily living such as dressing, bathing, feeding as well as ability to shop for food, drive, and work if the person is working. Inquiring about their daily nutrition intake can provide a point of reference on whether or not they take in an adequate amount of calories and protein in their diet. Asking about weight loss or whether or not their clothes are becoming too loose to wear may provide additional insight into their nutritional status. Symptoms such as shortness of breath, use of supplemental oxygen at home, or need for it during an acute hospitalization

can be useful when providing precautions for rehabilitation program in the treatment plan.

Pain can also be present. This may have several different etiologies and it is important to obtain a good pain history. This pain history typically includes information about the type of pain, location, onset, character, radiation, intensity, aggravating and alleviating factors, chronic versus acute, associated systemic factors, and treatments tried to date as well as their level of effectiveness. Common sources of pain in lung cancer patients include (a) postthoracotomy pain, (b) neuropathic pain due to peripheral neuropathy, radiculopathy (c) pain from a pathological fracture or impending fracture, (d) vertebral compression fracture secondary to metastatic disease to spine, and (e) RF related pain. It is not unusual for a patient to have a preexisting pain exacerbated by either lung cancer treatment or complication associated with the diagnosis. For example, a patient may have a preexisting history of lumbar spinal stenosis secondary to degenerative changes in the spine that is exacerbated by the presence of metastatic disease to the lumbar spine. The patient may present with localized low back pain or radiculopathy. If the patient was treated with radiation therapy to the lumbar spine and pelvic region, they may also experience pain from a radiation-related fracture.

Inquiring about cognitive function is important in patients with either known brain metastatic disease that was treated with radiation therapy and/or surgery or in those suspected of having brain metastatic disease. The impact on cognitive function can range from very subtle changes affecting their daily life and work to significant changes in which the person cannot perform activities of daily living and require assistance from family members or home health aides. It can even affect their ability to participate in clinical decision-making with respect to their care. It is also important to ask if the person is depressed and/or anxious and if present, are they currently being treated for it.

It is equally important to ask about the person's social support system. Is this a person whom has a wide network of family members and/or friends that are very involved in his/her life and care about the patient's well-being or does the person live alone with limited circle of friends and family to assist in care. A more limited social network can make it more difficult for the patient to take care of themselves or attend doctor and treatment appointments. It is important to ask the patient about their ability to perform activities of daily living and if unable to perform these activities who is available to assist and how much assistance is required. It is not unusual for rehabilitation clinicians

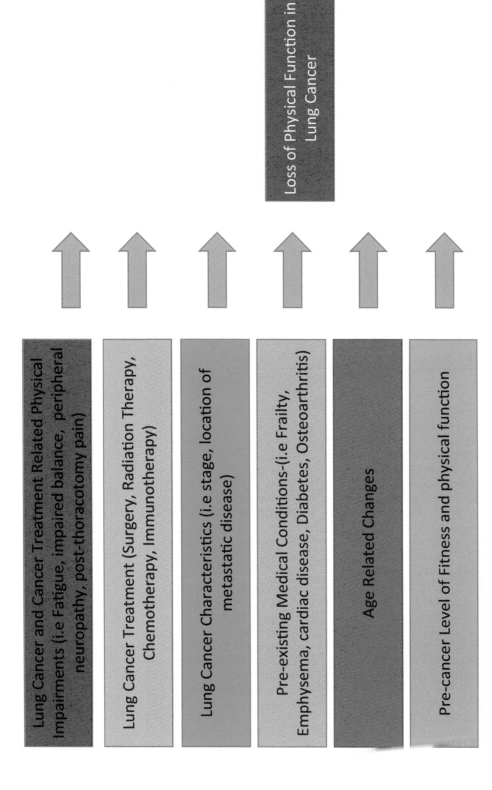

"Factors Contributing to Loss of Physical Function in Lung Cancer"

FIG. 3.1 Factors contributing to loss of physical function in lung cancer.

TABLE 3.1 Lung Cancer Assessment Checklist.	Yes	No
Fatigue		
Shortness of breath		
General weakness		
Poor appetite and nutrition		
Gastrointestinal symptoms—nausea, vomiting		
Postthoracotomy pain		
Peripheral neuropathy pain		
Musculoskeletal pain joint and muscle pain		
Risk of pathological fracture		
Cognitive impairment		
Depression/Anxiety		
Limited social support system		
Difficulty performing activities of daily living		
Difficulty walking		
Impaired balance and falls		

to evaluate and treat patients with lung cancer who are still working. If so, asking about the impact of the lung cancer and its treatment on ability to carry on their work is important. If there are limitations, contributing factors to those limitations may include fatigue, shortness of breath, pain, general weakness, or gastrointestinal symptoms such as nausea and vomiting associated with active cancer treatments. A review of the person's medications including medicines used to treat pain such as opioid medications, pregabalin, gabapentin, antidepressants, and steroid medications is useful since they can contribute to fatigue, general weakness, and cognitive impairment. It is important to review for possible drug—drug and drug—disease interactions.

It is also important to ask if the person with lung cancer is experiencing any falls or near-falls. An impaired balance can be due to leg muscle weakness, presence of peripheral neuropathy affecting the lower extremities, brain metastasis, as well as side effects of medications and cancer treatments. If there is an impaired balance, questions about use of assistive devices for ambulation at home or in the community or need to lean on others or objects can yield important information that can be used as part of the rehabilitation

treatment plan. If the person is deemed to be at an increased risk of falling in the home, follow-up inquiries about high risk environment such as the bathroom can be helpful to determine if there is a need for adaptive equipment such as tub seat or grab bars.

PHYSICAL EXAMINATION

The physical examination of the person with lung cancer should focus on specific complaints generated from the medical interview; however, it is important to also evaluate for other factors that can contribute to the development of physical impairments affecting self-care activities, work, and quality of life. The physical examination should include an evaluation of vital signs—ideally assessing for evidence of orthostatic changes as the person might be volume depleted as well as breathing rate and oxygenation level with pulse oximetry. The rehabilitation clinician should perform a general physical examination that includes an assessment of cardiopulmonary function as well as an assessment of the nervous and musculoskeletal systems. Typical components of the nervous system evaluation include general orientation, brief cognitive evaluation, sensory examination such as light touch, pinprick, vibration, proprioception, hot/cold perception, muscle stretch reflexes, motor strength of key muscle groups of the upper and lower extremities, and gait and balance/coordination evaluation. Assessment of the musculoskeletal system should include inspection and palpation of surgical scars, bones, muscles and soft tissues of the upper and lower extremities, and spine for tenderness. Active and passive range of motion testing in limbs not deemed to be at risk for imminent pathological fracture can provide additional useful information.

Patient reported outcome questionnaires can yield important self-reported information about the individual's level of physical function and ability to perform daily self-care as well as presence of fatigue for daily activities. Functional exams can also be included in the physical examination if the patient is deemed to be safe to perform them. Some examples include grip strength, timed up and go test, sit to stand, and balance tests.

MEDICAL RECORD REVIEW

A review of medical records of the patient is important. Useful information detailing the staging and treatment of the lung cancer is usually found in medical, surgical, and radiation oncology notes. In reviewing medical oncology notes, rehabilitation clinicians can obtain information about the cancer history and its treatment with systemic therapy. The medications used, number of treatment cycles, and any complications from the treatment that may have required a dose reduction or change in treatment plan can often provide important information regarding toxicities associated with these treatments.

Surgical reports and postsurgery hospitalization notes can identify location of the surgery, tissues removed, cancer as well as noncancer, and any complications associated with the surgery. Radiation therapy treatment plans and summaries of treatment can provide information on the type of radiation therapy used as well as the tissues affected by the radiation therapy. This information becomes important when assessing the patient with late effects of radiation therapy such as RF as well as possible sources of pain in areas that were exposed to radiation. Other helpful documentation to review includes notes of palliative care physicians, neuro-oncologists, pulmonologists, nutritionists, nursing staff, and mental health providers as applicable.

DIAGNOSTIC IMAGING AND LABORATORY TESTING

It is often useful to review pertinent diagnostic imaging studies and laboratory studies when available. This

information can then be used to establish precautions and guide the treatment plan in the rehabilitation medicine prescription. It is very useful if rehabilitation clinicians can review reports and/or images such as X-rays, bone scans, CT/MRI, and PET/CT scans. Information that can be found in these imaging studies can provide useful information about the location of the lung cancer in the lungs as well as in other parts of the body such as the spine, brain, femur, and humeri. The presence of skeletal involvement of the lung cancer can lead to discussions about risk of impending pathological fracture and strategies to minimize that risk during rehabilitation treatments. The presence of brain metastasis can lead to discussions about presence of cognitive or balance impairments. Laboratory tests of importance for rehabilitation clinicians include hemoglobin level for presence of anemia, platelet count for presence of thrombocytopenia, and white blood cell count for presence of infection. Liver and kidney function tests are also important to assess, especially as they pertain to decisions regarding prescribing medications for pain management.

CONCLUSION

Lung cancer patients often have complex and interconnecting physical impairments that can lead to loss of physical function and reduced quality of life. Rehabilitation clinicians providing care to this population should have a good understanding of the anatomy and pathophysiology of lung cancer, its treatment with surgery, systemic therapy and radiotherapy, and the toxicities and side effects associated with these treatments. Based on that fundamental knowledge, a holistic, multidisciplinary treatment plan can be created to treat the physical impairments and improve the level of function and quality of life of those affected by this type of cancer.

REFERENCES

1. Sattar H. *Fundamentals of Pathology*. Chicago: Pathoma LLC; 2018:86−98.
2. Jamal A, Miller K, Ma J, et al. Higher lung cancer incidence in young women than young men in the United States. *N Engl J Med*; 2018. https://www.nejm.org/doi/10.1056/NEJMoa1715907?url_ver=Z39.88-2003&rfr_id=ori%3Arid%3Acrossref.org&rfr_dat=cr_pub%3Dwww.ncbi.nlm.nih.gov. Accessed July 1, 2021.
3. Samet JM, Avila-Tang E, Boffetta P, et al. Lung cancer in never smokers: clinical epidemiology and environmental risk factors. *Clin Cancer Res*. 2009;15(18):5626−5645. https://doi.org/10.1158/1078-0432.ccr-09-0376.
4. Cancer among adults from exposure to secondhand smoke. In: *The Health Consequences of Involuntary Exposure*

to Tobacco Smoke: A Report of the Surgeon General. U.S. Dept. of Health and Human Services, Public Health Service, Office of the Surgeon General; 2006.

5. Celis MDE, Mosenifar MDZ, Diaz-Mendoza MDJ. *Lung Anatomy: Overview, Gross Anatomy, Microscopic Anatomy*; 2017. https://emedicine.medscape.com/article/1884995-overview#a1. Accessed July 1, 2021.

6. Gilroy A, MacPherson B, Schünke M, et al. *Atlas of Anatomy*. 3rd ed. New York: Thieme Publishers; 2016:116–129.

7. Takahashi N, Chen HY, Harris IS, et al. Cancer cells Co-opt the neuronal redox-sensing channel TRPA1 to promote oxidative-stress tolerance. *Cancer Cell*. 2018;33(6). https://doi.org/10.1016/j.ccell.2018.05.001, 985–1003.e7.

8. Feng SH, Yang ST. The new 8th TNM staging system of lung cancer and its potential imaging interpretation pitfalls and limitations with CT image demonstrations. *Diagn Interv Radiol*. 2019;25(4):270–279.

9. Tan WW, Huq S. Non-small cell lung cancer (NSCLC). In: *Practice Essentials, Background, Pathophysiology*; July 15, 2021. https://emedicine.medscape.com/article/279960-overview. Accessed July 15, 2021.

10. Oberg C, Folch E, Santacruz JF. Management of malignant airway obstruction. *AME Med J*. 2018;3:115.

11. Powell CA, Halmos B, Nana-Sinkam SP. Update in lung cancer and mesothelioma 2012. *Am J Respir Crit Care Med*. 2013;188(2):157–166. https://doi.org/10.1164/rccm.201304-0716UP.

12. Li B. *Zhonghua jie he he hu xi za zhi = Zhonghua jiehe he huxi zazhi = Chinese J Tuberc Respir Dis*. 1998;21(12):735–738.

13. Yun YH, Kim YA, Min YH, et al. Health-related quality of life in disease-free survivors of surgically treated lung cancer compared with the general population. In: *Medscape Drugs & Diseases - Comprehensive Peer-Reviewed Medical Condition, Surgery, and Clinical Procedure Articles with Symptoms, Diagnosis, Staging, Treatment, Drugs and Medications, Prognosis, Follow-Up, and Pictures*; 2012. https://reference.medscape.com/medline/abstract/22470076. Accessed July 1, 2021.

14. Brunelli A, Kim AW, Berger KI, Addrizzo-Harris DJ. Physiologic evaluation of the patient with lung cancer being considered for resectional surgery: diagnosis and management of lung cancer: American College of Chest Physicians evidence-based clinical practice guidelines. *Chest*. 2013; 143(5):e166S–e190S.

15. Brunelli A, Xiumé F, Refai M, et al. Evaluation of expiratory volume, diffusion capacity, and exercise tolerance following major lung resection: a prospective follow-up analysis. *Chest*. 2007;131(1):141–147.

16. Wu M-T, Pan H-B, Chiang AA, et al. Prediction of postoperative lung function in patients with lung cancer: comparison of quantitative CT with perfusion scintigraphy. *Am J Roentgenol*. 2002;178(3):667–672.

17. Campisi A, Bertolaccini L, Luo J, Franco S, Fang W. Management of medical complications after pneumonectomy. *Shanghai Chest*. 2020:4. n. pag. Web. 1 Sep. 2021.

18. Shapiro M, Swanson SJ, Wright CD. Predictors of major morbidity and mortality after pneumonectomy utilizing the society for thoracic surgeons general thoracic surgery database. discussion 934-5 *Ann Thorac Surg*. 2010;90(3): 927–934. https://doi.org/10.1016/j.athoracsur.2010.05.041.

19. Alloubi I, Jougon J, Delcambre F, Baste JM, Velly JF. Early complications after pneumonectomy: retrospective study of 168 patients. *Interact Cardiovasc Thorac Surg*. 2010;11(2): 162–165. https://doi.org/10.1510/icvts.2010.232595.

20. Thomas A, Cox G, Sharma R, et al. Gemcitabine and paclitaxel associated pneumonitis in non-small cell lung cancer: report of a phase I/II dose-escalating study. *Eur J Cancer*. 2000;36(18):2329–2334.

21. Kreuter M, Vansteenkiste J, Herth FJ, et al. Impact and safety of adjuvant chemotherapy on pulmonary function in early stage non-small cell lung cancer. *Respiration*. 2014;87(3):204–210.

22. Berthod G, Lazor R, Letovanec I, et al. Pulmonary sarcoid-like granulomatosis induced by ipilimumab. *J Clin Oncol*. 2012;30(17):e156–159.

23. Kainthola A, Haritwal T, Tiwari M, et al. Immunological aspect of radiation-induced pneumonitis, current treatment strategies, and future prospects. *Front Immunol*. 2017;8:506.

24. Tsoutsou PG, Koukourakis MI. Radiation pneumonitis and fibrosis: mechanisms underlying its pathogenesis and implications for future research. *Int J Radiat Oncol Biol Phys*. 2006;66(5):1281–1293.

25. Frey KA, Gross MD, Hayman JA, et al. Changes in global function and regional ventilation and perfusion on SPECT during the course of radiotherapy in patients with non-small-cell lung cancer. *Int J Radiat Oncol Biol Phys*. 2012; 82(4):e631–e638.

26. Jaén J, Vázquez G, Alonso E, León A, Guerrero R, Almansa JF. Changes in pulmonary function after incidental lung irradiation for breast cancer: a prospective study. *Int J Radiat Oncol Biol Phys*. 2006;65(5):1381–1388.

27. Rawat S, Kumar G, Puri A, Sharma MK, Kakria A, Kumar P. Correlation of six-minute walk test, pulmonary function test and radiation pneumonitis in the management of carcinoma of oesophagus: a prospective pilot study. *J Radiother Pract*. 2011;10(3):191–199.

28. Hershman DL, Lacchetti C, Dworkin RH, et al. Prevention and management of chemotherapy-induced peripheral neuropathy in survivors of adult cancers: American Society of Clinical Oncology clinical practice guideline. *J Clin Oncol*. 2014;32(18):1941–1967.

29. Stubblefield MD. *Cancer Rehabilitation: Principles and Practice*. Springer Publishing Company; 2018.

30. Dirks-Naylor AJ, Griffiths CL. Glucocorticoid-induced apoptosis and cellular mechanisms of myopathy. *J Steroid Biochem Mol Biol*. 2009;117(1–3):1–7.

FURTHER READING

1. Cristian A, Batmangelich S, Ahmed MA. *Physical Medicine and Rehabilitation Patient-Centered Care: Mastering the Competencies*. New York, NY: Demos Medical; 2015.

CHAPTER 4

Assessment, Treatment, and Rehabilitation of Bone and Spinal Metastasis in Lung Cancer

LISA MARIE RUPPERT, MD • HANNA OH, MD

BACKGROUND

Bone is a frequent and early site of metastases for patients with lung cancer. Literature reports that 20%−40% of lung cancer patients will develop bone metastases and that up to 80% of these osseous lesions will be diagnosed during the initial metastatic work up.[1,2] The spine is the most common site of bony metastases (40%−50%) followed by the ribs (20%−27%).[3]

Osseous metastases produce some of the most feared and debilitating complications of the disease, including pain, pathologic fractures, and spinal cord compromise.[3] These complications are frequently referred to as skeletal-related events (SREs) and are associated with impaired mobility, reduced quality of life, poor prognosis, and increased health care costs.[4,5] Treatment of SREs should involve a multidisciplinary team of medical oncologists, surgeons, physiatrists, and pain specialists to provide comprehensive oncologic management while optimizing the patient's functional status and quality of life.

PATHOPHYSIOLOGY OF OSSEOUS METASTASES

Although the mechanisms underlying osseous metastases are yet to be fully understood, evidence suggests that the bone microenvironment contributes to lung cancer's bone tropism. This is particularly true of bones rich in red marrow and trabecular bone, such as the vertebral bodies, ribs, pelvis, and long bones.[2,6]

For patients with lung cancer, most osseous metastases occur through hematogenous spread.[1] Direct extension of primary lung tumors may also lead to bone metastases. An example of this is paravertebral apical lung tumors which can directly invade adjacent vertebrae.[5]

Bone metastases from lung cancer may be osteolytic or mixed osteolytic/osteoblastic. Osteolytic lesions result in more significant bone destruction than bone formation, and osteoblastic lesions result in bone deposition without the breakdown of old bone first. Both lytic and blastic lesions alter the typical bone architecture and can result in deformity or pathologic fracture.[7] In the spine, these pathologic fractures can lead to instability by increasing strain on the spine's support elements, including muscles, tendons, ligaments, and joint capsules. They can also result in retropulsion of fractured bone fragments into the epidural space causing spinal cord compression.[7]

Spinal column metastases may directly extend into the epidural space resulting in spinal epidural metastases.[5] Paravertebral apical lung tumors, such as Pancoast tumors, may also result in epidural metastases through direct extension into adjacent vertebrae or growth through the neuroforamen to enter the epidural space.[8] These metastases may result in nerve root or spinal cord compression with injury to axons and myelin. They may also result in vascular compromise of spinal arteries and the epidural venous plexus, leading to injury through cord ischemia or infarction.[7]

EPIDEMIOLOGY
Bone Metastases

Approximately 30%−70% of bone metastases are associated with lung cancer,[2] with nonsmall cell lung cancer (NSCLC) being the third most common cause of bone metastases. Osseous metastases are found in 20%−40% of lung cancer patients at the time of diagnosis and are a frequent extrapulmonary site of recurrence, particularly for patients with NSCLC.[1,2,9] It is more common for patients to be diagnosed with multiple

Lung Cancer Rehabilitation. https://doi.org/10.1016/B978-0-323-83404-0.00003-1

bony metastatic lesions than oligometastases.[9,10] The most common site of osseous metastases in lung cancer is the spine, followed by the ribs and pelvis.[3] Spinal metastases are evenly distributed along the length of the spinal column; however, some lung cancer series have shown a disproportional propensity for the thoracic spine.[8]

Spinal Epidural Metastasis

Spinal epidural metastasis refers to tumor growth into the epidural space, anywhere along the spinal column. These metastases can cause epidural spinal cord compression (ESCC) through mechanical injury to axons and myelin and spinal cord ischemia/infarction via compression of spinal arteries and the epidural venous plexus.[8] While spinal epidural metastasis occurs in 5%–10% of cancer patients overall, 30% of lung cancer patients have one or more noncontiguous epidural lesions at the time of presentation[11,12] which may or may not be symptomatic.[8] Lung carcinoma is the cancer type most often identified in patients for whom spinal epidural metastases is the presenting feature of a previously undiagnosed neoplasm.[12] Most epidural involvement occurs in the thoracic and lumbosacral regions[13] and generally extends over 1–2 spinal segments.[8] The prognosis for patients with spinal epidural disease ranges from months to years depending on cancer type.[13]

Intramedullary Spinal Cord Metastasis

Intramedullary spinal cord metastasis represents <5% of total spinal cord lesions and typically occurs in the setting of extensive metastatic disease.[7,14] Lung cancer is the most common source of intramedullary spinal cord metastases, accounting for more than 50% of cases.[15,16] This type of metastatic disease is more prevalent in small cell lung cancer (SCLC) than NSCLC. Intramedullary metastases are theorized to arise from hematogenous spread[16] and can occur as a solitary lesion in the spinal cord. The cervical spine, a vascular-rich area, tends to be the most common site.[17] Prognosis is typically poor, with mortality common within 3 months.[18]

Intradural Extramedullary Spinal Metastasis (Leptomeningeal Disease)

Leptomeningeal disease (LMD) is more common in SCLC than NSCLC.[19] Patients with SCLC with LMD typically have widely disseminated disease, and approximately half of this population also has brain metastases.[20] Similar to epidural metastases, LMD is thought to occur through hematogenous spread or direct extension.[7] LMD typically occurs at the base of the brain or along the cauda equina and can result in cord compression and vascular compromise. Vascular compromise in this setting can result not only in cord ischemia but subarachnoid hemorrhage, particularly in those on anticoagulation.[7] Like intramedullary metastases, the prognosis for LMD is poor, often limited to months.[18]

SKELETAL-RELATED EVENTS

Osseous metastases cause morbidity, leading to possible pain, weakness, and SREs.[21] These SREs can include pain, hypercalcemia, pathological fracture, spinal cord compression, and radiation-induced bony injury. In a population-based cohort study of 29,720 patients with lung cancer in Demark, 6% were diagnosed with bone metastasis within 1 year of their initial diagnosis. Half of those with bone metastasis also experienced at least one SRE within 1 year of their bone metastasis diagnosis.[22]

Pain

Bone pain is one of the most common types of pain cancer patients experience. Most patients initially experience intermittent and dull aches, becoming more severe and constant as the disease progresses. Bone pain intensifies during movement, can be accompanied by fever, and increases in severity at night.[9]

Pain from bone metastasis can be attributed to tumor cells causing osteolysis, leading to the release of pain mediators such as endothelin.[23] Periosteal irritation and nerve damage are secondary effects of bony destruction which can also cause pain.[24] Treatment of pain from osseous metastases requires a multimodal approach with tumor-targeted treatments, such as local surgery, radiation therapy, systemic therapies, analgesics, bone-targeted therapies, and adjuvant agents such as steroids.[9]

This pain is referred to as "tumor-related pain" or "biologic pain" in the spine. Biologic pain typically occurs at night and is thought to be related to nocturnally reduced endogenous steroid secretion. Biologic pain typically responds well to anti-inflammatory medications, which may help distinguish this pain from other types of back pain. Radiation therapy is often incorporated to treat biologic pain with good results.[10]

Hypercalcemia

Hypercalcemia in malignancy can result from bony destruction, with osteolytic metastases present in 80% of cases. A common sequela of squamous cell lung cancer, hypercalcemia, can lead to fatigue, anorexia, constipation, impaired renal function, and altered mental status.[21] Hypercalcemia in malignancy is associated with a poor prognosis, with approximately 50% of patients dying within 30 days of this diagnosis.[25] Stewart describes mild hypercalcemia to be a serum calcium level of 10.5−11.9 mg per deciliter (2.6−2.9 mmol per liter), moderate hypercalcemia a level of 12.0−13.9 mg per deciliter (3.0−3.4 mmol per liter), and severe hypercalcemia a level of 14.0 mg per deciliter (3.5 mmol per liter) or greater. Treatment includes aggressive hydration, calciuresis with diuretics, and initiation of intravenous bisphosphonates, which inhibit bone resorption.[26]

Pathologic Fractures

When metastatic lesions invade bone, the load-bearing ability can become impaired, resulting in painful microfractures. Pathologic fractures most commonly occur in ribs and vertebrae.

Mirels' criteria (Table 4.1) is a scoring system used to determine if surgical intervention is needed to stabilize long bone structures affected by metastatic disease. It includes imaging assessment of the lesion site, nature of the lesion, size of the lesion, and presence of pain. Lesion sites include the upper extremity, lower extremity, and peritrochanteric area of the femur. Lesion types include blastic, mixed, or lytic. Lesion size is expressed as a fraction of cortical thickness, classified by lesion/cortex ratios of <1/3, 1/3 to 2/3, and >2/3. Each characteristic is scored from 1−3 based on the severity.[27]

Mirels recommends prophylactic surgical fixation for a lesion with an overall score of ≥9. Radiotherapy and observation are recommended for a lesion scoring ≤7.[13]

In 2010, the Spine Oncology Study Group (SOSG) created the Spinal Instability Neoplastic Score (SINS) to serve as a prognostic tool for surgical evaluation and decision-making for patients with spinal metastases and concerns of instability. It scores six variables: location of the lesion, characterization of pain, type of bony lesion, radiographic spinal alignment, degree of vertebral body destruction, and involvement of posterolateral spinal elements (Table 4.2). Scores range from a minimum of 0 to a maximum of 18. Scores 7−12 are associated with potential instability, while 13−18 denote instability. SOSG recommends surgical consultation for all patients with SINS >7.[28]

Spinal Cord Compression

Metastatic spinal cord compression is one of the most feared SREs in lung cancer. Symptoms associated with cord compression depend on the spinal segments and spinal tracts involved. Patients may experience weakness, sensory impairments, and bowel and bladder dysfunction. Anterior cord, posterior cord, Brown−Sequard, central cord, conus medullaris, and cauda equina patterns have been described.[13]

Radiation-Induced Bony Injury

Radiation therapy intended to treat metastasis to bone can lead to adverse reactions, including radiation osteitis, osteoradionecrosis, and insufficiency fractures.[20,29] The pathophysiology of these sequelae is only partly understood and thought to be related to a decline in bone marrow cells in the treated tissue and impaired bone remodeling.[30−32] Multiple factors play a role in the risk and likelihood of developing radiation-induced bony injuries, including radiation dose and fractionation and target tissue exposure. Irradiated bone can appear osteopenic about 1 year after treatment.[33] Radiation osteitis, a radiologic finding of a mottled appearance of bone with coarse trabeculation, occurs 2−3 years after radiation therapy.[34] Osteoradionecrosis is often associated with facial bones but can occur in any bone subject to radiation. It is considered a nonhealing bone that persists at least 3 months after radiation and can lead to pain and impaired mobility. Radiation-induced insufficiency fractures are stress fractures that occur under everyday

TABLE 4.1
Mirels' Criteria for Diagnosing Impending Pathologic Fractures.

Variable	SCORE		
	1	2	3
Site	Upper limb	Lower limb	Peritrochanter
Pain	Mild	Moderate	Functional
Lesion	Blastic	Mixed	Lytic
Size	<1/3	1/3−2/3	>2/3

Adapted from Mirels H. Metastatic disease in long bones: A proposed scoring system for diagnosing impending pathologic fractures. *Clin Orthop Relat Res.* 1989:S4−13, 2003.

TABLE 4.2
Spinal Instability Neoplastic Score (SINS) System Total Score 0–6: Stable Total Score 7–12: Potentially Unstable Total Score 13–18: Unstable a SINS of >7 Warrants Surgical Consultation to Assess for Spine Instability.

Component	Score
LOCATION	
Junctional (O–C2; C7-T2; T11-L1; L5-S1)	3
Mobile spine (C3-6; L2-4)	2
Semirigid (T3-10)	1
Rigid (S2–S5)	0
MECHANICAL PAIN	
Yes	3
No	2
Pain-free lesion	1
BONE LESION	
Lytic	2
Mixed (lytic/blastic)	1
Blastic	0
RADIOGRAPHIC SPINAL ALIGNMENT	
Subluxation/translation present	4
Deformity (kyphosis/scoliosis)	2
Normal	0
VERTEBRAL BODY COLLAPSE	
>50% collapse	3
<50% collapse	2
No collapse with >50% body involved	1
None of the above	0
POSTEROLATERAL INVOLVEMENT	
Bilateral	3
Unilateral	1
None of the above	0

Adapted from Fisher CG, DiPaola CP, Ryken TC, et al. A novel classification system for spinal instability in neoplastic disease: an evidence-based approach and expert consensus from the Spine Oncology Study Group. *Spine.* 2010;35(22):E1221–E1229.

physiologic loads applied to bone weakened by radiation. Sacral fractures from pelvic radiation are the most frequent insufficiency fractures reported in the literature.[35]

DIAGNOSTIC EVALUATION
Imaging Studies
X-ray (Plain Films, Radiograph)
Radiographs can be helpful in the assessment of pathologic fractures. They can also help determine whether metastatic lesions are osteolytic, osteoblastic, or mixed. Unfortunately, X-rays have limitations. For a destructive lesion in the trabecular bone to be recognized, it must be > 1 cm in diameter with a loss of ~50% of the bone mineral content.[5] Plain films are also insensitive when assessing for paraspinal masses and epidural disease, as they are difficult to visualize.[36] Pedicle erosion can be seen on radiographs, which is a red flag for epidural disease[37] (Figs. 4.1 and 4.2).

Computed Tomography
Computed tomography (CT) scan is a convenient tool for the initial evaluation of fracture risk in a long bone given its accessibility and low cost.[38] CT scans are particularly useful in localizing lesions for biopsy, allowing for tissue diagnosis in the setting of metastatic disease. They are, however, limited in use when evaluating for treatment response in the bone due to difficulty in differentiating between metabolically active versus inactive bony lesions (Figs. 4.3 and 4.4).

Myelogram
A myelogram can be performed alongside other imaging modalities such as CT scan, magnetic resonance imaging (MRI), or radiographs. Contrast dye is injected into the spinal column during a myelogram to visualize the spinal cord, subarachnoid space, and adjacent structures. CT myelograms are sensitive to changes in bone density and bony metastases. CT myelography is preferred when MRI is unavailable. Before MRI technology, myelograms assisted in diagnosing spinal epidural metastases. There are risks with myelography, including infection, bleeding, and iatrogenic neurologic injury.[39]

Magnetic Resonance Imaging
MRI with contrast of the spine is considered the most sensitive imaging modality and preferred when cord compression is suspected. Not only can bony involvement and epidural disease be assessed, but intramedullary tumors and LMD can also be potentially visualized.[40,41,42] MRI can also help evaluate the cause of a vertebral compression fracture identified on radiograph[5] (Fig. 4.5).

Vertebral body involvement is best visualized using T1-weighted or STIR images, whereas the degree of ESCC and presence of paraspinal tumors are best assessed using axial T2-weighted and T1-weighted

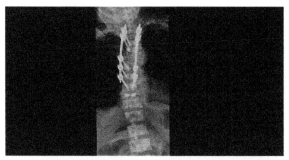
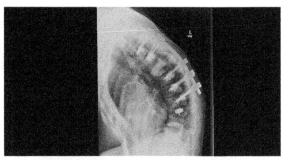

FIG. 4.1 Plain radiographs of patient of a 66-year-old female with NSCLS showing diffuse skeletal metastatic disease involving the axial and appendicular skeleton, kyphosis, postsurgical appearance status postposterior and fusion with bilateral rods, and transpedicular screws spanning T4-T10 and T11 kyphoplasty.

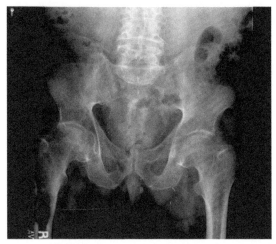

FIG. 4.2 XR Pelvis showing lytic lesion right subtrochanteric femur in 85-year-old male with extensive metastatic disease.

postcontrast images.[43] A total spine MRI is helpful to assess for asymptomatic noncontiguous lesions in patients with lung cancer.[8]

Positron Emission Tomography

Positron emission tomography (PET) uses fluorodeoxy-glucose (FDG) to detect the presence of tumors based on metabolic activity. 18F-FDG-PET/CT is the most sensitive modality for assessing osteolytic and bone marrow metastases. PET-CT can help differentiate tumors from benign lesions.[44] In patients with newly diagnosed bony metastases of unknown origin (FDG)-PET/CT is often the first choice for imaging workup.[45,46] It is also the most accurate way of assessing for treatment response in hypermetabolic bone metastasis by using quantitative assessment of FDG uptake immediately before, during, and after therapy. Compared to bone scintigraphy, PET imaging has

superior diagnostic accuracy, higher spatial resolution, and shorter imaging times[5] (Figs. 4.6 and 4.7).

Typically, untreated lytic lesions demonstrate greater FDG uptake than osteosclerotic metastases.[5] The use of PET-CT to distinguish between worsening sclerosis and response to disease progression is limited as the appearance of a sclerotic area of bone could represent cancer progression or reflect healing within a lesion that was not large enough to visualize on prior imaging studies. Obtaining tumor markers in conjunction with PET-CT can be helpful in this setting.[47]

Laboratory Studies

Laboratory studies, including calcium levels and alkaline phosphatase (ALP), should be monitored. Calcium levels assess for hypercalcemia, the most common metabolic derangement seen in cancer patients.[26] Serum ALP, a serum marker of bone turnover and mineralization, is a diagnostic marker for the presence of bone metastases.[48] Elevation of ALP with osteolytic bone lesions is due to local bone formation. Alternatively, in osteoblastic bone metastasis, elevations are due to activation of local osteoblasts.[49] Elevated serum ALP is correlated with poor prognosis in the setting of bone metastasis.[2]

TREATMENT

A multidisciplinary approach is essential in determining treatment for lung cancer patients with bone and spine involvement. A good illustration of this need is the NOMS (neurologic, oncologic, mechanical stability, and systemic disease) framework used in spinal metastases. The neurologic and oncologic elements determine surgical indications and the best approach to radiation therapy. Spinal mechanical instability alone is an indication for surgical intervention if a patient can tolerate surgery. Finally, the systemic disease component

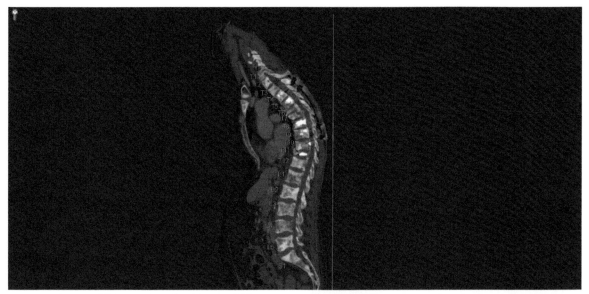

FIG. 4.3 CT total spine of a 66-year-old female with NSCLC showing postoperative changes including cemented posterior fusion of T4-T5 and T8-T10 with T11 kyphoplasty. Moderate to severe compressions of T6, T7, and T11 with mild height loss of T8 and borderline mild height loss of T10. Retropulsion/ventral epidural extension at T7 and retropulsion and left ventral epidural disease at T11 (ESCCS 1B). Multilevel mixed sclerotic and lytic lesions.

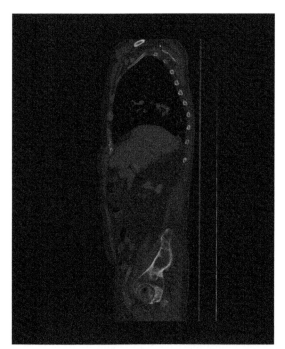

FIG. 4.4 CT chest/abdomen/pelvis showing mixed lytic and sclerotic osseous metastases in the pelvis of an 85-year-old male with extensive metastatic disease.

considers the extent and impact of a patient's systemic disease on treatment outcomes and tolerance.[13]

Systemic Treatment

For patients with lung cancer, systemic treatment varies based on cancer type, the extent of osseous involvement, and the presence or absence of extraskeletal metastases. Resistance to systemic treatments can occur, necessitating changing treatment programs to regain control of the disease.[5]

Surgical Intervention

The goals of surgical treatment are to address pain and preserve function, prevent impending fractures, and stabilize pathologic fractures. While pathological fractures are a clear indication for surgery, treatment for impending fractures is more complicated and requires consideration of multiple factors such as the behavior of the primary tumor/disease in the bone and efficacy of available treatments.[5]

In addition to SINS, NOMS, and Mirels' classification systems previously mentioned, other systems that assist in surgical decision-making are the Tokuhashi and Tomita scoring systems. Tokuhashi et al. created a scoring system based on six parameters for the prognostic assessment of patients with metastasis: general medical condition, number of extraspinal metastases,

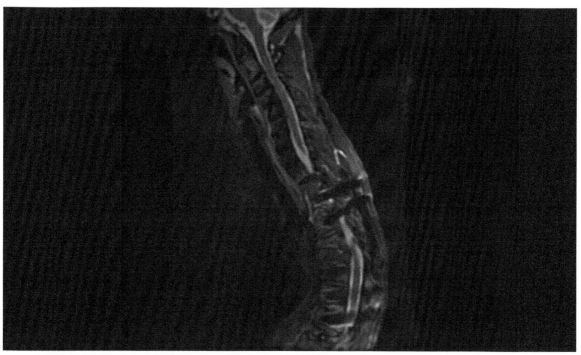

FIG. 4.5 MRI T2-weighted image showing cemented posterior fusion of T4-T5 and T8-T10 with T11 kyphoplasty. Unchanged severe compression of T6 and moderate compression of T7 and T10, mild left ventral epidural extension at T7 (ESCCS 1B), and diffuse osseous involvement in a 66-year-old female with history nonsmall cell lung cancer with NSCLC with innumerable brain metastases, LMD, bone, and nodal disease.

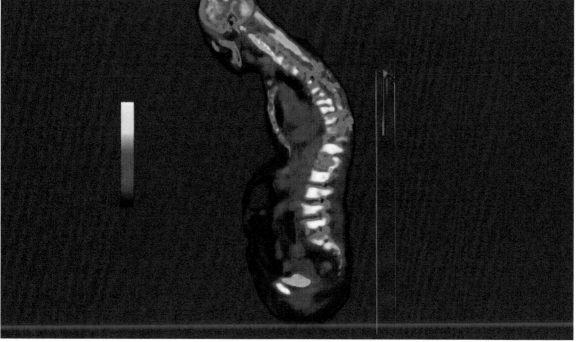

FIG. 4.6 FDG PET/CT of a 66-year-old female with NSCLC which shows mixed changes in FDG avid osseous lesions in the sternum and spine.

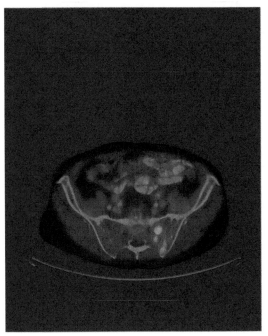
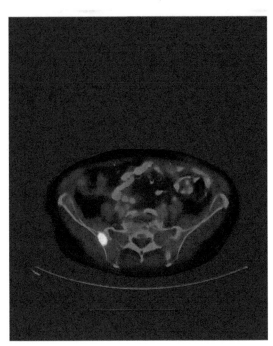

FIG. 4.7 FDG PET/CT showing increased uptake in the pelvis in 85-year-old male with extensive metastatic disease.

number of vertebral metastases, presence of visceral metastases, primary tumor type, and neurologic deficits.[50] Tomita et al. proposed a more precise strategy in which the scoring system uses three prognostic factors: grade of malignancy, visceral metastases, and bone metastasis.[51]

Long Bones

Surgical treatment for metastatic bone disease and a pathological fracture in long bone aims to provide a stable and secure fixation that allows immediate weight-bearing and restoration of function and will outlast the patient. Radiation therapy often follows surgical intervention to decrease the risk of disease progression.[52] The best method of reconstruction remains controversial among surgeons. Some prefer an en bloc resection with endoprosthetic replacement, while others advocate for less invasive intralesional procedures using reconstruction nails or other osteosynthetic devices with or without the adjunct of cement.[53]

En bloc resection with endoprosthetic reconstruction is used for both curative and palliative treatment. It prevents local complications but is associated with infections, aseptic loosening of hardware, and mechanical failure. Intralesional procedures are less invasive but

associated with higher implant failure rates within the first year, persistent pain, and local tumor progression.[54] Surgical scoring scales, patient tolerance, life expectancy, and functional status ultimately drive decision making.

Prophylactic stabilization for an impending fracture is preferred to surgical fixation after a pathologic fracture has occurred as outcomes such as functional recovery and surgical complications are overall better (Fig. 4.8). For example, patients who undergo surgery for impending pathologic fractures of the femur have a shorter hospital stay, greater likelihood of resuming support-free ambulation, and greater likelihood of discharge home rather than a rehabilitation setting when compared to patients who undergo surgery after pathologic fracture of the femur.[55]

Based on Mirels' criteria, prophylactic surgery is generally recommended for lesions ≥30 mm in greatest dimension, lytic destruction of ≥50% of the cortex of a long bone, and persistent pain.[56] Prophylactic fixation surgeries typically utilize synthetic implants such as plates, screws, and intramedullary nails to restore the function of the affected limb with a less invasive procedure than an endoprosthetic reconstruction.[53]

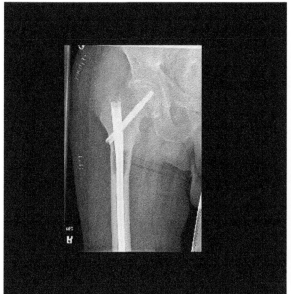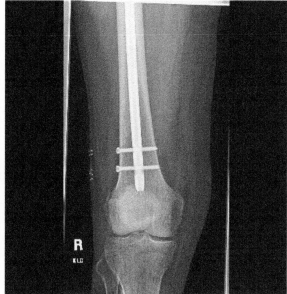

FIG. 4.8 XR Femur showing right femur fixation utilizing an intramedullary nail with two distal interlocking screws and dynamic hip screw prophylactic for concerns of impending fracture in 85-year-old male with extensive metastatic disease. Unchanged subtrochanteric lytic lesion.

Cementoplasty is a minimally invasive procedure in which Polymethylmethacrylate bone cement is injected percutaneously into a region of damaged bone, particularly in patients ineligible for surgical reconstruction.[57] Cazzato et al. concluded that percutaneous long bone cementoplasty is most effective in the upper limbs for pain relief and when the largest dimension of the lesion is < 3 cm.[58] Its use is not without adverse events. Documented adverse events include "bone cement implantation syndrome," characterized by hypoxia, hypotension, cardiovascular collapse, and increased risk of pulmonary embolism.[59] In addition, tumor recurrence can also occur postprocedure, necessitating further surgery or alternative means of pain control.[60]

Treating teams may consider regional techniques such as thermal ablation, cryotherapy, and embolization for tumor debulking in addition to surgery.[61] Cryoablation impairs cell membrane integrity using argon gas, causing cell death,[62] whereas embolization induces tumor necrosis by occluding feeding vessels. These ablative techniques can also be helpful for pain relief.[63]

Any type of surgical intervention does carry risks which can include instrument failure, respiratory complications, DVT/PE, wound infections, and worsening of neurologic symptoms.[59,64]

Spine
Pathologic Fractures and Instability
Spine stabilization and instrumentation is required in the setting of pathologic fractures of the vertebral body and/or retropulsion of fragments into the spinal cord (Fig. 4.1).[39]

Spinal Epidural Metastases and Cord Compression
Spinal cord compression from epidural spinal metastasis is a medical emergency.

Steroids, particularly dexamethasone, are generally started as soon as a diagnosis of cord compression is made.[8] Separation surgery is a surgical technique often employed for cord compression. During separation surgery, the spinal cord is decompressed, spinal fluid space is reconstituted, and the spinal column is stabilized using long screw rod instrumentation fusion. Tumors in the paraspinal musculature and vertebral body may not be fully resected. Instead, the goal of separation surgery is to decompress the cord and allow for radiation therapy.[65] A separation of 2–3 mm is needed between the tumor and spinal cord to deliver treatment of stereotactic radiosurgery (SRS) without radiation toxicity to the spinal cord.[66]

Less invasive surgical procedures include screw-rod instrumentation, percutaneous cement augmentation, pedicle screw fixation, and conjoined SRS. Treatment of acute spinal cord compression is aimed toward pain control, decreasing tumor burden, and preserving spinal stability and neurologic function.[67]

Radiation Therapy
Long Bones
Radiation therapy treats symptomatic appendicular bone lesions by achieving local tumor control and treating pain. Symptomatic pain improves with a reduction of tumor size and surrounding inflammation.[68] A typical treatment plan for palliative radiation to a long bone lesion is 80 Gy in a single fraction or 20−30 Gy in 5−10 fractions.[61] After radiation therapy, pain relief typically occurs quite quickly, with more than 50% of responders reporting improvement with 1−2 weeks.[69]

In a Phase II study at MD Anderson Cancer Center, single-fraction SBRT (stereotactic body radiotherapy) was noninferior to standard multifractionated radiotherapy for pain control and local disease control for bony nonspine lesions. Patients in this study received either 12 Gy or 16Gy to bony sites.[70] Supporting these findings, a systemic review in 2019 concluded that studies reported higher rates of pain relief following SBRT than conventional RT for treatment of bone metastases.[71]

Spine
Radiation to the spine is typically fractionated into small doses over days to weeks. However, those with a reduced life expectancy typically have a shorter, more truncated schedule.[39] A fractionated radiation treatment plan is generally 30−40 Gy in 10−15 days to target 1−2 vertebral bodies above and below the lesion.[8] Patients with SCLC tend to have better responses to radiation than those with NSCLC.[72] Most patients with intramedullary spinal cord metastasis have improved neurologic function after a standard fractionated radiation plan.[16]

SRS is a precise form of radiation therapy delivered as a single fraction. Typically, the use of SRS is restricted to tumors confined to bone or with minimal epidural impingement.[73] All patients treated with SRS for spinal epidural metastasis should be followed regularly to monitor for recurrence. Yamada et al. describe a 3-year recurrence rate of only 4 in 413 patients treated with SRS for spine malignant tumors.[74]

As described previously, radiation can cause adverse effects on bone. Radiation therapy can also cause radiation-induced nerve injury, plexopathy, and myelopathy. Risk of radiation-induced myelopathy is correlated to the total radiation dose delivered, dose delivered per fraction, and length of spinal cord irradiated. The timing between courses of radiation therapy and concurrent treatment with chemotherapy reportedly also affects the occurrence and severity of radiation-induced myelopathies.[75,76] Acute transient radiation myelopathy, hypothesized to result from demyelination of the dorsal columns, is more common than chronic progressive radiation myelopathy (CPRM), typically occurring 1−29 months after completion of radiation treatment. CPRM can occur 9−15 months after treatment. CPRM, classically characterized by a latent period during which the patient is asymptomatic, is associated with a painless insidious onset of neurologic deficits, worsening steadily over time. These include ascending weakness and sensory impairments.[77]

The Pallis criteria for diagnosing CPRM state that the radiation field must include the spinal cord, the primary neurologic deficit must be within the segment of the cord exposed, and other spinal cord lesions must be ruled out before making the diagnosis.[78]

Side effects like dysphagia and diarrhea may occur with radiation when large portions of the gastrointestinal tract are in the treatment field.[39]

Pain Management/Palliative Care
A multidisciplinary team of health care subspecialists including neuro/orthopedic surgeons, radiation oncologists, medical oncologists, physiatrists, and pain specialists is integral for oncologic decision-making and managing symptoms such as pain to improve a patient's quality of life. In practice, pain management for osseous metastases involves interventional pain procedures, oral medications, physical/occupational therapy, bracing, and complementary medicine approaches.[79]

While radiation therapy is the preferred method for localized bone pain, patients may have widespread disease and pain necessitating pain medications for improved quality of life and overall pain relief. The World Health Organization (WHO) set guidelines in 2018 for analgesia of cancer pain, "to relieve pain to a level that allows for an acceptable quality of life".[80]

Medication management of pain symptoms includes nonsteroidal antiinflammatory drugs (NSAIDs), steroids, antiepileptic medications, opioids, and tricyclic antidepressants (Table 4.3).[13] Approximately 70% of patients with NSCLC with bony metastasis require opioids for pain relief. Use of bisphosphonates, which block osteoclast activity and inhibit bone resorption, and denosumab, a RANK ligand inhibitor, may also

TABLE 4.3
Medications for Cancer Pain.

Medicine Group	Medicine Class	Examples
Nonopioids	Paracetamol NSAIDS (non-steroidal antiinflammatory drugs)	Paracetamol oral tablets, liquid, rectal suppositories, IV Ibuprofen oral tablets and liquid Ketorolac oral tablets and IV Acetylsalicylic acid oral tablets and rectal suppositories
Opioids	Weak opioids	Codeine oral tablets, liquid, and IV Tramadol oral tablets and liquid
	Strong opioids	Morphine oral tablets Hydromorphone oral tablets, liquid, and IV Oxycodone oral tablets and liquid Fentanyl IV, transdermal patch, transmucosal lozenge Methadone oral tablet, liquid, and IV
Adjuvants	Steroids	Dexamethasone oral tablet and IV Methylprednisolone oral tablets and IV Prednisolone oral tablets
	Antidepressants	Amitriptyline oral tablets Venlafaxine oral tablets
	Anticonvulsants	Carbamazepine oral tablets and IV Gabapentin oral tablet and liquid
	Bisphosphonates	Zoledronate IV
	RANKL inhibitor	Denosumab

2018 WHO Guidelines for the Pharmacological and Radiotherapeutic Management of Cancer Pain in Adults and Adolescents recommend that NSAIDs, paracetamol, and opioids should be used either alone or in combination depending on pain severity and clinical assessment, for pain control in adults and adolescents with cancer. They make no recommendation for or against the use of antidepressants and anticonvulsants for cancer-related neuropathic pain. For patients with bone metastases, they recommend the use of bisphosphonates to prevent and treat bone pain. Data from Fallon M, Giusti R, Aielli F, et al. Management of cancer pain in adult patients: ESMO Clinical Practice Guidelines. *Ann Oncol.* 2018; 29(Suppl 4):iv166–iv191. "WHO Guidelines for the Pharmacological and Radiotherapeutic Management of Cancer Pain in Adults and Adolescents. Geneva: World Health Organization; 2018".

help treat pain from osseous metastases.[81] Zoledronic acid was associated with 30%–40% reduced risk of SRE in a retrospective analysis by Hatoum et al.[82] Consideration and discussion of side effect profiles and potential medication interactions are essential when prescribing any oral medications.[83]

Interventional procedures such as kyphoplasty and vertebroplasty may play a role in treating pain in the setting of pathologic compression fractures.[84] Vertebroplasty involves polymethylmethacrylate injection, a biological cement, into the bone via percutaneously inserted needles under radiologic guidance, whereas kyphoplasty uses a high-pressure balloon to create a cavity within the vertebral body, with subsequent use of a biological cement. Minimally invasive radiofrequency ablation and vertebroplasty or kyphoplasty in combination reduce tumor mass and stabilizes the vertebral body.[61] Other interventional procedures considered in pain management include joint injections, peripheral nerve blocks, and ablative treatments.[79,85] Finally, for patients with more complex

or diffuse pain symptoms, spinal cord stimulation or intrathecal drug delivery may be offered.[79]

PHYSIATRIST ASSESSMENT
Physiatrists can play an integral role on a multidisciplinary oncologic team to diagnose functional and neurologic deficits from bone metastases, treat mobility impairments, and prevent further medical complications.[79]

Clinical Presentation
When obtaining a history in patients with metastatic lung cancer and known osseous metastases, including spine involvement, it is crucial to ask about pain patterns and assess for the presence of neurologic deficits.

Long Bones
Pain is often the presenting symptom of bone or spine metastases. Pain from bone metastases is usually worse at night, which is the opposite pattern of pain from

degenerative disease. Localized tenderness is usually present. Any sudden worsening of pain in long bones should raise suspicion of a pathologic fracture or enlarging bony lesion.[86]

Spine

For patients with spinal metastases, there are three classic pain types described in the literature. These include biologic, radicular, and mechanical pain.[10] Localized pain is characterized as a deep gnawing or aching pain. Radicular pain occurs with tumor compression of nerve roots and is typically described as sharp, shooting, or stabbing in nature following a dermatomal pattern. Mechanical pain varies with position or activity, characteristically occurring with transitional movements or axial loading of the spine. Mechanical pain can be indicative of impending or established spinal instability.[7] Localized pain may precede the development of neurologic impairments by weeks to months for patients with epidural cord compression.[7]

Patients with spinal epidural metastases can also present with neurologic deficits such as weakness, sensory impairments, bowel and bladder dysfunction, balance impairments, and ataxia depending on the location of spinal cord involvement.[87]

Physical Examination
Long Bone

There are no formal guidelines for performing a physical examination or manual muscle testing on patients with suspected metastatic bony lesions. Providers must take caution to limit the risk of pathologic fractures as these lesions can compromise bone integrity. Patients may endorse pain with weight-bearing if there is a lesion in a lower extremity weight-bearing bone or with lifting if the upper extremity is involved.

Spinal Metastases

A focused physical examination is crucial to assess pain symptoms, neurologic status, and spinal stability.[10] Pain that worsens with movement and axial loading during the examination should raise a flag for the examiner to consider imaging to assess spine stability. Of note, when the thoracolumbar spine is involved, patients may have pain when asked to lay supine due to spine extension causing an unstable kyphosis.[67]

Further examination should include evaluation of strength, sensation, tone, reflexes, and sphincter function. Overall, it should mirror the ISNCSCI (International Standards for Neurological Classification of Spinal Cord Injury) examination used in traumatic spinal cord injuries. Although not validated to determine neurologic prognosis, the initial ISNSCI examination helps establish the diagnosis of myelopathy, determine a neurologic level of injury (NLI), and guide functional assessments.[88] Follow-up ISNCSI examinations can help detect changes in neurologic status and guide diagnostic workup for recurrence or disease progression when present.

Physical examination of skin is essential during physiatrist assessment as patients with impaired sensation, limited mobility, and bowel or bladder incontinence are at increased risk of skin breakdown. Attention should be paid to common areas for pressure injuries, including the heels, sacrum, ischium, and gluteal folds.[89]

REHABILITATION EFFORTS

Whether patients are in a restorative, supportive, or palliative stage of oncologic treatment, rehabilitation efforts can assist in relieving symptoms, preventing medical complications, and improving quality of life.[64,90]

Precautions

Oncologists, surgeons, radiation oncologists, and other health care team members should discuss any potential mobility or activity precautions with patients with bone metastases.

Long Bone

Providers prescribing physical therapy or physical activity must be aware of locations of bony disease to ensure that prescription is appropriate and does not lead to further injury.[87]

Literature shows that physical therapy and activity are beneficial for patients with metastatic cancer. In a study on patients with prostate cancer and bone metastases, Galvao et al. found that aerobic, resistance, and flexibility exercise programs led to physical function and strength improvements while still avoiding loading bones with metastatic involvement.[91] If there is a high risk for fracture, consider modalities such as neuromuscular electrical stimulation (NMES) to promote muscle strength.[92]

When the spinal column is involved, additional spine precautions are necessary, which can vary based on the location of spine involvement. Typically, patients are counseled to limit excessive spinal flexion, extension or rotation, and limit lifting to no more than 10 pounds. As a result of these precautions, the 2017 International Spine Oncology Consortium reports on multidisciplinary management of spinal metastases recommended a physical medicine and rehabilitation consultation for patients with neurologic impairments due to spine involvement to optimize function and independence.[85]

Certain patients may benefit from the use of braces to maintain these precautions. In addition, patients may benefit from evaluation/prescription for a wheelchair, as their primary method of mobility, and durable medical equipment (DME) such as shower benches and commodes to ensure safety with self-care when precautions are in place.[11]

Symptom-Specific Management

Pain is one of the most common symptoms of osseous and spinal metastases. Determining its underlying etiology is pivotal to management. In addition to the oncologic, medication, and interventional management previously mentioned, conservative options are available for treatment, including postural bracing, physical therapy, and modalities.[7]

Consider postural bracing for spine metastasis as management for nonsurgical or residual mechanical pain. Custom or commercial orthotics, chosen based on a patient's needs, provide improved spinal alignment and postural correction. Also, they can serve as a reminder for patients to adhere to spinal precautions.[85] Similarly, patients requiring nonweight bearing status while pending surgical stabilization may find pain relief with an offloading brace.[7,11]

Physical modalities including heat, cold, electrical stimulation, and ultrasound play a role in the pain management plan. Caution must be used with their application over areas with sensory loss to prevent injury. Given these modalities can promote increased blood flow, caution should also be taken as there is a risk of promoting disease spread.[7]

Neurologic Impairments

The pattern and level of neurologic impairments reflect the location of metastatic involvement. Management of these impairments includes targeted physical and occupational therapy and evaluation/prescription for bracing and adaptive equipment. Examples of braces include ankle-foot orthoses for lower extremity weakness, multipodus boots to prevent or treat ankle contractures secondary to increased tone, disuse, or flaccidity, and wrist hand orthoses to maintain neutral wrist positioning. Family education and needed home modifications are essential aspects to review to ensure safety with any DME prescribed.[13]

Patients with spinal cord compression may develop spasticity. When mild, spasticity can be treated conservatively with stretching and bracing. Oral antispasmodic medications or localized chemo denervation

procedures (botulinum toxin injections) are often utilized for more severe symptoms. Intrathecal administration of baclofen may also be considered for the management of severe spasticity involving multiple extremities.[7,90]

Functional Impairments

Physical and occupational therapy play an essential role in the management of functional impairments. Physical therapy for bone and spinal metastases should include exercises to reduce fall risk, improve muscle strength, improve sensation, maintain joint range of motion, and ensure safe transfers and mobility. It should also include education on maintaining mobility precautions.[7]

Prognosis plays a significant role in determining realistic functional goals of physical therapy. For patients with a poor prognosis, efforts focus on teaching caregivers techniques for tasks such as transfers, rather than focusing on long-terms goals of regaining strength for independent tasks. Energy conservation techniques, passive ROM, relaxation, and guided imagery are a few techniques incorporated at this stage.[87]

In addition to mobility impairments, cancer survivors are significantly more likely to have one or more limitations in activities of daily living (ADLs).[87] Occupational therapy is crucial to assist patients in learning compensatory techniques for ADLs if they have pain or weight-bearing restrictions in an extremity due to a long bone lesion or neurologic impairments from spinal cord compression. In addition, they can provide recommendations on adaptive equipment for self-care and education to caregivers when assistance is needed.

Skin

As previously mentioned, patients with mobility and sensory impairments are at high risk of developing skin breakdown and pressure injuries. If skin breakdown is present, physiatrists may provide wound care recommendations. In addition, they may provide counseling on pressure-relieving techniques, skin hygiene, and optimal nutrition for both pressure injury management and prevention.[64]

Neurogenic Bowel Dysfunction

Bowel dysfunction can lead to impaired emptying/constipation and incontinence episodes. Physiatrists can improve a patient's quality of life by developing a bowel program to ensure adequate bowel emptying and limit incontinence episodes. Patients with upper motor neuron hyperreflexic bowel patterns may benefit from a program of stool softeners, oral stimulants, and suppositories to result in a timed daily bowel movement. Patients with lower motor neuron hyporeflexic bowel patterns typically benefit from bulking agents to ensure formed stool for timed manual removal. Many patients with cancer, including those undergoing oncologic treatment, may have cytopenias such as neutropenia and thrombocytopenia, which require caution with stimulation and use of suppositories or enemas.[11]

Neurogenic Bladder Dysfunction

Anticholinergic agents are helpful in patients who have detrusor overactivity (upper motor neuron pattern), whereas cholinergic medications and techniques such as Crede and double void can help patients prone to retention from detrusor hypocontracility.[13] An intermittent catheterization program or temporary indwelling catheter may be needed if a patient continues to have symptoms of urinary retention or high postvoid residuals despite these treatments.[13] Pelvic floor therapy focusing on pelvic/sphincter muscle retraining and sensory awareness may assist both bowel and bladder management plans.

Cardiovascular Dysfunction

Orthostatic hypotension, due to reduced sympathetic efferent activity and reduced vasoconstriction, may occur in individuals with spinal cord compression depending on the region of involvement. Treatment of orthostatic hypotension may include ensuring adequate hydration, use of compression stockings and abdominal binders, and pharmacologic treatments such as midodrine and salt tablets.[11]

Autonomic dysreflexia (AD), a well-known medical emergency in traumatic spinal cord injuries above the level of T6, can also occur with spinal cord injury from metastatic disease. Triggered by a noxious stimulus below the NLI, AD results in sympathetic overactivity below the NLI and unopposed parasympathetic tone above. Pain from metastases and tumor response to treatment are potential triggers for AD in the cancer setting. Treatment involves identifying and neutralizing any clear triggers, such as an over distended bladder, tight-fitting clothing, bowel constipation, or pain. If symptoms do not resolve with these interventions, pharmacologic treatment with short-acting, rapid-onset medications (nifedipine, captopril) may be trialed.[13]

ROLE OF INPATIENT REHABILITATION

Long Bone

Like rehabilitation for hip arthroplasty for degenerative processes or other orthopedic procedures, patients undergoing surgery for pathologic fractures or impending fractures often require acute inpatient rehabilitation. Mobility limitations from postoperative pain, range of motion restrictions, or weight-bearing limitations require patients to learn new techniques for mobility, transfers, and performance of ADLs. Studies such as one by Bunting and Shea suggest that rehabilitation efforts are safe, reporting an incidence of 1 out of 96 patients developing a pathologic long bone fracture during physical therapy.[93]

If patients cannot tolerate upwards of 3 hours of therapy per day, participation in subacute rehabilitation can improve a patient's endurance and tolerance for activity and optimize safety before returning home. When considering inpatient rehabilitation, place attention on the timing of upcoming oncologic treatment and the potential for radiation therapy.

Spine

Patients with spinal involvement and resultant myelopathy may benefit from acute inpatient rehabilitation if aligned with their goals, treatments, and life expectancy.[13] Ruff et al. found that patients with spinal cord compression from epidural metastases who participated in a 2-week course of inpatient rehabilitation had improved pain, less depression, and better life satisfaction than historical cohorts that did not receive inpatient rehabilitation.[13] Of note, if acute inpatient rehabilitation is deemed appropriate in this setting, it should be conducted in a dedicated spinal cord injury unit.

Rehabilitation efforts may also occur at home with a home-based physical and occupational therapy program or in outpatient therapy facilities.

DISCUSSIONS ON PROGNOSIS AND SURVIVAL

Consistent communication between all care team members (patient, family, medical/surgical/radiation oncology, and rehabilitation) is essential for discussing prognosis, survival, treatment goals, and functional expectations for patients with metastatic lung cancer. Studies in the oncology literature show that a growing number of patients want to know about and understand their cancer diagnosis, chances of cure, and details about treatment side effects. In addition, these studies have shown that gratitude, peace of mind, positive attitude, reduced anxiety, and better adjustment are benefits individuals experienced from having been told their prognosis, even if the prognosis was poor.[94]

CONCLUSION

Treatment of bone and spinal lesions for patients with metastatic lung cancer requires a multidisciplinary team of medical oncologists, surgeons, physiatrists, and pain specialists to provide comprehensive oncologic management while optimizing the patient's functional status and quality of life.

REFERENCES

1. Kuchuk M, Addison CL, Clemons M, et al. Incidence and consequences of bone metastases in lung cancer patients. *J Bone Oncol.* 2013;2:22–29.
2. Zhang L, Gong Z. Clinical characteristics and prognostic factors in bone metastases from lung cancer. *Med Sci Monit.* 2017;23:4087–4094.
3. Greenberger JS. The pathophysiology and management of spine metastasis from lung cancer. *J Neuro Oncol.* 1995;23:109–120.
4. Schulman KL, Kohles J. Economic burden of metastatic bone disease in the U.S. *Cancer.* 2007;109:2334–2342.
5. Coleman R, Hadji P, Body JJ, et al. Bone health in cancer: ESMO clinical practice guidelines. *Ann Oncol.* 2020;31:1650–1663.
6. Hiraga T. Bone metastasis: interaction between cancer cells and bone microenvironment. *J Oral Biosci.* 2019;61:95–98.
7. Ruppert LM. Malignant spinal cord compression: adapting conventional rehabilitation approaches. *Phys Med Rehabil Clin N Am.* 2017;28:101–114.
8. Dropcho EJ. Neurologic complications of lung cancer. *Handb Clin Neurol.* 2014;119:335–361.
9. Zajaczkowska R, Kocot-Kepska M, Leppert W, et al. Bone pain in cancer patients: mechanisms and current treatment. *Int J Mol Sci.* 2019;20.
10. Bilsky M, Smith M. Surgical approach to epidural spinal cord compression. *Hematol Oncol Clin N Am.* 2006;20:1307–1317.
11. Schiff D, O'Neill BP, Suman VJ. Spinal epidural metastasis as the initial manifestation of malignancy: clinical features and diagnostic approach. *Neurology.* 1997;49(2):452–456.
12. Schiff D. Spinal cord compression. *Neurol Clin.* 2003;21(1):67–viii.
13. Ruppert LM, Reilly J. Metastatic spine oncology: symptom-directed management. *Neurooncol Pract.* 2020;7:i54–i61.
14. Sung WS, Sung MJ, Chan JH, et al. Intramedullary spinal cord metastases: a 20-year institutional experience with a comprehensive literature review. *World Neurosurg.* 2013;79(3–4):576–584.
15. Dam-Hieu P, Seizeur R, Mineo JF, et al. Retrospective study of 19 patients with intramedullary spinal cord metastasis. *Clin Neurol Neurosurg.* 2009;111(1):10–17.
16. Schiff D, O'Neill BP. Intramedullary spinal cord metastases: clinical features and treatment outcome. *Neurology.* 1996;47(4):906–912.
17. Kim DC, UK S, Bilsky M. *Tumors of the Spine.* 1st ed. Philadephia, PA: Elsevier Health Sciences; 2008

18. Grem JL, Burgess J, Trump DL. Clinical features and natural history of intramedullary spinal cord metastasis. *Cancer.* 1985;56(9):2305–2314.
19. Chamberlain MC, Kormanik P. Carcinoma meningitis secondary to non-small cell lung cancer: combined modality therapy. *Arch Neurol.* 1998;55(4):506–512.
20. Seute T, Leffers P, ten Velde GP, et al. Leptomeningeal metastases from small cell lung carcinoma. *Cancer.* 2005;104(8):1700–1705.
21. Coleman RE. Clinical features of metastatic bone disease and risk of skeletal morbidity. *Clin Cancer Res.* 2006;12(20 Pt 2):6243s–6249s.
22. Cetin K, Christiansen CF, Jacobsen JB, et al. Bone metastasis, skeletal-related events, and mortality in lung cancer patients: a Danish population-based cohort study. *Lung Cancer.* 2014;86(2):247–254.
23. Ghilardi JR, Röhrich H, Lindsay TH, et al. Selective blockade of the capsaicin receptor TRPV1 attenuates bone cancer pain. *J Neurosci.* 2005;25(12):3126–3131.
24. Coleman RE. Skeletal complications of malignancy. *Cancer.* 1997;80(8 Suppl):1588–1594.
25. Ralston SH, Gallacher SJ, Patel U, et al. Cancer-associated hypercalcemia: morbidity and mortality. Clinical experience in 126 treated patients. *Ann Intern Med.* 1990;112(7):499–504.
26. Stewart AF. Clinical practice. Hypercalcemia associated with cancer. *N Engl J Med.* 2005;352(4):373–379.
27. Mirels H. Metastatic disease in long bones: a proposed scoring system for diagnosing impending pathologic fractures. *Clin Orthop Relat Res.* 1989:S4–S13.
28. Fisher CG, DiPaola CP, Ryken TC, et al. A novel classification system for spinal instability in neoplastic disease: an evidence-based approach and expert consensus from the Spine Oncology Study Group. *Spine.* 2010;35(22):E1221–E1229.
29. Dalinka MK, Mazzeo Jr VP. Complications of radiation therapy. *Crit Rev Diagn Imag.* 1985;23(3):235–267.
30. Daldrup-Link HE, Henning T, Link TM. MR imaging of therapy-induced changes of bone marrow. *Eur Radiol.* 2007;17(3):743–761.
31. Daldrup HE, Link TM, Blasius S, et al. Monitoring radiation-induced changes in bone marrow histopathology with ultra-small superparamagnetic iron oxide (USPIO)-enhanced MRI. *J Magn Reson Imag.* 1999;9(5):643–652.
32. Shah KN, Racine J, Jones LC, Aaron RK. Pathophysiology and risk factors for osteonecrosis. *Curr Rev Musculoskelet Med.* 2015;8(3):201–209.
33. Howland WJ, Loeffler RK, Starchman DE, et al. Postirradiation atrophic changes of bone and related complications. *Radiology.* 1975;117(3 Pt 1):677–685.
34. Bluemke DA, Fishman EK, Scott Jr WW. Skeletal complications of radiation therapy. *Radiographics.* 1994;14(1):111–121.
35. Oh D, Huh SJ. Insufficiency fracture after radiation therapy. *Radiat Oncol J.* 2014;32(4):213–220.
36. Kienstra GE, Terwee CB, Dekker FW, et al. Prediction of spinal epidural metastases. *Arch Neurol.* 2000;57(5):690–695.

37. Batjer HH, Loftus CM. *Textbook of Neurological Surgery: Principles and Practice.* Phila Pa: Lippincott Williams; 2003.

38. Shie P, Cardarelli R, Brandon D, Erdman W, Abdulrahim N. Meta-analysis: comparison of F-18 Fluorodeoxyglucose-positron emission tomography and bone scintigraphy in the detection of bone metastases in patients with breast cancer. *Clin Nucl Med.* 2008;33(2): 97−101.

39. Mut M, Schiff D, Shaffrey ME. Metastasis to nervous system: spinal epidural and intramedullary metastasis. *J Neuro Oncol.* 2005;75(1):43−56.

40. Khasraw M, Posner JB. Neurological complications of systemic cancer. *Lancet Neurol.* 2010;9(12):1214−1227.

41. Portenoy RK, Lipton RB, Foley KM. Back pain in the cancer patient: an algorithm for evaluation and management. *Neurology.* 1987;37(1):134−138.

42. van der Sande JJ, Kröger R, Boogerd W. Multiple spinal epidural metastases; an unexpectedly frequent finding. *J Neurol Neurosurg Psychiatry.* 1990;53(11):1001−1003.

43. Bilsky MH, Laufer I, Fourney DR, et al. Reliability analysis of the epidural spinal cord compression scale. *J Neurosurg Spine.* 2010;13(3):324−328.

44. Laufer I, Lis E, Pisinski L, et al. The accuracy of [(18)F]fluoro-deoxyglucose positron emission tomography as confirmed by biopsy in the diagnosis of spine metastases in a cancer population. *Neurosurgery.* 2009;64(1):107−114.

45. D'Addario G, Felip E, ESMO Guidelines Working Group. Non-small-cell lung cancer: ESMO clinical recommendations for diagnosis, treatment and follow-up. *Ann Oncol.* 2009;20(Suppl 4):68−70.

46. Budak E, Yanarateş A. Role of ^{18}F-FDG PET/CT in the detection of primary malignancy in patients with bone metastasis of unknown origin. *Rev Española Med Nucl Imagen Mol.* 2020;39(1):14−19.

47. Ryan CJ, Shah S, Efstathiou E, et al. Phase II study of abiraterone acetate in chemotherapy-naive metastatic castration-resistant prostate cancer displaying bone flare discordant with serologic response. *Clin Cancer Res.* 2011;17(14):4854−4861.

48. Coleman JE. Structure and mechanism of alkaline phosphatase. *Annu Rev Biophys Biomol Struct.* 1992;21: 441−483.

49. Karhade AV, Thio QCBS, Kuverji M, et al. Prognostic value of serum alkaline phosphatase in spinal metastatic disease. *Br J Cancer.* 2019;20(6):640−646.

50. Tokuhashi Y, Matsuzaki H, Oda H, et al. A revised scoring system for preoperative evaluation of metastatic spine tumor prognosis. *Spine.* 2005;30(19):2186−2191.

51. Tomita K, Kawahara N, Kobayashi T, et al. Surgical strategy for spinal metastases. *Spine.* 2001;26(3):298−306.

52. Eastley N, Newey M, Robert A. Skeletal metastases - the role of the orthopaedic and spinal surgeon. *Surg Oncol.* 2012;21(3):216−222.

53. Wedin R, Bauer HC. Surgical treatment of skeletal metastatic lesions of the proximal femur. *J. Bone Jt Surgery Br.* 2005;87-B(12):1653−1657.

54. Bischel OE, Suda AJ, Böhm PM, Lehner B, Bitsch RG, Seeger JB. En-bloc resection of metastases of the proximal femur and reconstruction by modular arthroplasty is not only justified in patients with a curative treatment option-an observational study of a consecutive series of 45 patients. *J Clin Med.* 2020;9(3):758.

55. Ward WG, Holsenbeck S, Dorey FJ, Spang J, Howe D. Metastatic disease of the femur: surgical treatment. *Clin Orthop Relat Res.* 2003;415(Suppl):S230−S244.

56. Willeumier JJ, van der Linden YM, van de Sande MAJ, et al. Treatment of pathological fractures of the long bones. *EFORT Open Rev.* 2017;1(5):136−145.

57. Anselmetti G. Osteoplasty: percutaneous bone cement injection beyond the spine. *Semin Intervent Radiol.* 2010; 27(02):199−208.

58. Cazzato RL, Buy X, Eker O, et al. Percutaneous long bone cementoplasty of the limbs: experience with fifty-one non-surgical patients. *Eur Radiol.* 2014;24(12):3059−3068.

59. Herrenbruck T, Erickson EW, Damron TA, et al. Adverse clinical events during cemented long-stem femoral arthroplasty. *Clin Orthop Relat Res.* 2002;395:154−163.

60. Krishnan CK, Kim HS, Yun JY, et al. Factors associated with local recurrence after surgery for bone metastasis to the extremities. *J Surg Oncol.* 2018;117(4):797−804.

61. Saravana-Bawan S, David E, Sahgal A, et al. Palliation of bone metastases-exploring options beyond radiotherapy. *Ann Palliat Med.* 2019;8(2):168−177.

62. Laredo JD, Chiras J, Kemel S, et al. Vertebroplasty and interventional radiology procedures for bone metastases. *Joint Bone Spine.* 2018;85(2):191−199.

63. Kurup AN, Callstrom MR. Ablation of skeletal metastases: current status. *J Vasc Intervent Radiol.* 2010;21(8 Suppl): S242−S250.

64. Raj VS, Lofton L. Rehabilitation and treatment of spinal cord tumors. *J Spinal Cord Med.* 2013;36(1):4−11.

65. Moulding HD, Elder JB, Lis E, et al. Local disease control after decompressive surgery and adjuvant high-dose single-fraction radiosurgery for spine metastases. *J Neurosurg Spine.* 2010;13(1):87−93.

66. Laufer I, Iorgulescu JB, Chapman T, et al. Local disease control for spinal metastases following "separation surgery" and adjuvant hypofractionated or high-dose single-fraction stereotactic radiosurgery: outcome analysis in 186 patients. *J Neurosurg Spine.* 2013;18(3):207−214.

67. Bilsky MH, Laufer I, Matros E, Yamada J, Rusch VW. Advanced lung cancer - aggressive surgical therapy vertebral body involvement. *Thorac Surg Clin.* 2014;24(4): 423−431.

68. Yu HH, Hoffe SE. Beyond the conventional role of external-beam radiation therapy for skeletal metastases: new technologies and stereotactic directions. *Cancer Contr.* 2012;19(2):129−136.

69. Agarwal JP. The role of external beam radiotherapy in the management of bone metastases. *Clin Oncol.* 2006;18: 747−760.

70. Nguyen QN, Chun SG, Chow E, et al. Single-fraction stereotactic vs conventional multifraction radiotherapy for pain relief in patients with predominantly nonspine bone metastases: a randomized phase 2 trial. *JAMA Oncol.* 2019;5(6):872−878.

71. Spencer KL, van der Velden JM, Wong E, et al. Systematic review of the role of stereotactic radiotherapy for bone metastases. *J Natl Cancer Inst.* 2019;111(10):1023−1032.

72. Rades D, Veninga T, Stalpers LJ, et al. Outcome after radiotherapy alone for metastatic spinal cord compression in patients with oligometastases. *J Clin Oncol.* 2007;25(1): 50−56.

73. Ryu S, Rock J, Jain R, et al. Radiosurgical decompression of metastatic epidural compression. *Cancer.* 2010;116(9): 2250−2257.

74. Yamada Y, Cox BW, Zelefsky, et al. An analysis of prognostic factors for local control of malignant spine tumors treated with spine radiosurgery. *J Rad Oncol.* 2011;82(2): S132−S133.

75. Mauch PM. Treatment of metastatic cancer of bone. In: *Cancer Principles and Practice Onology.* Lippincott co. Phil.; 2018.

76. Perez ca, Brady LW. *Principals and Practices of Radiation Oncology.* Lipincott. Phil.; 1987:650−683.

77. Hammack JE. Spinal cord disease in patients with cancer. *Continuum.* 2012;18(2):312−327.

78. Goldwein JW. Radiation myelopathy: a review. *Med Pediatr Oncol.* 1987;15(2):89−95.

79. Glare PA, Davies PS, Finlay E, et al. Pain in cancer survivors. *J Clin Oncol.* 2014;32:1739−1747.

80. *WHO Guidelines for the Pharmacological and Radiotherapeutic Management of Cancer Pain in Adults and Adolescents.* Geneva: World Health Organization; 2018, 1: Introduction.

81. Rossi A, Gridelli C, Ricciardi S, de Marinis F. Bone metastases and non-small cell lung cancer: from bisphosphonates to targeted therapy. *Curr Med Chem.* 2012;19(32): 5524−5535.

82. Hatoum HT, Lin SJ, Guo A, et al. Zoledronic acid therapy impacts risk and frequency of skeletal complications and follow-up duration in prostate cancer patients with bone metastasis. *Curr Med Res Opin.* 2011;27(1):55−62.

83. Hendriks LE, Hermans BC, van den Beuken-van Everdingen MH. Effect of bisphosphonates, denosumab, and radioisotopes on bone pain and quality of life in patients with non-small cell lung cancer and bone metastases: a systematic review. *J Thorac Oncol.* 2016;11:155−173.

84. Gerszten PC, Germanwala A, Burton SA, et al. Combination kyphoplasty and spinal radiosurgery: a new treatment paradigm for pathological fractures. *J Neurosurg Spine.* 2005;3(4):296−301.

85. Spratt DE, Beeler WH, de Moraes FY, et al. An integrated multidisciplinary algorithm for the management of spinal metastases: an International Spine Oncology Consortium report. *Lancet Oncol.* 2017;18:e720−e730.

86. Sun JM, Ahn JS, Lee S, et al. Predictors of skeletal-related events in non-small cell lung cancer patients with bone metastases. *Lung Cancer.* 2011;71:89−93.

87. Guo Y, Ngo-Huang AT, Fu JB. Perspectives on spinal precautions in patients who have cancer and spinal metastasis. *Phys Ther.* 2020;100(3):554−563.

88. Singh Chhabra H, ed. *ISCoS Textbook on Comprehensive Management of Spinal Cord Injuries.* 1st ed. New Delhi: Wolters Kluwer; 2015.

89. Consortium for Spinal Cord Medicine Clinical Practice Guidelines. Pressure ulcer prevention and treatment following spinal cord injury: a clinical practice guideline for health-care professionals. *J Spinal Cord Med.* 2001; 24(Suppl 1):S40−S101.

90. Kirshblum S, O'Dell MW, Ho C, et al. Rehabilitation of persons with central nervous system tumors. *Cancer.* 2001;92:1029−1038.

91. Galvão DA, Taaffe DR, Spry N, et al. Exercise preserves physical function in prostate cancer patients with bone metastases. *Med Sci Sports Exerc.* 2018;50(3):393−399.

92. Crevenna R, Kainberger F, Wiltschke C, et al. Cancer rehabilitation - current trends and practices within an Austrian University Hospital Center. *Disabil Rehabil.* 2020;42(1): 2−7.

93. Bunting RW, Shea B. Bone metastasis and rehabilitation. *Cancer.* 2001;92(4 Suppl):1020−1028.

94. Fichtenbaum J, Kirshblum S, Ruppert L, et al. Prognosis disclosure in spinal cord injury. *PM R.* 2017;9:76−82.

CHAPTER 5

Lung Cancer in the Palliative Care Setting: Successes, Challenges, and Opportunities for Collaboration

SULEYKI MEDINA, MD • EILEEN R. SLAVIN, DO, MPH

INTRODUCTION

The World Health Organization (WHO) defines Palliative Care as "an approach that improves the quality of life of patients and their families facing the problem associated with life-threatening illness, through the prevention and relief of suffering by means of early identification and impeccable assessment and treatment of pain and other problems, physical, psychosocial, and spiritual."[1]

Palliative Medicine provides additional support for the relief of pain, nonpain symptoms, and stress associated with serious illness. These services can be delivered by primary care physicians or oncologists (Primary Palliative Care) or by specialized Palliative Medicine teams. Specialty Palliative Care teams are comprised of palliative care–certified physicians, nurses, social workers, chaplains, and individuals from other disciplines who work together with a patient's primary team in an integrated fashion to deliver comprehensive care.

Palliative Medicine clinicians specialize in pain management (cancer-related pain) and nonpain symptom management (i.e., management of chemotherapy-induced peripheral neuropathy, nausea, vomiting, diarrhea, appetite disturbances, constipation, fatigue, insomnia, and mood disorders). The Palliative Medicine team also provides psychosocial and spiritual support to patients, families, and caregivers. The team collaborates with social workers and chaplains to provide counseling, education, respite, and bereavement care.

Palliative Medicine specialists also elicit patients' illness understanding and prognostic awareness. Patients' end-of-life preferences are carefully elicited and documented in the electronic medical record through the process of Advance Care Planning. Near the end-of-life, Palliative Care teams facilitate and support patients' and their families' decision to enroll in hospice care, and can ease the transition from receiving aggressive treatment to focusing solely on comfort.

These specialists also work hand-in-hand with the other specialties—medical oncology, radiation oncology, surgical oncology, physical medicine, and rehabilitation—not only to understand the patient's illness, goals, and overall prognosis; but to provide optimal symptom control and relief of suffering.

Palliative Care delivered early on in the course of a serious illness (ex. cancer) can improve patients' symptoms, satisfaction with care, and quality of life (QOL). Other benefits of early palliative care (EPC) interventions include increased patient and family level of understanding of what to expect as disease progresses and death approaches; relief of pain and other symptoms; increased family and caregiver support; decreased crises and health care utilization (i.e., 911 calls, emergency department visits, and hospitalizations); improved QOL; and sometimes survival (possibly due to decreased toxicity from tumor directed therapies).

Palliative care is often categorized as synonymous to hospice, and although the field of Palliative Care did evolve from the modern hospice movement, there are distinguishing factors among the two. While hospice is a "palliative care only" approach, palliative care begins at the time of diagnosis of a serious illness and can be delivered alongside curative or life prolonging therapies. In order to receive hospice in the United States, a patient must have a certified prognosis of less than 6 months if the illness runs its natural course. In addition, once enrolled in hospice, a patient agrees to forfeit insurance coverage for their "hospice-qualifying diagnosis." Finally, while receiving hospice care, a patient must forego "curative" or life prolonging

Lung Cancer Rehabilitation, https://doi.org/10.1016/B978-0-323-83404-9.00009-8

therapies, whereas palliative care services are appropriately delivered concurrently with all appropriate disease modifying treatments (ex. chemotherapy). Most importantly, palliative care is provided based on patient and family needs (independent of prognosis). It is also appropriate at any stage of serious illness from disease onset to bereavement for families.

Both palliative care and hospice care are underutilized in the United States. According to the Center to Advance Palliative Care, as of 2017, only 48% of Medicare deaths are preceded by hospice care. Among enrollees, 54% receive hospice care for less than 30 days, and 28% receive hospice care for a week or less.

Palliative care has become an integral part of the care of cancer patients. In the case of lung cancer patients, it is now recognized that integrative models of palliative care and oncology care in the management of advanced lung cancer patients can improve QOL and even survival when incorporated early on in the disease trajectory.

There are many palliative care needs in the advanced lung cancer population. Common symptoms reported by these patients include pain, dyspnea, cough, fatigue, depression, and anxiety.[2] Patients with lung cancer have also been found to have higher levels of psychological distress compared with other cancers.[2] In turn, higher levels of emotional and psychological distress are associated with increased symptom burden.[2] The goals of palliative care are to improve QOL, which is diminished by both disease related factors and toxicities from disease modifying therapies. Palliative care interventions aim to improve QOL by ensuring the provision of impeccable symptom management and psychosocial support.

LUNG CANCER EPIDEMIOLOGY

In 2018, lung cancer occurred in approximately 2.1 million patients worldwide and caused an estimated 1.8 million deaths worldwide.[3] It remains the leading cause of cancer-related death in adults. In the United States, lung cancer occurs in about 234,000 patients and causes over 154,000 deaths annually.[4] In the United States and other industrialized nations, it is primarily caused by exposure to tobacco products (ex. cigarette smoke). In other parts of the word, air pollution and cigarette smoke are likely the causative agents.

In the United States, nonsmall cell lung cancer (NSCLC) accounts for the majority (85%) of the cases, with the remainder as mostly small cell lung cancer (SCLC). For the majority of patients, the diagnosis is made late at stages (III and IV at presentation), where survival is poor, with an overall 5 year survival of 9.5%−16%.[5]

Treatment and long-term outcomes of lung cancer depend on the extent of disease at presentation, a patient's overall health status, as well as a patient's performance status. Most cases remain incurable. Treatment modalities include surgery, chemotherapy, radiation therapy, as well as targeted therapy and immunotherapy. Palliative care can be provided to patients with serious illness and their caregivers, regardless of the intent of their treatments: supportive/palliative (aimed at improving QOL only) or with curative intent.[2] For these reasons, the role of Palliative Care in the management of these patients has gained importance in recent years.

INTEGRATED INTERDISCIPLINARY PALLIATIVE CARE ALONGSIDE STANDARD ONCOLOGIC CARE IN THE MANAGEMENT OF NONSMALL CELL LUNG CANCER PATIENTS

Palliative care supports the best possible QOL for patients with serious and complex illnesses (such as lung cancer) by optimizing assessment and screening early on and incorporating symptom management strategies when most needed.

Given the threats to QOL presented by this illness, the effects of Palliative Care delivery in the lung cancer population have been the focus of significant research efforts.[2] It is well established that early integration of Palliative Care in standard oncologic care improves QOL, depression, anxiety, and satisfaction with care. There are several studies supporting the role of Palliative Care in the medical management of lung cancer patients.[2]

The ENABLE trial utilized four weekly educational sessions in Palliative Care, followed by monthly telephone follow ups, demonstrating an improvement in QOL for patients with advanced cancer.[2] In the ENABLE II trial, patients with advanced cancer received early subspecialty Palliative Care consultations along with monthly follow-up interventions. This study also showed improvement in overall survival, and improvement in caregiver depression scores and stress burden.[2] A landmark study by Temel et al. randomized 151 patients with advanced NSCLC to receive early Palliative Care (EPC) plus standard oncology care or standard oncology care (SOC) alone. EPC was associated with improved QOL, fewer depressive symptoms, less aggressive end-of-life care, and longer lengths of stay on hospice compared to standard oncology care alone. In addition, median overall survival in the EPC group was 11.6 months compared to 8.9 months in the standard oncology care arm $(P = .02)$.[6] A trial led by Bakitas et al. of 322 pts, including 117 advanced lung cancer patients, randomized to usual oncologic care or usual care plus an advanced practice nurse led palliative care intervention showed improvement in QOL and mood.[6] Zimmerman et al. led a randomized control trial of newly diagnosed advanced cancer patients with an estimated prognosis of 6—24 months at a single tertiary center. The study evaluated consultation with follow up with Palliative Care team versus standard of care, found improved QOL at the end-of-life, and improved satisfaction with care. In a retrospective analysis of a large cohort of patients diagnosed with advanced lung cancer, an improved survival was noted if a Palliative Care visit occurred between 31 and 365 days after diagnosis.[2] The study also showed reduced likelihood of death in an acute care setting.

The American Society of Clinical Oncology (ASCO) recommends that patients (and their caregivers) receiving treatment for advanced lung cancer receive palliative care services within 8 weeks of diagnosis. However, referral patterns will likely depend on the availability of these services, given a shortage in the Palliative Care workforce. It is not unreasonable to refer lung cancer patients to Palliative Care when needs arise (ex. patient is experiencing pain and/or other debilitating symptoms). For patients with minimal symptoms and access to tumor-directed therapies, a Palliative Care referral can be reserved until worsening of symptoms or disease progression. Additional criteria guiding Palliative Care referrals include a life expectancy of less than 1 year and poor performance status (ECOG score of 3 or higher).

Several conceptual models for the integration and delivery of Palliative Care exist. They have been conceptualized by Hui et al. as follows[2]:

1. The onco-centric or solo practice model—oncologists manage all patient symptoms and provide oncologic care
2. The congress model—oncologists refer patients to specialists who focus on symptom control
3. The integrated care model—oncologists make early referrals to specialty Palliative Care, and supportive care is provided by both the oncology and the palliative care teams in tandem.

The integrated model likely offers more support to oncology providers (and patients alike), as well as more comprehensive care to each patient than the congress model, which relies upon multiple subspecialty consultations.[2]

Despite the benefits of the integrated Palliative Care model, opinions guided by personal biases and misconceptions regarding the role of Palliative Care (from both providers' and patients' perspectives) have led to delay of Palliative Care referrals to the advanced lung cancer population. In addition, the challenges of a limited Palliative Care task force have diminished the access to Palliative Care services for every patient who has advanced cancer. A potential solution to this problem may lie in introducing the concept of Primary Palliative Care in efforts to deliver comprehensive care to this patient population.

One strategy to enhance the delivery of Primary Palliative Care includes incorporating dedicated education on Palliative Care within oncology training. Because increasing the Palliative Care task force can take decades of investment from governments and health care systems, coming up with new and innovative ways of improving Primary Palliative Care and its intersection with Specialty Palliative Care will also become essential.[2] Distress screening and patient-reported outcomes (PROs) can potentially bridge the gap of integrating oncologic care and palliative care.

Distress screening, which has been mandated by the National Comprehensive Cancer Network (NCCN) since 1997, can provide an opportunity to bridge the gap between oncologic care and palliative care. Distress is defined by the NCCN as "a multifactorial unpleasant experience of psychological (i.e., cognitive, behavioral, and emotional), social, spiritual, and/or physical nature that may interfere with the ability to cope effectively with cancer, its physical symptoms, and its treatment."[2]

Patient-reported outcomes (PROs) have become an important outcome of interest in clinical practice. PROs provide information on the physical and mental health of a patient from a patient's perspective, as opposed to a clinician's report. "Basch et al. found that integrating PROs into the routine care of patients with advanced cancer led to a statistically significant improvement in overall survival in a single tertiary care center." Patients randomized to PRO intervention had longer overall survival and were also able to tolerate continuation of chemotherapy for longer periods of time, compared to control patients. The study outcomes suggested that the use of PROs may have allowed providers to identify and manage treatment-related adverse effects more effectively and timely.[2]

Systematic reviews have also shown that PROs help improve patient and provider communication, and increase patient satisfaction. Another trial with Stage IIA—IV lung cancer patients receiving web-based monitoring of PROs reported significantly increased overall survival. PROs can also potentially guide the appropriate timing of referrals to Palliative Care as they are used to monitor symptom burden.[2] Given that currently recognized unmet needs in the advanced lung cancer population have not been fully addressed by present models of integrating palliative care and oncologic care, it is possible that PROs may provide an opportunity to integrate these two specialties, thereby improving cancer care and symptom management in this population.

ASSESSMENT OF PATIENTS—THE PALLIATIVE CARE APPROACH

A comprehensive assessment using a multidimensional approach is essential to the management of cancer patients with advanced lung cancer. Uncontrolled symptoms, including pain, fatigue, and dyspnea among others, often result in worsening well-being, psychological symptoms, and ultimately worsening QOL for patients and their families. Symptom assessment tools are widely available in the field of Palliative Care to ensure timely screening and diagnosis of symptoms, resulting in their timely management. The palliative care domains important to assess are physical symptoms, performance status; psychological/psychiatric symptoms; and social and economic needs of the patient, family, caregiver; religious, spiritual, and existential issues.[7]

Validated tools such as the NCCN Distress Thermometer are effective in screening for untreated distress in the physical, social, or psychological domains. Patients can rate distress from 0 to 10 and designate particular areas of concern which may merit a palliative care consultation.[8]

The Edmonton Symptom Assessment Scale (ESAS) and the Memorial Symptom Assessment Scale (MSAS) are reliable, validated tools used to assess physical symptoms in the clinical setting. The ESAS assesses 10 common symptoms (pain, fatigue, nausea, depression, anxiety, drowsiness, shortness of breath, appetite, feeling of well-being, and other symptoms) over the past 24 hrs.[7] Symptom assessment by means of these tools can be administered at subsequent clinic visits, can guide treatment decisions, and assess QOL. Performance status tools used in Palliative Care include the Eastern Cooperative Oncology Group (ECOG) and the Palliative Performance Scale (PPS), among others. The ECOG Performance Status has been validated in patients with cancer and correlate with survival. For example, an ECOG score of greater than three is associated with survival of 3 months or less.[8]

Tools to assess psychological, psychiatric, and cognitive domains include ESAS (Edmonton Symptom Assessment Scale), MDAS (Memorial Delirium Assessment Scale), and the PHQ-9 (Patient Health Questionnaire). The FICA (faith, importance, community, action) is a validated tool to assess the spiritual domain.[7] The CAGE Alcohol Questionnaire (Cut, Annoyed, Guilty, and Eye) is used regularly in the assessment of chemical coping.

ROLE OF TELEMEDICINE IN PALLIATIVE CARE

Telemedicine provides a virtual means to support face-to-face clinical care and can include video conferencing or digital information (imaging, reports, and other resources) that can be accessed on demand. Telemedicine can also include patient education and self-care resources.[9] Studies have shown improved patient and health care provider satisfaction with telemedicine.[10] Several factors have contributed to the increase in telemedicine usage for health care delivery including a predicted shortage of oncologic providers, an aging population, and the absence of available services in rural areas. Telemedicine has other benefits too, including increased cost savings and the opportunity for interprofessional collaboration. Since health care providers do not have to travel to clinics or patient homes, there is more clinical time available for an increased number of encounters.[11]

Telemedicine has played an essential role in the delivery of health care services to oncology patients particularly when there is limited availability of medical care.[9] Patients with serious medical conditions are frequently faced with the decision to choose costly emergency medical services when their condition worsens.[11] Many outpatient clinics are also not able to accommodate patients after hours. Poor physical health and limited social support present additional obstacles to obtaining health care resources. Calton et al. 2020 conducted a telephone-based survey among a small number of palliative care patients from a quaternary urban medical center receiving telemedicine visits, half of whom were cancer patients, and their caregivers. The results of the survey were very positive, with nearly all patients reporting that they would have another telemedicine visit if it was offered to them.[12] The patients reported ease of use of the telemedicine services as 97% and 100% of caregivers "felt comfortable discussing sensitive topics by telemedicine."

Studies have demonstrated that telemedicine communication provides an equivalent level of care to in-person medical services in specialties other than Palliative Care.[10] Telephone-based interventions have been successful at improving QOL and lowering depression symptoms in newly diagnosed lung cancer patients. The benefits also extend to the patients' family members as telemedicine appointments allow increased opportunities for engagement while reducing travel time to appointments. One study by Chua et al. 2019 is currently investigating the effectiveness of telemedicine to improve QOL outcomes, end-of-life preferences, and length of stay in hospice. The intervention will include a telehealth-based early Palliative Care (EPC) intervention study arm and an in-person intervention study arm in 20 major cancer centers throughout the United States. The hope is to determine the applicability of using telemedicine for advanced Palliative Care patients and enhancing the ability to reach communities with limited care access. Another multicenter trial which aims to study the effectiveness of early integrated telehealth Palliative Care compared to in-person Palliative Care in a cohort of patients with advanced NSCLC is currently ongoing.[13] This study will examine various aspects of palliative care including improvement of QOL and mood symptoms, communication about end-of-life care preferences, and patient/caregiver satisfaction with telehealth. These patients will be followed at 3-month time increments after being randomized to either the monthly in-person palliative care visits or telehealth monthly visits.

Current events have also necessitated the use of telemedicine to augment the direct communication which is essential to Palliative Care services.[14] The COVID-19 pandemic has made in-person communication difficult due to restrictions surrounding in-person visitation. Palliative care has changed drastically to accommodate for the intimate nature of end-of-life care. Telemedicine has allowed patients to virtually address psychosocial issues, symptom management, goals of care, and bereavement to isolated patients and their family members. One interdisciplinary team at the VA Affairs healthcare system in Washington state developed a workgroup to implement quality improvement changes in a business model format with the intention of delivering health care services without minimizing human contact. They developed a formal operating procedure to teach communication strategies, technology modalities, and end-of-life care to stakeholders throughout the health care system.

Many studies are ongoing in the field of telemedicine including randomized controlled trials and pilot programs that are expanding access to care in rural areas.[13] More data will aid health care providers on the effectiveness of telemedicine and Palliative Care delivery, as the need for this service continues to grow. This research will also benefit the lung cancer population.[10]

PHYSICAL SYMPTOM MANAGEMENT
Pain Management
Pain is defined as "an unpleasant sensory and emotional experience associated with actual or potential tissue injury or damage. The intensity of pain varies with the degree of injury, disease, or emotional impact".[15] Pain is one of the main symptoms experienced by cancer patients during both curative and palliative therapy. Numerous national and international surveys have found that 30%–50% of cancer patients in active therapy and as many as 60%–90% with advanced disease have pain.[7] Although pain management and the alleviation of suffering are core clinical competencies for all clinicians treating seriously ill patients, in reality pain is frequently undertreated. There are many barriers to pain management, which include physician's limited knowledge, decreased availability of opioid medications, governmental regulations, physicians' fear of regulations, diversion of medications, and fear of addiction.[7]

In 2016, the American Society of Clinical Oncology (ASCO) issued a statement reflecting that cancer patients should be largely exempt from measures taken to halt the epidemic of opioid abuse and addiction, on the grounds that cancer patients are a "special population." Their statement also reflected that cancer patients should be exempt from regulations that limit their access to appropriate medical opioid therapy given the unique nature of cancer, its treatment, and potentially the lifelong adverse health effects from having had cancer. ASCO also recognized the need to balance public health concerns regarding abuse and misuse of prescription opioids with the need to ensure access to appropriate pain management to cancer patients and survivors. Emphasis should be placed on safe opioid prescribing principles including appropriate utilization, storage, and disposal of prescription pain medications. Regularly consulting your state's prescription monitoring program, which enables clinicians to access patients' controlled substance prescription history, was also highly recommended.[16]

Pain syndromes are generally divided into two categories: acute versus chronic/persistent. Pain that occurs in the acute setting is mainly related to cancer therapeutic interventions. Chronic or persistent pain is subdivided into nociceptive (*somatic* vs. *visceral*) and neuropathic. *Nociceptive* pain is associated with ongoing tissue damage. *Somatic* pain occurs as a result of activation of cutaneous and deep tissue receptors and it is roughly described as sharp, well localized, throbbing, and gnawing. *Visceral* pain results when distention, stretching, and inflammation activate nociceptors. It is described as dull, poorly localized, cramping, or pressure. Neuropathic pain is described as tingling, shooting, stabbing, burning, electric like, and numb, and results from damage to nerves.[7] Persistent pain continues beyond the expected time of healing, or for at least 3–6 months. The etiology is usually multifactorial.

Breakthrough pain is common in cancer patients and is defined by Yennuranjalingam and Bruera as a "transitory exacerbation of pain that occurs on a background of otherwise stable persistent pain." Breakthrough pain may be caused by activity or end-of-dose failure (a situation in which a patient experiences pain before their medication therapeutic time is expected to end); it can also occur spontaneously.[7]

The intensity of pain should be measured on a 0 (no pain) to 10 (extreme severe pain) scale, and this intensity should be quantified over time to identify any underlying patterns and to assess treatment efficacy. Mild levels of pain (less than 4/10) are not disabling and allow a more normal function and engagement. Moderate pain levels of 4/10 to 6/10 on a 10-points scale tend to interfere with normal function and sleep, while severe pain levels of 7/10 to 10/10 significantly affect the patient's ability to perform instrumental activities of daily living (IADLs). Alternatives for self-reporting of pain include thermometers and face scales. The scale should be personalized to the appropriate individual. For patients with moderate to severe cognitive impairment, direct observational scales such as the Pain Assessment in Advanced Dementia Scale are very helpful. It is important to remember that psychological, social, spiritual, and financial problems can affect a patient's perception and tolerance of pain.[17]

Opioids are the basis for the management of cancer-related pain as they are the most effective and fastest acting analgesics to target this condition. The treatment of cancer-related pain should also involve a multidimensional approach that includes the optimization of non-opioid analgesics, non-pharmacologic treatments, and the expertise of specialists when necessary.[7]

There are no strict rules to follow when choosing between strong opioids (i.e., morphine, hydromorphone, methadone, fentanyl) to treat cancer-related pain. Generic morphine is a reasonable initial choice because of its efficacy, relatively low cost, familiarity by physicians, wide availability, and variety of formulations.

Initial choice of opioid therapy should also be guided by patient factors such as the presence of renal and hepatic dysfunction and older age.[17] Cancer pain management will be discussed in another chapter.

DYSPNEA

For patients with cancer, "breathlessness" or "dyspnea" is cited as the "most distressing symptom."[18] Dyspnea can occur in many forms but is essentially described as a discomfort associated with breathing and can occur even despite optimal medical and respiratory interventions. Dyspnea has a significant impact on QOL and is a poor prognostic indicator. The prevalence of breathlessness in cancer patients has been estimated to be between "20% and 70%." Due to the subjective nature of breathlessness, this symptom is often underestimated or overlooked. Physiological data including pulmonary function tests and vital signs do not necessarily correlate with the severity of breathlessness.

There are self-reported measurements such as the Numerical Rating Scale (NRS) and the modified Medical Research Council Breathlessness Scale that help clinicians measure breathlessness quality and its functional impact.[18] These tools can help estimate how breathlessness impacts social, psychological, financial, and spiritual aspects of a patient's life. Frequency, timing, and severity of episodes also need to be taken into consideration during evaluations.

Breathlessness can be treated in pharmacologic and nonpharmacologic ways.[18] Regardless of the treatment approach, the best way to treat breathlessness is to treat the underlying cause. Breathlessness can be attributed to cancer progression, complications from treatment, and/or from preexisting medical conditions such as Congestive Heart Failure (CHF) or Chronic Obsptructive Pulmonary Disease (COPD). Nonpharmacologic strategies to treat breathlessness include using a handheld fan, breathing retraining, and mobility aids. Using a handheld fan is a cost-effective, portable, and easy way for patients to obtain symptomatic relief. Patients are also not stigmatized by using a handheld fan. Some studies have shown a statistically significant improvement in breathlessness; however, some authors have called for larger studies with more diverse patient populations to further elucidate the effectiveness of using a handheld fan. Patients can also benefit from breath retraining. Patients can learn techniques to help them gain control over their breathing and combat altered breathing patterns such as accessory muscle use, apical breathing, and dynamic hyperinflation (defined as "when a breath is initiated prior to complete exhalation of the previous breath" and is a contributor to dyspnea in COPD).[19] Lastly, there is evidence in randomized crossover studies that patients with COPD who use a rollator "improve self-paced walking distance" in "both indoor and outdoor environments."

Pharmacologic therapies to relieve breathlessness typically include opioids or benzodiazepines. Opioids have been studied at length to relieve breathlessness. Though the mechanism of opioids in alleviating breathlessness is not completely understood, it is thought to be mainly related to depressing respiratory drive.[20,21] Clinically opioids may have some effectiveness in improving breathlessness though the overall evidence is lacking. For opioid naïve patients, one multicenter parallel group randomized controlled trial found that neither sustained release Oxycodone (20 mg/day) nor extended-release Oxycodone (5 mg every 8 h) provided immediate relief of breathlessness symptoms as compared to placebo over a 7-day period.[18] In some smaller crossover trials, opioid-tolerant patients receiving doses of immediate release morphine higher than their 4 h scheduled doses for pain management did not experience relief of breathlessness. Another small study found evidence in favor of greater symptom management for fentanyl buccal tablets as compared to morphine sulfate. One Cochrane review cited small sample sizes and the variability in outcome measures as a reason for limited analysis.[20] Benzodiazepines have also been examined in other Cochrane reviews, with varying starting doses and dosing strategies. One such review examined 8 diverse randomized controlled trials with 214 participants and did not find evidence for a beneficial effect on breathlessness for advanced cancer patients and for patients with advanced COPD.[22]

Other pharmacologic options for improving breathlessness have been explored. Corticosteroids have been used in some randomized controlled trials to examine their efficacy for relieving breathlessness. The evidence is present though inconclusive and larger trials are currently underway. Supplemental oxygen has not been shown to affect breathlessness in cancer patients in the palliative care setting. Lastly, since breathlessness can be tied to anxiety and depression, some studies have examined the effect of antidepressants on improving breathlessness. Sertraline was used in one large randomized controlled trial with no proven benefit.

Other effective strategies to treat breathlessness include a combination of pharmacologic and nonpharmacologic interventions. The Breathlessness Intervention Service is a complex and comprehensive plan to support patients with advanced cancers who experience breathlessness.[23] The team consists of Palliative Care trained medical personnel, occupational therapists, and physiotherapists who support the patient via in-person visits at their home and via telehealth. These experts provide counseling including safe and appropriate personalized exercise programs, positioning to reduce work of breathing, and emergency planning. A small Phase III single blind mixed method randomized controlled trial of 67 patients with advanced cancer who were randomized to receive Breathlessness Intervention Service versus the standard of care treatment after a 2-week period found a statistically significant reduction NRS scores. This study included 16 patients with lung cancer randomly assigned to the intervention group. The American Thoracic Society and European Respiratory Society have both noted the benefits of a pulmonary rehabilitation program for patients with lung cancer.[24] Since patients with cancer are often deconditioned due to their illness, appropriate exercise training can improve well-being and strength.[11,24] Lower limb training can specifically target quadriceps strength, enabling an improvement in balance, walking ability, and participation in ADLs therefore reducing breathlessness. Inspiratory muscle training can help with breathlessness but should be individually prescribed.

Additionally, complementary medicine interventions have been used in lung cancer patients experiencing breathlessness. Cannabinoids have not been studied in patients with lung cancer in the palliative care setting and have only been studied for use in COPD and in healthy volunteers to date. Acupuncture has been used for treatment of cancer-related symptoms. Acupuncture is thought to cause symptom relief due to endogenous opioid release. A pilot study by Bauml et al. 2016 enrolled 12 patients for a trial of acupuncture sessions delivered over a 10-week period with a primary endpoint of measuring changes in dyspnea severity.[25] Mean dyspnea scores as measured by the NRS were lessened in a statistically significant manner. Although the small sample size and lack of a control group limits interpretation of results, further work should explore the usefulness of acupuncture as a therapeutic tool. Additional research and multimodal approaches to manage breathlessness are needed to determine the best methods to reduce dyspnea in lung cancer patients in the the Palliative Care setting.

COUGH

Lung cancer patients have reported up to 27 different symptoms throughout the course of their illness.[26]

Lung cancer—related cough specifically has been identified by some researchers as an "unmet clinical need."[27] Clinicians frequently underestimate the impact that cough has on a patient's activities of daily living. Cough can impact a patient's social interactions, psychological health, and causes increased levels of anxiety. Cough severity and frequency is associated with poor QOL in lung cancer patients and is closely related to breathlessness and fatigue.[28] It is difficult to determine the exact prevalence of cough among lung cancer patients due to the multifactorial nature of cough.[27] Chronic cough can be caused by comorbidities, such as gastroesophageal reflux disease or asthma. It can also be a side effect of treatment for a cooccurring condition as is seen in patients with hypertension taking ACE inhibitors.[11] Acute cough can be caused by treatment for lung cancer as well as by cooccurring infection. Seven large studies, identified by Harle et al. 2012, identified a prevalence rate of cough that varied between 24.9% and 84% for patients at the time of their cancer diagnosis.[29]

There are several factors that must be taken into consideration when assessing patients for cough.[29] Cough is an unintended side effect of many lung cancer treatments including external beam radiotherapy and chemoradiotherapy. Increasing cancer survivorship has also meant that patients have more chronic symptomology. In general, cough is difficult to treat. Several cough assessment tools exist which examine both the severity and impact of cough on a patient's daily life. Severity includes frequency, intensity, and disruptiveness. Clinicians can use the Visual Analog Scale as a quick way to identify severity. Other available scales include the Leicester Cough Questionnaire and the Cough Specific Quality of Life Questionnaire. The Cough Severity Diary is another tool which measures disruptiveness, frequency, and severity specifically. This tool was found to be reliable, reproducible, and valid.

Previous studies have shown that patients undergoing surgery for lung cancer have worsening QOL scores.[26] In some cases, QOL scores return to normal within 3—6 months after surgery. At 4 months, postop cough was rated to be one of the most severe symptoms. Oksholm et al. looked at symptom variation and severity over time in patients undergoing surgery for lung cancer and found that cough severity initially improved at 1 month and then worsened at months 4 and 5 postoperatively. Patients who received adjuvant chemotherapy were 3.34 times more likely to report a higher severity rating for cough. The authors reported that cough has multiple etiologies which can vary over the course of a patient's illness.

There are several treatment strategies that can be used for cough.[29] Basic recommendations include benzonatate (100—200 mg po three times daily) for a mild cough that does not improve with breathing exercises, education, and counseling.[11] For a moderate to severe cough, a centrally acting opioid is recommended such as morphine 5 mg po every 4 hours and hydrocodone 10 mg po daily as an alternative to morphine. Molassiotis et al. 2010 have proposed a stepwise approach to treating cough. Their proposed ladder recommends the use of simple linctus/glycerol as a primary strategy. Treatment then escalates to the use of a steroid trial, opioids, local anesthetics, and experimental therapies. Improving cough is contingent upon adequate cancer treatment and proper management of comorbidities such as COPD and CHF. Smoking cessation is yet another way to augment available treatment strategies for cough. There are also nonpharmacological strategies which address psychological components of cough.[30] These evidence-based approaches include mindfulness and cognitive behavioral therapy.

FATIGUE

Fatigue is a common symptom reported by lung cancer patients and frequently coexists with other lung cancer related symptoms.[31] For cancer patients, fatigue can affect all stages of disease and can occur even during treatment.[32] Fatigue can take the form of tiredness, exhaustion, lack of energy, and an "inability to function." The NCCN defines fatigue as "a distressing, persistent, subjective sense of tiredness or exhaustion related to cancer or cancer treatment that is not proportional to recent activity and interferes with usual functioning." Several studies have demonstrated that cancer patients have lower QOL due to fatigue. Fatigue also affects psychosocial well-being. Patients may depend on others for assistance, which causes disruptions in the activities of daily living of caregivers and family members.

Cancer-related fatigue is subjective. Therefore, as many as 24 different definitions have been identified.[32] Not all definitions include an analysis of the functional impact of fatigue. A meta-analysis conducted by Al Maqbali et al. 2021 found that approximately 49% of cancer patients experience fatigue. The prevalence ranges from 11% to 99% in the literature which can be attributed to different cancer types and treatments, varying comorbidities, and the lack of homogeneity in an acceptable definition and measurement of fatigue. This meta-analysis found that female gender has a significant association with fatigue. There is also an association between fatigue and anxiety, depression, and other physical symptoms.

Cancer treatments also contribute to fatigue symptomology.[33] One study by Wang et al. found that among 64 patients receiving chemoradiation for curative treatment of NSCLC with Stage III unresectable disease, 25% had preexisting fatigue rated as a 5 on a 0—10 scale. This figure reached 40% of patients studied during chemoradiation treatment. Additionally, the patients rated fatigue as the most severe symptom that they experienced; a number that did not change even 5—6 weeks after completion of treatment. In this study, fatigue also had the highest predictive value for interference with daily activities.

Anemia, cytokine release, and cancer-associate cachexia contribute the patient's cancer-related fatigue.[34] Treating these abnormal physiologic processes associated with cancer may improve symptoms of fatigue.[11] Proinflammatory cytokines, and proteolysis-inducing factor, specifically produced by cytokines, affect the rate of muscle breakdown and lower muscle protein synthesis in cachexia.[34] Anemia is multifactorial in the palliative care patient, yet its role in fatigue may be overdiagnosed in this population.[11] There are no studies to date examining anemia in relation to advanced palliative cancer populations. Pain also plays a role in fatigue. Patients with uncontrolled pain may experience psychological distress and sleeping difficulties, thereby exacerbating fatigue.

A variety of pharmacologic and non-pharmacologic therapies are available to improve fatigue in lung cancer patients.[11] Some guidelines recommend the use of central nervous system stimulants to improve cancer-related fatigue.[35] In the literature, results are mixed. In a study of 298 patients with NSCLC not receiving chemoradiation in the 4 weeks prior to the start of the study randomized to receive modafinil 100 mg by mouth for 14 days and 200 mg by mouth for the remaining 14 days, versus a matched placebo, found no evidence that modafinil improved fatigue symptoms. Recent research by Wang et al. suggests that the anti-inflammatory properties of the tetracycline, minocycline, at a dose of 100 mg by mouth twice a day, may improve cancer-related fatigue in patients undergoing chemoradiation treatment for NSCLC.[36] Methylphenidate has been used historically for cancer-related fatigue, and a Cochrane systematic review from 2015 mentions a "superior effect" when compared to placebo.[37] A large meta-analysis conducted by Mustian et al. examined 113 studies using interventions from four major domains to treat cancer-related fatigue: exercise, psychological, and combined exercise and psychological. Their outcome was severity of cancer-related fatigue and their study population included over 11,000 patients with cancer. Though the effectiveness of treatment was based on many factors relating to the patients' cancer diagnosis and treatment, exercise and psychological interventions were superior to pharmaceutical interventions.

Physical activity can improve cancer-related fatigue although studies have demonstrated mixed results. Though evidence is limited, some observational studies have reported improved QOL and reduced all-cause mortality from cancer with physical activity interventions. Dhillon et al. 2017 randomized 112 Stage III/IV lung cancer patients to either an 8-week exercise intervention or usual care to examine if physical activity improved fatigue or QOL.[31] Results showed that while adherence to physical activity was high there were no significant differences in QOL and fatigue scores for those receiving the intervention. A meta-analysis of 16 studies by Nadler et al. 2019 found that among patients with metastatic cancer, improvement in QOL and fatigue scores were only seen in a small subset of patients.[38] There were no adverse safety events explicitly reported in all studies. More research is needed regarding the usefulness of physical activity interventions in lung cancer patients.

Several alternative therapies have been considered to improve cancer-related fatigue. One group in Italy has proposed the use of ozone therapy to alleviate symptoms of fatigue.[39] Research suggests that ozone derived from medical grade oxygen has therapeutic effects including "antioxidative responses," altering oxygenation in resting muscles, and can be used for hypoxemia. Tirelli et al. 2018 found that in a small number of lung cancer patients being treated in a palliative setting, over half reported relief of their fatigue symptoms on a Fatigue Severity Scale.

CACHEXIA

Cancer cachexia has a strong association with lung cancer.[40] Cachexia is a disorder that is characterized by a "loss of body weight with specific losses of skeletal muscle and adipose tissue." It is not related to malnutrition or starvation. There are several factors which contribute to cachexia which are driven by tumor-related changes and reduced oral intake. There is no unified definition for cancer-associated cachexia; however, a key feature appears to be a loss of skeletal muscle mass. Rates of cachexia among cancer patients are high in the palliative care setting which may be due to the advanced stage of disease. Other factors contributing to cachexia include gender, increased age, genetic risk factors, and catabolic effects from cancer treatment. Cancer-associated anorexia is a clinically different syndrome, although due its frequent co-occurrence with cachexia, there has been a combined definition recognized as the "anorexia—cachexia syndrome."[41] Anorexia is specifically the "loss of appetite or desire to eat." It is a contributor to decreased caloric intake and protein—calorie malnutrition.

No specific diagnostic criteria exist for cancer-associated cachexia.[40] Weight loss is usually one of the first clinical signs with a 5% weight loss being a "threshold of major risk of poor clinical outcome." Poor dietary intake plays a role in the development of cachexia. Records of dietary intake and measures of resting energy expenditure can help identify patients who are at risk. There are also laboratory markers which help identify patients at greater risk which include albumin, transthyretin, and CRP.

Controlling cachexia involves managing symptoms related to cachexia.[40] Optimal approaches suggested in the literature include a multimodal approach which is uniquely tailored to the individual.[42] Cachexia has not only physical effects, but also functional and psychological components. Patients will benefit from the assistance of an interdisciplinary team of oncologists, palliative care and rehabilitation physicians, psychologists, and nutritionists to treat the symptoms of cachexia. Early mobilization under care of a physiatrist can slow the breakdown of skeletal muscle which in turn helps reduce loss of physical functioning from cachexia. In patients with advanced cancer, a randomized controlled trial consisting of an 8-week exercise program versus usual care has been shown to improve physical performance.[43]

Adequate nutrition is the foundational treatment of cachexia.[40] Oral nutritional supplements are first-line therapy to provide micronutrient and macronutrient support. Identifying nutritional impact symptoms, such as nausea, pain, sore mouth, constipation, and diarrhea, is helpful to recognize at-risk patients and provide appropriate medical interventions and education regarding healthy eating.[42,44] These symptoms can exacerbate the effects of cachexia because they interfere with a patient's oral intake and absorption of nutrients. Appetite stimulants can also provide additional support to increase a patient's appetite. There are several other drug therapies which have demonstrated varied effects on outcomes such as lean muscle mass and bodyweight. Further research needs to be done to establish efficacy of these newer drug therapies.

DEPRESSION

Psychological distress is a significant cause of suffering among patients with advanced cancer and is highly associated with decreased QOL. Major depression has a point prevalence of 10%—20% in cancer patients, irrespective of cancer stage (11). Differentiating the causes of normative distress associated with illness from other psychiatric disorders is essential to the implementation of appropriate treatment plans and to prevent any further threats to patients' physical, psychological, social, and spiritual well-being.[17]

Depression is a significant distressing emotional experience for patients and their families. In the context of a serious illness such as cancer, it can be amplified by physical symptoms, fear of dying, family distress, and as death approaches.[17] It also decreases patient's ability to feel pleasure and connectedness.[8] Depression is also associated with decreased adherence to medical treatments, prolonged hospital stays, and reduced QOL. It is also an independent risk factor for suicide and requests for hastened death. Depression has been increasingly recognized to affect survival in several cancers. Symptoms of depression have been reported in up to 58% of patients with cancer. Rates of major depression range as high as 38% among these patients.[8] There are numerous risk factors for depression in cancer. The most important cancer-related factors include advanced stage of disease, poor performance status, and poor pain control.

Clinical depression is associated with feelings of hopelessness, helplessness, worthlessness, and guilt. Numerous symptom scales have been used to assess depression symptoms. A few commonly used instruments include the Hospital and Anxiety Depression Scale (HADS); the Beck Depression Inventory, Short Form (BDI-SF); and the Geriatric Depression Scale (GDS). In the cancer setting, there are multiple barriers to the assessment of depression in these patients, most notably time constraints and stigma concerning mental illness or weakness perceived by patients and families. Simple 1- or 2-item screening techniques are increasingly being used as they simplify the starting point in symptom assessment. Akizuki et al. described a 1-item survey initially tested in 275 patients and found it to correlate well with the Hospital Anxiety and Depression Scale (HADS) (r = 0.66) and the Distress Thermometer (r = 0.71).

Because many of the symptoms of severe illness overlap with symptoms of depression (fatigue, anorexia, sleep disturbance, poor concentration, social withdrawal, hopelessness), consultation with an experienced psychiatrist ± psychologist may be helpful in complex situations.

The need to medically treat depression depends on its intensity, persistence, and disruption of basic life functioning. Treatment should be considered when these effects dominate other emotions and interfere with the ability to enjoy other aspects of life. Assessment and treatment of adjustment disorders, depression, and anxiety are discussed elsewhere in this book.

SPIRITUAL AND EXISTENTIAL DISTRESS

A life-threatening illness, in particular a cancer diagnosis, brings about emotional, psychological, cognitive, physical, and spiritual well-being concerns.[45] Patients can experience existential distress at every stage of their disease through palliation to the end-of-life. Because lung cancer has a poor prognosis, there is an essential need for clinical focus on end-of-life interventions. Due to increased patient care loads and the fact that some health care providers have their own death-related anxiety; this can be a challenging task. In addition, patients who feel alone in their suffering often experience alienation and regret, and a higher level of existential distress. This can also possibly contribute to suicidal ideation. Those patients who overcome existential demands can use the end-of-life period as a time of psychological growth and to deepen bonds between their loved ones.

Despite some advances in treatment therapies of late-stage lung cancer, there is little known about how to prolong life or drastically improve patients' QOL.[46] The literature suggests therefore that QOL and other topics relating to palliative care should be initially discussed when developing a plan of care at diagnosis. One such topic affecting QOL is depression. Depression and depressive symptoms are associated with a cancer diagnosis and in terminal illness. Poorer QOL is tied to depressive symptoms particularly in patients who have functional decline, uncontrolled pain, and other severe symptoms. Patients with life-threatening illnesses have reported that social, emotional, and existential topics are just as important as receiving treatment for symptoms such as pain. Some research has examined the role that spiritual well-being plays in QOL.[47] Lee 2021 identified that symptom clusters such as appetite loss, dyspnea, pain, and fatigue mediate the relationship between spiritual well-being and QOL for patients undergoing treatment for NSCLC. This presents an opportunity for caregivers to focus not only on spiritual concerns but also on controlling distressing physical symptoms in order to improve QOL.

There is a great need to address the spiritual aspect of care in those with advanced cancers though it is difficult to define and assess spiritual needs.[48,49] Approximately "86%–91%" of patients with advanced cancer report needing some level of spiritual support. Due to the close association between symptom management and existential distress, it is of particular interest to define "trajectories of social, psychological, and spiritual well-being" to develop health care interventions. One qualitative study by Murray et al. noted increasing isolation from family and friends due to not only the stigma of a cancer diagnosis, but also physical limitations that changed relationship dynamics. The authors noted that patients experienced increased psychological distress at four specific time points: the time of diagnosis, treatment cessation, disease progression, and the terminal stages of illness. Spiritual needs varied for patients depending on their faith background. Some patients found comfort in the "transition" and others experienced a "questioning of self-worth." There is an increasing need for multidisciplinary approaches to assist patients in all aspects of care because palliation plays an inevitable role in a lung cancer diagnosis.

Spiritual care is also very significant for caregivers of NSCLC patients since these individuals are involved in their loved one's day-to-day symptom management and provide psychological support.[50] Unfortunately, caregivers report high levels of "distress, fatigue, and sleep disturbances." There is an interdependence of care outcomes, as a sick or distressed caregiver may not be able to properly provide for a loved one, thereby increasing their levels of psychosocial distress. Examining various aspects of spirituality and mindfulness among lung cancer patients and their caregivers is an emerging area of research.

FAMILY AND CAREGIVER SUPPORT/ CAREGIVER BURNOUT

There has been a shift toward early integration of Palliative Care for patients with advanced cancers, as first demonstrated by Temel et al. 2010.[51] This work showed that among patients diagnosed with metastatic NSCLC who received EPC services, there was an improvement in QOL and reduced symptom burden. Caregivers and family members may also reap the benefits of EPC interventions. One meta-analysis examined the effectiveness of EPC on improving outcomes for lung cancer patients and their caregivers. They found that the caregivers' total distress and depression were reduced; however, there were no changes observed in anxiety levels or QOL. This trend continued at both 3- and 6-months before the death of the cancer patient. Another positive effect of EPC for patients with lung cancer is increased social support.[52] Palliative care physicians provide support to patients via counseling and symptom management, which complement their oncologic care. This added layer of support also decreases caregiver burden which, in turn, may improve patient's well-being.

Family and caregiver support is a crucial element of the patient's cancer experience.[53] One small study in Greece found a negative correlation with pain and anxiety in relation to having a sense of family support in a cohort of 101 lung cancer patients. This evidence underscores the importance of family support in improving QOL for patients. Some studies note a high level of depression, anxiety, irritability, guilt, and anger among caregivers of cancer patients.[54] This also extends to poorer social functioning and spiritual well-being. The interdependent nature of the caregiver and patient relationship provides an opportunity for intervention. In one study which examined 190 lung cancer patients and their caregivers at various stages on the cancer continuum, semistructured interviews were conducted to determine the extent of depressive symptomatology and the quality of the family environment. Spousal caregivers were found to have higher depressive symptoms. This group found a relationship between a patient's rating of "low cohesiveness," "low expressiveness," and "higher conflict" of the family dynamic being associated with higher levels of depression in the caregiver. The importance of family communication is also relevant in a Palliative Care setting.[55] Family meetings are frequently employed to improve collaboration and communication between palliative care patients and their families, and can assist with goals of care and symptom management.

Despite research examining caregiver psychological distress during a patient's illness, there is a paucity of data regarding the experiences of bereaved caregivers.[56] Some studies have reported high levels of depression and anxiety for up to 2 years after a patient's death. Since caregivers provide end-of-life care for patients with advanced cancers, it is reasonable to assert that they experience their own substantial distress. One study found that 30% and 43% of caregivers reported depression and anxiety respectively during bereavement. There was also an association between depression and anxiety experienced by caregivers and the physical and psychological distress that patients endure at the end of life. This study underscores the importance of providing support to caregivers to potentially enhance their "self-efficacy" and lower their "psychological distress."

ADVANCE CARE PLANNING

Understanding patients' goals in the context of their cancer diagnosis enhances the clinician's ability to align the care that is delivered to patients with what is most important to them. Frequent discussions about patients' goals, values, and what matters to them also promote good decision-making, patient-centered care, and earlier end-of-life planning.[57] These high quality discussions are often missing in the process of completing an advance directive (AD), which is a document a patient completes while still in possession of decisional capacity, and reflects how treatment decisions should be made on her or his behalf in the event she or he loses the capacity to make such decisions".[57] Different types of ADs are used in clinical practice today. These include health care power of attorney or durable power of attorney for health care, which only allows designation of a surrogate/proxy decision maker, excluding specific details about wishes for care; living wills, FIVE Wishes, Physician Orders for Life Sustaining Treatment, which comprises physician orders regarding cardiopulmonary resuscitation and other medical interventions including antibiotics and artificial nutrition and hydration. Out of hospital DNR (do not resuscitate) forms prevent unwanted resuscitations of terminally ill patients living at home or in a hospice facility.[8]

The advance care planning (ACP) process extends beyond completing an AD because it stresses ongoing conversations among patients, their families, caregivers, and health care providers. It reflects on the exploration of goals, values, beliefs, illness understanding, medical care/treatment options, and plans for the future. It also promotes the documentation of these conversations in the electronic medical record. Ideally, these conversations are integrated into routine care and are often revisited/ongoing throughout the disease trajectory or natural course of the illness. They should also be held during important transition points such as prior to embarking on a potentially life-threatening or risky treatment or procedure (i.e., a new chemotherapy regimen, high-risk surgery) and in the presence of evidence-based indicators for limited life expectancy (i.e., cancer patient progressing on all antitumor regimens). A patient's primary care physician or a specialist such as an oncologist who has been following a patient longitudinally for their cancer treatment is the most appropriate person to initiate ACP discussions. ACP discussions are associated with higher satisfaction with medical care, as well as lower risks of stress, anxiety, and depression. ACP is also associated with better patient outcomes.

END OF LIFE

Despite significant progress in the development of cancer therapeutics, in most cases, lung cancer remains incurable and progressive. Due to its inherently poor prognosis, it is essential that oncologists, as well as every health care professional caring for lung cancer patients, become familiar with the needs of these patients as they are facing the end of life.

The National Council of Palliative Care in the United Kingdom defines end-of-life care as care that helps patients facing progressive, incurable illness live as well as they can, until they die. End-of-life care is also defined as care that enables palliative care needs of both patients and families to be identified and met; care that includes management of pain and nonpain symptom management; and care that addresses psychological, social, and spiritual concerns.[5]

Presently there is no consensus on the timeframe for end of life. In the United Kingdom, the General Medical Council (GMC) guidance refers to patients approaching the end-of-life when they are likely to die within the next 12 months. Alternatively, in the United States, Medicare defines the need for hospice care at the end-of- life as the last 6 months of life.[5]

Excellent end-of-life care entails that health care professionals respect the dignity of patients and their families, and that patients' wishes be respected. It also entails that the care received by patients is consistent with their choices or values and that their right to refuse treatments be respected. Finally, it is essential that patients are provided access to Palliative Care and Hospice Services.

Despite increased access to hospice and palliative care services, there are presently significant barriers to the provision of quality end-of-life care. The most significant barrier is lack of meaningful communication among patients and medical oncologists. Oncologists presently engage in limited conversations with their patients regarding prognosis, expectations as disease progresses, and end-of-life preparation.[5] Studies have shown that less than one third of oncologists have end-of-life discussions with their patients.[5] Unfortunately, the literature also shows that failure to engage in these discussions is associated with an increase use of chemotherapy and ICU care in the last month of life.[5] The perceived duty from health care professionals to preserve life at all costs has also been identified as a barrier. Furthermore, advances in medical technology and life prolonging interventions make it inherently difficult to find the right balance between quantity of life and QOL. Fears and doubts about using sedative medications that may potentially hasten death; discomfort with decision-making in regards to withholding and withdrawing life-sustaining treatments (cardiopulmonary resuscitation, ventilator support, artificial nutrition, and hydration); and fear of medico legal action against physicians are also barriers to end-of-life care.

Apart from engaging in excellent communication and dialogue with patients and their families, recognizing when death is near can facilitate the mobilization of services required to deliver compassionate end-of-life care. There are significant events that precede death, often by several months. These events may include increased occurrence of infections, more frequent hospitalizations, less time between hospital trips, and multisystem complications.[58] At this stage, patients may also withdraw from loved ones and the public and may show decreased interest in socialization. Weeks prior to death, one can expect patients to sleep more.[58] Patients may also experience shortness of breath, increased confusion, and develop decreased tolerance to food.[58] More medications (increased doses and/or frequency of medication doses) may be required to ease symptom burden. Days prior to death patients may experience labored breathing, fevers, restlessness, and decreased food and fluid intake.[58] In the final hours of life, a patient's skin becomes mottled, perspiration increases, breathing changes occur, and awareness decreases.[58] The signs and symptoms of imminent death include terminal secretions (death rattle), mandibular breathing, cyanosed extremities, and pulselessness.[59]

As patients reach the final stages of their illness, opportunities may arise for patients to engage in reflection, life review, priorities, and goal setting. Examples of important priorities reported by patients as their lives come to an end include[60]:

1. Receiving adequate symptom management
2. Achieving spiritual peace
3. Having their affairs in order
4. Strengthening relationships with loved ones
5. Finding meaning and a sense of purpose in their lives
6. Bringing closure to personal affairs
7. Reviewing beliefs, values, and hopes

As patients reach the final stages as life, it is important that clinicians help patients and families balance a sense of hope while discussing end-of-life preparation. It is also important that clinicians focus on what can be done for patients, as opposed to what is not possible. It is also recommended that hope be reframed from hope for a cure, to hope for more time, and from hope for symptom relief, to hope for a comfortable and dignified death. Patients should be assured that if hospice care is desired, that the hospice team will demonstrate a caring attitude, will guide them and their families in the transition to the end of life, and will help them achieve their goals to provide closure as life comes to an end.

TRANSITION TO HOSPICE

Transition to hospice, or shifting care from an aggressive approach to a comfort-based approach, is appropriate when a patient's cancer has progressed despite multiple lines of treatments or when treatments are no longer desired or accomplishing patients' goals. It is also appropriate when profound decline in performance status precludes patients from receiving any more disease-directed therapies. Hospice may also be appropriate for patients who are looking to focus on QOL, rather than quantity of life.

Prognostic indicators such as performance status, form important inclusion criteria for hospice admission. For example, patients spending >50% of their time sitting or lying down have an estimated prognosis of 3 months or less, and are thus eligible for hospice.[61] Survival time also tends to decrease as additional physical symptoms develop. An ECOG score of 2–3 and a PPS score of 70% or less are generally supportive of hospice eligibility as well.[61] Patients scoring 70% or lower on the PPS are unable to carry on normal activity or perform normal work.[61] They are unable to move or ambulate and may spend more than 50% of their time in a bed or a chair. They may also exhibit significant evidence of disease, have reduced nutritional intake, and are likely able to perform only limited self-care.[61] Generally, patients are eligible for hospice if their disease presents with metastasis at diagnosis. They are also eligible if they experience progression of disease from an earlier stage of disease to metastatic disease. Progressive decline in spite of the best disease directed treatments or patients' refusal to continue disease directed therapies also support hospice eligibility.[61]

The Medicare Hospice Benefit covers 100% of the cost of care related to the hospice eligible diagnosis. Medicaid coverage will vary by states. The hospice benefit includes four levels of care[61]:

1. Routine home care—homecare provided at patients' residences
2. Continuous home care—provides nursing care up to 24 hrs at the bedside when medically necessary to manage acute symptoms

3. Inpatient hospice care—provided in a free-standing inpatient unit or contract bed in a hospital or nursing facility, is provided to patients whose symptoms cannot be adequately managed at home.
4. Respite care—provides up to five consecutive days of respite to patients' caregivers.

Hospice covers all professional services, ancillary supplies, and equipment related to the patient's hospice diagnosis, level of care, and location.

CONCLUSION

Palliative Care is a philosophy of care that advocates for medical interventions that enhance the QOL of patients and families facing life-limiting illnesses through the prevention and relief of suffering. Palliative Care specialists have additional expertise in managing distressing physical and psychological symptoms (ex. pain, fatigue, anxiety, dyspnea, nausea, etc.); in building rapport and relationships with patients and caregivers; in breaking bad news and managing expectations; in exploring goals of care/treatment goals; and educating about illness and prognosis, among others. Specialty Palliative Care is delivered in an interdisciplinary fashion in collaboration with physicians, nurses, chaplains, pharmacists, social workers, and individuals of various disciplines who work alongside patients' primary managing team. The American Society of Clinical Oncology recommends integration of Palliative Care in standard oncologic care early on in the treatment of patients with metastatic cancer and or high symptom burden. There are multiple studies supporting the role of EPC in the medical management of lung cancer patients, given reported benefits in enhanced QOL and mood. In addition, patients receiving EPC are less likely to receive aggressive care at the end-of-life and can benefit from longer survival compared to patients who receive standard oncologic care alone. It is of high importance to continue to educate medical professionals caring for patients with advanced lung cancer, given the needs and challenges these patients face near the end of their lives. It is important to provide additional emotional, psychological, social, and spiritual support, as these patients often experience extraordinary suffering as a result of progressive disease, heavy symptom burden, and poor QOL. It is essential that advanced lung cancer patients have access to hospice care, whereby they and their families are more likely to receive more dignified and compassionate end-of-life care.

REFERENCES

1. www.who.int/cancer/palliative/definition/en.
2. Tan I, Ramchandran K. The role of palliative care in the management of patients with lung cancer. *Lung Cancer Manag.* 2020:LMT39. https://doi.org/10.2217/lmt-2020-0016.
3. Mannino DM. *Cigarette Smoking and Other Possible Risk Factors for Lung Cancer;* February 18, 2021. UpToDate https://www.uptodate.com/contents/cigarette-smoking-and-other-possible-risk-factors-for-lung-cancer.
4. Deffebach ME, Humphrey L. *Screening for Lung Cancer;* October 4, 2021. UpToDate https://www.uptodate.com/contents/screening-for-lung-cancer.
5. Lim RBL. End-of-life care in patients with advanced lung cancer. *Ther Adv Respir Dis.* 2016;10(5):455−467. https://doi.org/10.1177/1753465816660925.
6. King JD, Eickhoff J, Traynor A, Campbell TC. Integrated onco-palliative care associated with prolonged survival compared to standard care for patients with advanced lung cancer: a retrospective review. *J Pain Symptom Manag.* 2016;51(6):1027−1032. https://doi.org/10.1016/j.jpainsymman.2016.01.003.
7. Yennuranjalingam S, Bruera E. *Oxford American Handbook of Hospice and Palliative Medicine.* Oxford University Press; 2011.
8. Goldstein NE, Morrison RS. *Evidence-based Practice of Palliative Medicine.* Elsevier; 2013.
9. Chua IS, Zachariah F, Dale W, et al. Early integrated telehealth versus in-person palliative care for patients with advanced lung cancer: a study protocol. *J Palliat Med.* 2019;22(S1):S7−S19. https://doi.org/10.1089/jpm.2019.0210.
10. Sirintrapun SJ, Lopez AM. Telemedicine in cancer care. In: *ASCO Educational Book.* American Society of Clinical Oncology; 2018:540−545.
11. Grant H, Lustbader D. In: Bruera E, Higginson IJ, Von Gunten CF, Morita T, eds. *Textbook of Palliative Medicine and Supportive Care.* CRC Press; 2021.
12. Calton B, Shibley WP, Cohen E, et al. Patient and caregiver experience with outpatient palliative care telemedicine visits. *Palliat Med Rep.* 2020;1(1):339−346. https://doi.org/10.1089/pmr.2020.0075.
13. Watts KA, Malone E, Dionne-Odom JN, et al. Can you hear me now? Improving palliative care access through telehealth. *Res Nurs Health.* 2020;44:226−237. https://doi.org/10.1002/nur.22105.
14. Ritchey KC, Foy A, McArdel E, Gruenewald DA. Reinventing palliative care delivery in the era of COVID-19: how telemedicine can support end of life care. *Am J Hospice Palliat Med.* 2020;37(11):992−997. https://doi.org/10.1177/1049909120948235.
15. Bruera E, Dalal S. *The MD Anderson Supportive and Palliative Care Handbook.* 5th ed. USA: UT Printing & Media Services. The University of Texas Health Science Center at Houston; 2008.
16. Moryl N, Hadler R, Koranteng L. Pharmacologic pain management in the cancer patient. In: Stubblefield MD, ed. *Cancer Rehabilitation: Principles and Practice.* Springer Publishing; 2019:564−575.
17. Periyakoil V, Denney-Koelsch E, White & P, Zhuvosky D. *Primer of Palliative Care.* 7th ed. American Academy of Hospice and Palliative Medicine; 2019.
18. Hui D, Maddocks M, Johnson MJ, et al. Management of breathlessness in patients with cancer: EMSO clinical practice guidelines. *EMSO Open.* 2020;5:1−13. https://doi.org/10.1136/esmoopen-2020-001038.
19. Soffler MI, Hayes MM, Schwartzstein RM. Respiratory sensations in dynamic hyperinflation: physiological and clinical applications. *Respir Care.* 2017;62(9):1212−1223. https://doi.org/10.4187/respcare.05198.
20. Barnes H, McDonald J, Smallwood N, Manser R. Opioids for the palliation of refractory breathlessness in adults with advanced disease and terminal illness (review). *Cochrane Database Syst Rev.* 2016;3:1−103. https://doi.org/10.1002/14651858.CD01008.pub2.
21. Mahler DA. Opioids for refractory dyspnea. *Expet Rev Respir Med.* 2013;7(2):123−135. https://doi.org/10.1586/ers.13.5.
22. Simon ST, Higginson IJ, Booth S, Harding R, Weingartner V, Bausewein C. Benzodiazepines for the relief of breathlessness in advanced malignant and non-malignant diseases in adults (review). *Cochrane Database Syst Rev.* 2016;10:1−60. https://doi.org/10.1002/14651858.CD007354.pub.3.
23. Farquhar MC, Prevost AT, McCrone P, et al. Is a specialist breathlessness service more effective and cost-effective for patients with advanced cancer and their carers than standard care? Findings of a mixed-method randomized controlled trial. *BMC Med.* 2014;12(194):1−13. https://doi.org/10.1186/s12916-014-0194-2.
24. Spruit MA, Singh SJ, Garvey C, et al. An official American Thoracic Society/European Respiratory Society statement: key concepts and advancements in pulmonary rehabilitation. *Am J Respir Crit Care Med.* 2013;188(8):e13−e64. https://doi.org/10.1164/rccm.201309-1634ST.
25. Bauml J, Haas A, Simone CB, et al. Acupuncture for dyspnea in lung cancer: results of a feasibility trial. *Integr Cancer Ther.* 2016;15(3):326−332. https://doi.org/10.1177/1534735415624138.
26. Oksholm T, Rustoen T, Cooper B, et al. Trajectories of symptom occurrence and severity from before through five months after lung cancer surgery. *J Pain Symptom Manag.* 2015;49(6):995−1015. https://doi.org/10.1016/j.jpainsymman.2014.11.297.
27. Harle A, Molassiotis A, Buffin O, et al. A cross sectional study to determine the prevalence of cough and its impact in patients with lung cancer: a patient unmet need. *BMC Cancer.* 2020;20(9):1−8. https://doi.org/10.1186/s12885-019-6451-1.
28. Molassiotis A, Smith JA, Mazzone P, Blackhall F, Irwin RS. Symptomatic treatment of cough among adult patients with lung cancer: CHEST guideline and expert panel report. *Chest.* 2017;151(4):861−874. https://doi.org/10.1016/j.chest.2016.12.028.

29. Harle ASM, Blackhall F, Smith JA, Molassiotis A. Understanding cough and its management in lung cancer. *Curr Opin Support Palliat Care*. 2012;6(2):153−162. https://doi.org/10.1097/SPC.0b013e328352b6a5.

30. Booth S, Johnson MJ. Improving the quality of life of people with advanced respiratory disease and severe breathlessness. *Breathe*. 2019;15(3):198−215. https://doi.org/10.1183/20734735.0200-2019.

31. Dhillon HM, Bell ML, van der Ploeg HP, et al. Impact of physical activity on fatigue and quality of life in people with advanced lung cancer: a randomized controlled trial. *Ann Oncol*. 2017;28:1889−1897. https://doi.org/10.1093/annonc/mdx205.

32. Al Maqbali M, Al Sinani M, Al Naamani Z, Al Badi K, Tanash MI. Prevalence of fatigue in patients with cancer: a systematic review and meta-analysis. *J Pain Symptom Manag*. 2021;61(1). https://doi.org/10.1016/j.jpainsymman.2020.07.037, 167−189.e14.

33. Wang XS, Fairclough DL, Liao Z, et al. Longitudinal study of the relationship between chemoradiation therapy for non-small cell lung cancer and patient symptoms. *J Clin Oncol*. 2006;24(27):4485−4491. https://doi.org/10.1200/JCO.2006.07.1126.

34. Stewart GD, Skipworth RJE, Fearon KCH. Cancer cachexia and fatigue. *Clin Med*. 2006;6(2):140−143. https://doi.org/10.7861/clinmedicine.6-2-140.

35. Spathis A, Fife K, Blackhall F, et al. Modafinil for the treatment of fatigue in lung cancer: results of a placebo-controlled, double-blind, randomized trial. *J Clin Oncol*. 2014;32(18):1882−1888. https://doi.org/10.1200/JCO.2013.54.4346.

36. Wang XS, Qiuling S, Mendoza T, et al. Minocycline reduces chemoradiation-related symptom burden in patients with non-small cell lung cancer: a phase II randomized trial. *Int J Radiat Oncol Biol Phys*. 2020;106(1):100−107. https://doi.org/10.1016/j.ijrobp.2019.10.010.

37. Mücke M, Mochamat M, Cuhls H, et al. Pharmacologic treatments for fatigue associated with palliative care. *Cochrane Database Syst Rev*. 2015;5:1−76. https://doi.org/10.1002/14651858.CD006788.pub3.

38. Nadler MB, Desnoyers A, Langelier DM, Amir E. The effect of exercise on quality of life, fatigue, physical function, and safety in advanced solid tumor cancers: a meta-analysis of randomized control trials. *J Pain Symptom Manag*. 2019;58(5). https://doi.org/10.1016/j.jpainsymman.2019.07.005, 899−908.e7.

39. Tirelli U, Cirrito C, Pavanello M, Del Pup L, Lleshi A, Berretta M. Oxygen-ozone therapy as support and palliative therapy in 50 cancer patients with fatigue − a short report. *Eur Rev Med Pharmacol Sci*. 2018;22:8030−8033.

40. Baracos VE, Martin L, Korc M, Guttridge DC, Fearon KCH. Cancer-associated cachexia. *Nat Rev Dis Prim*. 2018;4:1−18. https://doi.org/10.1038/nrdp.2017.105.

41. Del Ferraro C, Grant M, Koczywas M, Dorr-Uyemura LA. Management of anorexia-cachexia in late stage lung cancer patients. *J Hospice Palliat Nurs*. 2012;14(6):1−12. https://doi.org/10.1097/NJH.0b013e31825f3470.

42. Maddocks M, Hopkinson J, Conibear J, Reeves A, Shaw C, Fearon KCH. Practical multimodal care for cancer cachexia. *Curr Opin Support Palliat Care*. 2016;10:298−305. https://doi.org/10.1097/SPC.0000000000000241.

43. Oldervoll LM, Loge JH, Lydersen S, et al. Physical exercise for cancer patients with advanced disease: a randomized controlled trial. *Oncologist*. 2011;16(11):1649−1657. https://doi.org/10.1634/theoncologist.2011-0133.

44. Jain R, Coss C, Whooley P, Phelps M, Owen DH. The role of malnutrition and muscle wasting in advanced lung cancer. *Curr Oncol Rep*. 2020;22:53−63. https://doi.org/10.1007/s11912-020-00916-9.

45. Lehto RH. The challenge of existential issues in acute care: nursing considerations for the patient with a new diagnosis of lung cancer. *Clin J Oncol Nurs*. 2012;16(1):E4−E11. https://doi.org/10.1188/12.CJON.E1-E8.

46. Adorno G, Wallace C. Preparation for the end of life and life completion during late-stage lung cancer: an exploratory analysis. *Palliat Support Care*. 2017;15:554−564. https://doi.org/10.1017/S1478951516001012.

47. Lee MK. Interactions of spiritual well-being, symptoms, and quality of life in patients undergoing treatment for non-small cell lung cancer: a cross sectional study. *Semin Oncol Nurs*. 2021;37:1−7. https://doi.org/10.1016/j.soncn.2021.151139.

48. Sun V, Kim JY, Irish TL, et al. Palliative care and spiritual well-being in lung cancer patients and family caregivers. *Psycho Oncol*. 2016;25(12):1448−1455. https://doi.org/10.1002/pon.3987.

49. Murray SA, Kendall M, Grant E, Boyd K, Barclay S, Sheikh A. Patterns of social, psychological and spiritual decline toward the end of life in lung cancer and heart failure. *J Pain Symptom Manag*. 2007;34(4):393−402. https://doi.org/10.1016/j.jpainsymman.2006.12.009.

50. Cho D, Kim S, Durrani S, Liao Z, Milbury Z. Associations between spirituality, mindfulness, and psychological symptoms among advanced lung cancer patients and their spousal caregivers. *J Pain Symptom Manag*. 2021;61(5). https://doi.org/10.1016/j.jpainsymman.2020.10.001, 898−908.e1.

51. Kochovska S, Ferreira DH, Luckett T, Phillips JL, Currow DC. Earlier multidisciplinary palliative care intervention for people with lung cancer: a systematic review and meta-analysis. *Transl Lung Cancer Res*. 2020;4:1699−1709. https://doi.org/10.21037/tlcr.2019.12.18.

52. Irwin KE, Greer JA, Khatib J, Temel JS, Pirl WF. Early palliative care and metastatic non-small cell lung cancer: potential mechanisms of prolonged survival. *Chron Respir Dis*. 2012;10(1):35−47. https://doi.org/10.1177/1479972312471549.

53. Lekka D, Pachi A, Zafeiropoulos G, et al. Pain and anxiety versus sense of family support in lung cancer patients. *Pain Res Treat*. 2014:1−7. https://doi.org/10.1155/2014/312941.

54. Siminoff LA, Wilson-Genderson M, Baker S. Depressive symptoms in lung cancer patients and their family

caregivers and the influence of the family environment. *Pscyhooncology.* 2010;19(12):1285–1293. https://doi.org/10.1002/pon.1696.

55. Forbat L, Cert PG, Francois K, O'Callaghan K, Kulikowski K. Family meetings in inpatient specialist palliative care: a mechanism to convey empathy. *J Pain Symptom Manag.* 2018;55(5):1253–1259. https://doi.org/10.1016/j.jpainsymman.2018.01.020.

56. El-Jawahri A, Greer JA, Park ER, et al. Psychological distress in bereaved caregivers of patients with lung cancer. *J Pain Symptom Manag.* 2021;61(3):488–494. https://doi.org/10.1016/j.jpainsymman.2020.08.028.

57. Silveira MJ. *Advance Care Planning and Advance Directives;* October 12, 2021. UpToDate https://www.uptodate.com/contents/advance-care-planning-and-advance-directives.

58. Kramlinger M. Making the most of the time we have left: caring for a loved one at life's end. VITAS Healthcare.

59. Morita T, Ichiki T, Tsunoda J, Inoue S, Chihara S. A prospective study on the dying process in terminally ill cancer patients. *Am J Hosp Palliat Care.* 1998;15:217–222. https://doi.org/10.1177/104990919801500407.

60. Irwin SA, Fairman N, Hirst JM, Siegel JD, Montross-Thomas L. *Essential Practices in Hospice and Palliative Medicine: UNIPAC 2: Psychiatric, Psychological, and Spiritual Care.* 5th ed. American Academy of Hospice and Palliative Medicine; 2017.

61. VITAS Healthcare. *Hospice Eligibility Guidelines for End-Stage Cancer Patients;* (n.d.). https://www.vitas.com/for-healthcare-professionals/hospice-and-palliative-care-eligibility-guidelines/hospice-eligibility-guidelines/oncology.

FURTHER READING

1. Mustian K, Alfano CM, Heckler C, et al. Comparison of pharmaceutical, psychological, and exercise treatments for cancer related fatigue a meta-analysis. *JAMA Oncol.* 2017;3(7):961–968. https://doi.org/10.1001/jamaoncol.2016.6914.

CHAPTER 6

Psychosocial Distress and Anxiety in Lung Cancer

LYNN KIM, OTD, OTR/L • VANESSA MONIQUE YANEZ, MSOT, OTR/L •
VINITA KHANNA, LCSW, MPH, ACHP-SW, OSW-C • SHERRY HITE, MOT, OTR/L

BACKGROUND

In the last decade, there has been a growing awareness of the importance of psychosocial screening and intervention as part of comprehensive cancer care. The negative effects of psychosocial distress and anxiety on health outcomes have been increasingly reported in the literature. Current research shows that survivors of lung cancer are at greater risk for psychosocial distress than other cancers. In order to standardize care across cancer centers, several regulatory bodies have published guidelines for screening, assessment, and management of psychosocial concerns with the provision of clinical pathways to guide clinical practice in efforts to standardize care across oncology centers and equip health care professionals with the tools necessary to implement these recommendations into everyday practice.

DEFINING DISTRESS AND ANXIETY

Cancer-related distress and anxiety span across a range of emotions and may fluctuate throughout an individual's disease course. Distress is defined as a subjective experience that can cause disturbances in an individual's quality of life and is defined as "a multifactorial unpleasant experience of a psychological, social, spiritual, and/or physical nature that may interfere with the ability to cope effectively with cancer, its physical symptoms, and its treatment." 1 Symptoms of anxiety, such as excessive worrying and fear, are often described as a normal and an adaptive reaction to cancer. When gone unchecked, these symptoms may develop into prolonged and intense worrying and fear, impacting daily functioning and may be classified as a psychological disorder.

DISTRESS AND ANXIETY IN THE LUNG CANCER POPULATION

Lung cancer accounts for nearly 25% of cancer deaths in women and men, more than breast, colon, and prostate combined.[2] People with lung cancer have been identified as having greater distress than other cancers, at rates as high as 43.5%,[3] due to most cases being diagnosed at advanced stages with increased physical and psychological symptom burden.[4] Increased psychological distress has also been correlated to lung cancer, suicidal ideation, hopelessness, low quality of life, and poor body image.[5]

The prevalence of lung cancer and the high likelihood of encountering these individuals during the rehabilitation process necessitate the pressing need for health care professionals to increase their awareness and knowledge of the signs and symptoms of distress and anxiety and include screening, assessment, and intervention into standard practice. To illustrate its critical importance within routine care, distress screening has been increasingly considered the "sixth vital sign," along with pain, temperature, pulse, respiration, and blood pressure.[6]

Routine assessment of psychosocial distress allows individuals and health care professionals to regularly communicate about sources of distress throughout the continuum of care, especially with survivors being more likely than ever to undergo treatments, such as chemotherapy, surgery, radiation, and immunotherapy, which may trigger distress and anxiety at various time points along their care continuum, including at diagnostic workup, active treatment, advanced stage and metastatic disease, and end-of-life. When unaddressed, distress can reduce the quality of life and impact cancer survivorship, with the potential for decreased compliance with therapies and exacerbation of symptom burden.[4]

Lung Cancer Rehabilitation. https://doi.org/10.1016/B978-0-323-83404-9.00019-0

PSYCHOSOCIAL NEEDS OF THE LUNG CANCER POPULATION

While certain triggers for distress and anxiety may be more common or generalizable to the larger oncology population, there are certain triggers specific to the lung cancer population which must be considered to provide the most holistic and individualized care possible.

Lung Cancer Stigma

A majority of individuals with lung cancer (95%) report feeling stigmatized by their disease, leading to shame, guilt, and fear of discrimination.[7,8] Research on lung cancer stigma has indicated associations between lung cancer stigma and internal self-blame, perceived self-infliction, impaired patient–clinician communication, limited engagement in prevention and early detection interventions, poor self-esteem, and mental maladjustment.[7,9,10] Furthermore, lung cancer stigma was a strong predictor in delayed medical help-seeking behavior after symptom onset, which is a critical issue in a diagnosis with such a high mortality rate and exponential disease growth.[10]

Impact on Treatment Adherence

Studies have shown that underlying distress or anxiety can inhibit progress and even impact treatment adherence. It has been suggested that adherence to screenings can be impacted by lack of awareness of screening benefits, screening fatigue, financial costs, and proximity to referral centers.[11] It is vital for the multidisciplinary team to further evaluate the possible underlying causes of noncompliance, such as health literacy levels, lack of understanding of the potential impact on quality of life, and psychosocial concerns. A full biopsychosocial assessment of a patient is warranted in order to capture a complete profile of an individual and aid in joint decision-making processes between the provider and the patient. Health care professionals should make efforts to identify predictors of intentional or unintentional nonadherence and sources of distress to ensure patient understanding of the necessity of such treatments. A study analyzing motivations for nonadherence to lung cancer screening in the military population found that a majority of patients were lost to follow-up due to communication difficulties, and recommendations were made to improve contact via multiple avenues.[11] This example of unintentional nonadherence due to perceived lack of follow-up demonstrates how improving efficiency and communication in our health care systems can lead to improved care for patients.

Advanced Lung Cancer and End of Life

Patients with advanced cancer have reported high levels of distress due to feelings of hopelessness, impaired emotional functioning, and body image distortions.[5] Furthermore, many individuals with end-stage lung cancer capitulate to their disease while also experiencing poor quality of life, despite the medical advancements in lung cancer care.[12] When addressing the goals of care for individuals with advanced lung cancer, providers must recognize when the focus of treatment should be aggressive life-sustaining measures versus symptom management and preparation of the patient and family for a progressive and inevitable decline.[12] Maintaining clear and honest lines of communication can help aid in joint decision-making in order to ensure that proper palliative care is provided to patients who are at very high risk for distress and severe psychological symptoms.

Immunotherapy and Targeted Therapy

Advancements in the treatment of lung cancer have resulted in populations with longer periods of disease control despite metastatic disease.[13] This emerging population of survivors living beyond their original prognoses faces a unique set of challenges, including persistent toxicities related to treatment, uncertainty surrounding prognosis, and scan-related anxiety.[13] Furthermore, individuals with long-term clinical trial participation have reported negative quality of life due to frequent surveillance and the need for regular hospital attendance.[13] A comprehensive qualitative study looking at the lived experiences of lung cancer patients on immunotherapy identified several themes among this cohort of survivors, some of which included the liminal experience of living in limbo as well as the lack of established and practical information on immunotherapies from providers.[14] Providers are encouraged to increase their awareness of the known impact of immunotherapy and target therapies in order to weigh the values of treatment as it relates to quality of life.[14]

Fear of Recurrence

Fear of recurrence (FCR) is a prevalent psychological burden that may manifest as a normal response to cancer to a pathological response. The potential ramifications of an availability of treatment options and increased survival rates include an increase in psychological burden over a prolonged period of time due to fear of disease recurrence. Long-term treatment and psychosocial care are warranted in order to ensure positive adjustment and improved quality of life during and after treatment. A systematic review analyzing factors affecting FCR across different cancer populations found strong associations between FCR and younger age, physical symptoms, and poor mental health—related quality of life.[15] The direct impact of distress on FCR still needs to be studied in the literature. However, maintaining honest and open lines of communication and providing adequate follow-up care must be implemented to help patients navigate potential challenges with symptom management and the trajectory of treatment.

Caregiver Distress

Caregivers play a pivotal role in the promotion of symptom management and provision of psychosocial support for individuals with lung cancer. In addition to providing instrumental care and support, caregivers are often tasked with clinical responsibilities, including postsurgical drain management, administration of medication, and assistance with activities of daily living. However, the psychosocial needs of the caregiver may often be overlooked, as care for the patient is prioritized. It is important to consider that caregiver burden and distress can be affected more by the patient's quality of life than the stage of the cancer.[16] Many caregivers of patients with lung cancer have reported significant distress due to the uncertainty of their role as a caregiver and how to manage an uncertain future.[17]

Caregiver burden and distress can increase over time as disability increases with progressive disease or intensified symptom burden. In order to ensure that the needs of caregivers are met as they progress with the patient along the continuum of care, all members of the interdisciplinary team are recommended to provide caregiver support and actively engage caregivers at all levels of care in order to train and equip them with the skills needed to care for their loved ones effectively. Health care professionals may establish welcoming atmospheres for caregivers to encourage open communication to discuss special needs and identify areas for more support.

SCREENING FOR DISTRESS

Screening as Preventive Medicine

The goal of preventive medicine, as defined by the American Board of Medical Specialties, is to promote health and well-being and prevent disease, disability, and death.[18] Screening should be viewed as a powerful preventive tool in health care in order to increase awareness of the prevalence of distress while identifying methods to reduce distress. The National Comprehensive Cancer Network (NCCN), the Institute of Medicine,

and the American Society of Clinical Oncology (ASCO) have made recommendations for the inclusion of screening, assessment, follow-up, and treatment of psychosocial distress as a quality care standard in routine cancer care. The U.S. Preventive Services Task Force recommends screening patients in clinical practices that have systems in place to ensure precise diagnosis, efficient treatment, and follow-up care.

The unique dynamic of lung cancer and the stigma associated with lung cancer symptoms and diagnosis necessitates the need to integrate early and regular screening of psychosocial distress and anxiety into routine care regardless of practice setting, size and type of institution, or patient prognosis. Screening for distress at or near the time of diagnosis and rescreening throughout the treatment continuum may provide increased opportunities to address the consequences of psychosocial concerns and improve quality of life. By preventing and reducing distress and anxiety, health care professionals can take positive steps toward reducing the "human cost of cancer" by addressing not only medical, but also psychosocial, psychiatric, financial, emotional, and spiritual concerns.[19]

Oncology Stakeholders and Standards for Distress Screening

American College of Surgeons Commission on Cancer

The American College of Surgeons (ACOS) Commission on Cancer (COC) is a consortium of professional organizations that publish requirements for accreditation of cancer clinics and establish standards to support high-quality, comprehensive cancer care. The COC publication, *Optimal Resources for Cancer Care: 2020 Standards*, provides accreditation requirements for psychosocial distress screening, such as the availability of psychosocial services on-site or by referral and the requirement to report findings of psychosocial distress screenings to the institution's cancer committee.[20]

The COC provides a list of requirements to support the policies and procedures of implementing a comprehensive psychosocial distress screening in cancer programs, to measure compliance with accreditation standards, and to guide the identification of the psychological, social, financial, and behavioral issues which may affect the patient's treatment plan and outcomes.[20] Cancer programs are recommended to carefully assess their program's size, resources, location, and patient population in order to determine the feasibility of implementing these standards.[20]

The COC requires at least one distress screening during the first course of treatment, with additional screenings to be administered at the discretion of the health care provider.[20] The mode of administration must be determined by the site, and adequate training must be provided to medical staff responsible for administering and interpreting the screening results. The use of standardized and validated instruments or tools is recommended. If moderate or severe distress is identified, it is crucial to follow-up via direct contact in order to confirm screening results and identify appropriate follow-up care and referrals.[20]

The National Comprehensive Cancer Network

The NCCN's Guidelines for Distress Management provides an overview of the evidence in support of early and regular distress screening, as well as a comprehensive consensus of evidence-based screening and treatment methods.[1] The NCCN's Distress Management Panel established Standards of Care for Distress Management with principles for implementing these standards in line with the recommendations put forth by the American College of Surgeons Commission on Cancer (NCCN) (Fig. 6.1).

Quality Oncology Practice Initiative

Another effort to improve the standard of cancer care is the ASCO's Quality Oncology Practice Initiative.[21] This quality assessment program was launched in 2002 and includes measures that have been developed by a team of oncologists and quality experts with the goal of providing a standard methodology for practice, evaluating oncology practices, and fostering improvement in the management of physical and psychological issues within outpatient oncology settings. The International Association for the Study of Lung Cancer track is also available within the QOPI-related Measures and is available to all international practices with abstraction for nonsmall cell lung cancer (NSCLC) and small cell lung cancer.

The QOPI Certification Program Standards require documentation of initial psychosocial assessment in the medical record and subsequent action. Psychosocial documentation may include a distress and anxiety screening, patient self-report of distress or anxiety, or medical record documentation regarding patient coping, adjustment, depression, distress, anxiety,

---

NCCN Standards of Care for Distress Management

- Distress should be recognized, monitored, documented and treated promptly at all stages of the disease and in all settings.
- Screening should identify the level and nature of the distress.
- Ideally, patients should be screened for distress at every medical visit as a hallmark of patient-centered care. At a minimum, patients should be screened to ascertain their level of distress at the initial visit, at appropriate intervals, and as clinically indicated, especially with changes in disease status.
- Distress should be assessed and managed according to clinical practice guidelines.
- Interdisciplinary institutional committees should be formed to implement standards for distress management.
- Educational and training programs should be developed to ensure that health care professionals and certified chaplains have knowledge and skills in the assessment and management of distress.
- Licensed mental health professionals and certified chaplains experienced in the psychosocial aspects of cancer should be readily available as staff members or by referral.
- Medical care contracts should include adequate reimbursement for services provided by mental health professionals.
- Clinical health outcomes measurements should include assessment of the psychosocial domain.
- Patients, families, and treatment teams should be informed that distress management is an integral part of total medical care and includes appropriate information about psychosocial services in the treatment center and in the community.
- The quality of distress management programs/services should be included in institutional continuous quality improvement projects.

FIG. 6.1 NCCN standards of care for distress management. (Adapted with permission from the NCCN Guidelines for Distress Management V.4.2021© 2021 National Comprehensive Cancer Network, Inc. All rights reserved. The NCCN Guidelines and illustrations hererin may not be reproduced in any form for any purpose without the express written permission of the NCCN.)

emotional status, family support and caregiving, coping style, cultural background, and socioeconomic status.[21] It is recommended to conduct reassessments at regular intervals to capture potential psychosocial changes which can occur over time. Sites may also establish policies or written procedures to describe workflows and parameters for referral processes in order to streamline clinical practice.[21] For example, some key timepoints which may warrant reassessments are the start of each new cycle of chemotherapy or a transition to the next level of care.

Implementation of Psychosocial Screening in Lung Cancer Care

Regular and standardized distress screening is recommended in cancer care settings to address the known risk factors for psychosocial distress in the lung cancer population. The prevalence of distress and cancer-related mortality in the lung cancer population warrants the need to gather more information on predictors of distress in this population to ensure that all needs are met.[22]

Prior to utilizing a screening tool, it is crucial to obtain a thorough understanding of the patient's biopsychosocial profile to identify potential risk factors for distress. A patient's profile may include medical history, social history, psychiatric history, drug/alcohol history, faith system/spirituality, cognitive concerns, and physical issues. Multiple disciplines may contribute to the documentation of the patient's profile in order to ensure that complete and accurate information is obtained.

After obtaining the patient's profile, screening can be conducted to obtain a standardized report of the patient's current distress level. Distress screening can be performed periodically by various designated disciplines through different communication pathways, such as face-to-face appointments, phone calls, and electronic methods.

The increase in distress screening must then be followed by effective follow-up evaluation, referrals, and clinical pathways to address the resulting increase in the volume of needs to be addressed. It is important that every team member involved in the screening and treatment process communicate their involvement in order to consolidate care and improve interdisciplinary collaboration efforts.

Recommendations for Distress Screening Programs

The Screening for Psychosocial Distress Program was a national 2-year training and implementation support program developed and implemented in 2014 to support institutions and cancer care clinicians in meeting compliance with the ACOS COC's psychosocial distress screening standards.

As a result of this program, researchers organized a comprehensive list of optimal implementation strategies to aid other institutions in implementing successful distress screening programs[23]:

- Getting buy-in of key stakeholders in the institution, including administration, clinical staff, and information technology
- Building supportive clinician relationships between two or more clinicians who can sustain the program
- Creating an oncology interdisciplinary psychosocial committee to establish policies and monitor compliance
- Developing a distress screening policy to formalize distress screening processes
- Training staff to increase knowledge and skills about psychosocial distress and maintain a standardized, comprehensive approach to distress screening
- Selecting a distress screening tool, such as the NCCN Distress Thermometer (DT)
- Establishing a referral network and resource list to ensure that all patient needs will be met
- Following up in the event of a significant distress screening score and documenting all distress screening processes to ensure compliance with institutional policies and guidelines

Suggested Screening Tools
The NCCN Distress Thermometer and Problem List

Regular and standardized screening for distress is recommended by the NCCN. The DT had previously been developed and empirically validated for this purpose. The NCCN DT and Problem List is a freely available tool for screening distress on a simple scale of 0 (no distress) to 10 (extreme distress).[1] The patient is prompted to indicate the number that describes their overall level of distress over the past week on a 0–10 scale, and then identify sources of distress listed on the 39-item Problem List, including problems unrelated to cancer. The DT has been validated for use in a variety of settings with good sensitivity and specificity. It is easy to administer and empowers the clinician to facilitate appropriate psychosocial support and referrals.

The Patient Health Questionnaire-4

Kroenke et al.[24] found that anxiety had a substantial impact on functioning, especially when comorbid with depression, which further emphasizes the importance of screening both anxiety and depression. In 2009, the Patient Health Questionnaire-4 (PHQ-4) was validated as an efficient, ultrabrief screening tool to address both anxiety and depression, as these mood disorders are frequently comorbid.[24] It consists of the PHQ-2 for depression, which is a short version of the 9-item PHQ-9, and the Generalized Anxiety Disorder-2 (GAD-2) for anxiety, which is a short version of the 7-item GAD-7. The brief and efficient nature of the assessment lends itself to use in busy clinical settings or as part of a more comprehensive evaluation process to identify the need for further referrals or interventions.[24,25] As such, it is intended for use as a screener and not as a diagnostic tool. An elevated score is an indication for mental health referrals and further evaluation into clinical disorders of anxiety and/or depression.[24,25] Because each individual institution has various workflow processes in place, it is crucial to

identify the clinical pathways needed to address further referrals triggered by the results of these screenings and assessments prior to administration. Institutions would need to determine the appropriate timing of administration of screenings as well (Fig. 6.2).

Suicide Risk

Cancer-associated suicide rate has been found to be nearly twice that of the general population in the United States, with suicide risk highest in individuals with lung cancer.[26] Risk factors associated with increased suicide risk were related to an advanced stage of disease at the time of diagnosis, long disease course, unpredictable disease course, history of psychiatric illness, and the specific anatomic site of the cancer.[26] Individuals with lung malignancies, specifically those with poor tumor prognostic features, metastatic disease, and small cell lung carcinoma, were found to be at the

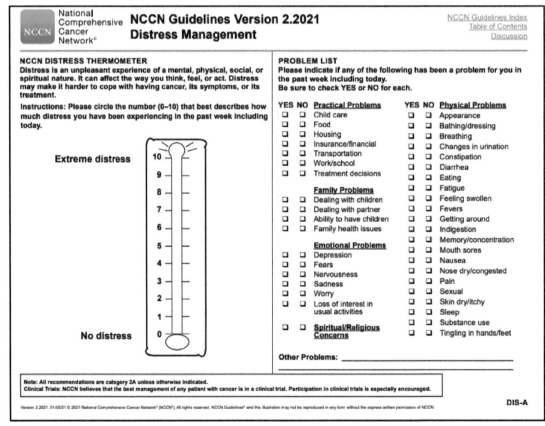

FIG. 6.2 NCCN distress thermometer and problem list. (Reprinted with permission from the NCCN Guidelines for Distress Management V.4.2021© 2021 National Comprehensive Cancer Network, Inc. All rights reserved. The NCCN Guidelines and illustrations hererin may not be reproduced in any form for any purpose without the express written permission of the NCCN.)

highest risk for suicide, with a risk of 5.1 times higher within the first 3 months of diagnosis (Table 6.1).[26,27]

High rates of anxiety and depression reported immediately after a lung cancer diagnosis have been associated with higher suicide risk, in addition to decreased knowledge about disease prognosis, sensations of guilt, poor support systems, or other personal factors.[27] The known psychosocial factors associated with suicide risk in the lung cancer population warrant improved screening methods with appropriate follow-up care for comprehensive assessment and treatment of psychiatric disorders. Health care providers must increase efforts to educate patients early on in diagnosis in order to build therapeutic alliances and engage in decision-making around treatment.

Several assessment tools exist to help inform clinical judgment and aid in broaching this sensitive topic with patients. The Columbia-Suicide Severity Rating Scale is a well-established and validated assessment that can be used to assess suicidal thinking in patients and can be utilized in various clinical settings.[28] The National Institute of Mental Health (NIH) Ask Suicide-Screening Questions (ASQ) tool is a very brief assessment of four questions that can be utilized in medical settings and help providers identify individuals at risk for suicide.[29] The NIH recommends that any patient who screens positive for suicide risk should receive a brief suicide safety assessment in order to determine the need for a more comprehensive mental health evaluation.[29]

Though there has been an increase in screening for depression and suicidal thoughts, the methods by which these issues are handled vary based on the facility and the available resources.[26] Screening is recommended at the earliest possible screening point, and facilities must determine their respective workflows regarding referral processes and feasibility of follow-up care.

INTERVENTIONS FOR PSYCHOLOGICAL DISTRESS AND ANXIETY

Follow-up care and referrals are crucial and mandated components of ensuring proper and thorough psychosocial support for individuals experiencing distress. Upon completion of a standardized screening, health care providers must interpret results and determine

TABLE 6.1
Screening Instruments for Distress and Anxiety.

SCREENING INSTRUMENTS FOR DISTRESS AND ANXIETY

Instrument	Measures	Scales	Scoring
NCCN distress thermometer[1]	General distress	1 item, 11-point likert scale	≥4 indicates moderate-to-severe distress
The patient health Questionnaire-4 (PHQ-4)	Anxiety and depression	4 item, 4 point likert scale	Score ≥3 on depression subscale and/or score ≥3 on anxiety subscale is positive, indicates need for mental health referral and further evaluation
Generalized anxiety Disorder-7 (GAD-7)	Anxiety	7-item questionnaire on 4-point scale	5 mild anxiety; 10 moderate anxiety; 15 severe anxiety; ≥10 further evaluation recommended
Symptom distress scale	Symptom-related distress	13-item, 5-point likert scale	≥25 moderate distress; ≥33 severe distress
Edmonton symptom severity scale revised (ESAS-r)	Symptom-related distress	9-item, 10-point scale	3–4 moderate/severe intensity of symptoms; 6–7 severe intensity of symptoms
Hospital anxiety and depression scale (HADS)	Anxiety and depression	14-item scale	8–10 borderline, 11–21 abnormal

the appropriate referral processes to address the specific source(s) of distress. Providers must also understand how to triage and address distress as it arises during patient encounters along the continuum of lung cancer care. All members of the cancer rehabilitation team must maintain a sense of vigilance in identifying the risk factors for distress specific to their subspecialties, as the nature of distress can be multifactorial and require a multimodal approach to intervention. Recent research shows support for psychosocial interventions for distress management, especially in light of the known psychosocial burdens and risk factors identified within the lung cancer population.

Pharmacological Interventions

For a comprehensive approach to intervention, various types of psychotropic medications can help manage symptoms of depression and anxiety. Prior to prescribing psychotropic medications, the NCCN Guidelines for Distress Management recommends a psychological or psychiatric evaluation that includes an assessment of the nature of the distress, such as interpersonal problems, psychological/psychiatric history, use of medications, substance abuse disorder, and other physical symptoms. For anxiety disorders, psychotherapy is recommended as the first-line treatment with subsequent treatment with psychotropic medication, such as antidepressants, benzodiazepines, and antipsychotics.[1] Individuals with preexisting anxiety disorders may require adjustment of medications, as lung cancer diagnosis may exacerbate illness. As with any prescription for medication, it is crucial to consider the potential adverse effects of specific psychotropic drugs, such as cardiac side effects with some antidepressants and antipsychotics. The NCCN recommends dose reduction with benzodiazepines due to the known side effects and risks, including memory difficulties, confusion, ataxia leading to falls, and addiction.

Cognitive-Behavioral Therapy

Cognitive-behavioral interventions are commonly referred to as the gold standard for psychosocial concerns in various patient populations. Cognitive-behavioral therapy, or CBT, is an intervention approach focused on reframing cognitive distortions and facilitating adaptive coping responses by engaging individuals in interpersonal skills training and relaxation skills training.[30,31] This intervention may significantly impact individuals with lung cancer, especially given the psychosocial burden associated with this diagnosis specifically due to the high symptom burden, the stigma of lung cancer, and associated negative feelings and thoughts of shame, guilt, and fear.[32]

CBT has been found to have moderate to large improvements in personal benefits and decreased health-related stigma after a 6-week CBT program which included instruction in cognitive restructuring, problem-solving, communication, relaxation, and activity—rest cycle training.[8] CBT to treat anxiety as a result of breathlessness has also been found to improve quality of life, dyspnea, and depressive symptoms when administered in conjunction with training in relaxation and meditation.[30] The findings of these studies suggest that cognitive-behavioral interventions may provide benefits with reducing symptoms and improving the overall quality of life.

Psychoeducation

Psychoeducation includes information about the disease, details about treatment methods and anticipated side effects, strategies to manage symptoms, or other resources. Psychoeducation can be delivered in a variety of different modes, including group or individual sessions, dyadic partnerships with caregiver involvement, telehealth or teleconferencing, email, or phone calls. The provision of resources, such as written information or even video education, can be included to enhance patient learning. Psychoeducation grounded in self-determination theory can provide guidance and education to patients and their caregivers in order to empower them to manage their disease, guide decision-making, relieve uncertainty, and facilitate psychosocial adaptation to illness.

A multifaceted psychoeducational intervention with information on nutrition, exercise, and relaxation techniques for newly diagnosed lung cancer patients found that the intervention group had improved management of side effects, increased protein intake, decreased depressive symptoms, and improved overall performance status.[33] Another psychosocial intervention grounded in self-determination theory studied the impact of an intervention group with a dyadic approach toward lung cancer patients and their caregivers in minimizing psychosocial distress by providing tailored manuals addressing self-care, stress and coping, symptom management, effective communication, problem-solving, and maintaining and enhancing relationships.[34] Study results demonstrated significant improvements in psychosocial indices, including depression, anxiety, and caregiver burden.[34] Research supports these interventions to help patients and their caregivers navigate the challenges of lung cancer together.[34]

Research suggests that psychoeducation may be combined with other interventions as well.

Psychoeducation combined with psychotherapy has been found to have significant decreases in depressive symptom symptoms in lung cancer patients, suggesting that psychoeducation may be an effective intervention to utilize in conjunction with other interventions such as symptom management.[35] Psychotherapy alone, however, did not yield significant effects for depressive symptoms.[35]

Complementary Therapies: Mind—Body Practices

There is growing awareness of the benefits of mind—body practices as complementary treatments to manage distress and other side effects of cancer and cancer treatment.[36] Mind—body practices are defined as practices that promote health and well-being by focusing on the mind, brain, body, and behavior. These practices, such as Yoga and Tai Chi, are referred to complementary therapies versus alternative treatments as the term "complementary treatment" refers to evidence-based techniques, whereas "alternative medicine" refers to unproven methods, which lack data to support its benefit. Other synonymous terms to complementary therapies include "integrative medicine" or "integrative oncology." Current literature supports the use of certain mind—body practices to improve emotional distress in persons with lung cancer.

Mindfulness-Based Stress Reduction

Meditation is an ancient practice defined as a "moment-to-moment present awareness with an attitude of nonjudgment, acceptance, and openness."[37] In general, meditative practices share a similar purpose of increasing a person's awareness and connection between the mind and the body. Meditative practices have been incorporated into clinical settings to reduce emotional distress, as well as symptoms of anxiety and depression.

In a randomized control study with the primary outcome of psychological distress in persons with lung cancer, the intervention group included an 8-week, group-based MBSR program in addition to standard care, whereas the control group included care as usual.[38] The results suggest that persons with lung cancer benefited from the MBSR program and showed improvements in emotional distress, mindfulness skills, self-compassion, rumination, and quality of life. In a mixed-method study by Van den Hurk et al.,[25] the aim was to understand the feasibility and effectiveness of MBSR. Although no significant changes were observed in emotional distress, participants and their caregivers reported positive feelings and a decline in

caregiver burden. Although some studies are promising, additional research is needed to support MBSR in the lung cancer population.

Tai Chi

Tai Chi is an ancient mind—body practice evolving from China and incorporates meditation, breathing, and movement.[31] There are many clinical studies that support this mind—body practice to improve an array of health issues, from cardiovascular problems to psychosocial well-being.[39] Research studies specific to lung cancer are limited, but a study by Wang et al.[39] is supporting the use of Tai Chi in this population. In a 16-week Tai Chi intervention, 32 postthoracotomy patients with NSCLC survivors showed decreases in cortisol levels and the percentage of Type 2 cytokine-producing cells, suggesting that Tai Chi might be helpful in postsurgical lung cancer patients.[39]

Yoga

Yoga is another ancient mind—body practice that involves breathing, postures, meditations, and movement. This practice is considered a low-impact exercise that focuses on a person's breath, and this emphasis on chest expansion can be beneficial for individuals diagnosed with lung cancer.[40] A pilot study by Medysky et al.[41] found that a 12-week Yoga program for lung cancer patients was safe, modestly feasible, and efficacious as seen by improvements in physical and psychosocial symptoms, including decreased depressive symptoms, increased grip strength, and body flexibility, and improved quality of life. In a recent feasibility study, another 12-week Yoga program for cancer patients and their partners showed improved physical and psychosocial symptoms.[42] These studies suggest that low-intensity Yoga may be a complementary approach to cancer care with potential physical and psychosocial benefits in the lung cancer population.

Spirituality

Spirituality is broadly defined as a connection to a higher being or greater than oneself with or without a commitment to a faith or religious affiliation.[43] With a multipronged approach to emotional distress, spirituality is acknowledged as an important contributing factor to psychosocial well-being and quality of life. This is also reflected in the NCCN DT, which includes concerns with spirituality in their list of potential problems.[1]

A referral to chaplaincy care can be made for further chaplaincy assessment, which includes, but is not limited to, concerns with lack of meaning/purpose, concerns about dying/death, conflicts between religious beliefs and recommended treatment, grief/loss, and interpersonal conflict regarding spiritual/religious beliefs and practices.[1] Based on assessment results, the chaplain may administer interventions such as spiritual/existential care and counseling, spiritual/existential rituals, and meditation or prayer.[1] The chaplain may also refer the patient to another health care professional such as a mental health professional or palliative care services.[1]

To further understand the relationship between spirituality and emotional distress, a study by Gudenkauf et al. [44] examined 865 newly diagnosed lung cancer survivors. Participants completed the Functional Assessment of Chronic Illness Therapy Spiritual Well-Being, and the Short-Form-8 for emotional distress within a year of their diagnosis and then a year later. The results showed a relationship between spirituality and a lower prevalence of emotional distress at baseline and 1 year later, suggesting that spirituality may be a protective factor for psychological well-being in lung cancer survivors.

Caregiver Support and Education

Caregiver burden and distress can increase over time with an increased disability as a result of high symptom burden and progressive lung cancer. A study found benefits in an interdisciplinary palliative care intervention that addressed various quality of life domains within an individualized program for patients with lung cancer and their family caregivers.[17] Within the various quality of life domains, including physical well-being, psychological well-being, social well-being, and spiritual well-being, caregivers identified their most significant needs as fatigue, worry and fear, communication, and meaning in life.[17] These caregivers were engaged in educational sessions guided by their self-selected quality of life domains and were assisted in developing an individualized palliative care plan, including information on self-management of lifestyle and assistance with symptom management for their family member.[17]

Family caregivers of lung cancer patients have endorsed significant psychosocial distress even after surgery.[45] Transitions of care, such as transitioning from hospital to home, are critical time points to prioritize caregiver education and training. Efforts to meet caregiver needs must increase the caregiver's self-efficacy by involving them early on in the patient's care and engaging them in hands-on training when appropriate. To alleviate distress and decrease the impact on the quality of life of caregivers, rehabilitation professionals may address recommendations for durable medical equipment, symptom management strategies, transfer training, mobility skills, and hygiene techniques.[46]

A pilot study examining the feasibility of a personalized telehealth intervention for GI and lung cancer surgery patients and caregivers found that the interventions were feasible and acceptable.[47] Although this study primarily focused on physical interventions, psychological distress was also monitored and was found to have different trajectories between patients and their caregivers. Patients demonstrated mild distress preoperatively, with levels increasing prior to discharge from the hospital, and then improving 2−4 weeks after discharge. Caregiver distress levels were higher than patients prior to 2-week after discharge, but then gradually decreased. This study reinforces the importance of addressing psychological distress in both patients and their caregivers.

Telemedicine

Telehealth refers to the use of technology to communicate health information to patients and their caregivers.[48] With advances in technology, telehealth modalities have been shown to be feasible, safe, convenient, acceptable, and a reassuring approach to cancer care.[47,48,49,50] The delivery of interventions via telehealth or telemedicine must be considered for individuals with lung cancer, especially for those with advanced stage cancers who may experience debilitating treatment burdens that can limit follow-up medical care and decrease health self-management.[47,48,50] In a study by Kroll et al.,[50] psychosocial interventions in a group format were provided to women diagnosed with NSCLC with 92% of participants preferring online delivery and 44% reporting that telehealth services would have been similar to face-to-face interaction. Patients have also reported that telehealth services can improve access to care, coordination of services, and patient's competence, as well as reduce physical and social isolation.

IMPLICATIONS FOR CLINICAL PRACTICE
Rescreening

Rescreening for distress and anxiety at regular time points throughout the continuum of lung cancer care is vital in ensuring that psychosocial needs are being addressed. ASCO's Quality Oncology Practice Initiative (QOPI) Measure provides standards for rescreening at every line of therapy and every new admission. Practical application of these standards is dependent on the treatment setting, type of cancer, and resources available in the institution.[51] However, regardless of practice setting, the sense of urgency associated with lung cancer due to its high mortality rate and known risks for high distress may warrant even more frequent rescreening practices to ensure that concerns are addressed in a timely manner.

Resource Management

Health care professionals are encouraged to conduct a thorough evaluation to review the availability of resources in their respective facilities and assess the feasibility and capability of implementing screening and interventions. Improving the efficiency of service delivery is critical and can be achieved by leveraging the capabilities of the electronic medical record by embedding screenings and assessments into standard practice, incorporating distress screening into routine practice, creating clinical pathways to guide health care professionals on appropriate referral processes, and optimizing communication among members of the multidisciplinary team. It is crucial to realize that these practices can realistically be implemented in practice settings such as community hospitals and primary care centers, even if they may lack the resources present in larger comprehensive cancer centers.

Community Resources

Institutions are encouraged to conduct a scoping review of the resources available within their respective facilities and communities so that they can utilize their resources to the highest potential. Community resources can be leveraged as additional support for patients and their caregivers in the form of support groups, transportation resources, home health care, or financial assistance. Such examples of resources include the American Cancer Society, American Lung Association, CancerCare, and local government agencies. Many communities offer community-based programs at low or no cost, including educational classes, events, in-person or televideo groups, or counseling for cancer survivors and their caregivers. Furthermore, assisting patients to find community-based mental health providers based on insurance coverage or limited facility resources can link the patient to long-term support and ensure that these concerns are not lost to follow-up.

Unique Role of Rehabilitation

Rehabilitation professionals, including occupational therapy and physical therapy, are key members of the multidisciplinary care team. They often build close rapport with their patients due to frequent and consistent follow-up, deeper inquiries into personal life factors, and the establishment of therapeutic alliances. This intimate, regular contact with patients over time allows therapists to witness the direct impact of distress and anxiety on quality of life and may predispose the patient to disclose their psychosocial concerns. Therefore, rehabilitation professionals are recommended to maintain a heightened sense of vigilance and sensitivity to psychosocial distress when working with individuals with lung cancer so that they can achieve goal progression and improve the overall quality of life. They are encouraged to administer interventions within their scope of practice and make the appropriate referrals as needed.

CONCLUSION

Distress screening programs are not universal by design, as each practice setting must consider how distress screening can be incorporated into their practice based on variability in volume, availability of resources, and site culture. For this reason, the ACOS COC and the National Comprehensive Cancer Center established standards to guide cancer programs in establishing their own comprehensive distress screening programs and clinical pathways respective to the idiosyncrasies of their sites.

In order to effectively implement a comprehensive approach to distress and anxiety in the lung cancer population, all health care professionals must heighten not only their awareness and knowledge of the pervasive need of mental health care but also their clinical acumen in the administration of screening, review of results, provision of resources, and referral to appropriate providers. A vigilant health care team acutely aware of the signs of and symptoms of distress and anxiety in the lung cancer population can proactively implement coordinated efforts to reduce the burden of lung cancer and promote improved quality of life for this underserved population.

REFERENCES

1. Referenced With Permission from the NCCN Guidelines® for Distress Management V.4.2021 © National Comprehensive Cancer Network, Inc. 2021. All rights reserved. Accessed 12 May 2021. Available online at: www.NCCN.org.NCCN. (makes no warranties of any kind whatsoever regarding their content, use, or application and disclaims any responsibility for their application or use in any way).
2. American Cancer Society. *Key Statistics for Lung Cancer.* Accessed 12 2021. https://www.cancer.org/cancer/lung-cancer/about/key-statistics.html.
3. Hurria A, Li D, Hansen K, et al. Distress in older patients with cancer. *J Clin Oncol.* 2009;27(26), 4361-4351.
4. Badger T, Lebaron VT, McCorkle R. Screening for emotional distress in older patients with lung cancer. *Oncol Nurse Ed.* 2010;24(4).

5. Diaz-Frutos D, Baca-Garcia E, Garcia-Foncillas J, Lopez-Castoman J. Predictors of psychological distress in advanced cancer patients under palliative treatments. *Eur J Cancer Care.* 2016;25(4):608–615.

6. Holland J, Watson M, Dunn J. The IPOS new International Standard of Quality Cancer Care: integrating the psychosocial domain into routine care. *Psycho Oncol.* 2011;20(7): 677–680.

7. Shen MJ, Hamann HA, Thomas AJ, Ostroff JS. Association between patient-provider communication and lung cancer stigma. *Support Care Cancer.* 2016;24(5):2093–2099.

8. Chambers SK, Baade P, Youl P, et al. Psychological distress and quality of life in lung cancer: the role of health-related stigma, illness appraisals and social constraints. *Psycho Oncol.* 2015;24(11):1569–1577.

9. Hamann HA, Ver Hoeve ES, Carter-Harris L, Studts JL, Ostroff JS. Multilevel opportunities to address lung cancer stigma across the cancer control continuum. *J Thorac Oncol.* 2018;13(8):1062–1075.

10. Carter-Harris L. Lung cancer stigma as a barrier to medical help-seeking behavior: practice implications. *J Am Assoc Nurse Pract.* 2015;27(5):240–245.

11. Seastedt P, Luca MJ, Antevil JL, et al. Patient motivations for non-adherence to lung cancer screening in a military population. *J Thorac Dis.* 2020;12(10):5916–5924.

12. Lim RBL. End-of-life care in patients with advanced lung cancer. *Ther Adv Respir Dis.* 2016;10(5):455–467.

13. Lai-Kwon J, Heynemann S, Flore J, et al. Living with and beyond metastatic non-small cell lung cancer: the survivorship experience for people treated with immunotherapy or targeted therapy. *J Cancer Survivorship.* 2021;15:392–397.

14. Park R, Shaw JW, Korn A, McAuliffe J. The value of immunotherapy for survivors of stage IV non-small cell lung cancer: patient perspectives on quality of life. *J Cancer Survivorship.* 2020;14:363–376.

15. Crist JV, Grunfeld EA. Factors reported to influence fear of recurrence in cancer patients: a systematic review. *Psycho Oncol.* 2013;22:978–986.

16. Borges EL, Franceschini J, Costa LHD, Fernandes ALG, Jamnik S, Santoro IL. Family caregiver burden: the burden of caring for lung cancer patients according to the cancer stage and patient quality of life. *J Bras Pneumol.* 2017; 43(1):18–23.

17. Borneman T, Sun V, Williams AC, et al. Support for patients and family caregivers in lung cancer: educational components of an interdisciplinary palliative care intervention. *J Hospice Palliat Nurs.* 2015;17(4):309–318.

18. American Board of Medical Specialties: About Preventive Medicine; (n.d.). Retrieved June 7, 2021, from: https://www.acpm.org/about-acpm/what-is-preventive-medicine/.

19. Andersen BL, DeRubeis RJ, Berman BS, et al. Screening, assessment, and care of anxiety and depressive symptoms in adults with cancer: an American Society of Clinical Oncology guideline adaptation. *J Clin Oncol.* 2014; 32(15):1605–1619.

20. *Optimal Resources for Cancer Care: 2020 Standards.* Chicago, IL: Commission on Cancer; 2021.

21. ASCO QOPI Certification Program Standards Manual. *Required Processes and Documentation to Meet Certification Standards and Elements.* Version 6.1.2018. American Society of Clinical Oncology; 2018.

22. Graves KD, Arnold SM, Love CL, Kirsh KL, Moore PG, Passik SD. Distress screening in a multidisciplinary lung cancer clinic: prevalence and predictors of clinically-significant distress. *Lung Cancer.* 2007;55(2):215–224.

23. Ercolano E, Hoffman E, Tan H, Pasacreta N, Lazenby M, McCorkle R. Managing psychosocial distress comorbidity: lessons learned in optimizing psychosocial distress screening program implementation. *Oncology.* 2018; 32(10):488–493.

24. Kroenke K, Spitzer RL, Williams JBW, Lowe B. An ultra-brief screening scale for anxiety and depression: the PHQ-4. *Psychosomatics.* 2009;50(6):613–621.

25. Lowe B, Wahl I, Rose M, et al. A 4-item measure of depression and anxiety: validation and standardization of the Patient Health Questionnaire-4 (PHQ-4) in the general population. *J Affect Disord.* 2010;122(1–2):86–95.

26. Rahouma M, Kamel M, Abouarab A, et al. Lung cancer patients have the highest malignancy-associated suicide rate in USA: a population-based analysis. *Ecancermedicalscience.* 2018;12:859.

27. Urban D, Rao A, Bressel M, Neiger D, Solomon B, Mileshkin L. Suicide in lung cancer: who is at risk? *Chest.* 2013;144(4):1245–1252.

28. Posner K, Brown GK, Stanley B, et al. The Columbia-Suicide Severity Rating Scale: initial validity and internal consistency findings from three multisite studies with adolescents and adults. *Am J Psychiatr.* 2011;168: 1266–1277.

29. Ask Suicide-Screening Questions (ASQ) Toolkit: National Institute of Mental Health; (n.d.). Retrieved June 9, 2021, from: https://www.nimh.nih.gov/research/research-conducted-at-nimh/asq-toolkit-materials/.

30. Greer JA, MacDonald JJ, Vaughn J, et al. Pilot study of a brief behavioral intervention for dyspnea in patients with advanced lung cancer. *J Pain Symptom Manag.* 2015; 50(6):854–860.

31. Lehto RH. Psychosocial challenges for patients with advanced lung cancer: interventions to improve well-being. *Lung Cancer.* 2017;8:79–90.

32. Major B, O'Brien LT. The social psychology of stigma. *Annu Rev Psychol.* 2005;56:393–421.

33. Tian J, Jia LN, Cheng ZC. Relationships between patient knowledge and the severity of side effects, daily nutrient intake, psychological status, and performance status in lung cancer patients. *Curr Oncol.* 2015;22(4):e254–e258.

34. Badr H, Smith CB, Goldstein NE, Gomez JE, Redd WH. Dyadic psychosocial intervention for advanced lung cancer patients and their family caregivers: results of a randomized pilot trial. *Cancer.* 2015;121(1):150–158.

35. Hsieh CC, Hsiao F. The effects of supportive care interventions on depressive symptoms among patients with lung cancer: a metaanalysis of randomized controlled studies. *Palliat Support Care.* 2017;15:710–723.

36. Deng GE, Rausch SM, Jones LW, et al. Complementary therapies and integrative medicine in lung cancer: diagnosis and management of lung cancer: American College of Chest Physicians evidence-based clinical practice guidelines. *Chest*. 2013;143(5):e420S–e436S.

37. Van den Hurk DG, Schellekens MP, Molema J, Speckens AE, van der Drift MA. Mindfulness-based stress reduction for lung cancer patients and their partners: results of a mixed methods pilot study. *Palliat Med*. 2015; 29(7):652–660.

38. Schellekens MPJ, van den Hurk DGM, Prins JB, et al. Mindfulness-based stress reduction added to care as usual for lung cancer patients and/or their partners: a multicentre randomized controlled trial. *Psycho Oncol*. 2017;26(12): 2118–2126.

39. Wang R, Liu J, Chen P, Yu D. Tai chi exercise decreases the percentage of type 2 cytokine-producing cells in postsurgical non-small cell lung cancer survivors. *Cancer Nurs*. 2013;36(4):e27–34.

40. Fuerst ML. Yoga benefits lung cancer patients & their caregivers. *Oncol Times*. 2017;39(22):63.

41. Medysky ME, Sullivan DR, Tyzik A, Thomas CR, Winters-Stone KM. Feasibility and acceptability of yoga to improve psychosocial and physical function among patients with lung cancer: a pilot study. *J Clin Oncol*. 2020;38(15): e24068.

42. Sullivan DR, Medysky ME, Tyzik AL, Dieckmann NF, Denfeld QE, Winters-Stone K. Feasibility and potential benefits of partner-supported yoga on psychosocial and physical function among lung cancer patients. *Psycho Oncol*. 2019;30:789–793.

43. Puchalski CM, Vitillo R, Hull SK, Reller N. Improving the spiritual dimension of whole person care: reaching national and international consensus. *J Palliat Med*. 2014; 17(6):642–656.

44. Gudenkauf LM, Clark MM, Novotny PJ, et al. Spirituality and emotional distress among lung cancer survivors. *Clin Lung Cancer*. 2019;20(6):e661–e666.

45. Kim JY, Sun V, Raz DJ, et al. The impact of lung cancer surgery on quality of life trajectories in patients and family caregivers. *Elsevier*. 2016;101:35–39.

46. Yadav R. Rehabilitation of surgical cancer patients at University of Texas M.D. Anderson Cancer Center. *J Surg Oncol*. 2007;95:361–369.

47. Lafaro KJ, Raz DJ, Kim JY, et al. Pilot study of a telehealth perioperative physical activity intervention for older adults with cancer and their caregivers. *Support Care Cancer*. 2019; 28(8):3867–3876.

48. Cox A, Lucas G, Marcu A, et al. Cancer survivors' experience with telehealth: a systematic review and thematic synthesis. *J Med Internet Res*. 2017;19(1):e11.

49. Head BA, Studts JL, Bumpous JM, et al. Development of a telehealth intervention for head and neck cancer patients. *Telemed e-Health*. 2009;15(1):44–52.

50. Kroll JL, Higgins H, Snyder S, et al. Feasibility of a group-based telehealth psychosocial intervention for women with non-small cell lung cancer (NSCLC). *Cancer Epidemiol Prev Biomarkers*. 2021;30(4):803.

51. Buxton D, Lazenby M, Daugherty A, et al. Distress screening for oncology patients: practical steps for developing and implementing a comprehensive distress screening program. *ACCC*. 2014 (OI).

CHAPTER 7

Lung Cancer Survivorship

PATRICK MARTONE, DO • ELISA ALPERT, MD • J. ANTHONY GARCIA, DO

SURVIVORSHIP

The number of cancer survivors is estimated to continue to grow given advancements in detection and treatment of cancer. Survivorship begins from the time of diagnosis and lasts throughout one's life, and thus is ideally integrated into the cancer care continuum. Survivorship includes not only the patient, but family members/caregivers as well. Survivorship broadly includes the principles and practices of surveillance for recurrence of disease/primary cancers, treatment of long-term and late effects of cancers and its treatments, physical health promotion, and emotional well-being.[1]

While the overall survival rates for lung cancer have improved with the use of screening modalities and a decline in smoking rates, the overall survival rate for lung cancer is estimated to be 19%. However, this varies greatly based upon the time of detection. In those patients diagnosed with localized stage disease, the survival rate is 57%. For those diagnosed with metastatic disease, the 5-year survival rate is 5%. Future rates of survivorship will likely continue to be impacted by the implementation of early detection programs, such as the ones utilizing low-dose computed tomography (CT) for screening.[2]

Cancer survivorship includes multidisciplinary care involving different specialists and practitioners with a patient-centered approach to treatment. An essential component of survivorship care is following clinical practice guidelines for detection of malignancy as well as screening for late effects of treatment. Comprehensive survivorship teams can include a primary care physician, nurse, oncologist, psychologist, rehabilitation team, dietician, and other specialists. Primary care physicians or speciality trained nurses can act as the coordinating providers during survivorship care. These coordinators can then refer survivors to specialized care that is required to address their symptoms such as neuropsychology, cardiology, neurology, endocrinology, and rehabilitation specialists.[3]

Primary care physicians and oncologists may provide preventative care services and screening for cancer recurrence including routine history and physical exams at visits. Physiatrists and other rehabilitation professionals may act on the team to identify physical and cognitive impairments in lung cancer survivors.[4] Palliative care teams can also be utilized in survivorship care to manage persistent pain after disease-directed treatment and taper opioids to mitigate the risk of opiate misuse.[5]

Survivorship visits for lung cancer patients can include the use of survivorship care plans. These care plans can be used to communicate and coordinate care between providers and assist patients in navigating their future care. A summary of previous treatment should include the cancer stage and diagnosis, contact information for previous providers, surgeries, chemotherapies and/or radiation received, and on-going toxicities. Follow-up care plans have information related to clinic visits and continued diagnostic surveillance testing, emotional and financial resources, smoking cessation, and other information promoting a healthy lifestyle and diet.[6]

(See figure: Lung Cancer Survivorship Care Plan and ASCO Cancer Treatment and Survivorship Care Plan).[6,32,33]

Survivorship Key Points

- The number of survivors is estimated to grow given advancements in lung cancer detection and treatment.
- Survivorship includes not only the patient, but family members and caregivers as well.
- Survivorship includes surveillance for recurrence, treatment of long-term/late effects of cancer and its treatments, promotion of physical health and emotional well-being.
- Cancer survivorship includes multidisciplinary care involving different specialists and practitioners with a patient-centered approach to treatment.
- Survivorship care plans can be used to communicate and coordinate care between providers and assist patients in navigating their future care.

Lung Cancer Rehabilitation. https://doi.org/10.1016/B978-0-323-83404-9.00016-5

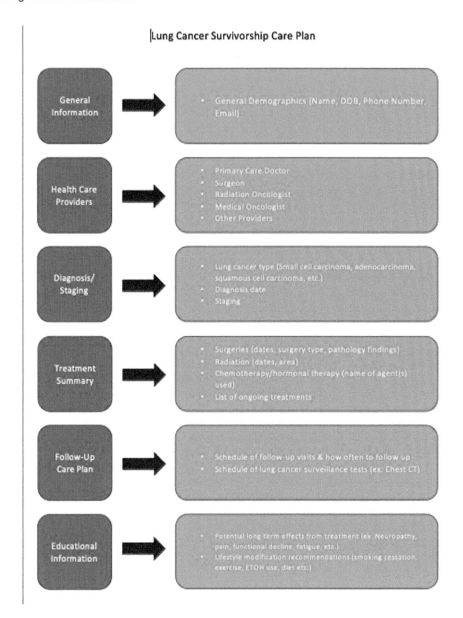

Lung Cancer Survivorship Care Plan

General Information →
- General Demographics (Name, DOB, Phone Number, Email)

Health Care Providers →
- Primary Care Doctor
- Surgeon
- Radiation Oncologist
- Medical Oncologist
- Other Providers

Diagnosis/Staging →
- Lung cancer type (Small cell carcinoma, adenocarcinoma, squamous cell carcinoma, etc.)
- Diagnosis date
- Staging

Treatment Summary →
- Surgeries (dates, surgery type, pathology findings)
- Radiation (dates, area)
- Chemotherapy/hormonal therapy (name of agent(s) used)
- List of ongoing treatments

Follow-Up Care Plan →
- Schedule of follow-up visits & how often to follow up
- Schedule of lung cancer surveillance tests (ex. Chest CT)

Educational Information →
- Potential long term effects from treatment (ex. Neuropathy, pain, functional decline, fatigue, etc.)
- Lifestyle modification recommendations (smoking cessation, exercise, ETOH use, diet etc.)

General Information	
Patient Name:	Patient DOB:
Patient phone:	Email:

Health Care Providers (Including Names, Institution)

Primary Care Provider:
Surgeon:
Radiation Oncologist:
Medical Oncologist:
Other Providers:

Treatment Summary	

Diagnosis

Cancer Type/Location/Histology Subtype: Non-Small Cell Lung Cancer	Diagnosis Date (year):
Stage: ☐I ☐II ☐III ☐Not applicable	

Treatment <u>Completed</u>

Surgery ☐ Yes ☐No	Surgery Date(s) (year):
Surgical procedure/location/findings:	

Radiation ☐ Yes ☐No	Body area treated:	End Date (year):

Systemic Therapy (chemotherapy, hormonal therapy, other) ☐ Yes   ☐No

Names of Agents Used	End Dates (year)
☐ Carboplatin	
☐ Cisplatin	
☐ Gemcitabine	
☐ Paclitaxel/Docetaxel	
☐ Pemetrexed	
☐ Vinorelbine	
☐ Other	

Persistent symptoms or side effects at completion of treatment: ☐ No ☐ Yes (enter type(s)) :

Treatment <u>Ongoing</u>

Need for ongoing (adjuvant) treatment for cancer   ☐ Yes ☐ No

Additional treatment name	Planned duration	Possible Side effects

Follow-up Care Plan	

Schedule of Clinical Visits

Coordinating Provider	When/How often

Cancer Surveillance or Other Recommended Tests		
Coordinating Provider	Test	How Often

Please continue to see your primary care provider for all general health care recommended for a (man) (woman) your age, including cancer screening tests. Any symptoms should be brought to the attention of your provider:
1. Anything that represents a brand new symptom;
2. Anything that represents a persistent symptom;
3. Anything you are worried about that might be related to the cancer coming back.

Possible late- and long-term effects that someone with this type of cancer and treatment may experience:
- Constipation
- Esophageal stricture
- Hearing loss
- Kidney problems
- Peripheral neuropathy or numbness and tingling
- Pneumonitis or inflammation of the lung (3-6 months after treatment)
- Pulmonary fibrosis or scarring
- Trouble with or painful swallowing

Cancer survivors may experience issues with the areas listed below. If you have any concerns in these or other areas, please speak with your doctors or nurses to find out how you can get help with them.

☐Anxiety or depression ☐Insurance ☐Sexual Functioning
☐Emotional and mental health ☐Memory or concentration loss ☐Stopping Smoking
☐Fatigue ☐Parenting ☐Weight changes
☐Fertility ☐Physical functioning ☐Other
☐Financial advice or assistance ☐School/work

A number of lifestyle/behaviors can affect your ongoing health, including the risk for the cancer coming back or developing another cancer. Discuss these recommendations with your doctor or nurse:

☐Alcohol use ☐Physical activity ☐Other
☐Diet ☐Sun screen use
☐Management of my medications ☐Tobacco use/cessation
☐Management of my other illnesses ☐Weight management (loss/gain)

Resources you may be interested in:
- www.cancer.net
- Other:

Other comments:

Prepared by: Delivered on:

- This Survivorship Care Plan is a cancer treatment summary and follow-up plan and is provided to you to keep with your health care records and to share with your primary care provider or any of your doctors and nurses.
- This summary is a brief record of major aspects of your cancer treatment not a detailed or comprehensive record of your care. You should review this with your cancer provider.

QUALITY OF LIFE IN LUNG CANCER SURVIVORSHIP

Quality of life in lung cancer survivors has been demonstrated to be worse than in that of the general population. Quality of life in lung cancer survivors can be impacted by physical functional decline, emotional distress, fatigue, pain, cough, and dyspnea. Dyspnea has been repeatedly demonstrated to be an important risk factor for poor quality of life. Mental distress is also an important correlate for a lower quality of life.[7] Identifying, rehabilitating, and improving all of these factors are important for improving survivorship and quality of life in this patient population.

Staging of cancer and treatment types can be important factors impacting quality of life. Surgical resections that are more extensive such as bilobectomy and pneumonectomy may negatively impact quality of life more so than compared to a lobectomy.[8] Furthermore, patients who undergo combined chemotherapy and radiation therapy may be more susceptible to toxicity resulting in increased symptom burden.

There are multiple measurement tools which can be used to evaluate quality of life specifically in the lung cancer population. The European Organization for Research and Treatment of Cancer (EORTC) LC-13 questionnaire provides a list of symptoms related to lung cancer and its treatments. The Functional Assessment of Cancer Therapy questionnaire (FACT-L) is a 41-item survey which covers general health status, in addition to site specific symptoms. Lastly, the Lung Cancer Symptom Scale (LCSS) involves patient and observer evaluation of symptoms.[9]

A survivorship model of care is important to address these quality of life concerns regarding long term surveillance, for recurrence of cancer, symptom management and treatment of other comorbidities. One example of this model involved a nurse practitioner (NP), providing the follow up care for thoracic cancer patients. These survivorship visits included surveillance for recurrence of cancer, assessment and management of effects of treatment, screening for second malignancies and health promotion (diet, exercise, smoking cessation, referrals to support groups and other specialists). This survivorship model of care successfully identified lung cancer recurrences/new lung cancers and provided an assessment and treatment for cancer associated medical and psychological issues which impact quality of life.[10]

Quality of Life in Lung Cancer Survivorship Key Points

- Quality of life in lung cancer survivors can be impacted by physical functional decline, emotional distress, fatigue, pain, cough, dyspnea and mental distress.
- Identifying, rehabilitating and improving all of these factors are important for improving survivorship and quality of life in this patient population.
- Staging of cancer and treatment types are important factors impacting quality of life.
- There are multiple measurement tools which can be used to evaluate quality of life specifically in the lung cancer population, including the EORTC LC-13, FACT-L, and LCSS.
- A survivorship model of care can help identify lung cancer recurrences/new lung cancers and provide an assessment and treatment for cancer-associated medical and psychological issues which impact quality of life.

TOBACCO CESSATION

Smoking cessation is an essential aspect of survivorship in lung cancer. This is crucial because individuals who continue to smoke after diagnosis of early stage lung cancer have been shown to have a higher risk of recurrence, a higher risk of second primary tumor, and a higher mortality rate.[11] Clinical practice guidelines generally recommend that all current smokers are advised to quit and for former smokers to remain abstinent.

There are many different strategies and modalities to approach smoking cessation. Patients should be asked about their tobacco use at each visit and be advised about the benefits of quitting and willingness to discuss cessation. A framework which can be used to facilitate these discussions include the "5 As": ask, advise, assess, assist, and arrange. Counseling on cessation can be performed through phone call quit-lines, group classes, or individualized counseling.

In addition to counseling, pharmacotherapy is another means to assist with smoking cessation. Nicotine replacement therapy can be performed with transdermal patches, lozenges, or gum. Bupropion is a non-nicotine alternative medication to assist in cessation and can also act as an antidepressant. Another alternative is to use varenicline which acts as a partial agonist to nicotinic acetylcholine receptors.[12]

Tobacco Cessation Key Points

Tobacco Cessation Key Points

- Individuals who continue to smoke after diagnosis of early stage lung cancer have been shown to have a higher risk of recurrence, a higher risk of second primary tumor, and a higher mortality rate.
- Patients should be asked about their tobacco use at each visit and be advised about the benefits of quitting and willingness to discuss cessation.
- In addition to counseling, pharmacotherapy is another means to assist with smoking cessation.

CANCER-RELATED PAIN

Cancer-related pain can be a significant factor impairing the quality of life of lung cancer survivors. Up to 45% of cancer patients will experience inadequate pain control and 40% of cancer survivors will still experience symptoms at 5 years post-treatment. Possible mechanisms for pain include the tumor itself or impingement upon adjacent tissue, obstruction of blood vessels, side effects from radiation and chemotherapeutic agents, and post-thoracotomy pain.[13] Therefore, methods for managing pain symptoms should be incorporated into survivorship.

Lung cancer survivors should be screened for common causes of pain in this population which can include chest wall pain, post-thoracotomy pain syndrome, myofascial pain, chemotherapy-induced peripheral neuropathy, and radiation therapy–related pain. Multimodal approaches can be utilized to manage these pain symptoms. The World Health Organization (WHO) Analgesic Ladder can be utilized as a tool by which pharmacologic management of pain can be prescribed in a stepwise fashion. Rehabilitation therapies can be incorporated into treatment plans for techniques such as myofascial release and stretching exercises. Additional interventional approaches to pain management can include peripheral injections or intercostal nerve blocks, thoracic nerve root/paravertebral procedures, and trigger point injections.[14]

Cancer-Related Pain Key Points

- Up to 45% of cancer patients will experience inadequate pain control and 40% of cancer survivors will still experience symptoms at 5 years post-treatment.
- Lung cancer survivors should be screened for common causes of pain in this population which can include chest wall pain, post-thoracotomy pain syndrome, myofascial pain, chemotherapy-induced peripheral neuropathy, and radiation therapy–related pain.

Cancer-Related Pain Key Points

- Multimodal approaches can be utilized to manage these pain symptoms, including pharmacological management, rehabilitation therapies, and interventional pain management.

FATIGUE

Cancer-related fatigue is one of the most prevalent symptoms in lung cancer patients, affecting up to 90% of lung cancer survivors.[15] It is defined as "a distressing and persistent sense of physical, emotional, and/or cognitive tiredness or exhaustion related to cancer and/or cancer treatment that is not proportional to recent activity and interferes with usual functioning."[16] Cancer-related fatigue can affect a patient's ability to perform activities of daily living and impacts quality of life.[17] Fatigue can be worsened by coexisting or associated symptoms such as dyspnea, depression, or other medical conditions. Many patients have a constellation of symptoms, in addition to fatigue, which are also worsened by surgery, chemotherapy, or radiation. Since fatigue has many correlated and contributing factors, fatigue screening and treatment should be addressed comprehensively and include screening for dyspnea and mood disorders as well as pain and sleep disturbance in lung cancer survivors.[18] Underlying mechanism of cancer-related fatigue include increased proinflammatory cytokines, angiogenic modulators, anemia, hormone effects due to disruption of the hypothalamic/pituitary/adrenal axis, and serotonin metabolism.[16]

Due to the high prevalence of cancer-related fatigue in lung cancer survivors, fatigue screening should be performed at initial diagnosis and throughout treatment and post-treatment visits. While there are many fatigue scales which can be used, a common screening technique uses the Visual Analog Scale (VAS). This scale ranges from 0 to 10 with 0 indicating no fatigue and 10 being the worst imaginable. In this scale, mild fatigue is rated 1–3 and indicates that fatigue does not impact activities of daily living. Patients can be reassured and advised on coping strategies. Patients with moderate to severe fatigue (4 or higher on the VAS) should have a more comprehensive fatigue evaluation. There are also many other scales which can be used to monitor and screen for cancer-related fatigue.

As fatigue is common in both cancer patients and the general population, a complete history, review of symptoms, physical exam, and evaluation should be done to assess for reversible or contributing causes of fatigue.

Medical conditions such as anemia, infection, organ dysfunction, hypothyroidism, and other medical conditions can also contribute. Factors such as pain, anxiety, depression, nutrition imbalance, activity level, and conditions including sleep disorders should also be addressed. Activity level can also play a role. Medical issues which can be treated or may be reversible include anemia and other organ system dysfunction. Hypothyroidism, hypogonadism, and sleep disorders such as insomnia, obstructive sleep apnea, and restless leg syndrome should also be evaluated.[19] Medications including pain medications and beta-blockers should also be reviewed for side effects. While sleep interventions such as sleep hygiene and relaxation techniques have shown mixed results in fatigue outcomes, they can be helpful in patients with sleep disorders. Cognitive Behavioral Therapy may also be helpful.[20]

Cancer-related fatigue is primarily treated with non-pharmacologic measures. Exercise is one of the primary treatments for fatigue.[21] Studies have shown best outcomes for patients who participate in at least 3–5 hours of moderate activity per week. Patients with recent surgery, significant deconditioning, or comorbidities can benefit from physical therapy or a supervised exercise program. Exercise can be used with caution in patients with bone metastasis, thrombocytopenia, and anemia. However, patients should be monitored for symptoms including fever or active infection. Exercise can increase functional capacity which can lead to a decrease in fatigue, while reduced activity can lead to weakness and decreased endurance. Aerobic exercise has shown the most benefit and an exercise program should be individualized based on the patient's age, gender, cancer, and fitness level.[16]

Mindfulness approaches including psychosocial treatment, yoga, and acupuncture have also been shown to be beneficial in cancer-related fatigue. Studies have had mixed results on the benefit of psychostimulants in treating fatigue; however, if reversible conditions have been addressed and nonpharmacological treatments do not adequately relieve symptoms, then a trial of a psychostimulant is recommended. Initial studies on methylphenidate showed benefit; however, the effect may be dose dependent and more beneficial in patients with severe fatigue symptoms. Modafinil has also shown mixed results; while glucocorticoids can also improve fatigue and quality of life scores, but is limited by long term side effects.[20]

Fatigue Key Points

- Cancer-related fatigue is one of the most prevalent symptoms in lung cancer patients, affecting up to 90% of lung cancer survivors.
- A comprehensive history, physical exam, and assessment should be performed to assess for reversible/contributing causes of fatigue. Such contributing factors include anemia, infection, organ dysfunction, hypothyroidism, pain, anxiety, malnutrition, deconditioning, poor sleep, or medication side effects.
- The VAS is commonly used to screen and assess for fatigue severity.
- Cancer-related fatigue is primarily treated with nonpharmacologic measures such as exercise.
- Exercise can increase functional capacity which can lead to a decrease in fatigue.
- Mindfulness approaches including psychosocial treatment, yoga, and acupuncture have also been shown to be beneficial in cancer-related fatigue.
- Studies have had mixed results on the benefit of psychostimulants in treating fatigue; however, if conservative management does not adequately relieve symptoms then a trial of a psychostimulant is recommended.

DYSPNEA

Dyspnea is the sense of breathlessness or otherwise termed air-hunger and can be a distressing symptom in lung cancer survivors. Dyspnea, along with other symptoms previously mentioned (i.e., fatigue, depression, anxiety), can impact quality of life and function. The management and treatment of dyspnea is multifactorial and should address physical and emotional components utilizing pharmacological and nonpharmacological approaches.

Evaluation of dyspnea should begin with identifying if there are any reversible causes such as pleural effusions, asthma, pneumonia, or pulmonary embolism. Also, management of chronic conditions such as chronic obstructive pulmonary disease and heart failure should be optimized. Pharmacologic approaches can include consideration of the use of opiates, short-acting benzodiazepines (for dyspnea related to anxiety), systemic corticosteroids (for inflammatory conditions), and bronchodilators. Airflow interventions can include supplemental oxygen for patients who are experiencing hypoxemia, and directing airflow via a fan to the cheek. Physical therapeutic approaches should address posture training, breathing techniques (such as pursed lips), abdominal breathing, timed breathing, and relaxation training.[22] Exercise is another strategy which can be utilized to improve dyspnea in lung cancer survivors. There are many approaches to exercise in lung cancer survivors and thus exercise plans may be tailored to the individual, which could include resistance training, aerobic exercise, and breathing techniques.[18]

Dyspnea Key Points

- Evaluation of dyspnea should begin with identifying if there are any reversible causes such as pleural effusions, asthma, pneumonia, or pulmonary embolism. Also, management of chronic conditions such as chronic obstructive pulmonary disease (COPD) and heart failure should be optimized.
- The management and treatment of dyspnea is multifactorial and should address physical and emotional components utilizing pharmacological and nonpharmacological approaches.

PHYSICAL ACTIVITY

Exercise has been shown to benefit the general population in many ways, and these benefits also extend to lung cancer survivors. Exercise is a nonpharmacological intervention which has a benefit on fatigue, quality of life, strength, fitness, and psychological health. Lung cancer patients may often be sedentary pre-diagnosis, and symptoms from lung cancer or co-existing conditions may contribute to low adherence to exercise programs. In order to increase likelihood of participation, an exercise program should be flexible, easy to start, and progress gradually. While many patients are limited by physical symptoms, a comprehensive customized approach based on a patient's physical status and preferences can increase participation.[16]

Pulmonary rehabilitation programs have been shown to have a positive effect on function, exercise capacity, and symptoms such as dyspnea. Up to 66% of lung cancer survivors do not meet recommended activity guidelines of 150 min of moderate or 75 min of vigorous intensity activity weekly, with strength training and stretching. Patients that do meet the recommended activity level have higher quality of life scores.[23]

There are several proposed mechanisms for how physical activity and exercise can influence lung cancer outcomes. It is proposed that exercise affects chronic inflammation and improves modulation of insulin and glucose and may also impact oxidative stress and immune function. Exercise may increase pro-inflammatory cytokine levels and natural killer cell infiltration into tumors. In mice studies, wheel running was found to decrease tumor volume. In a 16-week long prospective randomized study of postsurgical patients with Non-small Cell Lung Carcinoma (NSCLC) performing tai chi, the tai chi arm was shown to have increased proliferation of mononuclear cells, with increased cytotoxicity in lung cancer cells. Natural killer cells, natural killer T-cells, and CD11c cells were also higher in the tai chi group. Studies have also shown a more stable ratio of T-lymphocytes and cortisol levels in patients status-post chemotherapy who started resistance exercise.[16]

Exercise may improve cancer-related fatigue due to modulation of these biological mechanisms. There have been observational studies which have shown an inverse relationship between physical activity and fatigue, with moderate to vigorous activity associated with fewer symptoms. For example, Janssen et al. completed a study which included a program for 50 lung cancer patients participating in exercise 3 times per week. After 12 weeks, fatigue, quality of life, and cardiopulmonary fitness had significantly improved scores. Benefits were noted especially if initiated early after surgery. While other studies have shown a less clear benefit of exercise, they did not show worsening of fatigue with exercise intervention.[16]

Quality of life impairment is long lasting in lung cancer survivorship, regardless of the type of treatment.[23] However, exercise can limit this impact. A longitudinal study of 107 patients with lung cancer demonstrated a direct correlation between quality of life and time dedicated to walking activities. The benefit of exercise was shown to be of benefit both during and after treatment. A retrospective study on 82 patients with lung cancer included an exercise program including relaxation, respiratory training, cough training, and lower extremity exercise found increases in Forced Vital Capacity (FVC) and Forced Expiratory Volume-1 (FEV1) as well as decreased Diffusing Capacity for Carbon Monoxide (DLCO). Peak oxygen consumption and the 6 min walk test can assess cardiopulmonary fitness, which is an independent predictor for survival in lung cancer.[16]

Physical activity and exercise can be of benefit in patients with psychological distress. Exercise may modulate monoamine and cortisol levels which benefit patients with anxiety and depression. While studies on sleep have been mixed, some studies have shown improvement in subjective and objective sleep quality after initiating a home based exercise program.[16]

Physical Activity Key Points

- Exercise is a non-pharmacological intervention which has a benefit on fatigue, quality of life, strength, fitness, and psychological health. While many patients are limited by physical symptoms, a comprehensive customized approach based on a patient's physical status and preferences can increase participation.
- Pulmonary rehabilitation programs have been shown to have a positive effect on function, exercise capacity, and symptoms such as dyspnea. Studies show that exercise affects chronic inflammation and improves modulation of insulin and glucose, and may also impact oxidative stress and immune function. Additionally, exercise may increase proinflammatory cytokine levels and natural killer cell infiltration into tumors.
- Exercise may modulate monoamine and cortisol levels which benefit patients with anxiety and depression, in addition to improving sleep quality.

PSYCHOLOGICAL IMPACT

A significant number of lung cancer patients can have psychological distress and this number is generally greater than that of other cancer disease types. For example, in one study, 43% of lung cancer patients demonstrated psychological distress compared to a 35% prevalence rate among other cancer sites.[24] Psychologic distress can have an impact on quality of life and perception of symptom burden. Survivors can frequently experience symptoms of anxiety and depression. Furthermore, these needs are often unmet. Addressing this component of survivorship can help to improve quality of life in this patient population.[25]

Screening tools for depression and mental health can be effective at detecting these symptoms in lung cancer survivors. Assessment tools such as the Patient Health Questionnaire-9 (PHQ-9) and Generalized Anxiety Disorder-7 (GAD-7) can be utilized to detect these symptoms.[26] Multimodal interventions can be effective in treating symptoms of emotional distress. Mechanisms such as progressive muscle relaxation and education on self-management of symptoms can help to reduce anxiety. Education on coping skills to not only patients, but caregivers as well, can help to reduce depressive symptoms.[25]

Psychological Impact Key Points

- Psychologic distress such as anxiety and depression can have an impact on quality of life and perception of symptom burden.

Psychological Impact Key Points

- Studies show a larger prevalence of psychological distress in lung cancer patients when compared to other cancer types.
- Screening tools such as the PHQ-9 and GAD-7 can be effective at detecting depression and anxiety, respectively, in lung cancer survivors.
- Multimodal interventions can be effective in treating symptoms of emotional distress.

NUTRITION

Nutrition is an important factor to consider in lung cancer survivorship. Malnutrition is a common problem more prevalent with aging and can contribute to sarcopenia and frailty syndromes. In cancer patients over age 65, the malnutrition rate has been estimated to be between 23% and 66%, with even higher rates noted in lung cancer patients.[27,28] Since the mean age at diagnosis of lung cancer is over 70 years,[28] many patients at risk for lung cancer are already at risk for malnutrition and its sequela.[28] Higher rates of malnutrition occur in patients with more severe disease or who are undergoing chemotherapy, immunotherapy, or radiotherapy. Malnutrition contributes to sarcopenia, an age-related progressive loss of skeletal muscle mass and strength caused by an imbalance between protein synthesis and breakdown. Many adults do not consume the recommended amount of protein and may also have decreased uptake of amino acids needed for protein synthesis. Sarcopenia occurs in approximately 43% of NSCLC and 52% of Small Cell Lung Cancer (SCLC) patients.[27] Sarcopenia and cancer-related sarcopenia can coexist leading to an increased fall risk, disability, and decreased quality of life.[28]

Cancer-related sarcopenia may be caused by altered cytokines, systemic inflammation, energy imbalance, and loss of adipose tissue. This higher inflammatory state with increased weakness and decreased overall function can lead to poorer outcomes. Performance status and body composition can influence disease severity and mortality in lung cancer patients. Patients with NSCLC treated with Programed Cell Death Protein 1 inhibitors without sarcopenia at baseline have been shown to have better progression free survival. In lung cancer patients receiving chemotherapy, early nutritional intervention can counteract weight loss and sarcopenia; however, many patients still do not reach recommended dietary intake. Nutritional interventions include improving caloric intake, ensuring adequate protein, and supplementation.[28]

Cancer and cancer treatment can contribute to decreased food intake and metabolic changes which increase inflammation and catabolism leading to weight loss. Nutrition and exercise play an important role in minimizing the cycle of malnutrition and frailty. Early nutrition intervention with dietary counseling has been shown to prevent weight loss and preserve muscle mass by improving adequate calorie and protein intake and the use of supplements as needed.

Supplementation with eicosapentaenoic acid (EPA) and polyunsaturated fatty acids (PUFA) improves weight and muscle mass in advanced NSCLC patients. In observational studies, PUFA consumption increases body weight and is thought to decrease inflammation. Ghrelin receptor agonists have also shown the ability to increase lean body mass in patients with inoperable non-small cell lung cancer and cachexia. The Dietary Approaches to Stop Hypertension (DASH) diet is also associated with reduced mortality in lung cancer. Components of plant foods are associated with a reduction in inflammation.[28]

Nutrition Key Points[28]

- In cancer patients over age 65, the malnutrition rate has been estimated to be between 23% and 66%, with even higher rates noted in lung cancer patients. Higher rates of malnutrition occur in patients with more severe disease or who are undergoing chemotherapy, immunotherapy, or radiotherapy.
- Sarcopenia, an age-related progressive loss of skeletal muscle mass and strength, occurs in approximately 43% of NSCLC and 52% of SCLC patients, predisposing patients to increased fall risk, disability, and decreased quality of life.
- In lung cancer patients receiving chemotherapy, early nutritional intervention can counteract weight loss and sarcopenia.
- Nutritional interventions include improving caloric intake, ensuring adequate protein and supplementation.
- Supplementation with EPA and polyunsaturated fatty acids (PUFAs) improves weight and muscle mass in advanced NSCLC patients.
- The DASH diet is also associated with reduced mortality in lung cancer.

ROLE OF SURVIVORSHIP AND RETURN TO WORK

Many lung cancer survivors may have financial, social, intellectual, or other reasons to return to work during or after lung cancer treatment. While most cancer patients have medical insurance at time of diagnosis, 15% of cancer patients experience financial hardship due to their disease. Lung cancer is particularly associated with negative employment implications. Many patients take extended time off of work due to the mental and physical effects of their disease, in addition to the time required for treatment and recovery.[29]

While there are several potential barriers to return to work, a survivorship service can play a role in optimizing a patient's ability to return to work or other desired activity. Cancer survivorship practitioners should discuss with patients work-related issues during survivorship visits. Environmental and modifiable work accommodations should be identified in order to match the work demand with the survivors' physical and mental capabilities. Vocational rehabilitation can be utilized to enhance a survivor's quality of life to meet the demands of work.[30]

SURVEILLANCE AND PREVENTATIVE HEALTH

An essential component of survivorship includes routine follow-up and close monitoring of patients with a previous history of lung cancer. Even with advances in treatment modalities, recurrence rates or secondary cancers still pose a risk to lung cancer survivors. Unlike other cancer types which can rely on serum markers, lung cancer requires other means of surveillance. Risk of recurrence varies depending on stage of initial disease. For example, in non-small cell lung cancer, stage IIIA patients have a higher rate of recurrence and a greater rate of distant metastasis when compared to earlier staged disease types.[31]

Close surveillance, as recommended by the American Society of Clinical Oncology (ASCO), endorses a careful history and physical exam at routine intervals. In patients with curatively treated stage I–III NSCLC and SCLC, patients should undergo imaging surveillance every 6 months for the first 2 years and annually thereafter.

Imaging should be performed with diagnostic chest CT, with inclusion of the adrenals. Imaging is preferred with contrast during the first 2 years posttreatment. Low-dose screening chest CT can be utilized after the first 2 years.[32]

Surveillance and Preventative Health Key Points

- An essential component of survivorship includes routine follow-up and close monitoring of patients with a previous history of lung cancer.
- Close surveillance, as recommended by ASCO, endorses a careful history and physical exam at routine intervals.
- In patients with curatively treated stage I–III NSCLC and SCLC, patients should undergo imaging surveillance every 6 months for the first 2 years and annually thereafter.

CHALLENGES FACING DELIVERY OF SURVIVORSHIP SERVICES FOR LUNG CANCER SURVIVORS

There are many challenges in providing survivorship services for lung cancer survivors. Due to the complexities of some patients, care may need to be shared between many providers including oncology and primary care to adequately manage comorbidities and a patient's overall health condition, especially in older patients. Survivorship care faces some of the same challenges as delivery of care for all lung cancer patients, which can include symptom burden causing functional limitation. Many patients have poor quality of life and high symptom burden due to dyspnea, pain, and/or anxiety. These symptoms may make it difficult for patients to attend appointments including medical visits and physical therapy. The rise of telehealth and virtual or home care options may assist in overcoming some of these challenges. Providing a care plan includes clearly defined roles, a summary of treatments, effects from treatment, future plans for testing, scheduled visits, and lifestyle counseling which can assist patients and caregivers in navigating survivorship. Documenting these factors in a clear way is important, and who provides the documentation may vary based on site.[33] The time required to prepare these care plans can often be a limiting factor; however, time-based billing and reimbursement for time spent counseling may allow physicians to be reimbursed for these services.

CONCLUSION

Lung cancer patients having undergone treatment for their malignancy are impacted by many factors (dyspnea, pain, fatigue, mood disorders) which can impair their quality of life. Survivorship is utilized to identify and treat these impairments to improve physical and mental function. In addition, survivorship also includes the prevention and surveillance of future cancers. Incorporating these survivorship principles into practice is essential to promoting optimum health in lung cancer survivors.

REFERENCES

1. Shapiro CL. Cancer survivorship. *N Engl J Med*. 2018; 379(25):2438–2450.
2. Siegel RL, Miller KD, Jemal A. Cancer statistics, 2020. *CA Cancer J Clin*. 2020;70:7–30. https://doi.org/10.3322/caac.21590.
3. Loonen JJ, Bliijlevens NM, Prins J, et al. Cancer survivorship care: person centered care in a multidisciplinary shared care model. *Int J Integrated Care*. 2018;18(1).
4. Smith SR, Reish AG, Andrews C. Cancer survivorship: a growing role for physiatric care. *PM R*. 2015;7.
5. Goodlev ER, Discala S, Darnall BD, Hanson M, Petok A, Silverman M, et al. Managing cancer pain, monitoring for cancer recurrence, and mitigating risk of opioid use disorders: a team-based, interdisciplinary approach to cancer survivorship. *J Palliat Med*. 2019;22(11):1308–1317.
6. Mayer DK, Nekhlyudov L, Snyder CF, Merrill JK, Wollins DS, Schulman LN. American Society of Clinical Oncology clinical expert statement on cancer survivorship care planning. *J Oncol Prac*. 2014;10(6):345–351.
7. Hechtner M, Eichler M, Wehler B, et al. Quality of life in NSCLC survivors—a multicenter cross-sectional study. *J Thorac Oncol*. 2019;14(3):420–435.
8. Yang P, Cheville AL, Wampfler JA, et al. Quality of life and symptom burden among long-term lung cancer survivors. *J Thorac Oncol*. 2012;7(1):64–70.
9. Gridelli C, Perrone F, Nelli F, Ramponi S, De Marinis F. Quality of life in lung cancer patients. *Ann Oncol*. 2001; 12:S21–S25.
10. Huang J, Logue AE, Ostroff JS, et al. Comprehensive long-term care of patients with lung cancer: development of a novel thoracic survivorship program. *Ann Thorac Surg*. 2014;98(3):955–961.
11. Parsons A, Daley A, Begh R, Aveyard P. Influence of smoking cessation after diagnosis of early stage lung cancer on prognosis: systematic review of observational studies with meta-analysis. *Br Med J*. 2010;340.
12. Steliga MA, Yang P. Integration of smoking cessation and lung cancer screening. *Transl Lung Cancer Res*. 2019; 8(Suppl 1):S88.
13. Rausch SM, Gonzalez BD, Clark MM, et al. SNPs in PTGS2 and LTA predict pain and quality of life in long term lung cancer survivors. *Lung Cancer*. 2012;77(1):217–223.
14. Hochberg U, Francisca Elgueta M, Perez J. Interventional analgesic management of lung cancer pain. *Front Oncol*. 2017;7:17.
15. Hung R, Krebs P, Coups EJ, et al. Fatigue and functional impairment in early-stage non-small cell lung cancer survivors. *J Pain Symptom Manag*. 2011;41(2):426–435. https://doi.org/10.1016/j.jpainsymman.2010.05.017.
16. Avancini A, Sartori G, Gkountakos A, et al. Physical activity and exercise in lung cancer care: will Promises Be fulfilled? *Oncologist*. 2020;25(3):e555–e569. https://doi.org/10.1634/theoncologist.2019-0463. Epub 2019 Nov 26. PMID: 32162811; PMCID: PMC7066706.
17. Ebede CC, Jang Y, Escalante CP. Cancer-related fatigue in cancer survivorship. *Med Clin N Am*. 2017;101(6): 1085–1097. https://doi.org/10.1016/j.mcna.2017.06.007. Epub 2017 Aug 25. PMID: 28992856.
18. Henshall CL, Allin L, Aveyard H. A systematic review and narrative synthesis to explore the effectiveness of exercise-based interventions in improving fatigue, dyspnea, and depression in lung cancer survivors. *Cancer Nurs*. 7/8 2019;42(4):295–306.
19. Escalante CP, Manzullo EF. Cancer-related fatigue: the approach and treatment. *J Gen Intern Med*. 2009;24(Suppl 2):S412–S416. https://doi.org/10.1007/s11606-009-1056-z.

20. Berger AM, Mooney K, Alvarez-Perez A, et al. Cancer-related fatigue. Version 2.2015 *J Natl Compr Cancer Netw*. 2015;13(8):1012−1039. https://doi.org/10.6004/jnccn.2015.0122.

21. Mitchell Sandra A, Hoffman AJ, et al. Putting evidence into practice: an update of evidence-based interventions for cancer-related fatigue during and following treatment Weisbrod fatigue evidence-based practice. *Clin J Oncol Nurs*. 2014;18.

22. Hui D, Bohlke K, Bao T, et al. Management of dyspnea in advanced cancer: ASCO guideline. *J Clin Oncol*. 2021; 39(12):1389−1411.

23. Vijayvergia N, Shah PC, Denlinger CS. Survivorship in non-small cell lung cancer: challenges faced and Steps forward. *J Natl Compr Cancer Netw*. 2015;13(9): 1151−1161. https://doi.org/10.6004/jnccn.2015.0140. PMID: 26358799; PMCID: PMC5450910.

24. Zabora J, BrintzenhofeSzoc K, Curbow B, Hooker C, Piantadosi S. *Psycho Oncol*. 2001;10(1):19−28.

25. Yates P, Schofield P, Zhao I, Currow D. Supportive and palliative care for lung cancer patients. *J Thorac Dis*. 2013;5(Suppl 5):S623.

26. Rajapakse P. An Update on survivorship issues in lung cancer patients. *World J Oncol*. 2021;12(2−3):45.

27. Nascimento CM, Ingles M, Salvador-Pascual A, Cominetti MR, Gomez-Cabrera MC, Viña J. Sarcopenia, frailty and their prevention by exercise. *Free Radic Biol Med*. 2019;132:42−49. https://doi.org/10.1016/j.freeradbiomed.2018.08.035. Epub 2018 Aug 31. PMID: 30176345.

28. Nigro E, Perrotta F, Scialò F, et al. Food, nutrition, physical activity and Microbiota: which impact on lung cancer? *Int J Environ Res Publ Health*. 2021;18(5):2399. https://doi.org/10.3390/ijerph18052399. PMID: 33804536; PMCID: PMC7967729.

29. Nekhlyudov L, Walker R, Ziebell R, Rabin B, Nutt S, Chubak J. Cancer survivors' experiences with insurance, finances, and employment: results from a multisite study. *J Cancer Surviv*. 2016;10(6):1104−1111. https://doi.org/10.1007/s11764-016-0554-3. Epub 2016 Jun 9. PMID: 27277896.

30. Chow, Loon S, Su Ting A, Su TT. Development of conceptual framework to understand factors associated with return to work among cancer survivors: a systematic review. *Iran J Public Health*. 2014:391−405.

31. Lou F, Sima CS, Rusch VW, Jones DR, Huang J. Differences in patterns of recurrence in early-stage versus locally advanced non-small cell lung cancer. *Ann Thorac Surg*. 2014;98(5):1755−1761.

32. Schneider BJ, Ismaila N, Aerts J, et al. Lung cancer surveillance after definitive curative-intent therapy: ASCO guideline. *J Clin Oncol*. 2020;38(7):753−766.

33. Pozo CLP, Morgan MAA, Gray JE. Survivorship issues for patients with lung cancer. *Cancer Control*. 2014:40−50. https://doi.org/10.1177/107327481402100106.

CHAPTER 8

Exercise and Lung Cancer

SUZANNE GUTIÉRREZ TEISSONNIERE, MD • HANNA OH, MD

Lung cancer is the leading cause of cancer-related death worldwide.[1] Since the 1980s, multiple studies and organizations have demonstrated the benefit of exercise intervention and physical activity in oncology patients.[2] Although there is limited large-scale research regarding its benefits in lung cancer patients, engaging in exercise or physical activity has been found to be safe and is still strongly recommended.[3–5] The 2018 Physical Activity Guidelines Advisory Committee Scientific report (PAGAC) concluded there is moderate evidence that engaging in moderate to vigorous exercise may reduce risk or lower incidence for several cancer types, including lung cancer.[6] Nevertheless, there are other studies showing insufficient evidence because of smoking status as a confounding variable.[7,8] Most patients diagnosed with lung cancer have been described as sedentary.[9] In fact, the PAGAC report also found moderate evidence in at least two meta-analyses that increased sitting time may lead to increased risk of lung cancer.[10–12]

While the American College of Sports Medicine (ACSM) Cancer Roundtable in 2018 reported benefit of exercise and physical activity in many cancer types,[13] the guidelines found limited evidence regarding the benefits of exercise in lung cancer, and no clear guidelines on the type and intensity of recommended exercise.[14] Exercise intervention has been reported to work across multiple organ systems to improve cardiopulmonary fitness, offset treatment side effects, and improve health-related quality of life (HRQoL) in individuals with cancer.[15] The American Cancer Society and ACSM recommend avoiding inactivity and suggest that patients with cancer should engage in regular physical activity; specifically, they recommend at least 150 min per week of moderate aerobic activity, or 75 min of vigorous aerobic activity, with flexibility and strength exercise two or three times per week.[13] The 2018 ACSM guidelines further recommend that exercise prescription should be individualized by addressing health-related outcomes and accounting for special considerations in order to promote adherence and limit dropout.[16] Thus, tailoring exercise programs for patients diagnosed with lung cancer may improve the current low adherence and high dropout rates seen in a variety of studies mainly due to prediagnosis reduced fitness level and impairments related to cancer and its treatments.[15]

Surgery is known to be a major cause of morbidity and mortality in lung cancer, even leading to at least 25% of postoperative complications,[17,18] thus resulting in increased health care costs. Baseline cardiopulmonary fitness provides diagnostic and prognostic information. Peak oxygen consumption (VO_{2peak}) is an independent predictor of survival, and inversely related to perioperative and postoperative complications.[19,20] Studies have demonstrated that $VO_{2\ peak}$ or exercise tolerance is reduced in patients with lung cancer throughout the continuum of care.[19,21] Since lung cancer patients with lower exercise tolerance have worse surgical outcomes, chemotherapy response, and overall survival,[22] it will be instrumental to better understand what types of exercise programs are most beneficial for these patients.

There are multiple studies that assess physical activity among patients with cancer, while others seek to specify the benefits of exercise. To clarify, Caspersen et al. described physical activity as "a bodily movement by skeletal muscles that results in energy expenditure," while exercise is physical activity that is planned, structured, and repetitive with the goal to obtain or maintain physical fitness.[23]

CONTRIBUTORS TO DECREASED EXERCISE CAPACITY

Exercise tolerance or capacity is directly affected by patient's age, comorbidities, and previous exercise fitness, but the decline is accelerated by the tumor burden, its pathophysiology, and the treatment-related side effects.[24,25] Factors that may affect the exercise tolerance or capacity in patients with lung cancer should be evaluated when determining the best exercise setting and prescription for the individual patient (see Fig. 8.1).

Exercise capacity, a term used to describe the physical fitness of an individual, is defined as "the maximal

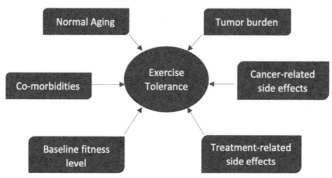

FIG. 8.1 Factors that may affect the exercise tolerance or capacity in patients with lung cancer.

capacity of an individual to perform aerobic work or maximal oxygen consumption."[26] For patients with lung cancer, exercise capacity is typically measured by field-based functional tests (e.g., the Six-Minute Walk Test (6MWT)), or laboratory-based exercise tests (e.g., cardiopulmonary exercise test to measure peak oxygen uptake (VO_{2peak}).

Baseline Fitness Level

Many patients with lung cancer do not meet the World Health Organization (WHO) exercise guidelines which recommend moderate-intensity aerobic exercise of at least 150 min per week.[9,13] Increased exercise capacity and physical activity levels in this patient population are associated with improved HRQoL.[27]

Currently, in nonsmall cell lung cancer (NSCLC), 6MWT is the most frequently reported assessment of exercise capacity.[28] Poor exercise capacity, as measured by the 6mWT, is a predictor of poor prognosis in advanced NSCLC and chronic obstructive pulmonary disease (COPD).[29,30]

A study by Granger et al. found that individuals with NSCLC were engaged in significantly less physical activity compared to aged-matched healthy peers. Only 60% of those diagnosed with NSCLC were meeting WHO physical activity guidelines, and had a subsequent decline in physical activity, functional capacity, and strength after diagnosis, unfortunately.[9]

Normal Aging

There is a known normal decline in exercise capacity that occurs with aging, and concomitantly, most people diagnosed with lung cancer are over the age of 65.[31]

Comorbidities

Many patients with lung cancer also have coexisting lung diseases, in which exercise tolerance is already reduced due to cardiopulmonary impairments.[32] These may include preexistent smoking history, COPD, asbestos-related lung disease, pulmonary fibrosis, and cardiac disease.[33] COPD is present concomitantly in 73% of men and 53% of women with newly diagnosed primary lung cancer.[34]

Cancer-Related and Treatment-Related Side Effects

Lung cancer, as well as cancer treatment, can cause weight loss, anemia, pulmonary dysfunction, and dyspnea, which can further negatively impact exercise capacity.[35] Moreover, all therapeutic management may further affect the pulmonary function.[36–38]

While lung resection has the best treatment survival outcomes in early-stage lung cancer, patients continue to have worsening physical fitness, respiratory function, and quality of life after surgery.[39,40] The presence of a tumor mass, together with related surgical procedures, may affect the respiratory system by reducing diffusion capacity. Chemotherapy-induced anemia, radiation-induced pneumonitis, and lung resection-related impairment are frequently seen and likely contribute to dyspnea and fatigue.[41,42]

Most patients affected by advanced lung cancer experience cachexia (69%) or sarcopenia (47%).[43] Sarcopenia is associated with reduced survival and is highly prevalent (47%) in patients with stage III and IV disease treated with chemotherapy.[44] Cachexia is defined as a multifactorial syndrome characterized by an ongoing loss of skeletal mass, with or without loss of fat mass, that cannot be fully reversed by conventional nutritional support and leads to progressive functional impairment.[45] It occurs in up to one-third of patients with stage III and IV lung cancer.[46] Patients with lung cancer may also suffer from muscle dysfunction due to disease-related metabolic disorders and side effects of chemotherapy.[47] Muscle mass has been shown to be a predictor of all-cause mortality.[24]

For those undergoing treatment, impaired cardiac function may also be secondary to thoracic radiation, cardiac side effects of chemotherapy, and anemia. Chemotherapeutic agents and radiotherapy may have cardiac side effects, decreased blood cell populations, and worsened vascular function.[48] Patients who have received >30–35 Gy exposure to the chest wall are at risk for radiation-associated heart damage which can include radiated-induced injury to the myocardium, coronary arteries, and valves, resulting in diastolic dysfunction.[49]

All these contributors not only limit a patient's exercise capacity but can also limit their ability to participate in activities of daily living (ADLs). Quality of life is also limited by direct effects of cancer progression such as fatigue, dyspnea, weight loss, pain, as well as effects of cancer treatment, which have the potential to be barriers to exercise.[50,51] One-third of patients with lung cancer attribute their disease as the major limitation to performing ADLs.[52]

PATHOPHYSIOLOGY

Many studies have investigated the antitumorigenic potential of exercise. Primary hypotheses regarding the benefits of exercise in cancer revolve around the idea of controlling chronic low-grade inflammation and the modulation of metabolic dysregulation substances (e.g., insulin, glucose, and insulin-like growth factors) and sex hormones. Exercise could also have an impact on oxidative stress and immune-related function which can modify and alter the tumor environment.[53] Exercise may also improve cancer-related fatigue by reducing overall symptom severity.[54]

The molecular mechanisms behind the benefits and the influence physical activity and exercise has on lung cancer outcomes continue to be an area of research. Malignant cells are known to have the ability to activate the hypoxia-inducible factor 1-alpha (HIF-1α) pathway to promote angiogenesis through proangiogenic factors, mainly via VEGF-α.[55] While it is still unclear how exercise modulates angiogenesis in an oncological setting, a study in mice showed that mice undergoing daily high-intensity interval training after tumor cell injection had 2.5-fold higher mRNA levels of VEGF-α compared to sedentary mice. This also correlated with a reduction of their tumor mass.[56] Cancer cells also utilize an ability to escape apoptosis and cell death. Exercise may play a role in stabilizing p53, avoiding downregulation, to affect oncogenesis.[57]

Pederson et al., in another mouse model, concluded that exercise may have an antitumorigenic impact by playing a role in increasing proinflammatory cytokine levels in the tumor microenvironment. They found that exercise, via wheel-running, in mice, not only reduced tumor volume but also lead to an upregulation of proinflammatory cytokines such as IL-1a and inducible nitric oxide synthase.[58] In humans, a prospective randomized study by Chen et al. demonstrated that postsurgical NSCLC patients who participated in 16 weeks of tai chi training promoted proliferation of peripheral blood mononuclear cells when compared to a control group. The patients who exercised also had an increase in circulating NK cell percentage and natural killer T cells when compared to the control group.[59]

BENEFITS OF EXERCISE

The benefits of exercise have been studied in breast and colon cancer, with large trials showing reduced mortality in both.[60,61] The reasons are likely multifactorial, due to adaptations in cardiac function (e.g., increased cardiac output), vascular function (e.g., increased anti-inflammatory activity), and increased muscle strength which contribute to improvements in exercise capacity following exercise training.[48]

Peak oxygen consumption (VO_{2peak}) is the gold standard assessment of cardiopulmonary fitness, which is an independent predictor of mortality in noncancer populations.[62] In advanced NSCLC, VO_{2peak} exercise testing is a noninvasive, safe and relatively inexpensive test that provides clinically relevant information.[25] Jones et al. advocate that VO_{2peak} is a strong independent predictor of survival in NSCLC, in conjunction with other traditional markers of prognosis. In their prospective study of 398 patients with potentially resectable NSCLC, they found an inverse association between VO_{2peak} and all-cause mortality.[63] While performance status has been demonstrated to be a strong predictor of survival in NSCLC, it is often a subjective assessment by a health care professional.[64] Adequate exercise capacity is critical for maintaining functional independence.[48] A patient's performance status and functional independence measures are often important considerations when forming an oncologic treatment plan. Patients with advanced lung cancer with borderline performance status (e.g., Eastern Cooperative Oncology Group rating of >2) experience high treatment-related toxicity and morbidity.[65]

The pathophysiology behind the improved outcomes associated with exercise in the lung cancer patient population is still being investigated, but such benefit may be linked with the known association between exercise and improved COPD symptoms, as many patients with lung cancer have chronic lung conditions.[34] Pulmonary rehabilitation has been shown to improve symptoms associated with COPD, as well as physical activity and quality of life.[66]

It has been generally observed that patients with lung cancer can safely participate in physical activity at any stage of the disease and its treatment.[3-5] Statements from the American Thoracic Society and the European Respiratory Society concluded that pulmonary rehabilitation has the potential to reduce dyspnea, as well as improve both exercise capacity and quality of life.[66] While Temel et al. did not observe an improvement in muscle strength, patients had a significant reduction of lung cancer symptoms (FACT-L) in a 12-week hospital-based combined endurance and muscle strength training intervention (NSCLC stage III/IV).[67] Preliminary cohort studies in advanced NSCLC indicate that exercise training improves exercise capacity and muscle force.[68] Tarumi et al. investigated the changes in respiratory function because of a perioperative intensive pulmonary rehabilitation program in patients with NSCLC who underwent induction chemoradiotherapy. Among a group of 82 patients with NSCLC IIB-IV stage, significant increase in forced expiratory volume in the first second (FEV1) and forced vital capacity were observed after a 10-week program.[69] Similarly, a Cochrane review has demonstrated that exercise training improves functional exercise capacity in patients following lung resection for early-stage NSCLC but found that exercise does not improve HRQoL.[70] However, indirectly, exercise has been shown to reduce cancer-related fatigue and can improve sleep quality in cancer survivors.[71,72]

Prehabilitation

The treatment for early-stage lung cancer (stages I and II) is surgery. Patients with COPD already have an increased surgical risk. Lung resection for lung cancer is associated with activity reduction at 1 month and reduced functional health status and worse pain scores at 6 months.[73] Therefore, many exercise-based studies have been focused on preoperative and postoperative exercise programs to optimize functional recovery.

However, in the first year after surgery, patients usually experience an increase in pulmonary parameters that may be attributed to compensatory mechanisms, such as the expansion of the remaining lobes and vascular tissues.[74,75]

Small trials in 2007 and 2014 showed that preoperative exercise training increased 6 minute walk distance (6 MWD), increased VO2, and improved quality of life (QoL) before surgery.[76] Promising studies have been completed in prehabilitation with goal of reducing

morbidity, improving physical and psychological function, and decreasing hospital readmissions.[77]

Advantages of home-based preoperative programs include greater flexibility and convenience for patients, low time consumption, and are overall cheaper than outpatient physical therapy.[78]

A Cochrane review concluded that prehabilitation prior to surgical resection resulted in a 67% reduction in the number of postoperative pulmonary complications and hospital length of stay.[79] Following this review, a prehabilitation program involving high-intensity interval training showed significant short-term improvements in preoperative exercise capacity.[80]

Restorative Rehabilitation

Results of postoperative exercise programs in NSCLC patients have been mixed, finding improvements in walking distance, but no change in strength or QoL.[81,82] Henke et al. performed a randomized controlled trial (RCT) in advanced-stage lung cancer patients receiving inpatient chemotherapy; implementing daily endurance training and every-other-day strength training, the group noted improvements in physical function scores, self-reported symptoms (pain, neuropathy, cognitive functioning, and dyspnea), and exercise tolerance.[83] Pulmonary rehabilitation has been effective for improving dyspnea in lung cancer.[84]

Early postoperative supervised exercise has been reported to be safe, feasible, and to improve exercise capacity and muscle strength.[85] The European society of thoracic surgery recommends that high-risk patients who are being treated with curative intent surgery should be referred to rehabilitation for general symptom management, with high-risk being defined as those with predicted postoperative (PPO) FEV1 or PPO diffusion capacity of the lung for carbon monoxide 60% and O2 max 10 mL/kg/min or 35%.[86] Regarding preference for exercise or physical activity, survey studies have been performed to further assess patient's preferences for exercise, which showed walking as a preferred form for physical activity.[87] The American College of Chest Physicians (CHEST) recommends exercises focused on cough suppression as an alternative or addition to pharmacological intervention for persistent cough.[88]

Quist et al. found that starting exercise early in the postoperative course is associated with greater reductions in cancer-related fatigue.[89]

Palliative Rehabilitation

In an RCT by Cheville et al. of patients with stage IV cancer, a home-based exercise program was shown to improve mobility, fatigue, and sleep quality.[90] In a survey study performed by the same group, patients with late-stage cancers endorsed that highly structured, nondaily activity-oriented exercise programs were unappealing and poorly accepted by this population without careful planning and implementation.[91] They concluded that patients in the late stages of cancer appear to conceptualize the relationships among their exercise behaviors, cancer, symptoms, and overall well-being in ways that are largely uninformed by professional caregivers. They recommended health care providers to prescribe home exercise programs that incorporate the daily activities of patients, who will then take part in it with a higher level of acceptance.

Limitations to exercise in the palliative setting include an inability to attend hospital-based programs due to mobility impairments and decreased energy.[92] However, patients who had been able to participate in a hospice-based exercise program endorsed a sense of regaining control and improvement in strength and balance.[93]

BARRIERS TO EXERCISE

Progression of symptoms in lung cancer has been referred to as the dyspnea spiral, where once patients develop shortness of breath, then activity is avoided, functional capacity declines, and dyspnea also worsens.[94] A common reason, among patients and providers, for avoiding exercise or physical activity in patients with advanced lung cancer is that patients are considered "too sick" for physical activity.[94] However, patients with a higher symptom burden may benefit most from exercise. Education to both clinicians and patients is key. Jensen et al. showed that >90% of patients with advanced cancer can perform some type of exercise or physical therapy.[95] Temel et al. reported that less than half of those recruited in an exercise trial were able to complete the exercise training intervention.[67] Similarly, Andersen et al. noted >50% drop out rate despite patients being found to have improved exercise tolerance when completing the intervention.[96] Aside from medical and health limitations, factors such as exercise preference and social implications have also been demonstrated to influence patient participation in a physical activity program.[97] Poor adherence to exercise programs limits its possible efficacy.

Patients with cancer may also feel self-conscious in an exercise environment, such as community gyms, where they are exercising next to healthy peers. In an assessment of patients with inoperable metastatic lung cancer, Kartolo et al. found that patients who have smoking history, history of COPD, and no exercise history had lower motivation to exercise.[51]

Psychological distress and sleep disorders are also common in patients with lung cancer, which may also limit the patient's motivation. It is thus extremely important to enhance patient's education regarding the benefits of exercise and adapt programs to their functional or sickness level.

The limited reimbursement for cancer rehabilitation and out-of-pocket expenses not covered by insurance may discourage patients from exercising.[98] Additional larger studies with structured interventions and predefined endpoints would be beneficial to further validate the need for individualized exercise and rehabilitation programs that would adapt to the patient's need, encourage adherence, and result in increased availability of such programs.

Exercise Precautions

Numerous studies have demonstrated the positive effects of exercise to the overall health and well-being of cancer patients and survivors. The ACSM Preparticipation Health Screening (updated for 2015 and beyond) recommends appropriate medical clearance for patients with any metabolic disease and sedentary lifestyle. Thus, emphasizing on special precautions is important to ensure the overall safety of patients while engaging in physical activity and/or exercise.

While multiple studies have assessed safety of various exercise intensities and timing of interventions, many studies have shown a high dropout rate and the fact that patients with lung cancer are sedentary.[67,96,99] Unfortunately, inactivity can spiral into a cycle of decreased muscle mass, weakness, deconditioning, further limiting a patient's ability to maintain an HRQoL, tolerate cancer treatment, or participate in physical activity.[100,101] Frailty is associated with falls, increased hospitalizations, and mortality.[102] Given the medical complexity and fragility of these patients, it is imperative to better understand the cardiopulmonary fitness of these patients, disease staging, side effects of current and prior cancer treatments, and comorbidities in order to develop a safe yet effective exercise program.

Considerations such as load and intensity of training are difficult to generalize to the lung cancer patient population due to varying oncologic sequelae. Stigt et al. noted increased pain and other limitations among lung cancer patients with an early postoperative physical activity regimen.[103] Special considerations in this oncologic population include reduced activity tolerance, fatigue, oxygen dependence, cardiovascular complications related to disease and its treatment, low blood values, bone pain, and gait disturbance due to neuropathy (see Fig. 8.2).

Cardiopulmonary	Fatigue, oxygen dependence, cardiac complications related to chemotherapy and radiotherapy, reduced pulmonary function
Neurological	Neuropathy, gait disturbance, brain metastases, spine metastases
Musculoskeletal	Arthralgia related to certain treatment, Postsurgical chest wall pain, reduced muscle mass (sarcopenia, cachexia)
Bone Health	Bone and spine Metastases
Psychology/ Behavioral	Increased anxiety, depression and sleep disorder, reduced motivation
Vascular	Edema, thrombosis risk
Other	Poor nutrition, weight loss, anemia
Exercise/ activity level	Reduced activity tolerance

FIG. 8.2 Cancer-related and treatment-related special considerations in patients with lung cancer.

While home-based programs are cost-effective, having a physical therapy guided exercise session can optimize technique and safety.[22] Patients with extreme fatigue and low cardiorespiratory fitness should only be recommended for low intensity exercise training.[104] Monitoring and checking vital signs, collaborating with cardiology, and assessing need for an echocardiogram may be warranted in patients who have received cardiotoxic chemotherapy or received thoracic radiation. In addition, assessing for edema and other signs for heart disease are also warranted, to check for symptoms of cardiac dysfunction.[105]

Bone metastases are common in lung cancer, and can result in pain, fracture, spinal cord compression, and other skeletal-related events.[106] Weight-bearing activities can have the benefits of improving mobility and improving bone density, but among patients with known bone metastases, caution must be taken as mobility can be challenging due to pain and fracture risk. Impairment-driven cancer rehabilitation: an essential component of quality care and survivorship.[107] Patients may need to offload affected limbs due to fracture risk, using assistive devices or orthoses for safe mobility.

FUTURE DIRECTIONS

Exercise therapy represents a low-cost way to improve cancer-related and treatment-related symptoms, as well as potentially outcomes in lung cancer. Results from a survey by Philip et al. showed that most patients desire physical activity advice from a physician before starting cancer treatment.[108] While the lack of consensus makes clinical recommendations for physical activity and exercise challenging, utilizing guidance from physical and occupational therapists, as well as expertise from cancer rehabilitation providers, can be instrumental in better assessing patient's functional limitations.

Cancer rehabilitation and exercise programs emphasizing on specific considerations related to lung cancer and its treatments should be created and further studied in larger research studies. This patient population is heterogenous given multiple comorbidities, dynamic health status, and treatment-related side effects. All of these details need to be considered when starting a physical activity or exercise program. An interdisciplinary team may consist of nutritionists, physical therapists, occupational therapist, speech therapists, psychologists, surgeons, oncologists, case managers, exercise physiologists, and cancer rehabilitation physicians. Nutritional counseling may help address sarcopenia and muscle wasting. A social worker or psychologist may play a role in behavioral adaptations such as smoking cessation.[85] Optimized collaboration between oncologists, cancer rehabilitation physicians, and exercise specialists may assist in creating exercise programs that fit patient's needs.

Telehealth care is being used increasingly to provide monitoring and home-based exercise programs to postoperative patients.[109,110] Further adaptability of implementing telemedicine options, as well as activity trackers, should be investigated.

SAMPLE EXERCISE PRESCRIPTIONS
Sample 1

Patient background: 75-year-old woman with COPD not on home oxygen, 50 pack-year smoking history, with newly diagnosed left lung tumor found to be NSCLC, pending surgery for partial lung resection. She has had a recent 20-pound weight loss, decreased activity due to fatigue, and dyspnea.

Indication: Optimize aerobic conditioning prior to lung surgery.

Precautions: falls, risk for desaturation (hold for activity/exercises where O_2 saturation drops below 90%)

Rx: endurance training, gait and balance training, core and hip girdle strengthening, and teach breathing techniques that will be useful in the immediate postoperative period.

Sample 2

Patient background: 75-year-old gentleman with metastatic small cell lung cancer, s/p left hip hemiarthroplasty 2 weeks ago for pathologic femur fracture, pending starting radiation therapy to the area as well. He has chemotherapy-induced peripheral neuropathy, previously systemically treated with cisplatin and etoposide 1 year ago. He has had radiation treatment at T3-5, L5, left lower ribs, and right humerus at all his known sites of bony metastasis. Overall, his activity tolerance has been limited by cancer-related fatigue and postoperative pain.

Indication: Optimize mobility in the setting of left hemiarthroplasty.

Precautions: falls, sensory, spine, left posterior hip.

Rx: gait and balance training, core and hip girdle strengthening, energy conservation techniques, transfer training with caregiver support, and family training.

REFERENCES

1. Bray F, Ferlay J, Soerjomataram I, et al. Global cancer statistics 2018: globocan estimates of incidence and mortality worldwide for 36 cancers in 185 countries. *CA Cancer J Clin.* 2018;68:394–424.
2. Winningham ML, MacVicar MG, Burke CA. Exercise for cancer patients: guidelines and precautions. *Phys Sportsmed.* 1986;14:125–134.
3. Janssen SM, Abbink JJ, Lindeboom R, Vliet Vlieland TP. Outcomes of pulmonary rehabilitation after treatment for non-small cell lung cancer stages I to IIIa: an observational study. *J Cardiopulm Rehabil Prev.* 2017;37(1):65–71.
4. Spruit MA, Janssen PP, Willemsen SC, et al. Exercise capacity before and after an 8-week multidisciplinary inpatient rehabilitation program in lung cancer patients: a pilot study. *Lung Cancer.* 2006;52:257–260.
5. Jastrzebski D, Zebrowska A, Rutkowsdi S, et al. Pulmonary rehabilitation with a stabilometric platform after thoracic surgery: a preliminary report. *J Hum Kinet.* 2018;65:79–87.
6. Physical Activity Guidelines Advisory Committee. *Physical Activity Guidelines Advisory Committee Scientific Report.* Washington, DC: U.S. Department of Health and Human Services; 2018.
7. Letizmann MF, Koebnick C, Abnet C, et al. Prospective study of physical activity and lung cancer by histologic type in current, former, and never smokers. *Am J Epidemiol.* 2009;169(5):542–553.
8. Brenner D, Yannitsos D, Farris M, Johansson M, Friedenreich C. Leisure-time physical activity and lung cancer risk: a systematic review and meta-analysis. *Lung Cancer.* 2016;95:17–27.
9. Granger CL, McDonald CF, Irving L, et al. Low physical activity levels and functional decline in individuals with lung cancer. *Lung Cancer.* 2014;83(2):292–299.
10. Schmid D, Leitzmann MF. Television viewing and time spent sedentary in relation to cancer risk: a meta-analysis. *J Natl Cancer Inst.* 2014;106(7):dju098.
11. Shen D, Mao W, Liu T, et al. Sedentary behavior and incident cancer: a meta-analysis of prospective studies. *PLoS One.* 2014;9(8):e105709.
12. Wang A, Qin F, Hedlin H, et al. Physical activity and sedentary behavior in relation to lung cancer incidence and mortality in older women: the Women's Health Initiative. *Int J Cancer.* 2016;139(10):2178–2192.
13. Schmitz KH, Courneya KS, Matthews C, et al. American College of Sports Medicine roundtable on exercise guidelines for cancer survivors. *Med Sci Sports Exerc.* 2010;42:1409–1426.
14. Hung R, Krebs P, Coups EJ, et al. Fatigue and functional impairment in early-stage non-small cell lung cancer survivors. *J Pain Symptom Manag.* 2011;41(2):426–435.
15. Jones LW, Eves ND, Haykowsky M, Freedland SJ, Mackey JR. Exercise intolerance in cancer and the role of exercise therapy to reverse dysfunction. *Lancet Oncol.* 2009;10(6):598–605.
16. Campbell K, Winters-Stone KM, Wiskemann J, et al. Exercise guidelines for cancer survivors: consensus statement from international multidisciplinary roundtable. *Med Sci Sports Exerc.* 2019;51(11):2375–2390.
17. Muehling BM, Halter GL, Schelzig H, et al. Reduction of postoperative pulmonary complications after lung surgery using a fast-track clinical pathway. *Eur J Cardio Thorac Surg.* 2008;34(1):174–180.
18. Pinto A, Faiz O, Davis R, et al. Surgical complications and their impact on patients' psychosocial well-being: a systematic review and meta-analysis. *BMJ Open.* 2016;6(2):e007224.
19. Loewen GM, Watson D, Kohman L, et al. Preoperative exercise VO2 measurement for lung resection candidates: results of Cancer and Leukemia Group B Protocol 9238. *J Thorac Oncol.* 2007;2(7):619–625.
20. Bobbio A, Chetta A, Carbognani P, et al. Changes in pulmonary function test and cardio-pulmonary exercise capacity in COPD patients after lobar pulmonary resection. *Eur J Cardio Thorac Surg.* 2005;28(5):754–758.
21. Degraff Jr AC, Taylor HF, Ord JW, et al. Exercise limitation following extensive pulmonary resection. *J Clin Oncol.* 1965;44:1514–1522.
22. Bade BC, Thomas DD, Scott JB, Silvestri GA. Increasing physical activity and exercise in lung cancer: reviewing safety, benefits, and application. *J Thorac Oncol.* 2015;10(6):861–871.
23. Caspersen CJ, Powell KE, Christenson GM. Physical activity, exercise, and physical fitness: definitions and

distinctions for health-related research. *Publ Health Rep.* 1985;100(2):126−131.

24. Avancini A, Sartori G, Gkountakos A, et al. Physical activity and exercise in lung cancer care: will promises be fulfilled? *Oncol.* 2020;25:e555−e569.

25. Jones LW, Eves ND, Mackey JR, et al. Safety and feasibility of cardiopulmonary exercise testing in patients with advanced cancer. *Lung Cancer.* 2007;55(2):225−232.

26. Fleg JL, Piña IL, Balady GJ, et al. Assessment of functional capacity in clinical and research applications: an advisory from the Committee on Exercise, Rehabilitation, and Prevention, Council on Clinical Cardiology, American Heart Association. *Circulation.* 2000;102(13):1591−1597.

27. Sloan JA, Cheville AL, Liu H, et al. Impact of self-reported physical activity and health promotion behaviors on lung cancer survivorship. *Health Qual Life Outcome.* 2016;14(1):66.

28. Granger CL, McDonald CF, Parry SM, et al. Functional capacity, physical activity and muscle strength assessment of individuals with non-small cell lung cancer: a systematic review of instruments and their measurement properties. *BMC Cancer.* 2013;13:135.

29. Dajczman E, Wardini R, Kasymjanova G, Préfontaine D, Baltzan MA, Wolkove N. Six-minute walk distance is a predictor of survival in patients with chronic obstructive pulmonary disease undergoing pulmonary rehabilitation. *Cancer Res J.* 2015;22(4):225−229.

30. Kasymjanova G, Correa JA, Kreisman H, et al. Prognostic value of the six-minute walk in advanced non-small cell lung cancer. *J Thorac Oncol.* 2009;4(5):602−607.

31. Edbrooke L, Granger CL, Denehy L. Physical activity for people with lung cancer. *Aust J Gen Pract.* 2020;49(4):175−181.

32. Ross RM. ATS/ACCP statement on cardiopulmonary exercise testing. *Am J Respir Crit Care Med.* 2003;167:1451. author reply 1451.

33. Leduc C, Antoni D, Charloux A, Falcoz PE, Quoix E. Comorbidities in the management of patients with lung cancer. *Eur Respir J.* 2017;49.

34. Loganathan RS, Stover DE, Shi W, Venkatraman E. Prevalence of COPD in women compared to men around the time of diagnosis of primary lung cancer. *Chest.* 2006;129:1305−1312.

35. Wang JS, Abboud RT, Wang LM. Effect of lung resection on exercise capacity and on carbon monoxide diffusing capacity during exercise. *Chest.* 2006;129(4):863−872.

36. Linhas A, Campainha S, Conde S, et al. Changes in pulmonary function in lung cancer patients after thoracic surgery. *J Thorac Oncol.* 2017;12:S611−S612.

37. Lopez Guerra JL, Gomez DR, Zhuang Y, et al. Changes in pulmonary function after three-dimensional conformal radiotherapy intensity-modulated radiotherapy, or proton beam therapy for non-small cell lung cancer. *Int J Radiat Oncol Biol Phys.* 2012;83:e537−e543.

38. Rivera MP, Detterbeck FC, Sacinski MA, et al. Impact of preoperative chemotherapy on pulmonary function tests in resectable early-stage non-small-cell lung cancer. *Chest.* 2009;135:1588−1595.

39. Brunelli A, Xiumé F, Refai M, et al. Evaluation of expiratory volume, diffusion capacity, and exercise tolerance following major lung resection: a prospective follow-up analysis. *Chest.* 2007;131(1):141−147.

40. Timmerman JG, Dekker-van Weering MGH, Stuiver MM, et al. Ambulant monitoring and web-accessible home-based exercise program during outpatient follow-up for resected lung cancer survivors: actual use and feasibility in clinical practice. *J Cancer Surviv.* 2017;11(6):720−731.

41. Pujol JL, Quantin X, Chakra M. Cardiorespiratory fitness in patients with advanced non-small cell lung cancer: why is this feature important to evaluate? Can it be improved? *J Thorac Oncol.* 2009;4(5):565−567.

42. Feinstein MB, Krebs P, Coups EJ, et al. Current dyspnea among long-term survivors of early-stage non-small cell lung cancer. *J Thorac Oncol.* 2010;5(8):1221−1226.

43. Srdic D, Plestina S, Sverko-Peternac A, et al. Cancer cachexia, sarcopenia and biochemical markers in patients with advanced non-small cell lung cancer—chemotherapy toxicity and prognostic value. *Support Care Cancer.* 2016;24(11):4495−4502.

44. Baracos VE, Reiman T, Mourtzakis M, Gioulbasanis I, Antoun S. Body composition in patients with non-small cell lung cancer: a contemporary view of cancer cachexia with the use of computed tomography image analysis. *Am J Clin Nutr.* 2010;91(4):1133S−1137S.

45. Fearon K, Strasser F, Anker SD, et al. Definition and classification of cancer cachexia: an international consensus. *Lancet Oncol.* 2011;12(5):489−495.

46. Edbrooke L, Aranda S, Granger CL, et al. Multidisciplinary home-based rehabilitation in inoperable lung cancer: a randomised controlled trial. *Thorax.* 2019;78(8):787−796.

47. Nattenmuller J, Wochner R, Muley T, et al. Prognostic impact of CT-quantified muscle and fat distribution before and after first line-chemotherapy in lung cancer patients. *PLoS One.* 2017;12:e0169136.

48. Lakoski SG, Eves ND, Douglas PS, Jones LW. Exercise rehabilitation in patients with cancer. *Nat Rev Clin Oncol.* 2012;9(5):288−296.

49. Bovelli D, Plataniotis G, Roila F, ESMO Guidelines Working Group. Cardiotoxicity of chemotherapeutic agents and radiotherapy-related heart disease: ESMO Clinical Practice Guidelines. *Ann Oncol.* 2010;21(Suppl 5):v277−v282.

50. Iyer S, Taylor-Stokes G, Roughley A. Symptom burden and quality of life in advanced non-small cell lung cancer patients in France and Germany. *Lung Cancer.* 2013;81(2):288−293.

51. Kartolo A, Cheng S, Petrella T. Motivation and preferences of exercise programmes in patients with inoperable metastatic lung cancer: a need assessment. *Support Care Cancer.* 2016;24(1):129−137.

52. Granger CL, Parry SM, Edbrooke L, et al. Improving the delivery of physical activity services in lung cancer: a qualitative representation of the patient's perspective. *Eur J Cancer Care.* 2019;28(1).

53. Ashcraft KA, Peace RM, Betof AS, et al. Efficacy and mechanisms of aerobic exercise on cancer initiation, progression, and metastasis: a critical systematic review of in vivo preclinical data. *Cancer Res.* 2016;76:4032−4050.

54. Cramp F, Byron-Daniel J. Exercise for the management of cancer-related fatigue in adults. *Cochrane Database Syst Rev.* 2012;11:CD006145.

55. Hanahan D, Weinberg RA. Hallmarks of cancer: the next generation. *Cell.* 2011;144:646−674.

56. Alves CRR, das Neves W, Tobias GC, et al. High intensity interval training slows down tumor progression in mice bearing Lewis lung carcinoma. *J Cachexia Sarcopenia Muscle.* 2018;1:60.

57. Higgins KA, Park D, Lee GY, et al. Exercise-induced lung cancer regression: mechanistic findings from a mouse model. *Cancer.* 2014;120:3302−3310.

58. Pedersen L, Idorn M, Olofsson GH, et al. Voluntary running suppresses tumor growth through epinephrine- and IL-6-dependent NK cell mobilization and redistribution. *Cell Metabol.* 2016;23:554−562.

59. Liu J, Chen P, Wang R, Yuan Y, Wang X, Li C. Effect of tai chi on mononuclear cell functions in patients with non-small cell lung cancer. *BMC Compl Alternative Med.* 2015; 15:3.

60. Peel JB, Sui X, Adams SA, Hébert JR, Hardin JW, Blair SN. A prospective study of cardiorespiratory fitness and breast cancer mortality. *Med Sci Sports Exerc.* 2009;41(4): 742−748.

61. Peel JB, Sui X, Matthews CE, et al. Cardiorespiratory fitness and digestive cancer mortality: findings from the aerobics center longitudinal study. *Cancer Epidemiol Biomarkers Prev.* 2009;18(4):1111−1117.

62. Myers J, Prakash M, Froelicher V, Do D, Partington S, Atwood JE. Exercise capacity and mortality among men referred for exercise testing. *N Engl J Med.* 2002; 346(11):793−801.

63. Jones LW, Watson D, Herndon 2nd JE, et al. Peak oxygen consumption and long-term all-cause mortality in non-small cell lung cancer. *Cancer.* 2010;116(20): 4825−4832.

64. Blanchon F, Grivaux M, Asselain B, et al. 4-year mortality in patients with non-small-cell lung cancer: development and validation of a prognostic index. *Lancet Oncol.* 2006; 7(10):829−836.

65. Johnson Z, Schiller. E1594 − a randomized phase III trial in metastatic non-small cell lung cancer (NSCLC) − outcome of PS 2 patients (Pts): an Eastern Cooperative Oncology Group Trial (ECOG). *Progr Proc Am Soc Clin Oncol.* 1999;18:461a.

66. Spruit MA, Singh SJ, Garvey C, et al. An official American Thoracic Society/European Respiratory Society statement: key concepts and advances in pulmonary rehabilitation. *Am J Respir Crit Care Med.* 2013;188(8):e13−e64.

67. Temel JS, Greer JA, Goldberg S, et al. A structured exercise program for patients with advanced non-small cell lung cancer. *J Thorac Oncol.* 2009;4(5):595−601.

68. Kuehr L, Wiskemann J, Abel U, Ulrich CM, Hummler S, Thomas M. Exercise in patients with non-small cell lung cancer. *Med Sci Sports Exerc.* 2014;46(4):656−663.

69. Tarumi S, Yokomise H, Gotoh M, et al. Pulmonary rehabilitation during induction chemoradiotherapy for lung cancer improves pulmonary function. *J Thorac Cardiovasc Surg.* 2015;149(2):569−573.

70. Cavalheri V, Tahirah F, Nonoyama M, Jenkins S, Hill K. Exercise training for people following lung resection for non-small cell lung cancer - a Cochrane systematic review. *Cancer Treat Rev.* 2014;40(4):585−594.

71. Chen HM, Tsai CM, Wu YC, et al. Effect of walking on circadian rhythms and sleep quality of patients with lung cancer: a randomised controlled trial. *Br J Cancer.* 2016;115:1304−1312.

72. Mustian KM, Alfano CM, Heckler C, et al. Comparison of pharmaceutical, psychological, and exercise treatments for cancer-related fatigue: a meta-analysis. *JAMA Oncol.* 2017;3(7):961−968.

73. Handy Jr JR, Asaph JW, Skokan L, et al. What happens to patients undergoing lung cancer surgery? Outcomes and quality of life before and after surgery. *Chest.* 2002; 122(1):21−30.

74. Kim HK, Lee YJ, Han KN, et al. Pulmonary function changes over 1 year after lobectomy in lung cancer. *Respir Care.* 2016;61:376−382.

75. Kim SJ, Lee YJ, Park JS, et al. Changes in pulmonary function in lung cancer patients after video-assisted thoracic surgery. *Ann Thorac Surg.* 2015;99:210−217.

76. Jones LW. Effects of presurgical exercise training on cardiorespiratory fitness among patients undergoing thoracic surgery for malignant lung lesions. *Cancer.* 2007;110:590−598.

77. Silver JK, Baima J. Cancer prehabilitation: an opportunity to decrease treatment-related morbidity, increase cancer treatment options, and improve physical and psychological health outcomes. *Am J Phys Med Rehabil.* 2013;92(8): 715−727.

78. Dalal HM, Zawada A, Jolly K, Moxham T, Taylor RS. Home based versus centre based cardiac rehabilitation: Cochrane systematic review and meta-analysis. *BMJ.* 2010;340:b5631.

79. Cavalheri V, Granger C. Preoperative exercise training for patients with non-small cell lung cancer. *Cochrane Database Syst Rev.* 2017;6(6):CD012020.

80. Licker M, Karenovics W, Diaper J, et al. Short-term preoperative high-intensity interval training in patients awaiting lung cancer surgery: a randomized controlled trial. *J Thorac Oncol.* 2017;12(2):323−333.

81. Arbane G. Effect of postoperative physical training on activity after curative surgery for non-small cell lung cancer: a multicentre randomised controlled trial. *Physiotherapy.* 2014;100:100−107.

82. Sterzi S. Post-operative rehabilitation for surgically resected non-small cell lung cancer patients: serial pulmonary functional analysis. *J Rehabil Med.* 2013;45:911−915.

83. Henke CC, Cabri J, Fricke L, et al. Strength and endurance training in the treatment of lung cancer patients in stages IIIA/IIIB/IV. *Support Care Cancer*. 2014;22(1):95–101.

84. Rivas-Perez H, Nana-Sinkam P. Integrating pulmonary rehabilitation into the multidisciplinary management of lung cancer: a review. *Respir Med*. 2015;109(4):437–442.

85. Sommer MS, Trier K, Vibe-Petersen J, et al. Perioperative rehabilitation in operable lung cancer patients (PRO-LUCA): a feasibility study. *Integr Cancer Ther*. 2016; 15(4):455–466.

86. Brunelli A, Kim AW, Berger KI, Addrizzo-Harris DJ. Physiologic evaluation of the patient with lung cancer being considered for resectional surgery: diagnosis and management of lung cancer, 3rd ed: American College of Chest Physicians evidence-based clinical practice guidelines. *Chest*. 2013;143(5 Suppl):e166S–e190S.

87. Leach HJ, Devonish JA, Bebb DG, Krenz KA, Culos-Reed SN. Exercise preferences, levels and quality of life in lung cancer survivors. *Support Care Cancer*. 2015;23: 3239–3247.

88. Molassiotis A, Smith JA, Mazzone P, Blackhall F, Irwin RS, Panel CEC. Symptomatic treatment of cough among adult patients with lung cancer: CHEST guideline and expert panel report. *Chest*. 2017;151:861–874.

89. Quist M, Sommer MS, Vibe-Petersen J, et al. Early initiated postoperative rehabilitation reduces fatigue in patients with operable lung cancer: a randomized trial. *Lung Cancer*. 2018;126:125–132.

90. Cheville AL, Kollasch J, Vandenberg J, et al. A home-based exercise program to improve function, fatigue, and sleep quality in patients with Stage IV lung and colorectal cancer: a randomized controlled trial. *J Pain Symptom Manag*. 2013;45(5):811–821.

91. Cheville AL, Dose AM, Basford JR, Rhudy LM. Insights into the reluctance of patients with late-stage cancer to adopt exercise as a means to reduce their symptoms and improve their function. *J Pain Symptom Manag*. 2012;44(1):84–94.

92. Oldervoll LM, Loge JH, Paltiel H, et al. Are palliative cancer patients willing and able to participate in a physical exercise program? *Palliat Support Care*. 2005;3(4):281–287.

93. Turner K, Tookman A, Bristowe K, Maddocks M. 'I am actually doing something to keep well. That feels really good': experiences of exercise within hospice care. *Prog Palliat Care*. 2016;24(4):204–212.

94. Bade BC, Brooks MC, Nietert SB, et al. Assessing the correlation between physical activity and quality of life in advanced lung cancer. *Integr Cancer Ther*. 2018;17(1):73–79.

95. Jensen W, Bialy L, Ketels G, Baumann FT, Bokemeyer C, Oechsle K. Physical exercise and therapy in terminally ill cancer patients: a retrospective feasibility analysis. *Support Care Cancer*. 2014;22:1261–1268.

96. Andersen AH, Vinther A, Poulsen LL, Mellemgaard A. Do patients with lung cancer benefit from physical exercise? *Acta Oncol*. 2011;50(2):307–313.

97. Granger CL, Connolly B, Denehy L, et al. Understanding factors influencing physical activity and exercise in lung cancer: a systematic review. *Support Care Cancer*. 2017; 25:983–999.

98. Haas BK, Kimmel G. Model for a community-based exercise program for cancer survivors: taking patient care to the next level. *J Oncol Pract*. 2011;7(4):252–256.

99. Cavalheri V, Jenkins S, Cecins N, et al. Exercise training for people following curative intent treatment for non-small cell lung cancer: a randomized controlled trial. *Braz J Phys Ther*. 2017;21:58–68.

100. Granger CL, Chao C, McDonald CF, Berney S, Denehy L. Safety and feasibility of an exercise intervention for patients following lung resection: a pilot randomized controlled trial. *Integr Cancer Ther*. 2013;12(3):213–224.

101. Humpel N, Iverson DC. Review and critique of the quality of exercise recommendations for cancer patients and survivors. *Support Care Cancer*. 2005;13(7):493–502.

102. Retornaz F, Monette J, Batist G, et al. Usefulness of frailty markers in the assessment of the health and functional status of older cancer patients referred for chemotherapy: a pilot study. *J Gerontol A Biol Sci Med Sci*. 2008;63(5): 518–522.

103. Stigt JA, Uil SM, van Riesen SJ, et al. A randomized controlled trial of postthoracotomy pulmonary rehabilitation in patients with resectable lung cancer. *J Thorac Oncol*. 2013;8(2):214–221.

104. Scott JM, Zabor EC, Schwitzer E, et al. Efficacy of exercise therapy on cardiorespiratory fitness in patients with cancer: a systematic review and meta-analysis. *J Clin Oncol*. 2018;36:2297–2305.

105. Maltser S, Cristian A, Silver JK, Morris GS, Stout NL. A focused review of safety considerations in cancer rehabilitation. *PM R*. 2017;9(9S2):S415–S428.

106. Coleman RE. Clinical features of metastatic bone disease and risk of skeletal morbidity. *Clin Cancer Res*. 2006; 12(20 Pt 2):6243s–6249s.

107. Silver JK, Baima J, Mayer RS. Impairment-driven cancer rehabilitation: an essential component of quality care and survivorship. *CA Cancer J Clin*. 2013;63(5):295–317.

108. Philip EJ, Coups EJ, Feinstein MB, Park BJ, Wilson DJ, Ostroff JS. Physical activity preferences of early-stage lung cancer survivors. *Support Care Cancer*. 2014;22(2): 495–502.

109. Dickinson R, Hall S, Sinclair JE, Bond C, Murchie P. Using technology to deliver cancer follow-up: a systematic review. *BMC Cancer*. 2014;14(1):311.

110. McLean S, Protti D, Sheikh A. Telehealthcare for long term conditions. *BMJ*. 2011;342:d120.

CHAPTER 9

Lung Cancer Book—Prehabilitation Chapter

JENNIFER BAIMA, MD

CASE STUDY

A 63-year-old woman with a 30-pack-year history of smoking presented with mid-back pain and was found to have 4 cm right upper lobe mass. She was diagnosed with T3N0 non-small cell lung carcinoma by CT-guided biopsy. She was offered chemoradiotherapy with curative intent. At her multidisciplinary evaluation, she complained of fatigue. CBC revealed hematocrit of 28, MCV of 71, and iron saturation of 3%. She was referred for prehabilitation.

On functional history, she could walk one flight of stairs without shortness of breath at physiatry evaluation. She was not exercising, but was willing to start with a walking program. She was counseled on smoking cessation and was able to wean off cigarettes. The dietician recommended iron supplementation and increased protein intake with examples of iron and protein-rich foods.

She started with a walk of half her 400 m driveway five times a week for the first week, and then was able to walk her whole driveway the second week, even during chemotherapy. She had to rest the third week when she started radiation. She went back to walking half the driveway the fourth week and the full driveway the fifth week. On the eighth week, she was able to walk down the street. By the twelfth week, she could walk one mile. After she finished radiation, she celebrated by walking 2 miles, five times per week. In the beginning, she hated the exercise. Then, her husband started joining her. They both felt better because he felt like that was something he could do to help and she slept better on the days that she walked. She is now in remission and enjoys walking up to 4 miles daily.

INTRODUCTION

A diagnosis of lung cancer carries immediate risks to health in addition to cancer mortality, such as perioperative surgical complications and toxicities of chemotherapy and radiation. More than in any other type of cancer, overall physical and lung function factors into the decision for the type of treatment administered. Improving aerobic function in patients with lung cancer not only improves quality of life, but may improve the efficacy of cancer treatment and prolong life expectancy.

Patients treated with surgery for lung cancer experience a decrease in physical activity.[1] Although types of recommended preoperative exercise are admittedly diverse, a Cochrane review showed that exercise interventions before lung cancer surgery may improve exercise capacity and lung function as well as reduce postoperative complications and hospital length of stay in patients with nonsmall cell lung cancer.[2]

COMMON PHYSICAL IMPAIRMENTS IN PREHABILITATION

In one sample of nonsmall cell lung cancer patients, fatigue was the most common symptom and was present in 100% of the 450 subjects.[3] Loss of appetite, shortness of breath, cough, pain, and blood in the sputum were the other common impairments. Fatigue is particularly amenable to exercise in cancer[4] and prehabilitation may be the best time to start before treatments that have fatigue as a known potential adverse effect.[5] Dietary consultation can be helpful for loss of appetite. Protein supplementation is of particular importance in improving outcomes in cancer.[6] Although shortness of breath can cause patients to be fearful of aerobic exercise,[7] exercise is a known panacea for dyspnea and smoking cessation has respiratory benefits.[8] The potential to decrease pain and expel respiratory secretions are other benefits of prehabilitation.

UNIMODAL AND MULTIMODAL PREHABILITATION

Prehabilitation is defined as "a process on the continuum of care that occurs between the time of diagnosis

Lung Cancer Rehabilitation. https://doi.org/10.1016/B978-0-323-83404-9.00017-7

and the beginning of acute treatment, includes physical and psychological assessments that establish a baseline functional level, identifies impairments, and provides targeted interventions that improve a patient's health to reduce the incidence and severity of current and future impairments."[9]

Surgical prehabilitation has the most evidence, and the most common form of unimodal prehabilitation is exercise.

Unimodal prehabilitation has been used for lung resection as early as 1997.[10] 32 patients with chronic obstructive pulmonary disease were randomized to perioperative exercise or no exercise. The exercise group had incentive spirometry and specific inspiratory muscle training starting 2 weeks before surgery and continuing for 3 months after. Those in the exercise group had better inspiratory muscle strength and lung function after surgery than those without that intervention. Another study extended the duration of preoperative rehabilitation to 4 weeks and measured the preoperative function of an intervention group compared to a control group that got only chest physiotherapy.[11] This more intensive whole body exercise intervention resulted in improved preoperative functional capacity and decreased postoperative pulmonary complications.[11] A third study showed that as little as 7 days of exercise may demonstrate a benefit in lung cancer patients.[12]

In addition to the previously mentioned Cochrane review, at least eight other reviews have examined perioperative function in patients with lung cancer. Preoperative physical therapy was recommended to last 2−4 weeks and should include both aerobic and strength training components.[13] Moderate or greater intensity was important.[14] Supervision and individualization were recommended.[15]

Five[13,15−18] of the reviews recommend preoperative and postoperative exercise interventions equally, while one[19] concluded that preoperative training is more beneficial for both preoperative and postoperative outcomes. One[14] of the five studies did note that postoperative exercise interventions require a longer training period to demonstrate efficacy. Proponents of prehabilitation suggest that not only is a shorter training period required to see benefit before surgery, but that patients are looking for an intervention to improve their outcomes during their waiting time for surgery.[20]

Authors of two of the reviews[18,21] that included metaanalysis found that preoperative exercise training may shorten hospital length of stay and reduce postoperative pulmonary complications. One described improved preoperative lung function[11] and the other[12] cited increased 6-minute walk distance. Both improved lung and overall function may be the mechanism for reduced length of stay and fewer pulmonary complications. The 6 min-walk test is less expensive and easier to measure than lung function, but may not affect the decision to offer surgery, which typically depends heavily on lung function and imaging.

A pulmonary rehabilitation program should ideally include both aerobic and strength training components with a duration of two to 4 weeks.[6] A 4-week graded aerobic program adding 10 minutes per week has been effective in improving the 6-minute walk test in subjects with lung cancer.[11] The rate of perceived exertion can be used to titrate exercise prescription.[22]

Although there are extensive data on the use of exercise in pulmonary prehabilitation, less is known about the other components recommended for successful multimodal prehabilitation.[5] These include nutrition, smoking cessation, psychologic support, and education. Authors of one review article[13] annotated which programs offered multimodal prehabilitation as opposed to unimodal, and this was only one out of the six studies. Exercise was the primary intervention of the unimodal studies and both aerobic and strength training were recommended.

The components of a multimodal prehabilitation program are best used together. For example, exercise is not going to be helpful if the patient does not get enough protein to increase muscle strength. Protein requirements are elevated in cancer. Oncology patients are recommended to consume between 1.2 and 2 gm/kg of protein daily.[6] Whey protein supplements can be particularly helpful postexercise.[6] Patients may be more amenable to dietary changes prior to starting treatments that can affect their appetite.

One pulmonary prehabilitation pilot program that included smoking cessation along with exercise and pharmacologic optimization demonstrated improved exercise capacity in subjects.[23] A review on smoking cessation before lung cancer surgery found six other studies on this topic, but could make no conclusion on benefit.[24] The biggest limitation is that subjects cannot be randomized to quit smoking before surgery. However, there is a plethora of evidence that smoking worsens outcomes in cancer.[25]

Psychologic prehabilitation has been studied in breast, colon, and prostate cancer patients.[26] Many cancer patients suffer psychological distress. Treating underlying mood disorders and cancer-associated adjustment disorders improves wound healing and pain.[26] Examples of psychologic prehabilitation include relaxation techniques and guided imagery.

Patient education is recommended in lung cancer, but outcomes of education as part of a prehabilitation program have not been specifically reported. One documented lung cancer rehabilitation program led by nursing includes the following educational topics: admission and discharge information, physiotherapy, pain management, nutrition, adjuvant treatment, smoking cessation, and information and support services.[27] In-person education is recommended over internet resources for a number of reasons, not the least of which is the readability level of these resources.[28]

Education components dovetail nicely with other components of multimodal prehabilitation. Nutrition may be more relevant to those at the extremes of body mass index, but smoking cessation may be of particular importance for many lung cancer patients. Psychologic prehabilitation may be more effective in those with comorbid mood disorders. Some prehabilitation programs also include optimization of cardiopulmonary or pain medications, correction of anemia, and alcohol cessation.[26] Funding for components other than exercise can be difficult to secure. The best strategy may be patient education as that is the least expensive and often already occurring through the nurse navigator or other team members. Integration of a nurse navigator, who performs the significant proportion of patient education, into the triage process in nonsmall cell lung cancer improves outcomes.[29]

PULMONARY PREHABILITATION IN PRACTICE

The prospective surveillance model in which rehabilitation professionals are involved from cancer diagnosis was developed in breast cancer, and is recommended for use in lung cancer.[30] Screening for impairments by a physiatrist, physical therapist, or occupational therapist early in the cancer care trajectory allows early intervention to document individual changes and improve outcomes. Exercise physiologists have extensive experience in implementing successful deconditioning programs, but are more prevalent in countries with universal health care systems.

In the United States, lung cancer rehabilitation is typical delivered by physiatrists, physical therapists, and occupational therapists. Nurse navigators, psychologists, exercise physiologists, geriatricians, anesthesiologists, and speech pathologists are also part of the cancer prehabilitation team. Incorporation of an exercise provider into the oncology team is the best option for success. When this is not available, referral to a physiatrist, physical therapist, or pulmonary rehabilitation program is the next best option.

Exercise tailored to the individual is best, but group exercise classes may be easier to establish due to the lower cost and allow for peer encouragement. If assessing a patient on an individual basis, the patient can be staged by Activity Measure for Post-Acute Care score to determine their individual exercise prescription.[30] Interventions will differ but are available for those with limited bed mobility and difficulty with transfers all the way through those who are nearly independent. Current exercise guidelines endorse the safety of any exercise over the absence of exercise in cancer.[31]

Barriers to physical activity in lung cancer from a patient perspective include symptoms, ability, motivation, and awareness.[32] Barriers to physical activity from a surgeon's perspective are travel, access to trained exercise professionals, comorbidities, and cost.[33] If barriers can be overcome, prehabilitation may afford lasting improvements.[34] An exercise program that a patient can do at home without equipment is the best place to start. Walking is low impact and inexpensive. A sample unimodal exercise prehabilitation is included in Table 9.1.

TABLE 9.1
Lung Cancer Prehabilitation Walking Exercise Program.

Week	Monday (min)	Tuesday (min)	Wednesday (min)	Thursday	Friday (min)	Saturday	Sunday (min)
1	10	10	10	Rest	10	Rest	10
2	15	15	10	Rest	15	Rest	15
3	20	20	20	Rest	20	Rest	20
4	25	25	25	Rest	25	Rest	25

This program can be changed to suit the patient's walking tolerance, but ten minutes of walking is a good starting Point in the absence of cardiolpulmonary exercise testing. The patient can record their progress and progress by 5–10 min a day or week as tolerated. Oxygen can be worn during work outs and this can be done indoors with a family member or a form of entertainment.
Current minutes per day walking: _____.

THE PREHABILITATION ASSESSMENT
Inclusion Criteria

- FEV1 and/or DLCO <80%
- comorbidities such as chronic obstructive pulmonary disease, tobacco use, obesity, malnutrition, diabetes, and/or hypertension
- patient desire for program
- one to 4 weeks available prior to intervention

Exclusion Criteria

- active or unstable coronary artery disease
- untreated vascular disease
- untreated thromboembolic disease
- altered mental status

Surgical resection is often the best option for survival in lung cancer. Assessment prior to lung cancer treatment typically includes pulmonary function testing (PFT), which should be available for review prior to prehabilitation. Patients with greater than 80% of predicted value of FEV1 (volume exhaled at the end of the first second) and DLCO (diffusing capacity of the lung for carbon monoxide) are typically deemed low risk and will not get further testing.[35] In general, FEV1 can decline 20%–40% after lobectomy and 40% –60% after pneumonectomy.[36] FEV1 or DLCO less than 40% suggests a higher risk for perioperative complications.[37] All lung cancer patients will have imaging as part of their work up. Taken together, PFTs and lung imaging correlate with immediate postoperative complications.[36] The patients in the at-risk group likely benefit more from prehabilitation, but may need to start at a lower level, such as 10 minutes of daily walking as outlined above.

Maximal oxygen capacity and physical fitness predict major postoperative and long-term complications.[36] Maximal oxygen is measured by cardiopulmonary exercise testing.[38] Although this is the gold standard for predicting perioperative mortality,[39] it is not available everywhere and the cost may be prohibitive. Lower cost tests of physical fitness include 6-minute walk, incremental shuttle walk, and stair climbing. Age and neuromuscular conditions may limit the patient's ability to perform these tests.

The 6-minute walk test is well tolerated during lung cancer treatment and has been associated with the following clinical outcomes: likelihood of respiratory failure, $V_{O_2}max$, postoperative complications, and survival (after both surgery and/or chemotherapy).[40] It has been used successfully to measure functional capacity even in subjects with advanced stage lung cancer. All that is required to execute this test is a timer and length of hallway to measure the distance walked in 6 min. This widely available assessment may have the most relevance to pulmonary prehabilitation in clinical practice where cardiopulmonary exercise testing is not easily accessible.

Although the shuttle walk test may correlate with outcomes in lung cancer, it is recommended to be used together with other parameters to improve the accuracy of results.[41] Patients with poor shuttle walk results may have better CPET results so some patients eligible for surgery could be missed if this test is used in isolation.[41] The test is performed by having the subject walk between two cones separated by 10 m at an incrementally increasing pace, stopping when they can no longer keep up.[42]

For the stair climbing test, the inability to climb two to three flights of stairs yields poor prognosis.[43] This test is performed by asking the subject to climb as many steps as possible supervised by a physician until exhaustion, shortness of breath, muscle fatigue, or chest pain.[43] It should not be performed in patients with recent myocardial infarction or known history of ischemic heart disease on effort. The critics of this test note the difficulty to generalize between size and number of stairs in a flight, resulting in limited reproducibility and disagreement on the number of flights that should be the cutoff value. However, it is highly accessible and low cost. It requires more energy than cycling and motivation to finish is higher. In a series of 640 subjects, less than 10% stopped climbing mid-flight (before they reached a landing).[43] Subjects who climbed more than 22 m in this series cost an average of $4174 less in hospital costs than those who did not reach 12m.[43] Remarkably, utilizing the stair climbing test allowed surgeons to operate on 73 of the 640 patients that were considered at prohibitive risk by their pulmonary function tests with a mortality rate within acceptable levels.[43]

For patients who cannot perform any physical test, risk estimation can be done by history. Being able to perform four METS or climb one flight of stairs, mow the lawn, or golf without a cart suggests fitness for surgery.[44] Questionnaires such as the Duke Activity Status Index can be used in lung cancer, but like many of the functional tests, it is not as accurate as cardiopulmonary exercise testing.[45] As with most physical activity, active or unstable coronary artery disease should be assessed and/or treated before physical activity.

COULD PREHABILITATION HAVE A ROLE IN LUNG CANCER SCREENING?

Lung cancer screening with low dose chest computed tomography (CT) has become increasingly available in the United States. Sarcopenia or decreased muscle mass is a known problem in cancer patients that can be observed on CT. Although sarcopenia has traditionally been measured by cross-sectional area of the iliopsoas,[46] it could theoretically be measured on chest CT by measuring the pectoralis muscles.[47] Sarcopenia is important to be aware of because it correlates with poor outcomes in several types of cancer, including lung.[48,49]

In stage I nonsmall cell lung cancer, sarcopenia was a predictor of poor prognosis.[50] Sarcopenia has been associated with increased fatigue and pain in nonsmall cell lung cancer patients.[51] Both cancer and sarcopenia have been associated with frailty in COPD,[52] which affects many lung cancer patients. The only evidence-based treatment for sarcopenia is exercise in the setting of proper nutrition.

STAKEHOLDER PERSPECTIVE

Both surgeons and patients prefer prehabilitation, so starting at the time of lung cancer screening, CT may increase the time available to participate. In a small sample of cardiothoracic surgeons, 91% said they would delay surgery to optimize patients for prehabilitation.[33] Potential benefits were described as improved exercise capacity, decreased length of stay, reduced postoperative complications, improved quality of life, and improved symptom management. In a larger sample of patients with different types of cancer, 32% would prefer to start their exercise before treatment.[53] That survey was done in 2002, before prehabilitation programs were even available. Authors who have implemented 20 such prehabilitation programs since then explain that patients are more motivated to participate when there is a fixed end date, such an established surgical date, rather than a more amorphous goal such as weight loss or increased function, before surgical reassessment.[54]

FUTURE DIRECTIONS IN PULMONARY PREHABILITATION

Telehealth may become increasingly important in areas where there is limited access to optimization prior to lung cancer treatment. In rural areas, patients may struggle with access to primary oncology care. Oncology consultation can now occur and chemotherapy can be administered with remote supervision.[55] Exercise treatments can be delivered along with this care to enhance treatment tolerance and compliance. Improved patient satisfaction in those who are elderly or homebound, even in the palliative care phase of cancer, has been demonstrated with telehealth.[56] A metaanalysis of eight studies of medical oncology care delivered by telephone

or web-based application showed improved quality of life in lung cancer patients.[57] Teleprehabilitation services could be modeled after these programs. This has been successfully accomplished during neoadjuvant therapy in pancreatic cancer.[58]

SUMMARY AND FUTURE DIRECTIONS

- Even as little as 1 week of prehabilitation can make a difference and some successful programs are only 2 weeks.
- Supervised, individualized multimodal prehabilitation with moderate intensity aerobic and strength training exercise may have the most benefit. Group exercise classes are cheaper and may be more easily established.
- Patients could be given a sample home walking program if no supervised program is available. Increasing by 10 minutes per week is based on evidence.[11]
- Education is likely already occurring at little to no additional cost.
- Integration into an established oncologic pathway such as screening or multidisciplinary assessment clinic is best to diminish barriers.
- Biomarkers may be used to measure the effect of exercise in the future. Exercise may change tumor gene expression. In breast cancer, exercise before surgery may improve biomarkers and gene expression.[59]
- Exercise may be used as part of cancer treatment. In colorectal cancer, exercise during chemotherapy and before surgery decreased the size of tumor on MRI.[60]

REFERENCES

1. Granger CL, Parry SM, Edbrooke L, Denehy L. Deterioration in physical activity and function differs according to treatment type in non-small cell lung cancer—future directions for physiotherapy management. *Physiotherapy*. 2016; 102(3):256—263.
2. Cavalheri V, Granger C. Preoperative exercise training for patients with non-small cell lung cancer. *Cochrane Database Syst Rev*. 2017;(6).
3. Iyer S, Roughley A, Rider A, Taylor-Stokes G. The symptom burden of non-small cell lung cancer in the USA: a real-world cross-sectional study. *Support Care Cancer*. 2014; 22(1):181—187.
4. Velthuis MJ, Agasi-Idenburg SC, Aufdemkampe G, Wittink HM. The effect of physical exercise on cancer-related fatigue during cancer treatment: a meta-analysis of randomised controlled trials. *Clin Oncol*. 2010;22(3): 208—221.
5. Santa Mina D, Brahmbhatt P, Lopez C, et al. The case for prehabilitation prior to breast cancer treatment. *PM R*. 2017;9(9):S305—S316

6. Carli F, Gillis C, Scheede-Bergdahl C. Promoting a culture of prehabilitation for the surgical cancer patient. *Acta Oncol*. 2017;56(2):128–133.

7. Giardino ND, Curtis JL, Andrei AC, et al. Anxiety is associated with diminished exercise performance and quality of life in severe emphysema: a cross-sectional study. *Respir Res*. 2010;11(1):1.

8. Pezzuto A, Carico E. Effectiveness of smoking cessation in smokers with COPD and nocturnal oxygen desaturation: functional analysis. *Clin Respir J*. 2020;14(1):29–34.

9. Silver JK, Baima J. Cancer prehabilitation: an opportunity to decrease treatment related morbidity, increase cancer treatment options, and improve physical and psychological health outcomes. *Am J Phys Med Rehabil*. 2013;92: 715Y727.

10. Weiner P, Man A, Weiner M, et al. The effect of incentive spirometry and inspiratory muscle training on pulmonary function after lung resection. *J Thorac Cardiovasc Surg*. 1997;113(3):552–557.

11. Morano MT, Araújo AS, Nascimento FB, et al. Preoperative pulmonary rehabilitation versus chest physical therapy in patients undergoing lung cancer resection: a pilot randomized controlled trial. *Arch Phys Med Rehabil*. 2013;94(1): 53–58.

12. Lai Y, Huang J, Yang M, Su J, Liu J, Che G. Seven-day intensive preoperative rehabilitation for elderly patients with lung cancer: a randomized controlled trial. *J Surg Res*. 2017;209:30–36.

13. Mainini C, Rebelo PF, Bardelli R, et al. Perioperative physical exercise interventions for patients undergoing lung cancer surgery: what is the evidence? *Sage Open Med*. 2016;4, 2050312116673855.

14. Pouwels S, Fiddelaers J, Teijink JA, Ter Woorst JF, Siebenga J, Smeenk FW. Preoperative exercise therapy in lung surgery patients: a systematic review. *Respir Med*. 2015;109(12):1495–1504.

15. Driessen EJ, Peeters ME, Bongers BC, et al. Effects of prehabilitation and rehabilitation including a home-based component on physical fitness, adherence, treatment tolerance, and recovery in patients with non-small cell lung cancer: a systematic review. *Crit Rev Oncol-Hematol*. 2017; 114:63–76.

16. Granger CL, McDonald CF, Berney S, Chao C, Denehy L. Exercise intervention to improve exercise capacity and health related quality of life for patients with non-small cell lung cancer: a systematic review. *Lung Cancer*. 2011; 72(2):139–153.

17. Crandall K, Maguire R, Campbell A, Kearney N. Exercise intervention for patients surgically treated for Non-Small Cell Lung Cancer (NSCLC): a systematic review. *Surg Oncol*. 2014;23(1):17–30.

18. Ni HJ, Pudasaini B, Yuan XT, Li HF, Shi L, Yuan P. Exercise training for patients pre-and postsurgically treated for non–small cell lung cancer: a systematic review and meta-analysis. *Integr Cancer Ther*. 2017;16(1):63–73.

19. Rodriguez-Larrad A, Lascurain-Aguirrebena I, Abecia-Inchaurregui LC, Seco J. Perioperative physiotherapy in patients undergoing lung cancer resection. *Interact Cardiovasc Thorac Surg*. 2014;19(2):269–281.

20. Ferreira V, Agnihotram RV, Bergdahl A, et al. Maximizing patient adherence to prehabilitation: what do the patients say? *Support Care Cancer*. 2018;26(8):2717–2723.

21. Sebio Garcia R, Yanez Brage MI, Gimenez Moolhuyzen E, Granger CL, Denehy L. Functional and postoperative outcomes after preoperative exercise training in patients with lung cancer: a systematic review and meta-analysis. *Interact Cardiovasc Thorac Surg*. 2016;23(3):486–497.

22. Eston R, Connolly D. The use of ratings of perceived exertion for exercise prescription in patients receiving β-blocker therapy. *Sports Med*. 1996;21(3):176–190.

23. Bobbio A, Chetta A, Ampollini L, et al. Preoperative pulmonary rehabilitation in patients undergoing lung resection for non-small cell lung cancer. *Eur J Cardio Thorac Surg*. 2008;33(1):95–98.

24. Schmidt-Hansen M, Page R, Hasler E. The effect of preoperative smoking cessation or preoperative pulmonary rehabilitation on outcomes after lung cancer surgery: a systematic review. *Clin Lung Cancer*. 2013;14(2):96–102.

25. Warren GW, Cummings KM. Tobacco and lung cancer: risks, trends, and outcomes in patients with cancer. *Am Soc Clin Oncol Educ Book*. 2013;33(1):359–364.

26. Scheede-Bergdahl C, Minnella EM, Carli F. Multi-modal prehabilitation: addressing the why, when, what, how, who and where next? *Anaesthesia*. 2019;74:20–26.

27. White J, Dixon S. Nurse led Patient Education Programme for patients undergoing a lung resection for primary lung cancer. *J Thorac Dis*. 2015;7(Suppl 2):S131.

28. Hansberry DR, White MD, D'Angelo M, et al. Lung cancer screening guidelines: how readable are internet-based patient education resources? *Am J Roentgenol*. 2018;211(1): W42–W46.

29. Zibrik K, Laskin J, Ho C. Integration of a nurse navigator into the triage process for patients with non-small-cell lung cancer: creating systematic improvements in patient care. *Curr Oncol*. 2016;23(3):e280.

30. Barnes CA, Stout NL, Varghese Jr TK, et al. Clinically integrated physical therapist practice in cancer care: a new comprehensive approach. *Phys Ther*. 2020;100(3): 543–553.

31. Campbell KL, Winters-Stone KM, Wiskemann J, et al. Exercise guidelines for cancer survivors: consensus statement from international multidisciplinary roundtable. *Med Sci Sports Exerc*. 2019;51(11):2375–2390.

32. Granger CL, Denehy L, Remedios L, et al. Barriers to translation of physical activity into the lung cancer model of care. A qualitative study of clinicians' perspectives. *Ann Am Thoracic Soc*. 2016;13(12):2215–2222.

33. Shukla A, Granger CL, Wright GM, Edbrooke L, Denehy L. Attitudes and perceptions to prehabilitation in lung cancer. *Integr Cancer Ther*. 2020;19, 1534735420924466.

34. Faithfull S, Turner L, Poole K, et al. Prehabilitation for adults diagnosed with cancer: a systematic review of long-term physical function, nutrition and patient-reported outcomes. *Eur J Cancer Care*. 2019;28(4):e13023.

35. Della Rocca G, Vetrugno L, Coccia C, et al. Preoperative evaluation of patients undergoing lung resection surgery: defining the role of the anesthesiologist on a multidisciplinary team. *J Cardiothorac Vasc Anesth.* 2016;30(2):530–538.

36. Licker M, Triponez F, Diaper J, Karenovics W, Bridevaux PO. Preoperative evaluation of lung cancer patients. *Curr Anesthesiol Rep.* 2014;4(2):124–134.

37. Beckles MA, Spiro SG, Colice GL, Rudd RM. The physiologic evaluation of patients with lung cancer being considered for resectional surgery. *Chest.* 2003;123(1), 105S-14S.

38. Win T, Jackson A, Sharples L, et al. Cardiopulmonary exercise tests and lung cancer surgical outcome. *Chest.* 2005;127(4):1159–1165.

39. Levett DZ, Jack S, Swart M, et al. Perioperative cardiopulmonary exercise testing (CPET): consensus clinical guidelines on indications, organization, conduct, and physiological interpretation. *Br J Anaesthesia.* 2018;120(3):484–500.

40. Ha D, Mazzone PJ, Ries AL, Malhotra A, Fuster M. The utility of exercise testing in patients with lung cancer. *J Thorac Oncol.* 2016;11(9):1397–1410.

41. Struthers R, Erasmus P, Holmes K, Warman P, Collingwood A, Sneyd JR. Assessing fitness for surgery: a comparison of questionnaire, incremental shuttle walk, and cardiopulmonary exercise testing in general surgical patients. *Br J Anaesthesia.* 2008;101(6):774–780.

42. Win T, Jackson A, Groves AM, et al. Relationship of shuttle walk test and lung cancer surgical outcome. *Eur J Cardio Thorac Surg.* 2004;26(6):1216–1219.

43. Brunelli A, Refai M, Xiumé F, et al. Performance at symptom-limited stair-climbing test is associated with increased cardiopulmonary complications, mortality, and costs after major lung resection. *Ann Thorac Surg.* 2008;86(1):240–248.

44. King MS. Preoperative evaluation. *Am Fam Physician.* 2000;62(2):387–396.

45. Li MH, Bolshinsky V, Ismail H, Ho KM, Heriot A, Riedel B. Comparison of Duke Activity Status Index with cardiopulmonary exercise testing in cancer patients. *J Anesth.* 2018;32(4):576–584.

46. Prado CMM, Lieffers JR, McCargar LJ, et al. Prevalence and clinical implications of sarcopenic obesity in patients with solid tumours of the respiratory and gastrointestinal tracts: a population based study. *Lancet Oncol.* 2008;9(7):629–635.

47. Kim EY, Kim YS, Park I, et al. Evaluation of sarcopenia in small-cell lung cancer patients by routine chest CT. *Support Care Cancer.* 2016;24(11):4721–4726.

48. Wilson RJ, Alamanda VK, Hartley KG, et al. Sarcopenia does not affect survival or outcomes in soft-tissue sarcoma. *Sarcoma.* 2015;2015.

49. Kim EY, Kim YS, Park I, Ahn HK, Cho EK, Jeong YM. Prognostic significance of CT-determined sarcopenia in patients with small-cell lung cancer. *J Thorac Oncol.* 2015;10(12):1795–1799.

50. Tsukioka T, Nishiyama N, Izumi N, et al. Sarcopenia is a novel poor prognostic factor in male patients with pathological Stage I non-small cell lung cancer. *Jpn J Clin Oncol.* 2017;47(4):363–368.

51. Bye A, Sjøblom B, Wentzel-Larsen T, et al. Muscle mass and association to quality of life in non-small cell lung cancer patients. *J Cachexia Sarcopenia Muscle.* 2017;8.

52. Limpawattana P, Putraveephong S, Inthasuwan P, Boonsawat W, Theerakulpisut D, Chindaprasirt J. Frailty syndrome in ambulatory patients with COPD. *Int J Chronic Obstr Pulm Dis.* 2017;12:1193.

53. Jones LW, Courneya KS. Exercise counseling and programming preferences of cancer survivors. *Cancer Pract.* 2002;10(4):208–215.

54. Shaughness G, Howard R, Englesbe M. Patient-centered surgical prehabilitation. *Am J Surg.* 2018;216(3):636–638.

55. Sabesan S, Larkins S, Evans R, et al. Telemedicine for rural cancer care in North Queensland: bringing cancer care home. *Aust J Rural Health.* 2012;20(5):259–264.

56. Worster B, Swartz K. Telemedicine and palliative care: an increasing role in supportive oncology. *Curr Oncol Rep.* 2017;19(6):37.

57. Pang L, Liu Z, Lin S, et al. The effects of telemedicine on the quality of life of patients with lung cancer: a systematic review and meta-analysis. *Therapeut Adv Chronic Dis.* 2020;11, 2040622320961597.

58. Sell NM, Silver JK, Rando S, Draviam AC, Santa Mina D, Qadan M. Prehabilitation telemedicine in Neoadjuvant surgical oncology patients during the novel COVID-19 coronavirus pandemic. *Ann Surg.* 2020;272(2):e81.

59. Ligibel JA, Dillon D, Giobbie-Hurder A, et al. Impact of a pre-operative exercise intervention on breast cancer proliferation and gene expression: results from the Pre-Operative Health and Body (PreHAB) Study. *Clin Cancer Res.* 2019;25(17):5398–5406.

60. West MA, Astin R, Moyses HE, et al. Exercise prehabilitation may lead to augmented tumor regression following neoadjuvant chemoradiotherapy in locally advanced rectal cancer. *Acta Oncol.* 2019;58(5):588–595.

CHAPTER 10

Cancer-Related Fatigue in Lung Cancer

JASMINE ZHENG, MD • BETTY CHERNACK, MD

INTRODUCTION

The American Society of Clinical Oncology (ASCO) reports that the majority of cancer patients will experience some amount of fatigue during their treatment course.[1] Fatigue can be due to the physical and psychological impacts of cancer and a consequence of cancer-associated treatments such as surgery, radiation, and chemotherapy.[2] Prevalence is reported to range from 25% to 99%,[3] with variability in reported numbers due to varying scales used to evaluate cancer-related fatigue (CRF), differences in quality of analysis and sampling strategies, and the inconsistencies in how fatigue may be experienced in different conditions.[4] Fatigue has a strong association to health-related quality of life.[5] Fatigue has a negative impact on patients' mood, sleep, and quality of life and unfortunately can persist beyond a few months.[3] Approximately two-thirds of those with CRF report that it is severe for at least 6 months, and one-third of those with CRF report that it persists for years after treatment conclusion.[6] In one telephone interview of cancer patients with a prior history of chemotherapy, fatigue was reported to be worse than pain, and disrupted day-to-day activity more than nausea, pain, or depression.[7]

Lung cancer is the second most common cancer among both men and women and the leading cause of cancer death.[8] The 5-year relative survival rate is estimated to only be 19%.[9] Compared to other cancer populations, patients with lung cancer not only have the highest amount of health and existential concerns, but also the greatest number of symptoms.[10] Despite the recent advances in lung cancer treatment, patients experience low quality of life, with fatigue continuing to be a distressing and frequent symptom in this group.[11] A study in 2015 cited relief from fatigue as the most common unmet need in lung cancer patients.[10]

Common treatments for lung cancer such as chemo-immunotherapy frequently lead to fatigue as a side effect.[12] As disease advances, fatigue symptoms typically increase in frequency and intensity as well.[11]

Importantly, symptoms such as fatigue, pain, dyspnea, and sleep disturbance have been related to poor outcomes,[11,13] with symptom burden possibly leading to treatment changes and discontinuation.[14] In addition, multiple studies have demonstrated fatigue to be significantly associated with physical functioning trajectory.[15] Thus, it is vital that clinicians not only recognize the pervasive nature of CRF in lung cancer, but also understand its pathophysiology and treatment options, to help patients maintain a good quality of life and to reduce symptoms that may ultimately affect their ability to tolerate treatments.

DEFINITIONS

The National Comprehensive Cancer Network (NCCN) defines CRF as "a distressing, persistent, subjective sense of physical, emotional, and/or cognitive tiredness or exhaustion related to cancer or cancer treatment that is not proportional to recent activity and interferes with usual functioning."[16] Similarly, the International Statistical Classification of Diseases and Related Health Problems 10th edition (ICD-10) criteria define CRF by presence of diminished energy, increased need for rest beyond what is expected by activity level, and related physical, emotional, and cognitive symptoms. These symptoms must have affected function and/or caused distress to the patient.[17,18] Frustratingly for patients, CRF does not simply resolve with sleep or rest.

When discussing fatigue, it is also worth noting the distinction between two types: peripheral and central fatigue. Peripheral fatigue is independent of the central nervous system and refers to the exhaustion of the neuromuscular and cardiopulmonary systems. Peripheral fatigue is believed to be due to reduction in glycogen stores, sarcolemmal excitability, or cardiopulmonary endurance.[19] Central fatigue refers to deficits in performance that is independent of muscle function, such as problems in memory, concentration, attention, and motivation. Patients may describe themselves as

Lung Cancer Rehabilitation. https://doi.org/10.1016/B978-0-323-83404-9.00001-3

having "brain fog" or "chemobrain," lacking the energy or motivation to begin or sustain tasks.[19] Identifying the types of fatigue a patient suffers from can allow the clinician to develop a more specific treatment plan for the patient.

MECHANISMS

Various mechanisms have been proposed to explain the etiology of CRF, and the development and persistence of CRF. Early and current research supports the idea that there are biological, psychosocial, and medical factors at play. Biological factors include cytokine dysregulation, hypothalamic–pituitary–adrenal (HPA) axis dysfunction, mitochondrial dysfunction, and genetic components.[3]

Cytokine Dysregulation and Inflammation

Inflammation can be triggered in a variety of ways in the lung cancer patient. Common treatments for lung cancer, including surgery, radiation, and chemotherapy, can result in inflammation due to the result of direct damage to tissues. Psychological stress can also increase inflammatory markers. In addition, cancer cells along with stromal and immune cells in the nearby tumor microenvironment, release proinflammatory cytokines.[20] These proinflammatory cytokines include IL-6, TNF-alpha, INF-gamma, and IL-1, the important players in peripheral immune activation. Altogether, these systemic inflammation changes can alter the body's protein and energy homeostasis.

The cytokine hypothesis of CRF has received the most attention and is based on research indicating that proinflammatory cytokines can elicit a change in the brain called the "sickness behavior." The sickness behavior includes changes such as decreased motor activity, social withdrawal, reduced oral intake, and cognitive alterations.[3] Treatment of cancer with cytokines has resulted in increase in fatigue, depressed mood, and sleep disturbances in human studies.[3] There is a strong association among inflammation and lung cancer. In NSCLC patients, high levels of Regulated on Activation, Normal T Cell Expressed and Secreted (RANTES) cytokine at diagnosis have been associated with greater severity of fatigue. Those with lower levels of plasma RANTES were associated with long-term survival, suggesting that those with higher levels of RANTES may experience more intense fatigue and have shorter survival time.[21] In a separate study of nonsmall cell lung cancer (NSCLC) patients undergoing combined radiation and chemotherapy, there was a simultaneous increase in symptom burden and in serum levels of IL-6,

sTNF-R1, and IL-10 at week 8. In addition, there was an association between worsening treatment-related symptoms and the amount of circulating proinflammatory cytokines.[22]

The increase in inflammation in cancer that then leads to CRF is a potential target for treatment. In fact, exercise and physical activity is believed to have a positive effect on chronic low-grade inflammation.[23] Exercise as a treatment will be further discussed later in this chapter.

Mitochondrial Dysfunction and Muscle Fatigue

ATP dysregulation due to impaired mitochondrial mechanisms is hypothesized to be another reason for fatigue in cancer patients. Skeletal muscle requires high levels of ATP for metabolism, and thus, there is an intricate relationship between mitochondrial function and muscle function, strength, and endurance.[24] Chemotherapies are known to target skeletal muscle, with particular predilection for mitochondria, leading to high oxidative stress and lower energy supplies. Muscle fatigue leads to the classic peripheral fatigue symptoms of weakness, reduced endurance, and decreased muscle power.

Proposed mechanisms for the long-term effects on skeletal muscle include damage to DNA that then hinders protein synthesis and cell processes; creation of free radicals that cause cell damage; reduced nuclear DNA transcription; and activation of mitochondrial death.[24] For example, doxorubicin, a chemotherapy used in lung cancer, increases radical oxygen species.[24] Platinum-derived chemotherapy agents, also used in lung cancer, may induce mutations in mitochondrial DNA that can lead to dysfunction and energy imbalances in skeletal muscle.[24] In a study of patients with NSCLC or gastrointestinal cancer, fatigue levels were negatively associated with skeletal muscle mass index.[25]

ATP infusion in patients with NSCLC demonstrated temporary improvements in fatigue and muscle strength.[26] Studies of exercise, including resistance training, found that physical activity is a significant modulator of skeletal muscle and may offset the detrimental effects of lung cancer and cancer treatment.[23] In addition, physical activity may modulate oxidative stress.[27]

Hypothalamic–Pituitary–Adrenal Axis Disruption

Disruption of the HPA axis has also been implicated in CRF. The HPA axis regulates the release of cortisol in response to stress. Cortisol plays a critical role in mediating energy and inflammation, inhibiting cytokine production.[28] Proinflammatory cytokines are stimulators of the HPA axis, and the HPA axis regulates cytokine production via a negative feedback loop. Chronic cytokine exposure results in decreased HPA axis stimulation. This can result in lower cortisol levels; studies have demonstrated the presence of hypocortisolemia in cancer and other chronic inflammatory conditions like rheumatoid arthritis and chronic fatigue syndrome.[29] In addition, lower cortisol levels can disrupt the circadian rhythm, which regulates behaviors such as sleep, body temperature, hormone secretion, and arousal.[29] In addition, cancer and its treatments can also directly alter endocrine pathways.[30]

Genetic Factors

Studies have shown an association between fatigue and various genotypes. In various cancer types, including lung cancer, patterns of fatigue have been associated with a variety of genetic findings. In lung cancer survivors, single nucleotide polymorphisms of IL-1β, IL-1RN, and IL-10 were significantly associated with fatigue levels.[19] In a separate study of NSCLC patients, the IL-8-T251A genotype was found to be associated with pain, depression, and fatigue. In early-stage NSCLC, genetic variants in the IL-10 receptor were significant for fatigue in women.[31]

Risk Factors

Psychosocial, behavioral, and medical factors may put patients at risk for development of CRF. Though much of the research on psychosocial and behavioral risk factors is in nonlung cancer populations, some of the information can likely be extrapolated to lung cancer patients.

Psychosocial and Behavioral

Higher levels of stress, anxiety, and loneliness are associated with fatigue.[20] In a survey study of patients with new diagnosis of lung cancer, approximately 33% of participants reported moderate to extreme amounts of emotional problems, which were significantly associated with reduced quality of life and greater fatigue levels, higher levels of pain, more dyspnea, and more dry coughing.[32] Greater lifetime stress exposure and severity may also be associated with circadian rhythm disruption, which was associated with fatigue. In contrast, those with high social attachment had characteristic changes in their cortisol rhythms, suggesting that social supports can be a buffer against stress or release of cortisol.[33] Other studies have shown that those

with impaired coping mechanisms and who catastrophize tend to have higher levels of fatigue.[34,35]

The relationship between depression and fatigue is not unidirectional, but both depression and fatigue are correlated in cancer populations.[3] In a study of 178 patients with advanced lung cancer, fatigue was the most frequently experienced symptom, but depression was cited by patients as having the greatest impact on their quality of life.[36] In a separate study that examined the effect of fatigue, anxiety, and depression on health-related quality of life in lung cancer patients, fatigue was the main explanatory variable for functional health-related quality of life. Anxiety, along with fatigue, was found to have strong explanatory power for emotional health-related quality of life, whereas depression had a weak power.[37]

SCREENING

CRF is underreported and subsequently undertreated.[38] Adequate screening is critical to identifying those patients who suffer from CRF and who may be at risk of developing CRF to ensure proper treatment is provided. It is recommended that screening for CRF occurs at the initial visit, at regular intervals throughout treatment, and as needed.

There is a lack of consensus on a primary fatigue screening tool and there is a dearth in research to show whether one screening tool is superior to another.[19] Assessment scales can be divided into unidimensional and multidimensional tools. Unidimensional assessment tools include scales such as the Cancer-related Fatigue Distress Scale, the Brief Fatigue Inventory, and the Visual Analog Scale.[39] Multidimensional tools, such as the Multidimensional Fatigue Symptom Inventory, Functional Assessment of Cancer Therapy-Fatigue Subscale Instrument, and the Cancer Fatigue Scale, are commonly used in clinical research.[39]

The NCCN recommends that once fatigue is identified, then determine the degree of fatigue over the last 7 days on a numeric scale (0–10), with mild (1–3), moderate (4–6), or severe fatigue (7–10).[16] Those with no fatigue or mild fatigue can be provided with education and basic management tips with ongoing evaluation at routine clinic visits. Patients with "red flags" such as new or worsening fatigue should be encouraged to reach out to their healthcare provider. Those who rate higher levels of fatigue or with moderate–severe fatigue should trigger a more extensive and thorough work-up of fatigue in addition to being provided with basic educational and management information (see Fig. 10.1).

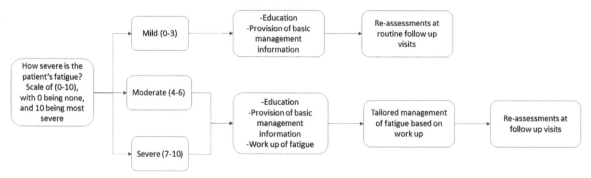

FIG. 10.1 Approach to the patient with fatigue.

APPROACH TO PATIENT WITH CRF

For patients with moderate to severe fatigue, a comprehensive clinical assessment including a focused physical examination, laboratory studies, and pertinent imaging is needed to provide optimal treatment.

History and Physical Examination

The first step to any clinical assessment is to obtain a comprehensive history from the patient. Clinicians should focus on onset of fatigue, duration, temporal pattern throughout the day, alleviating/aggravating factors, and whether the fatigue is getting worse or better over time. Since treatment approaches look to address any reversible causes of fatigue, it is important to review a patient's medications, supplements, past medical history, substance use, and nutritional intake as these can be common culprits. It is also important to note sleep patterns, possible stressors, and level of physical activity. Clinicians should remember to complete a full review of systems so as not to miss out on any underlying medically related contributors to fatigue. Determining current disease status (i.e., in remission, progression, etc.) and whether or not patient is actively receiving cancer-directed treatments such as chemotherapy or radiation is also important as these frequently contribute to fatigue level and have implications for individualized treatment approaches. Finally, clinicians should determine how fatigue is affecting a patient's quality of life and function, noting their current mobility status, and ability to perform Activities of Daily Living and social, leisure, and vocational pursuits.[1,40]

After a detailed history is obtained, a focused physical exam should be completed. For patient's general appearance, clinicians should note any apparent distress, frailty, or cachexia. Working from head to toes, clinicians should assess for dry mucous membranes (dehydration), conjunctival pallor (anemia), and angular cheilosis (vitamin deficiencies). On cardiopulmonary exam, clinicians should evaluate for tachycardia, arrhythmias, cyanosis, tachypnea, and accessory muscle use. A neurological exam can assess for polyneuropathy which may be contributing to fatigue as well as mental status which can reveal an underlying encephalopathy. A musculoskeletal exam should note any atrophy and include evaluation of overall strength with manual muscle testing. A flat or withdrawn affect noted on psychiatric exam may indicate underlying depression, another common contributor to fatigue.

Laboratory Studies

Specific laboratory studies can be helpful in determining potentially reversible underlying contributors to fatigue. A complete blood count with differential is useful in that it can assess for factors related to fatigue such as underlying infection or anemia. A comprehensive metabolic panel can reveal disturbances in sodium, calcium, potassium, magnesium, and glucose which can all contribute to low energy levels. Blood urea nitrogen and creatinine are important to rule out dehydration and renal insufficiency. Underlying hepatic dysfunction as noted by transaminitis and hyperbilirubinemia can also contribute to a patient's fatigue. Low albumin and total protein are markers of nutritional status. Studies such as HgbA1C and thyroid-stimulating hormone can rule out endocrine abnormalities.[1]

Other Diagnostic Testing

In conjunction with specific laboratory studies, focused imaging and other diagnostic testing can also provide the clinician with useful information pertaining to potential contributors to fatigue. Chest radiograph, computed tomography, and positron emission tomography can assess for progression of disease, overall disease burden, and infection, all of which have important implications for a patient's energy levels. Conversely, stable imaging when compared to prior studies allows clinicians to look for alternative causes of worsened fatigue. An echocardiogram and electrocardiogram can determine if poor cardiopulmonary reserve or arrhythmias are involved. Electromyography and nerve conduction studies can assess for underlying neuromuscular disorders.

Ultimately, a comprehensive history, physical examination, and diagnostic work-up are crucial to determining appropriate patient-centered treatment plans (see Fig. 10.2).

Differential Diagnosis

The differential diagnosis for patients with lung cancer who present with fatigue is vast. Fig. 10.3 highlights medical conditions that should be on the clinician's list of differential diagnoses.

TREATMENT

The first step in any treatment approach to a patient with lung cancer who presents with fatigue is to address any reversible contributing factors. Common culprits include sedating medications, poor nutrition, infection, uncontrolled pain, mood disorders, poor sleep, electrolyte or endocrine disturbances, and anemia.[39] If symptoms persist after addressing any easily reversible causes of fatigue, then there are a variety of nonpharmacologic and pharmacologic approaches that can be trialed.

Nonpharmacologic
Education and Counseling

Education and general counseling should be a key treatment intervention for patients with CRF. Patients should be taught how to recognize CRF including its natural history and temporal relation to specific cancer treatments such as chemotherapy and radiation. Clinicians should teach about energy conservation techniques, optimal sleep hygiene, diet, and exercise. Established energy conservation techniques include task delegation, appropriate pacing of activities, and avoiding multitasking. Cognitive behavioral therapy has been shown through high-quality studies to be an effective treatment strategy.[16,41] Patients can be directed to several websites that provide additional resources and educational material including the NCCN, National Cancer Institute, American Cancer Society, and the ASOC's patient information website *Cancer.Net.*

Exercise

Even just a few decades ago, lung cancer patients were advised to rest and limit physical activity. There is now growing evidence that exercise is not only safe for patients with mixed cancer types, but also beneficial for a variety of reasons, including the treatment of CRF.[42–45] In fact, a recent metaanalysis showed that exercise and psychological interventions are significantly better than any pharmacologic options currently being used to treat CRF.[46] The benefit of exercise has been shown to be helpful throughout the cancer continuum, from time of chemoradiation treatments to survivorship or through end of life. Even in the immediate postoperative time period following surgical resection in lung cancer patients, there has been notable improvements in CRF following an exercise program. A two-armed randomized controlled trial of 119 patients with operable NSCLC who initiated early postoperative rehabilitation had significant reduction in fatigue when compared with 116 patients randomized to a late rehabilitation group.[47]

While the majority of literature on exercise as a treatment for CRF is in the breast cancer population or mixed-cancer population, there are several studies and metaanalyses emerging for the lung cancer population. For patients with lung cancer specifically, a metaanalysis of nine prospective single group intervention studies which encompassed 192 participants with lung cancer supported exercise as an effective treatment intervention for CRF and further demonstrated that exercise is safe and feasible for the lung cancer population. Similar to other cancer diagnoses, the metaanalysis revealed no advantage on type or mode of exercise intervention utilized. The authors, however, did advise to interpret the results of their metaanalysis with caution as the studies included were small with total participants ranging between 9 and 29 patients.[48] A more recent review of the literature described multiple studies that supported exercise as an effective treatment intervention for CRF in the lung cancer population, but also noted multiple studies that did not show any significant benefit in reducing fatigue. The authors did note that none of the studies demonstrated that exercise exacerbated fatigue and highlighted the need for additional research.[23] Finally, in their metaanalysis of 14 studies with a total of 694 patients with lung cancer, Yang et al. showed home exercise programs significantly reduced CRF and the authors concluded that home-based exercise programs should routinely be recommended by clinicians and highlighted that they are inexpensive, convenient, and safe.[49]

Fatigue History

Fatigue Onset
Duration
Temporal pattern
Alleviating/Aggravating factors
Trajectory
Central versus peripheral fatigue

Current Medications

Are there pharmacologic agents with side effects that can exacerbate fatigue?
Is there a substance abuse history?

Sleep pattern

Is there a sleep disorder history?
Can sleep hygiene be optimized?

Nutrition

Is there adequate caloric intake?
Are there barriers to nutritional intake and absorption?

Functional History

Is the patient able to complete ADLs and IADLs independently?
What level of independence does the patient have in mobility?

Physical Exam

Assess:
General mobility in and out of the exam room and within the room
Level of distress at rest
Mucous membranes for dehydration
Conjunctival pallor
Rashes and lesions
Cyanosis, tachypnea, use of accessory muscles
Muscle atrophy, strength exam
Reflexes, balance, coordination, sensation
Mental status, executive function, affect

Diagnostic Tests

Check CMP, CBC, TSH, HgbA1c
Review and order pertinent tests such as body imaging, pulmonary function tests, sleep studies,
echocardiograms, electrocardiograms, nerve conduction studies

DEVELOP INDIVIDUALIZED PLAN FOR TREATMENT OF FATIGUE

FIG. 10.2 Suggested approach for the patient with CRF. *CBC, complete blood count; CMP, comprehensive metabolic panel; HgbA1c, hemoglobin A1c; TSH, thryoid stimulating hormone.*

Depression

Anxiety

Infection

Anemia

Dehydration

Electrolyte disturbances (hypokalemia, hyponatremia, hypercalcemia)

Malnutrition

Sedating medication

Illicit substances

Insomnia

Sleep apnea

Neuromuscular disorder

Chronic pain

FIG. 10.3 Differential diagnosis for the patient with CRF.

For the lung cancer population, it remains unclear what specific exercise type, intensity, and frequency is most beneficial. From studies in mixed cancer populations, there appears to be no significant difference between aerobic and resistive exercises in terms of treatment efficacy of CRF. A recent review of exercise interventions for patients with mixed cancers with CRF who were actively undergoing chemotherapy and/or radiation therapy found 13 systematic reviews, 4 guidelines, and 1 evidence summary with high-level evidence for exercise interventions. Based on the high-quality guidelines and metaanalysis review, the authors concluded that while a normal adult exercise intensity is safe for patients during cancer-directed treatments, it is important that all exercise treatment plans be individualized for each patient.[50] In order to individualize an exercise program for a patient, clinicians should note current physical condition, location of tumor(s) and site of surgery/radiation, including any activity restrictions, and most importantly, include frequent reevaluation of patient's response to exercise as his/her condition is likely to change depending on disease/treatment status. Safety considerations are also important. Clinicians must note any bone metastases, hematologic abnormalities such as thrombocytopenia, and brain metastases as exercise in these patients could lead to fracture, bleeding, and falls, respectively. The authors also emphasized that exercise should begin with shorter durations and lower intensity and increase progressively over time with a goal of reaching a normal adult exercise intensity level.[50]

Complementary and Integrative Medicine

There is emerging evidence that complementary and integrative medicine (CIM) treatments can be an effective adjuvant therapy to address CRF as well as a variety of other symptoms in lung cancer patients.[51] CIM approaches include yoga, acupuncture, mind–body modalities, and herbal medicine and have demonstrated variable clinical evidence of effectiveness in patients with lung CRF.

Traditional Chinese medicine (TCM) believes that the pathogenesis of CRF is related to a deficiency of qi and thus the mainstay treatment should aim to replenish qi. There are a variety of TCM injections (TCMJ) that are thought to act by replenishing qi and per TCM beliefs, can dispel knots, and relieve pain.[52] In the lung cancer–specific studies of their metaanalysis, Huang et al. found that the TCMJ group were superior to the control group in improving the fatigue status of CRF patients. Those with lung cancer also had statistically significant improved quality of life with TCMJ.[52]

In their metaanalysis, *Jang* et al. found that acupuncture has therapeutic potential for the management of CRF in mixed cancer survivors. There were 9 randomized controlled trials with a total of 809 participants that met their inclusion criteria. 6 of these studies reported significant improvement in fatigue with acupuncture when compared to control groups and the other three studies showed no significant difference between acupuncture and control groups. In their pooled estimates, Brief Fatigue Inventory scores were lower in true acupuncture versus sham acupuncture groups and in true acupuncture versus usual care.[53] The majority of the studies were conducted with breast cancer patients followed by mixed cancer diagnoses. Only one study was conducted exclusively with lung cancer patients. In this particular randomized, double-blind placebo-controlled pilot trial, acupuncture was found to be an effective treatment strategy for patients with NSCLC. A significant reduction in the Brief Fatigue Inventory score was observed in those patients who received active acupuncture twice weekly for 4 weeks when compared to those receiving placebo. Importantly, there was no increased risk of adverse events and the study demonstrated good compliance with acupuncture treatment.[54]

Herbal medicines are widely used for a variety of symptoms in the cancer population and may have potential therapeutic effects on fatigue. A metaanalysis of 12 RCTs with a total of 861 patients with lung cancer revealed improved fatigue level when herbal medicine was combined with conventional medicine when compared to conventional medicine alone. The authors concluded that herbal medicine can be beneficial for patients with lung cancer who experience fatigue as a part of a comprehensive treatment plan.[55]

There is evidence that yoga can improve CRF; however, the vast majority of the literature is found in the breast cancer population. One recent RCT of an 8-week yoga class intervention did include patients with different types of cancer and found that yoga effectively reduced fatigue; however, only 8%, or 13 patients, of the 159 total participants had lung cancer diagnoses, and those with breast cancer reported higher reduction in fatigue when compared with nonbreast cancer patients.[56]

Finally, there is evidence that a mindfulness-based approach can reduce fatigue in those with breast and mixed cancer,[57−59] but it is currently unclear whether these results can be generalized to the lung cancer population.

Pharmacologic Management

For lung cancer patients with moderate to severe fatigue that is refractory to nonpharmacologic treatments, judicious use of select pharmacologic agents can be considered. Despite limited and mixed evidence, the CNS stimulants methylphenidate and modafinil are often prescribed to patients to reduce CRF. In lung cancer populations specifically, modafinil has mixed evidence for efficacy. Spathis et al. found in their small pilot study of 20 patients with NSCLC that modafinil was well tolerated and resulted in rapid and clinically significant improvement in fatigue.[60] Conversely, a more recent and larger RCT of 160 patients with NSCLC found that modafinil had no effect on CRF although its use was associated with a clinically significant placebo effect. The authors concluded that modafinil should not be prescribed for lung cancer patients for the treatment of CRF.[61] It is important to note, however, that a large

randomized, placebo-controlled, double blind clinical trial of 631 patients with mixed cancer diagnoses on active chemotherapy did find that modafinil improved baseline fatigue in those with severe CRF.[62] Thus, despite lack of evidence in one RCT specific to lung cancer, modafinil can still be considered appropriate for a subset of lung cancer patients with severe fatigue who are currently undergoing active chemotherapy.

Methylphenidate, a central nervous system stimulant and widely used medication for attention deficit hyperactivity disorder, is the most studied pharmacologic agent used to treat CRF for mixed cancer diagnoses. In a metaanalysis of pharmacologic interventions for CRF, methylphenidate was found to significantly reduce fatigue severity. However, the authors noted that risks of anorexia, sleep disturbance, and arrhythmias may not outweigh the potential benefits.[63]

Corticosteroids can be an effective short-term treatment for patients with CRF as shown in a review of two placebo-controlled double blinded RCTs. Due to significant adverse effects of the long-term use of corticosteroids, however, this treatment approach should be limited to those with advanced incurable cancer who are approaching end of life.[64] See Table 10.1 for summary of pharmacologic options in treatment of CRF.

Proposed Multidimensional Treatment Approach

Based on existing ASCO, NCCN, and Canadian Association of Psychosocial Oncology clinical guidelines as well as anecdotally from clinical practice, the authors recommend a holistic, multidimensional treatment approach. These recommendations are outlined in Table 10.2.

ADDITIONAL CONSIDERATIONS
CRF and Prehabilitation

Prehabilitation is defined as the "process on the continuum of care that occurs between the time of cancer diagnosis and the beginning of acute treatment, includes physical and psychological assessments that establish a baseline function, identifies impairments, and provides targeted interventions that improve a patient's health to reduce the incidence and the severity of current and future impairments."[65] Prehabilitation programs for lung cancer may include exercise, nutrition changes, medication management, psychological assessments, and smoking cessation. Many of the current prehabilitation programs in lung cancer are directed toward those who are to undergo surgical resection of

TABLE 10.1
Pharmacologic Treatment for CRF.

Medication	Indication	Typical Dosing	Adverse Effects
Modafinil	Severe fatigue, during active cancer-directed treatment	100 mg daily for 3 days, followed by 200 mg daily	Headache, decreased appetite, abdominal pain, nausea, nervousness, rhinitis, back pain
Methylphenidate	Severe fatigue, palliative care/end of life setting	5 mg once to twice daily (given at 8 a.m. and 1 p.m.); can increase by 5 mg every 3 days up to 40 mg/day	Insomnia, headache, irritability, weight loss, decreased appetite, xerostomia, nausea, tachycardia
Dexamethasone	Fatigue, short duration (weeks); hospice	2–4 mg daily	Infection, weight gain, hyperglycemia, myopathy, avascular necrosis, peptic ulcer, edema, agitation

TABLE 10.2
Multidimensional Treatment Approach for CRF.

Address potential reversible contributing factors

Counsel patients on energy conservation and general fatigue management

Educational sessions on how to recognize CRF including natural history and temporal relation to specific cancer treatments

Exercise
Generally, we recommend moderate intensity physical activity of any type in any setting including aerobic, resistive, aerobic + resistive, yoga, and Tai Chi. Begin with shorter durations and low intensity and increase progressively over time. Goal 150 min per week
Consider lower intensity physical activity/chair-based home exercise programs for those at end of life
Consider a supervised exercise program for those with safety concerns such as thrombocytopenia, bone or brain metastases, weight bearing, or range of motion restrictions

Complementary and integrative medicine as adjunct therapy. Consider acupuncture and mindfulness

Cognitive behavioral therapy for those with underlying anxiety and/or depression

Judicious use of pharmacologic agents
Consider dexamethasone and methylphenidate for hospice population
Consider modafinil for those with severe fatigue currently receiving chemotherapy

their tumor; these patients typically have low cardiopulmonary fitness preoperatively.

Poor physical functional capacity prior to surgery is a predictor of morbidity and mortality postoperatively in lung surgery patients.[66] There is evidence to support the ability of exercise to improve functional capacity and lead to better outcomes, including reduced postoperative complications and shorter length of hospital stays.[67] A recent study that utilized yoga breathing found that patients who used this breathing technique preoperatively had short-term improvement in lung function.[68]

There is limited literature on the impact of prehabilitation on fatigue levels in lung cancer. However, in other studies looking at patient populations with respiratory disease, such as COPD, exercise has been shown to have a positive effect on fatigue.[69] In the breast cancer population, earlier rehabilitation interventions resulted in quicker return to baseline function[70] and stress reduction prior to surgery resulted in lower fatigue levels after surgery.[71] Additional research assessing the link between fatigue and prehabilitation in lung cancer will be useful, as prehabilitation may also be an underutilized opportunity to improve CRF.

Cancer-Related Fatigue at End of Life

Severe fatigue at the end of life can be highly distressing for patients with terminal lung cancer. Uncontrolled fatigue can limit mobility, functional status, and ability for patients to interact with their family and friends. Thus, even during the final days to weeks of life, effective treatment of CRF is essential to ensure the best quality of life possible for our patients with life-limiting disease. Home-based exercise programs have been successful in treating fatigue in patients with stage IV lung cancer. Home-based programs are ideal for those patients enrolled in hospice care as transportation of patients with terminal disease can be especially burdensome.[72] The ASCO guidelines recommend pharmacologic treatment of fatigue with methylphenidate and modafinil for those with advanced disease.[1] Finally, corticosteroids are often prescribed in the hospice setting as they can improve fatigue and a variety of other distressing symptoms and at least in the short term have no significant adverse effects.[64]

CONCLUSION

CRF is an extremely distressing experience that occurs in most lung cancer patients, impairing quality of life and even changing treatment course. Assessing for CRF in the lung cancer population throughout the cancer care continuum is critical to provide appropriate and timely education and treatment options. Diagnosis and treatment should follow a step-wise and multimodal approach, with reassessments of CRF over time as patients' cancer trajectories evolve.

REFERENCES

1. Bower JE, Bak K, Berger A, et al. Screening, assessment, and management of fatigue in adult survivors of cancer: an american society of clinical oncology clinical practice guideline adaptation. *J Clin Oncol.* 2014;32(17):1840.
2. Berger AM, Mitchell SA, Jacobsen PB, Pirl WF. Screening, evaluation, and management of cancer-related fatigue: ready for implementation to practice? *CA Cancer J Clin.* 2015;65(3):190–211.
3. Bower JE. Cancer-related fatigue—mechanisms, risk factors, and treatments. *Nat Rev Clin Oncol.* 2014;11(10):597.
4. Ma Y, He B, Jiang M, et al. Prevalence and risk factors of cancer-related fatigue: a systematic review and meta-analysis. *Int J Nurs Stud.* 2020:103707.
5. Yang P, Cheville AL, Wampfler JA, et al. Quality of life and symptom burden among long-term lung cancer survivors. *J Thorac Oncol.* 2012;7(1):64–70.
6. Fabi A, Bhargava R, Fatigoni S, et al. Cancer-related fatigue: ESMO clinical practice guidelines for diagnosis and treatment. *Ann Oncol.* 2020;31(6):713–723.
7. Curt GA, Breitbart W, Cella D, et al. Impact of cancer-related fatigue on the lives of patients: new findings from the fatigue coalition. *Oncologist.* 2000;5(5):353–360.
8. American Cancer Society. *Key statistics for lung cancer;* 2021. https://www.cancer.org/cancer/lung-cancer/about/key-statistics.html.
9. Siegel RL, Miller KD, Jemal A. Cancer statistics, 2019. *CA Cancer J Clin.* 2019;69(1):7–34.
10. Molassiotis A, Lowe M, Blackhall F, Lorigan P. A qualitative exploration of a respiratory distress symptom cluster in lung cancer: cough, breathlessness and fatigue. *Lung Cancer.* 2011;71(1):94–102.
11. Zhou L, Chen Q, Zhang J. Effect of exercise on fatigue in patients with lung cancer: a systematic review and meta-analysis of randomized trials. *J Palliat Med.* 2021;24(6):932–943.
12. Petrocchi S, Janssens R, Oliveri S, et al. What matters most to lung cancer patients? A qualitative study in Italy and Belgium to investigate patient preferences. *Front Pharmacol.* 2021;12:80.
13. Cheville AL, Novotny PJ, Sloan JA, et al. The value of a symptom cluster of fatigue, dyspnea, and cough in predicting clinical outcomes in lung cancer survivors. *J Pain Symptom Manag.* 2011;42(2):213–221.
14. Cleeland CS. Symptom burden: multiple symptoms and their impact as patient-reported outcomes. *J Natl Cancer Inst Monogr.* 2007;2007(37):16–21.
15. Medysky ME, Dieckmann NF, Winters-Stone KM, Sullivan DR, Lyons KS. Trajectories of self-reported physical functioning and symptoms in lung cancer survivors. *Cancer Nurs.* 2021;44(2):E83–E89.
16. Berger AM, Mooney K, Alvarez-Perez A, et al. Cancer-related fatigue, version 2.2015. *J Natl Compr Cancer Netw.* 2015;13(8):1012–1039. doi: 13/8/1012 [pii].
17. Cella D, Davis K, Breitbart W, Curt G. Fatigue Coalition. Cancer-related fatigue: prevalence of proposed diagnostic criteria in a United States sample of cancer survivors. *J Clin Oncol.* 2001;19(14):3385–3391.
18. World Health Organization. *ICD-11 (International Statistical Classification of Diseases and Related Health Problems, 11th Revision).* 2019. Geneva, Switzerland.
19. Gerber LH. Cancer-related fatigue: persistent, pervasive, and problematic. *Phys Med Rehabil Clin.* 2017;28(1):65–88.
20. Bower JE. The role of neuro-immune interactions in cancer-related fatigue: biobehavioral risk factors and mechanisms. *Cancer.* 2019;125(3):353–364.
21. Umekawa K, Kimura T, Kudoh S, et al. Plasma RANTES, IL-10, and IL-8 levels in non–small-cell lung cancer patients treated with EGFR-TKIs. *BMC Res Notes.* 2013;6(1):1–8.
22. Wang XS, Shi Q, Williams LA, et al. Inflammatory cytokines are associated with the development of symptom burden in patients with NSCLC undergoing concurrent chemoradiation therapy. *Brain Behav Immun.* 2010;24(6):968–974.
23. Avancini A, Sartori G, Gkountakos A, et al. Physical activity and exercise in lung cancer care: will promises be fulfilled? *Oncologist.* 2020;25(3):e555.

24. Yang S, Chu S, Gao Y, et al. A narrative review of cancer-related fatigue (CRF) and its possible pathogenesis. *Cells.* 2019;8(7):738.

25. Kilgour RD, Vigano A, Trutschnigg B, et al. Cancer-related fatigue: the impact of skeletal muscle mass and strength in patients with advanced cancer. *J Cachexia Sarcopenia Muscle.* 2010;1(2):177–185.

26. Agteresch HJ, Leij-Halfwerk S, Van Den Berg J, Hordijk-Luijk CH, Wilson J, Dagnelie PC. Effects of ATP infusion on glucose turnover and gluconeogenesis in patients with advanced non-small-cell lung cancer. *Clin Sci.* 2000; 98(6):689–695.

27. Ashcraft KA, Peace RM, Betof AS, Dewhirst MW, Jones LW. Efficacy and mechanisms of aerobic exercise on cancer initiation, progression, and metastasis: a critical systematic review of in vivo preclinical data. *Cancer Res.* 2016;76(14): 4032–4050.

28. Costanzo ES, Lutgendorf SK, Sood AK, Anderson B, Sorosky J, Lubaroff DM. Psychosocial factors and interleukin-6 among women with advanced ovarian cancer. *Cancer.* 2005;104(2):305–313.

29. O'Higgins CM, Brady B, O'Connor B, Walsh D, Reilly RB. The pathophysiology of cancer-related fatigue: current controversies. *Support Care Cancer.* 2018; 26(10):3353–3364.

30. Macciò A, Madeddu C. Inflammation and ovarian cancer. *Cytokine.* 2012;58(2):133–147.

31. Reyes-Gibby CC, Wang J, Spitz M, Wu X, Yennurajalingam S, Shete S. Genetic variations in interleukin-8 and interleukin-10 are associated with pain, depressed mood, and fatigue in lung cancer patients. *J Pain Symptom Manag.* 2013;46(2): 161–172.

32. Morrison EJ, Novotny PJ, Sloan JA, et al. Emotional problems, quality of life, and symptom burden in patients with lung cancer. *Clin Lung Cancer.* 2017;18(5):497–503.

33. Cuneo MG, Schrepf A, Slavich GM, et al. Diurnal cortisol rhythms, fatigue and psychosocial factors in five-year survivors of ovarian cancer. *Psychoneuroendocrinology.* 2017;84: 139–142. https://doi.org/10.1016/j.psyneuen.2017.06.019. https://www.sciencedirect.com/science/article/pii/S030645 3017300458.

34. Andrykowski MA, Schmidt JE, Salsman JM, Beacham AO, Jacobsen PB. Use of a case definition approach to identify cancer-related fatigue in women undergoing adjuvant therapy for breast cancer. *J Clin Oncol.* 2005;23(27):6613.

35. Jacobsen PB, Andrykowski MA, Thors CL. Relationship of catastrophizing to fatigue among women receiving treatment for breast cancer. *J Consult Clin Psychol.* 2004;72(2): 355.

36. Choi S, Ryu E. Effects of symptom clusters and depression on the quality of life in patients with advanced lung cancer. *Eur J Cancer Care.* 2018;27(1):e12508.

37. Jung JY, Lee JM, Kim MS, Shim YM, Zo JI, Yun YH. Comparison of fatigue, depression, and anxiety as factors affecting posttreatment health-related quality of life in lung cancer survivors. *Psycho Oncol.* 2018;27(2):465–470.

38. Vogelzang NJ, Breitbart W, Cella D, et al. Patient, caregiver, and oncologist perceptions of cancer-related fatigue:

39. Mohandas H, Jaganathan SK, Mani MP, Ayyar M, Rohini Thevi GV. Cancer-related fatigue treatment: an overview. *J Cancer Res Therapeut.* 2017;13(6):916–929. https://doi.org/10.4103/jcrt.JCRT_50_17.

40. Howell D, Keller-Olaman S, Oliver TK, et al. A pan-canadian practice guideline and algorithm: screening, assessment, and supportive care of adults with cancer-related fatigue. *Curr Oncol.* 2013;20(3):233–246. https://doi.org/10.3747/co.20.1302.

41. Bennett S, Pigott A, Beller EM, Haines T, Meredith P, Delaney C. Educational interventions for the management of cancer-related fatigue in adults. *Cochrane Database Syst Rev.* 2016;11. https://doi.org/10.1002/14651858.CD008144.pub2.

42. Schmitz KH, Courneya KS, Matthews C, et al. American College of Sports Medicine roundtable on exercise guidelines for cancer survivors. *Med Sci Sports Exerc.* 2010;42: 1409–1426.

43. Meneses-Echávez JF, González-Jiménez E, Ramírez-Vélez R. Supervised exercise reduces cancer-related fatigue: a systematic review. *J Physiother.* 2015;61(1):3–9. https://doi.org/10.1016/j.jphys.2014.08.019.

44. Tian L, Lu HJ, Lin L, Hu Y. Effects of aerobic exercise on cancer-related fatigue: a meta-analysis of randomized controlled trials. *Support Care Cancer.* 2016;24(2): 969–983. https://doi.org/10.1007/s00520-015-2953-9.

45. McNeely ML, Campbell KL, Rowe BH, Klassen TP, Mackey JR, Courneya KS. Effects of exercise on breast cancer patients and survivors: a systematic review and meta-analysis. *CMAJ.* 2006;175(1):34–41, 175/1/34 [pii].

46. Mustian KM, Alfano CM, Heckler C, et al. Comparison of pharmaceutical, psychological, and exercise treatments for cancer-related fatigue: a meta-analysis. *JAMA Oncol.* 2017; 3(7):961–968. https://doi.org/10.1001/jamaoncol.2016.6914.

47. Quist M, Sommer MS, Vibe-Petersen J, et al. Early initiated postoperative rehabilitation reduces fatigue in patients with operable lung cancer: a randomized trial. *Lung Cancer.* 2018;126:125–132. https://doi.org/10.1016/j.lungcan.2018.10.025.

48. Paramanandam VS, Dunn V. Exercise for the management of cancer-related fatigue in lung cancer: a systematic review. *Eur J Cancer Care.* 2015;24(1):4–14. https://doi.org/10.1111/ecc.12198. Epub 2014 Apr 10. PMID: 24720528.

49. Yang M, Liu L, Gan CE, et al. Effects of home-based exercise on exercise capacity, symptoms, and quality of life in patients with lung cancer: a meta-analysis. *Eur J Oncol Nurs.* 2020;49:101836. https://doi.org/10.1016/j.ejon.2020.101836. Epub 2020 Sep 17. PMID: 33120218.

50. Song J, Wang T, Wang Y, et al. Evaluation of evidence for exercise intervention in patients with cancer-related fatigue during chemoradiotherapy. *J Clin Nurs.* 2021;30(13–14): 1854–1862. https://doi.org/10.1111/jocn.15696. Epub 2021;8.

51. Finnegan-John J, Molassiotis A, Richardson A, Ream E. A systematic review of complementary and alternative

medicine interventions for the management of cancer-related fatigue. *Integr Cancer Ther.* 2013;12(4):276–290.

52. Huang Z, Zhang Q, Fan Y, et al. Effect of traditional Chinese medicine injection on cancer-related fatigue: a meta-analysis based on existing evidence. *Evid Based Complement Alternat Med.* 2020;2020:2456873. https://doi.org/10.1155/2020/2456873.

53. Jang A, Brown C, Lamoury G, et al. The effects of acupuncture on cancer-related fatigue: updated systematic review and meta-analysis. *Integr Cancer Ther.* 2020;19. https://doi.org/10.1177/1534735420949679.

54. Cheng CS, Chen LY, Ning ZY, et al. Acupuncture for cancer-related fatigue in lung cancer patients: a randomized, double blind, placebo-controlled pilot trial. *Support Care Cancer.* 2017;25(12):3807–3814. https://doi.org/10.1007/s00520-017-3812-7.

55. Kwon CY, Lee B, Kong M, et al. Effectiveness and safety of herbal medicine for cancer-related fatigue in lung cancer survivors: a systematic review and meta-analysis. *Phytother Res.* 2021;35(2):751–770. https://doi.org/10.1002/ptr.6860.

56. Zetzl T, Pittig A, Renner A, van Oorschot B, Jentschke E. Yoga therapy to reduce fatigue in cancer: effects of reminder e-mails and long-term efficacy. *Support Care Cancer.* 2021. https://doi.org/10.1007/s00520-021-06345-z.

57. van der Lee ML, Garssen B. Mindfulness-based cognitive therapy reduces chronic cancer-related fatigue: a treatment study. *Psycho Oncol.* 2012;21(3):264–272.

58. Lengacher CA, Reich RR, Post-White J, et al. Mindfulness based stress reduction in post-treatment breast cancer patients: an examination of symptoms and symptom clusters. *J Behav Med.* 2012;35(1):86–94. Epub 2011 Apr 20.

59. Hoffman CJ, Ersser SJ, Hopkinson JB, et al. Effectiveness of mindfulness-based stress reduction in mood, breast- and endocrine-related quality of life, and well-being in stage 0 to III breast cancer: a randomized, controlled trial. *J Clin Oncol.* 2012;30(12):1335. Epub 2012 Mar 19.

60. Spathis A, Dhillan R, Booden D, Forbes K, Vrotsou K, Fife K. Modafinil for the treatment of fatigue in lung cancer: a pilot study. *Palliat Med.* 2009;23(4):325–331. https://doi.org/10.1177/0269216309102614.

61. Spathis A, Fife K, Blackhall F, et al. Modafinil for the treatment of fatigue in lung cancer: results of a placebo-controlled, double-blind, randomized trial. *J Clin Oncol.* 2014;32(18):1882–1888. https://doi.org/10.1200/JCO.2013.54.4346.

62. Jean-Pierre P, Morrow GR, Roscoe JA, et al. A phase 3 randomized, placebo-controlled, double-blind, clinical trial of the effect of modafinil on cancer-related fatigue among 631 patients receiving chemotherapy: a university of rochester cancer center community clinical oncology program research base study. *Cancer.* 2010;116(14):3513–3520. https://doi.org/10.1002/cncr.25083.

63. Tomlinson D, Robinson PD, Oberoi S, et al. Pharmacologic interventions for fatigue in cancer and transplantation: a meta-analysis. *Curr Oncol.* 2018;25(2):e152–e167. https://doi.org/10.3747/co.25.3883.

64. Yennurajalingam S, Frisbee-Hume S, Palmer JL, et al. Reduction of cancer-related fatigue with dexamethasone: a double-blind, randomized, placebo-controlled trial in patients with advanced cancer. *J Clin Oncol.* 2013;31(25):3076–3082. https://doi.org/10.1200/JCO.2012.44.4661.

65. Silver JK, Baima J. Cancer prehabilitation: an opportunity to decrease treatment-related morbidity, increase cancer treatment options, and improve physical and psychological health outcomes. *Am J Phys Med Rehabil.* 2013;92(8):715–727.

66. Pouwels S, Fiddelaers J, Teijink JA, Ter Woorst JF, Siebenga J, Smeenk FW. Preoperative exercise therapy in lung surgery patients: a systematic review. *Respir Med.* 2015;109(12):1495–1504.

67. Shukla A, Granger CL, Wright GM, Edbrooke L, Denehy L. Attitudes and perceptions to prehabilitation in lung cancer. *Integr Cancer Ther.* 2020;19, 1534735420924466.

68. Barassi G, Bellomo RG, Di Iulio A, et al. Preoperative rehabilitation in lung cancer patients: yoga approach. In: *Rehabilitation Science in Context.* Springer; 2018:19–29.

69. McCarthy B, Casey D, Devane D, Murphy K, Murphy E, Lacasse Y. Pulmonary rehabilitation for chronic obstructive pulmonary disease. *Cochrane Database Syst Rev.* 2015;(2).

70. Cinar N, Seckin Ü, Keskin D, Bodur H, Bozkurt B, Cengiz Ö. The effectiveness of early rehabilitation in patients with modified radical mastectomy. *Cancer Nurs.* 2008;31(2):160–165.

71. Garssen B, Boomsma MF, de Jager Meezenbroek E, et al. Stress management training for breast cancer surgery patients. *Psycho Oncol.* 2013;22(3):572–580.

72. Cheville AL, Kollasch J, Vandenberg J, et al. A home-based exercise program to improve function, fatigue, and sleep quality in patients with stage IV lung and colorectal cancer: a randomized controlled trial. *J Pain Symptom Manag.* 2013;45(5):811–821. https://doi.org/10.1016/j.jpainsymman.2012.05.006.

CHAPTER 11

Sarcopenia and Frailty in Lung Cancer

JORDAN STUMPH, MD • FRANCHESCA KÖNIG, MD

INTRODUCTION

In 2020, lung cancer was the second most diagnosed cancer and the leading cause of cancer death worldwide causing an estimated 1.8 million deaths. This disease is broadly divided into two histologic subtypes: small cell (SCLC) and nonsmall cell lung cancer (NSCLCs). The clinical presentation of lung cancer is widely varied but often correlates with anatomic location of the tumor within the bronchial tree. Radiation, chemotherapy, surgery, and targeted therapy can all be employed as treatment options dependent upon many patient and tumor factors.[1] Unfortunately, lung cancer is often diagnosed in advanced stages leading to a high morbidity and mortality in this disease. Clinical outcomes in lung cancer are known to be associated with specific tumor-related factors such as histologic type, size of the tumor, nodal involvement, and evidence of metastases.[2] However, other host factors, such as sarcopenia and frailty status, have also demonstrated significant prognostication of morbidity and mortality among individuals with this malignancy. Sarcopenia is defined as the triad of loss of muscle mass or quality, reduced muscle strength, and impaired physical performance.[3] Frailty is described as a multidimensional syndrome characterized by vulnerability to minor stressors leading to an increased risk of adverse outcomes.[4] Both conditions ultimately predispose to functional decline, and thus are important to recognize in the clinical setting. Unlike intrinsic properties of an individual's lung cancer, sarcopenia and frailty are potentially modifiable. This makes both sarcopenia and frailty attractive targets for interventions that may lead to improved outcomes in this patient population. Physiatrists, particularly cancer rehabilitation specialists, are uniquely positioned to play a pivotal role in both the diagnosis and treatment of sarcopenia and frailty in patients with lung cancer.

DEFINITION OF SARCOPENIA

Sarcopenia is defined by the European Working Group on Sarcopenia in Older People 2 (EWGSOP2) as a "progressive and generalized skeletal muscle disorder that is associated with increased likelihood of adverse outcomes including falls, fractures, physical disability, and mortality."[5] According to EWGSOP2, the diagnosis of sarcopenia is probable when low muscle strength is detected, and it is confirmed when low skeletal muscle mass or skeletal muscle quality is demonstrated on imaging. Often, the proposed cut-off value for sarcopenia is appendicular skeletal muscle mass index (SMI) greater than two standard deviations below the sex-specific mean in healthy adults. If impairments of both muscle strength and quantity occur in conjunction with impaired physical performance, sarcopenia is qualified as severe. The EWGSOP2 definition of sarcopenia is just one of many definitions for this condition. Research in sarcopenia is evolving and thus many definitions have been proposed; most definitions involve some degree of loss of muscle mass, quality, strength, and performance. The latter two elements are important to remember. Without the findings of impaired muscle strength and function, an individual would be more appropriately diagnosed with malnutrition. Sarcopenia is not simply decreased muscle mass; it encompasses overall muscle function, thus more closely pertaining to the global function of the individual.[3]

Primary sarcopenia is a natural component of the aging process. Advanced age inevitably leads to decreased muscle mass and strength. This process often begins in the fourth or fifth decade of life and continues until death. Secondary sarcopenia arises in the setting of chronic inflammatory conditions such as cancer, physical inactivity, and inadequate macronutrient intake. Like sarcopenia, cancer is often a disease of aging. Thus, accounting for both primary and secondary sarcopenia, it is understandable why sarcopenia is highly prevalent in the cancer population. In fact, sarcopenia is now the hallmark component of the formal definition of cancer cachexia, a condition which has long been understood to negatively affect those afflicted with various malignancies.[6] Muscle mass decrements, however, predate most clinical signs of cancer cachexia. In other

Lung Cancer Rehabilitation. https://doi.org/10.1016/B978-0-323-83404-9.00012-8

words, sarcopenia is present prior to the weight loss and anorexia seen in cachexia. Therefore, it is essential to evaluate for the presence of sarcopenia in cancer patients prior to progression to clinical cachexia. It is additionally important to note that sarcopenia is not only present in underweight or thin individuals. Body mass index (BMI) has previously been used as a marker for nutritional status and function in cancer patients, but as the U.S. population becomes more obese, this measure has not been shown to accurately indicate muscle depletion. Loss of muscle mass is often present even when a patient's BMI is normal or elevated. The term sarcopenic obesity is used to describe this phenomenon of decreased muscle mass with concomitant elevated fat mass. Thus, there is no one phenotype for the sarcopenic patient; sarcopenia can be present in a cachectic 80-year-old lung cancer patient but can also be diagnosed in an overweight 60-year-old lung cancer patient.[7]

DEFINITION OF FRAILTY

In 2004, the American Geriatric Society defined frailty as "an excess vulnerability to stressors, with a reduced ability to maintain or regain homeostasis after a destabilizing event."[8] Continued insults in frailty lead to an eventual functional decline. It is known that decreased functional reserves increase the risk of hospitalization, falls, and disability in the geriatric population. In the cancer population, the added stressors of the disease itself and treatments such as surgery, chemotherapy, and radiation may ultimately prove too taxing for the frail patient. Thus, cancer can be seen as a "frailty stress test."

There are two main approaches of assessing frailty as a syndrome: the phenotypic definition and the accumulation of deficits definition. In the phenotypic definition, frailty is understood to be a physical condition. It is characterized by weight loss, exhaustion, weakness, slowness, and low physical activity. Three out of these five components must be present to deem an individual as "frail" using the phenotypic definition.[9] Conversely, an alternate approach to assessment of frailty is characterized by an accumulation of deficits. Using this approach, each additional medical symptom, functional impairment, psychosocial issue, and laboratory abnormality present in an individual increases their likelihood of frailty.[8] Most indices use between 30 and 70 variables to determine frailty. To be included, a variable must be "biologically sensible, accumulate with age, and does not saturate too early,"[10] meaning it is not too highly prevalent at a young age. Once a sum of deficits is determined, an individual can be classified as fit, prefrail, or frail with different cut-off values depending on which index of deficits is used.

With sarcopenia and frailty defined, it is evident that these two concepts are closely intertwined. However, it is important to distinguish these two discrete entities. Sarcopenia is a disease state of muscle, while frailty is a syndrome in which multiple physical and psychosocial domains decline over one's lifetime. Sarcopenia can contribute to frailty, but frailty has much broader implications.[11]

PREVALENCE OF SARCOPENIA AND FRAILTY

Due to the various definitions, populations, and cut-off values used when studying sarcopenia, there are broad ranges of prevalence reported in the literature. Sarcopenia is known to increase with age and with increased medical complexity. About 15% of healthy adults over age 45 and about 60% of adults over age 85 were found to be sarcopenic in one study. In another meta-analysis, the prevalence of EWGSOP-defined sarcopenia in community-dwelling adults was found to be in the range of 1%–29%. In that same meta-analysis, prevalence of sarcopenia in those living in long-term care centers ranged from 14% to 33%.[12] The prevalence of sarcopenia in individuals with non-small cell lung cancer (NSCLC) has been reported to be up to 50%, indicating that one of every two patients with NSCLC is sarcopenic.

As with sarcopenia, prevalence of frailty is contingent upon the definition employed and the index used for measurement. Drastically different prevalence of frailty within a population can be seen using various frailty assessment tools due to differences in items measured. One study that used a large sample from the National Health and Aging Trends Study noted that 15% of an elderly, community-dwelling population were frail and 45% were prefrail.[13] Frailty is more prevalent in women, racial and ethnic minorities, the elderly, and in low-income earners.[14] In the cancer population, rates of frailty are even higher. One systematic review of 2916 elderly cancer patients found that the median prevalence for frailty and prefrailty were 42% and 43%, respectively. Within the lung cancer population, frailty prevalence rates range from 13% to 68%.[15] Although the overall prevalence rates of sarcopenia and frailty are variable, these conditions significantly affect patients with lung cancer and should therefore be addressed routinely as part of their medical care.

PATHOPHYSIOLOGY OF SARCOPENIA IN LUNG CANCER

It is important to understand the pathophysiology of sarcopenia itself, both as a primary mechanism and secondarily to cancer. Almost all loss of skeletal muscle mass in sarcopenia is of Type II (fast twitch) muscle fibers, as opposed to Type I (slow twitch) fibers. There are a few underlying mechanisms that are thought to contribute to this loss of muscle mass. First, multiple components of the neurologic system can be affected over time leading to an effective neuropathic process of muscle loss. Additionally, aging is associated with changes in hormone production and sensitivity to those hormones; decreased testosterone, increase cortisol, decreased vitamin D, and insulin resistance can all contribute to sarcopenia.[16] These intrinsic changes along with other factors associated with aging, including immobility and poor nutrition lead to higher rates of sarcopenia in the elderly population. When thinking about cancer, the inflammatory nature of malignancy is what contribute to loss of muscle mass. Increased tumor necrosis factor-α, interleukin-6, interleukin-1, and CRP can lead to activation of cell-signaling pathways which lead to tissue degeneration.[17] Even a chronic low-grade inflammatory state related to aging can be implicated in sarcopenia, so it follows that the elevated inflammatory response and metabolic changes in cancer also lead to this condition.

MEASURING SARCOPENIA AND FRAILTY

Assessments for Frailty

It is pivotal to understand the multiple ways in which sarcopenia and frailty are measured. As previously discussed, frailty can be measured using tenets of the phenotypic definition or the accumulation of deficits definition. When considering the phenotypic definition of frailty, a clinician can assess a potentially frail individual using the Fried Frailty Index. Factors involved in this evaluation include unintentional weight loss of greater than 3 kg or greater than 5% of total body weight in 1 year, self-reported exhaustion via a questionnaire, weakness as measured by grip strength three times below the standard measure for the individual's sex and BMI, walking speed in the lowest quintile for age and height, and low physical activity measured by weekly energy expenditure as compared to those of the same sex.[18] While this evaluation can feasibly be completed during an office visit, its results may not be sensitive or specific enough to create a targeted intervention. One method of assessing an individual's accumulation of deficits is by using the frailty index. Originally

described by Rockwood and colleagues, the frailty index is a measure which assesses 70 unique clinical deficits. While the frailty index is more time consuming for a provider to administer, it is importantly more sensitive and specific in identifying deficits contributing to an individual's frailty status. Many simplified scales, including the Clinical Frailty Scale and the FRAIL scale, have been developed using tenets of the frailty index. The aim of these various scales is to allow for ease of administration in both research and clinical settings. Finally, the Comprehensive Geriatric Assessment (CGA) is another means to assess frailty and considers additional concerns such as an individual's cognition, functional status, nutritional status, emotional status, comorbidities, fall risk, and polypharmacy. The CGA is considered the "gold standard" in measuring frailty. Its comprehensive nature allows an evaluator to pinpoint which deficits need to be intervened upon to best address an individual's frailty. However, the CGA is the most time and resource-intensive of the described assessments. It is therefore often only utilized when there is a positive frailty screening test and additional information is needed to optimize a treatment plan.[19]

Frailty scales specific for individuals with cancer have also been developed. One such measure is the cancer-specific geriatric assessment. Although mostly used in research, this scale has been able to identify deficits even in patients with normal Karnofsky performance status. The G8 and Triage Risk Screening Tool (TRST1+) have been demonstrated to be strong tools in screening for frailty in elderly patients with cancer. Both have a good sensitivity, but poor negative predictive valude for frailty in this population. Accordingly, if there is high concern for frailty, this testing should still be followed by the "gold standard" CGA.[7] These assessments are often used in oncology practices with the aim of uncovering previously unrecognized biopsychosocial issues that may impact a patient's ability to successfully complete various treatments involved in cancer care.

Assessments for Sarcopenia

Like frailty, sarcopenia can also be measured in a myriad of ways. To identify individuals at risk for sarcopenia, a questionnaire (SARC-F) has been developed and validated for use in multiple populations. The SARC-F is named for the domains that it assesses: strength, walking, stair climbing, rising from a chair, and falls. Specifically, it is a self-reported measure of limitations in these domains. The specificity of this test is high, but it only has a low to moderate sensitivity. Thus, the SARC-F is likely to miss less severe cases, but correctly diagnose more serious cases of sarcopenia.[4]

However, compared to the imaging modalities discussed below, it may be the simplest and cheapest tool currently available to integrate into a wide variety of clinical practices (Figs. 11.1 and 11.2).

Imaging for Sarcopenia

Computed tomography (CT), magnetic resonance imaging (MRI), dual-energy X-ray absorptiometry scan (DEXA), musculoskeletal ultrasound (US), and bioelectrical impedance analysis (BIA) are all modalities used to assess the loss of muscle mass component of sarcopenia. BIA measures body composition by the rate at which low-voltage electrical current runs through the body. Fat mass impedes rate of travel, and thus slows the current. Using height, age, gender, and weight, BIA uses prediction equations to determine fat-free mass.[20] While both inexpensive and noninvasive, BIA is less sensitive and specific in diagnosing sarcopenia as compared to the gold standard imaging techniques described below. DEXA, regularly used to assess bone density, can also indirectly measure lean muscle mass, making it another method of identifying sarcopenia. However, DEXA is not often used for this purpose due to its low availability and high cost.

Musculoskeletal US is often used to assess muscle quality, thickness, and cross-sectional area. Recently, the SARCUS working group, a group that focuses on the standardization of musculoskeletal US, developed a consensus protocol for US assessment of 39 specific muscles. They determined standardized anatomical landmarks and measuring points for each muscle to assess its thickness, cross-sectional area, pennation angle, fascicle length, and echo-intensity. Cross-sectional area measured by musculoskeletal US has not shown any significant difference to that measured by MRI. Another strength of musculoskeletal US in assessing sarcopenia is that some measures have been shown to be related to muscle function. For example, muscle strength in elderly patients has been correlated with quadriceps muscle thickness and echo-intensity.[21] Although the SARCUS location standardization practices have been put in place, there is still often high operational variability between experienced and inexperienced scanners. Additionally, most studies in United States have been done on healthy subjects. This explains why there are not yet any standardized cut-off values for loss of muscle quality and mass. Thus, US is currently limited in its ability to fully evaluate sarcopenia.[22]

There are, however, some novel applications of US that may be useful when evaluating sarcopenia in the future. There methods include shear wave elastography, superb microvascular imaging, and contrast enhanced ultrasound. Shear wave elastography can detect increased muscle stiffness and fibrosis. Superb microvascular imaging identifies low flow microvascularization that is not currently visible with Color Doppler. This measure is often decreased in those with sarcopenia compared to healthy controls. Finally, contrast-enhanced US can be used to assess muscle perfusion, which can be impaired in sarcopenia. These measures, along with those currently used in US evaluations, may one day allow for better sensitivity and specificity of musculoskeletal US in evaluating sarcopenia.[23]

More commonly used forms of imaging, MRI and CT, are also used to measure decreased muscle mass in sarcopenia. While MRI may produce higher-quality imaging of muscle, the increased time and cost associated with it compared to CT scans make it the less preferred option. Additionally, CT scans are commonly used in oncologic cases for diagnostic purposes. Specifically, patients with lung cancer oftentimes already have chest and abdomen CT imaging readily available to assess for sarcopenia. For these reasons, CT scans are

Sarcopenia Component	Diagnostic Tool
Muscle Mass	Bioelectrical Impedance Analysis (BIA)
	Dual-Energy Absorptiometry Scan (DEXA)
	Musculoskeletal Ultrasound
	Computed Tomography (CT)
	Magnetic Resonance Imaging (MRI)
	Methyl-d3 creatine in fasting morning urine
Muscle Strength	Grip strength via handheld dynamometer
	30 second sit-to-stand
	Lower limb muscle strength
Physical Performance	Gait speed via 4-meter walk test
	Timed Up and Go (TUG)
	6 Minute Walk Test
	Stair Climb Test
	Short Physical Performance Battery (SPPB)

FIG. 11.1 Clinical assessment of sarcopenia.

Test	Components
Frailty Phenotype (Fried)	<ul><li>Weight loss of greater than 3 kilograms or greater than 5 percent of total body weight in one year</li><li>Self-reported exhaustion via a questionnaire</li><li>Weakness as measured by grip strength three times below the standard measure for the individual's sex and BMI</li><li>Walking speed in the lowest quintile for age and height</li><li>Low physical activity measured by weekly energy expenditure as compared to those of the same sex</li></ul>Scoring: 0= Robust 1-2= Pre-frail 3-5= Frail
Frailty index (Rockwood)	70 components including difficulty with ADLs, poor tone and coordination, falls, mood, neurologic, cardiovascular, and respiratory symptoms or diagnoses.
Clinical Frailty Scale	Most recent version is scored 1-9 from very fit to terminally ill. Worsening scores with presence of disease, impairment in activities, dependence on others for iADLs and/or ADLs
Frail scale	<ul><li>Fatigue (Are you fatigued?)</li><li>Resistance (Can you climb a flight of stairs?)</li><li>Ambulation (Can you walk one block?)</li><li>Illnesses (more than 5 underlying illnesses)</li><li>Loss of Weight (>5% body weight)</li></ul>Scoring: 0= Robust 1-2= Pre-frail 3-5= Frail
Comprehensive Geriatric Assessment	<ul><li>Functional status</li><li>Cognition</li><li>Emotional status</li><li>Nutritional status</li><li>Comorbidities</li><li>Polypharmacy</li><li>Geriatric syndromes (fall risk, delirium, urinary incontinence, dentition, visual, or hearing impairments)</li></ul>

FIG. 11.2 Clinical assessment of frailty.

the "gold standard" means of assessing sarcopenia in both the European and Asian guidelines, and CT is the most common modality of assessing sarcopenia in the lung cancer population in research studies. With this said, there is some discrepancy as to how sarcopenia is measured and what cut-off values are used for its diagnosis. L3 skeletal muscle index (L3SMI) is seemingly the most widely used sample to assess for sarcopenia.[7] This value is obtained by measuring the cross-sectional area (in cm^2) of the paraspinals, psoas major, rectus femoris, internal oblique, external oblique, and transverse abdominis muscles in two consecutive axial cuts at the L3 vertebral level. These two values are averaged and then divided by the square of the patient's height (in m^2) to determine the L3SMI.

Prado et al. proposed sex-specific cut-off values for sarcopenia within the lung and gastrointestinal cancer populations in a landmark study published in 2008. They determined that sarcopenia could be diagnosed in males with an L3SMI less than 52.4 cm^2/m^2 and in females with an L3SMI less than 38.5 cm^2/m^2. Updated cut-off values have been reported by Martin and colleagues due to the high prevalence of obesity in the Prado sample. Martin's cut-offs for L3SMI were 43.0 cm^2/m^2 in men with a BMI <25.0 kg/m^2, 53.0 cm^2/m^2 in men with a BMI ≥25.0 kg/m^2, and 41.0 cm^2/m^2 in women. While these values may be representative for an American or European population, multiple sources have since noted lower cut-off values for individuals of Asian descent. Therefore, there is still no "gold standard" for SMI cut-offs for sarcopenia. Furthermore, many studies use cross-sectional areas from other lumbar or even thoracic levels and additionally use different cut-off values (lowest quartile, etc.) when assessing for sarcopenia.[24,25] Lack of standardization in these measurements leads to discrepancy between studies, difficulty comparing results, and troubles when amalgamating data for meta-analyses.

Biomarkers for Sarcopenia

Biomarkers for assessing sarcopenia are limited, but one novel approach is now being studied. A noninvasive isotope dilution test has been developed which measures the concentration of methyl-d3 creatine in fasting morning urine. This test has demonstrated similar estimates of skeletal muscle mass when compared to values ascertained by MRI, but with lower cost and ease of administration. Currently issues with interindividual variability limit this test's use for diagnostics at this time, but with more research, methyl-d3 creatine may be used in the future when assessing for sarcopenia.[26]

Functional Assessments in Sarcopenia and Frailty

In addition to assessing muscle quantity and quality, it is critical to assess muscle strength to fully evaluate for sarcopenia (Fig. 11.3). Grip strength using a handheld dynamometer is one way to obtain a strength value. However, grip strength may be affected by concomitant medical conditions such as osteoarthritis of the hand or fingers, carpal tunnel syndrome, or prior stroke. A provider should note these possible confounding conditions and adjust the testing for strength as needed. For example, a 30 second sit to stand can be used in clinical practice as a proxy for lower extremity strength. This test measures the time it takes for an individual to rise from a seated position without using their upper extremities for assistance in 30 s.

The final component of sarcopenia that needs to be evaluated is physical performance. There are various functional tests that are used in the assessment of sarcopenic patients to assess muscle performance. Some examples of this include gait speed, the Timed-Up and Go (TUG), and the Short Physical Performance Battery (SPPB). A commonly used test for gait speed is the 4-meter walk test. The individual being tested is timed walking 4 m at their usual walking speed. EWGSOP2 uses the cut-off value of less than or equal to 0.8 m/s to signify severe sarcopenia. A 400-meter walk test can also be used to assess not only gait, but also endurance. Of note, gait speed can also be used as a frailty screening tool in patients 65 and over with cancer. In this population, gait speed less than 1 m/s on the 4-meter walk test denotes a patient who should complete a CGA for a full frailty evaluation. The TUG is a well-known test in the realm of physiatry. The TUG is performed by having an individual rise from a seated position, walk 3 m, walk back to the chair, and sit down. For this test, the EWGSOP2 designates any time greater than or equal to 20 s as being indicative of sarcopenia. As with strength testing, these functional tests can be affected by other underlying medical conditions. It is important to consider these comorbidities in the overall evaluation of both frailty and sarcopenia.

OUTCOMES

Prolonging survival and decreasing morbidity in the cancer population is of utmost importance to clinicians and researchers alike. Even with the advent of advanced treatment modalities, overall outcomes in individuals with lung cancer are still poor compared to those with other types of cancer. As current targeted treatments have shown insufficient improvement in lung cancer outcomes, many researchers have attempted to determine if sarcopenia and frailty can be used as prognostic

Test	Value Indicative of Sarcopenia
Grip strength	Women: <20 kg force
	Men: <30 kg force
30 second sit to stand	Women: <15 repetitions
	Men: <17 repetitions
4-meter walk test	Gait speed ≤ 0.8 m/s
Timed up and go (TUG)	Complete in <10.85 s
Short Physical Performance Battery (SPPB)	Score of > 8
	Scored from 0-12 (Balance, Gait Speed, and Chair Stand)

FIG. 11.3 Normative values for functional asessments in sarcoepnia and frailty.

factors for morbidity and mortality in various malignancies. It should come as no surprise that decreased functional reserves and impaired muscle function may increase complications in the cancer population. In fact, sarcopenia and frailty have been shown to correlate with poor prognosis in rectal, liver, esophageal, gastrointestinal, and renal cancer. Sarcopenia and frailty have also been studied extensively in the setting of lung cancer. Studies have explored how these conditions affect overall survival, disease-free survival, chemotherapy toxicity, and postoperative outcomes in lung cancer patients.

Surgery

In patients with resectable NSCLC, the first-line treatment is often surgical resection. Even with resection, there is a low 5-year survival rate for this subset of patients with lung cancer. In a large metaanalysis, surgically resected NSCLC patients with sarcopenia were shown to have a lower overall survival (61.1% vs. 74.2%) compared to those without sarcopenia. Results were even more striking for those patients with early-stage disease and sarcopenia versus those with early-stage disease without sarcopenia.[27] Although not found in the above metaanalysis, other studies have also demonstrated worsened disease-free survival for sarcopenic versus their nonsarcopenic counterparts after surgical resection for NSCLC.[28]

Postoperative complications were also found to occur more frequently in patients with lung cancer with sarcopenia than those without sarcopenia. This correlation also exists for individuals with gastrointestinal and hepatobiliary malignancies.[29,30] Common postoperative complications include prolonged air leak, pneumonia, and recurrent pleural effusions.[31] An increase in these postoperative complications was seen in both pneumonectomy and lobectomy for sarcopenic individuals. It is thought that increased an inflammatory response in patients with sarcopenia may be responsible for this phenomenon postoperatively.

Finally, continued surveillance for sarcopenia in the postoperative period is also crucial. One study found that even after curative resection of NSCLC, patients who developed sarcopenia in the 6-month postoperative period had a worse prognosis. This information may be helpful in identifying patients for interventions targeted to prevent or impede the development of sarcopenia.[32]

Chemotherapy and Immunotherapy

Evidence has also been found supporting the idea that frailty and sarcopenia increase morbidity and mortality in patients receiving chemotherapy. Wang et al. found that using a laboratory panel to diagnose frailty, there was a significantly worse chemotherapy tolerance and increased mortality in frail compared to nonfrail individuals with lung cancer.[33] Another study found that frail lung cancer patients, had higher odds of toxicity in the first cycle of chemotherapy than their nonfrail counterparts.[34] Cohen et al. also studied frailty's effects on an elderly cancer population receiving chemotherapy. Only 28.6% of this population of 500 individuals were diagnosed with lung cancer, and results were not separated by cancer subtype. Nonetheless, using a CGA-determined frailty status, the group found that frail and prefrail patients with cancer undergoing chemotherapy were more likely to discontinue chemotherapy and had increased hospitalization rates. There was no significant increased chemotherapy toxicity exhibited in this study.[35] In a population of Stage IV NSCLC patients on immunotherapy with nivolumab, overall outcomes were worse in sarcopenic compared to nonsarcopenic subjects.[22,25] Another metaanalysis reviewed outcomes in sarcopenic individuals with NSCLC taking immune checkpoint inhibitors. It demonstrated that positive pretreatment sarcopenic status was associated with decreased overall survival and worse immune checkpoint inhibitor treatment response.[36] Although many studies of sarcopenic patients have shown worse outcomes with chemotherapy and immunotherapy, it is important to note that there are other well-powered studies which have found no significant correlation between sarcopenia and toxicity or survival measures in the lung cancer population.

Understanding sarcopenia and frailty's poor prognostic effects in the lung cancer population is critical not only for oncologic providers, but all other clinician caring for this group. Due to worsened treatment-related outcomes and complications in the sarcopenic population, some have proposed that when frailty or sarcopenia deems a surgical or chemotherapeutic treatment option contraindicated, radiation therapy should be considered as a treatment option that maintains "a good balance between toxicity and results."[37] Sarcopenia or frailty status may lead others to consider palliative as opposed to therapeutic measures. As such, sarcopenia and frailty must be assessed and accounted for prior to solidifying treatment plans.

INTERVENTIONS

As the US population over age 65 is expected to more than double in size from 35 million in 2000 to 80 million in 2040, the incidence of frailty will undoubtedly increase as well. Due to the personal and economic burden that frailty imposes, it is important to consider ways to prevent and manage this condition. Individually tailored interventions should be implemented to improve and preserve independence, physical function, and cognition. The CGA can be used to identify which aspects of frailty to target to best address an individual's deficits. Various types of physical activity including resistance training, aerobic exercise, balance training, and combinations thereof have been evaluated in the frail population. However, there is significant variation in the literature regarding intensity, frequency, duration, and type of exercise implemented thus making the evidence for these interventions limited. Interventions focusing on nutritional supplementation, medication management, health education, and hormone supplementation have also been used to combat frailty.[38] One systematic review found that a combination of protein supplementation and strength exercise was the most effective and easiest to implement of the 38 combinations of interventions that it compared in delaying frailty.[39] While appetite stimulants such as dronabinol and megestrol have also been considered in the treatment of frailty, the prescribing provider should be aware of CNS side effects and increased risk for deep vein thrombosis, respectively.[40]

Like frailty, the primary treatments for sarcopenia are exercise, nutrition, and medications. As previously described, it is difficult to delineate the true effect of various exercise interventions as the intensity, frequency, duration, and type of exercise vary significantly from trial to trial in the current literature. However, systematic reviews have shown evidence of improved strength and muscle mass with an array of exercise interventions. The Sarcopenia and Physical fRailty IN older people: multicomponenT Treatment strategies (SPRINTT) study is an ongoing multicenter randomized controlled trial currently being performed in Europe. The aim of SPRINTT is to evaluate a long-term structured program involving physical activity, nutritional counseling, and a dietary intervention in preventing disability in patients with both frailty and sarcopenia over a 36-month period. This comprehensive trial may aid in creating a standardized program for frail and sarcopenic patients that can be used as a benchmark in the future.

There is minimal evidence for nutritional intervention alone as a treatment for sarcopenia; supplementation of protein, vitamin D, antioxidants, and polyunsaturated fatty acids have all been proposed as mechanisms to improve muscle mass and function in sarcopenic individuals. Studies have noted improvement in sarcopenia parameters with protein supplementation in addition to exercise. Other studies demonstrate that supplementation of essential amino acids such as leucine and β-hydroxy β-methylbutyric acid has some positive effect on muscle mass and function.[11] Early clinical trials for several pharmaceuticals have also shown promise in improving sarcopenia in lung cancer patients (Fig. 11.4). Anamorelin, a selective ghrelin receptor agonist, was shown to improve lean body mass in a Japanese cohort with advanced lung cancer. However, it did not demonstrate any improvement in the functional measures of handgrip strength or the 6-minute walk test in this population.[41] Espindolol, a nonselective beta-blocker, has exhibited improvement in weight and fat free mass in an advanced NSCLC cohort. Unlike Anamorelin, espindolol did demonstrate a significant improvement in handgrip strength.[42] Other novel medications such as myostatin inhibitors have shown early promise, but there is still a paucity of evidence for their clinical use at this time.[43]

One other consideration for combating both sarcopenia and frailty is addressing them prior to their onset. A large British study noted cumulative benefits of increased physical activity throughout mid-life on grip strength at age 60—64.[44] In other words, there is a strong correlation between staying active and maintaining functional muscle mass as one ages. While this may seem intuitive, it is important to note as prevention of sarcopenia and frailty may be more effective than remediation of these conditions. The preventative approach to sarcopenia and frailty management is promising as intervening at a younger age may make implementing a regular exercise routine and protein-rich diet more feasible. In a similar vein, prehabilitation interventions are being implemented in many cancer populations prior to surgery and chemotherapy. Silver describes

Medication	Mechanism of Action	Dosage
Anamorelin	Ghrelin Receptor Agonist	100 mg daily
Espindolol	Non-selective beta-blocker	10 mg twice a day
LY2495655 (LY)	Monoclonal Antibody- Myostatin Inhibitor	315 mg subcutaneous injection every 4 weeks

FIG. 11.4 Pharmaceuticals used for sarcopenia and frailty.

prehabilitation as "a process on the cancer continuum of care that occurs between the time of cancer diagnosis and the beginning of acute treatment and includes physical and psychological assessments that establish a baseline functional level, identify impairments, and provide interventions that promote physical and psychological health to reduce the incidence and/or severity of future impairments."[45] Many different prehabilitation programs have demonstrated improved functional outcomes after the intervention. They will continue to be developed and will be a mainstay of comprehensive cancer care for years to come.[46]

Developing targeted exercise regimens and therapy prescriptions to improve muscle mass and muscle function for sarcopenic and frail lung cancer patients are critical not only for quality of life, but also for overall morbidity and mortality. Additionally, as both sarcopenia and frailty require multimodal treatment approaches, coordination of care is of utmost importance for these individuals. Physiatrist's scope of training and practice make them well-suited to lead the management of sarcopenia and frailty in patients with cancer, including lung cancer. Knowing how and when to include specific physicians, nurses, physical therapists, occupational therapists, and nutritionists in a patient's medical or rehabilitative care is vital to improving patients' quality of life and disease outcomes.

CONCLUSION

Even with improvements in treatment, lung cancer was the malignancy that caused the highest mortality in 2020. The clinical and research communities are now attempting to target other modifiable factors which may contribute to increased morbidity and mortality in the lung cancer population. Sarcopenia and frailty are two such targets. Sarcopenia is a decrease in muscle quantity or quality with concurrent strength and/or physical performance impairment. Frailty is a multidimensional syndrome which increases vulnerability to stressors effectively leading to functional decline. There is a known high prevalence of both sarcopenia and frailty in the lung cancer population. Numerous clinical trials and metaanalyses have correlated the presence of sarcopenia and frailty with decreased overall and disease-free survival, increased chemotherapy toxicity, and increased postsurgical complications in patients with lung cancer. Interventions such as focused, individualized exercise programs, protein supplementation, and certain medications have been found to help delay or even reverse sarcopenia and frailty. Prehabilitation and other early interventions aimed at preventing these conditions may be beneficial to begin implementing

as the U.S. population ages. Cancer rehabilitation physicians are primed to manage both sarcopenia and frailty in the lung cancer population with the goal of improved quality of life and overall clinical outcomes for this vulnerable group of patients.

REFERENCES

1. Lemjabbar-Alaoui H, Hassan OU, Yang YW, Buchanan P. Lung cancer: biology and treatment options. *Biochim Biophys Acta.* 2015;1856(2):189–210. https://doi.org/10.1016/j.bbcan.2015.08.002.
2. Bray F, Ferlay J, Soerjomataram I, Siegel RL, Torre LA, Jemal A. Global cancer statistics 2018: GLOBOCAN estimates of incidence and mortality worldwide for 36 cancers in 185 countries [published correction appears in CA Cancer J Clin. 2020;70(4):313]. *CA Cancer J Clin.* 2018;68(6):394–424. https://doi.org/10.3322/caac.21492.
3. Collins J, Noble S, Chester J, Coles B, Byrne A. The assessment and impact of sarcopenia in lung cancer: a systematic literature review. *BMJ Open.* 2014;4(1):e003697. https://doi.org/10.1136/bmjopen-2013-003697.
4. Clegg A, Young J, Iliffe S, Rikkert MO, Rockwood K. Frailty in elderly people [published correction appears in Lancet. 2013 Oct 19;382(9901):1328]. *Lancet.* 2013;381(9868):752–762. https://doi.org/10.1016/S0140-6736(12)62167-9.
5. Cruz-Jentoft AJ, Bahat G, Bauer J, et al. Sarcopenia: revised European consensus on definition and diagnosis [published correction appears in Age Ageing. 2019 Jul 1; 48(4):601]. *Age Ageing.* 2019;48(1):16–31. https://doi.org/10.1093/ageing/afy169.
6. Fearon K, Strasser F, Anker SD, et al. Definition and classification of cancer cachexia: an international consensus. *Lancet Oncol.* 2011;12(5):489–495. https://doi.org/10.1016/S1470-2045(10)70218-7.
7. Baracos VE, Reiman T, Mourtzakis M, Gioulbasanis I, Antoun S. Body composition in patients with non-small cell lung cancer: a contemporary view of cancer cachexia with the use of computed tomography image analysis. *Am J Clin Nutr.* 2010;91(4):1133S–1137S. https://doi.org/10.3945/ajcn.2010.28608C.
8. Pamoukdjian F, Paillaud E, Zelek L, et al. Measurement of gait speed in older adults to identify complications associated with frailty: a systematic review. *J Geriatr Oncol.* 2015;6(6):484–496. https://doi.org/10.1016/j.jgo.2015.08.006.
9. Fried LP, Tangen CM, Walston J, et al. Frailty in older adults: evidence for a phenotype. *J Gerontol A Biol Sci Med Sci.* 2001;56(3):M146–M156. https://doi.org/10.1093/gerona/56.3.m146.
10. Song X, Mitnitski A, Rockwood K. Prevalence and 10-year outcomes of frailty in older adults in relation to deficit accumulation. *J Am Geriatr Soc.* 2010;58(4):681–687. https://doi.org/10.1111/j.1532-5415.2010.02764.x.
11. Gingrich A, Volkert D, Kiesswetter E, et al. Prevalence and overlap of sarcopenia, frailty, cachexia and malnutrition in older medical inpatients. *BMC Geriatr.* 2019;19(1):120. https://doi.org/10.1186/s12877-019-1115-1.

12. Cruz-Jentoft AJ, Landi F, Schneider SM, et al. Prevalence of and interventions for sarcopenia in ageing adults: a systematic review. Report of the International Sarcopenia Initiative (EWGSOP and IWGS). *Age Ageing*. 2014;43(6): 748−759. https://doi.org/10.1093/ageing/afu115.

13. Bandeen-Roche K, Seplaki CL, Huang J, et al. Frailty in older adults: a nationally representative profile in the United States. *J Gerontol A Biol Sci Med Sci*. 2015;70(11): 1427−1434. https://doi.org/10.1093/gerona/glv133.

14. Ofori-Asenso R, Chin KL, Mazidi M, et al. Global incidence of frailty and prefrailty among community-dwelling older adults: a systematic review and meta-analysis. *JAMA Netw Open*. 2019;2(8):e198398. https://doi.org/10.1001/jamanetworkopen.2019.8398.

15. Handforth C, Clegg A, Young C, et al. The prevalence and outcomes of frailty in older cancer patients: a systematic review. *Ann Oncol*. 2015;26(6):1091−1101. https:// doi.org/10.1093/annonc/mdu540. Epub 2014 Nov 17.

16. Kim TN, Choi KM. Sarcopenia: definition, epidemiology, and pathophysiology. *J Bone Metabol*. 2013;20(1):1−10. https://doi.org/10.11005/jbm.2013.20.1.1.

17. Ogawa S, Yakabe M, Akishita M. Age-related sarcopenia and its pathophysiological bases. *Inflamm Regen*. 2016; 36(17). https://doi.org/10.1186/s41232-016-0022-5.

18. Pao YC, Chen CY, Chang CI, Chen CY, Tsai JS. Self-reported exhaustion, physical activity, and grip strength predict frailty transitions in older outpatients with chronic diseases. *Medicine*. 2018;97(23):e10933. https://doi.org/ 10.1097/MD.0000000000010933.

19. Lee H, Lee E, Jang IY. Frailty and comprehensive geriatric assessment. *J Kor Med Sci*. 2020;35(3):e16. https:// doi.org/10.3346/jkms.2020.35.e16.

20. Aleixo GFP, Shachar SS, Nyrop KA, Muss HB, Battaglini CL, Williams GR. Bioelectrical impedance analysis for the assessment of sarcopenia in patients with cancer: a systematic review. *Oncologist*. 2020;25(2):170−182. https:// doi.org/10.1634/theoncologist.2019-0600.

21. Albano D, Messina C, Vitale J, Sconfienza LM. Imaging of sarcopenia: old evidence and new insights. *Eur Radiol*. 2020;30(4):2199−2208. https://doi.org/10.1007/s00330-019-06573-2.

22. Perkisas S, Bastijns S, Baudry S, et al. Application of ultrasound for muscle assessment in sarcopenia: 2020 SARCUS update. *Eur Geriatr Med*. 2021;12(1):45−59. https:// doi.org/10.1007/s41999-020-00433-9.

23. Hernández-Socorro CR, Saavedra P, López-Fernández JC, Lübbe-Vazquez F, Ruiz-Santana S. Novel high-quality sonographic methods to diagnose muscle wasting in long-stay critically ill patients: shear wave elastography, superb microvascular imaging and contrast-enhanced ultrasound. *Nutrients*. 2021;13(7):2224. https://doi.org/ 10.3390/nu13072224.

24. Kim EY, Kim YS, Park I, Ahn HK, Cho EK, Jeong YM. Prognostic significance of CT-determined sarcopenia in patients with small-cell lung cancer. *J Thorac Oncol*. 2015; 10(12):1795−1799. https://doi.org/10.1097/JTO.0000000000000690.

25. Matsuo Y. Sarcopenia is a potential factor for optimized treatment selection for elderly patients with early stage non-small cell lung cancer. *J Thorac Dis*. 2019;11(Suppl 3):S443−S445. https://doi.org/10.21037/jtd.2018.11.44.

26. Clark RV, Walker AC, Miller RR, O'Connor-Semmes RL, Ravussin E, Cefalu WT. Creatine (methyl-d3) dilution in urine for estimation of total body skeletal muscle mass: accuracy and variability vs. MRI and DXA. *J Appl Physiol*. 2018;124(1):1−9. https://doi.org/10.1152/japplphysiol. 00455.2016.

27. Deng HY, Hou L, Zha P, Huang KL, Peng L. Sarcopenia is an independent unfavorable prognostic factor of non-small cell lung cancer after surgical resection: a comprehensive systematic review and meta-analysis. *Eur J Surg Oncol*. 2019;45(5):728−735. https://doi.org/10.1016/ j.ejso.2018.09.026.

28. Deng HY, Zha P, Hou L, Huang KL. Does sarcopenia have any impact on survival of patients with surgically treated non-small-cell lung cancer? *Interact Cardiovasc Thorac Surg*. 2019;29(1):144−147. https://doi.org/10.1093/icvts/ ivz039.

29. Kawaguchi Y, Hanaoka J, Ohshio Y, et al. Sarcopenia predicts poor postoperative outcome in elderly patients with lung cancer. *Gen Thorac Cardiovasc Surg*. 2019;67(11): 949−954. https://doi.org/10.1007/s11748-019-01125-3.

30. Madariaga MLL, Troschel FM, Best TD, Knoll SJ, Gaissert HA, Fintelmann FJ. Low thoracic skeletal muscle area predicts morbidity after pneumonectomy for lung cancer. *Ann Thorac Surg*. 2020;109(3):907−913. https:// doi.org/10.1016/j.athoracsur.2019.10.041.

31. Lee J, Moon SW, Choi JS, Hyun K, Moon YK, Moon MH. Impact of sarcopenia on early postoperative complications in early-stage non-small-cell lung cancer. *Kor J Thorac Cardiovasc Surg*. 2020;53(3):93−103. https://doi.org/ 10.5090/kjtcs.2020.53.3.93.

32. Nakamura R, Inage Y, Tobita R, et al. Sarcopenia in resected NSCLC: effect on postoperative outcomes. *J Thorac Oncol*. 2018;13(7):895−903. https://doi.org/10. 1016/j.jtho.2018.04.035.

33. Wang Y, Zhang R, Shen Y, Su L, Dong B, Hao Q. Prediction of chemotherapy adverse reactions and mortality in older patients with primary lung cancer through frailty index based on routine laboratory data. *Clin Interv Aging*. 2019; 14:1187−1197. https://doi.org/10.2147/CIA.S201873.

34. Ruiz J, Miller AA, Tooze JA, et al. Frailty assessment predicts toxicity during first cycle chemotherapy for advanced lung cancer regardless of chronologic age. *J Geriatr Oncol*. 2019;10(1):48−54. https://doi.org/10.1016/j.jgo.2018.0 6.007.

35. Cohen HJ, Smith D, Sun CL, et al. Frailty as determined by a comprehensive geriatric assessment-derived deficit-accumulation index in older patients with cancer who receive chemotherapy. *Cancer*. 2016;122(24): 3865−3872. https://doi.org/10.1002/cncr.30269.

36. Wang J, Cao L, Xu S. Sarcopenia affects clinical efficacy of immune checkpoint inhibitors in non-small cell lung cancer patients: a systematic review and meta-analysis. *Int*

Immunopharm. 2020;88:106907. https://doi.org/10.1016/j.intimp.2020.106907.

37. Colloca G, Tagliaferri L, Capua BD, et al. Management of the elderly cancer patients complexity: the radiation oncology potential. *Aging Dis*. 2020;11(3):649−657. https://doi.org/10.14336/AD.2019.0616.

38. Dent E, Martin FC, Bergman H, Woo J, Romero-Ortuno R, Walston JD. Management of frailty: opportunities, challenges, and future directions. *Lancet*. 2019;394(10206):1376−1386. https://doi.org/10.1016/S0140-6736(19)31785-4.

39. Travers J, Romero-Ortuno R, Bailey J, Cooney MT. Delaying and reversing frailty: a systematic review of primary care interventions. *Br J Gen Pract*. 2019;69(678):e61−e69. https://doi.org/10.3399/bjgp18X700241.

40. Puts MTE, Toubasi S, Andrew MK, et al. Interventions to prevent or reduce the level of frailty in community-dwelling older adults: a scoping review of the literature and international policies. *Age Ageing*. 2017;46(3):383−392. https://doi.org/10.1093/ageing/afw247.

41. Katakami N, Uchino J, Yokoyama T, et al. Anamorelin (ONO-7643) for the treatment of patients with non-small cell lung cancer and cachexia: results from a randomized, double-blind, placebo-controlled, multicenter study of Japanese patients (ONO-7643-04). *Cancer*. 2018;124(3):606−616. https://doi.org/10.1002/cncr.31128.

42. Stewart Coats AJ, Ho GF, Prabhash K, et al. Espindolol for the treatment and prevention of cachexia in patients with stage III/IV non-small cell lung cancer or colorectal cancer: a randomized, double-blind, placebo-controlled, international multicentre phase II study (the ACT-ONE trial). *J Cachexia Sarcopenia Muscle*. 2016;7(3):355−365. https://doi.org/10.1002/jcsm.12126.

43. Cruz-Jentoft AJ, Sayer AA. Sarcopenia [published correction appears in Lancet. 2019 Jun 29;393(10191):2590]. *Lancet*. 2019;393(10191):2636−2646. https://doi.org/10.1016/S0140-6736(19)31138-9.

44. Dodds R, Kuh D, Aihie Sayer A, Cooper R. Physical activity levels across adult life and grip strength in early old age: updating findings from a British birth cohort. *Age Ageing*. 2013;42(6):794−798. https://doi.org/10.1093/ageing/aft124.

45. Silver JK, Baima J, Mayer RS. Impairment-driven cancer rehabilitation: an essential component of quality care and survivorship. *CA Cancer J Clin*. 2013;63(5):295−317. https://doi.org/10.3322/caac.21186.

46. Michael CM, Lehrer EJ, Schmitz KH, Zaorsky NG. Prehabilitation exercise therapy for cancer: a systematic review and meta-analysis. *Cancer Med*. 2021;10(13):4195−4205. https://doi.org/10.1002/cam4.4021.

CHAPTER 12

Nutritional Considerations in Lung Cancer Rehabilitation

MONICA DIAZ, RD/LDN, CPT • DOMINIQUE SYMONETTE, MS, RD/LDN, CNSC • HALEY R. APPEL, PA-C, MMS • ADRIAN CRISTIAN, MD, MHCM

INTRODUCTION

It has been estimated that about 235,760 people (119,100 men and 116.660 women) will be diagnosed with lung cancer in the United States in 2021.[1,2] 1 in 15 men and 1 in 17 women will be diagnosed with lung cancer in their lifetime with smokers having an increased risk compared to nonsmokers.[1,2] 541, 000 people in the United States have at some point in their lives been diagnosed with lung cancer.[1] According to the American Cancer Society, about 113,880 deaths (69,410 men and 62,470 women) will occur from lung cancer in 2021. Each year more people die of lung cancer than of breast, colon, and prostate combined.[2] There has been a steady decline in lung cancer diagnoses and lung cancer deaths by 50% for men and 1/3 for women[1,2] mostly from people quitting smoking and from advances in early detection and treatment.[2] Whereas smoking is responsible for 80% of lung cancer–related deaths, 20% of lung cancer deaths occur in people whom have never smoked. Family history as well as genetic factors may also have a role in development of lung cancer.[1,2] Lung cancer primarily occurs in people over the age of 65, with average age at diagnosis being about 70.[2] Approximately 30%−40% of lung cancers are diagnosed in people over the age of 70.[3,4] The 5-year survival rate for nonsmall cell lung cancer (NSCLC) is 63% for localized disease, 35% for regional disease, and 7% for distant disease. The 5-year survival rate for small cell lung cancer (SCLC) is 27% for localized disease, 16% for regional disease, and 3% for distant disease.[2]

Since lung cancer occurs primarily in older adults, frailty in this population can be common. Frailty has been characterized as a decline in functioning across multiple physiological systems. When compared to nonfrail patients, frail and prefrail patients have a higher risk of overall mortality and therapeutic toxicity.[3] It has been reported that more than half of older patients with cancer are frail at the time of cancer diagnosis, which in turn can increase the risk of inability to tolerate chemotherapy treatments, lead to postoperative complications and increased mortality.[3,5] Frailty can be associated with an increased risk of falls, disability and early mortality, postoperative complications, prolonged hospital length of stay, and substantially increased costs. It is important for clinicians to assess lung cancer patients before, during, and after the start of lung cancer treatments for key indicators of frailty such as weight loss, fatigue, weakness, and slow gait speed. Frail lung cancer patients may have significant other comorbidities such as coronary artery disease, heart failure, COPD, diabetes, and peripheral vascular disease that can affect ability to tolerate cancer treatments. Sarcopenia can also be present along with frailty and can be associated with increased risk of falls, disability, and prolonged hospitalizations and complications postsurgery and increased mortality.[6] The presence of sarcopenia can also reduce the benefits of immunotherapy.[7]

Nutrition and exercise are the cornerstones of mitigating frailty and sarcopenia in lung cancer patients. Prehabilitation is the time period between cancer diagnosis and start of cancer treatment. This is a unique opportunity to identify any preexisting physical impairments that could be exacerbated by cancer treatment such as impaired balance due to an underlying peripheral neuropathy and introduce rehabilitative interventions to minimize their impact. In addition, exercise, nutritional interventions, and psychosocial support can be initiated to improve the general physical and mental status of the individual. A generalized exercise program often includes a walking component as well as strength training of major muscle groups of the upper and lower extremities. For example, a 2 -week home-based

Lung Cancer Rehabilitation. https://doi.org/10.1016/B978-0-323-83404-9-00021-0

prehabilitation program that included aerobic and resistance exercises, respiratory training, nutritional counseling with whey protein supplementation, and psychological support achieved greater 6 min walking distance and peri-operative functional capacity in patients undergoing video-assisted thorascopic surgery lobectomy for lung cancer when compared to control group.[8] Prehabilitation is a safe intervention without any significant side effects reported for lung cancer patients. It can increase exercise capacity and significantly improve pulmonary function.[9]

Malnutrition is common in lung cancer patients. In one study, 51.1% of patients were undernourished, 23.9% were at risk for malnutrition, and only 25% showed a normal nutrition. Those that were well nourished evaluated their quality of life as better and those that were malnourished reported a decreased quality of life.[10] In this chapter, the focus is on the nutritional challenges and interventions in lung cancer patients. At end of this chapter, a case study is provided to illustrate the important role of nutritional interventions in the care of a lung cancer patient.

ESTIMATING NUTRITIONAL NEEDS FOR LUNG CANCER PATIENTS

Providing adequate calories is essential to maintain weight and/or prevent weight loss associated with lung cancer treatment or disease. During an initial nutritional assessment, energy and protein needs for lung cancer patients are assessed. Nutritional needs are recalculated, as needed, in all follow-up assessments.[11] Energy needs for patients with lung cancer can be estimated using the following parameters:

- 15 kcal/kg actual body weight for obese patients
- 20−25 kcal/kg actual body weight
- 25−30 kcal/kg actual body weight for non-ambulatory or sedentary adults
- 30−35 kcal/kg actual body weight for patients that are losing weight and/or malnourished
- 35 kcal/kg actual body weight and above for hypermetabolic or severely stressed patients, or for those with malabsorption. Avoid calorie provision above 35 kcal/kg prior to start of cancer treatment.[11]

The provision of adequate protein is essential for building and repairing cells and to reduce negative nitrogen balance. Protein needs for lung cancer patients are 1.2−1.5 gm/kg/day.[11]

The parameter that is used to calculate energy and protein needs is also dependent on the dietitian's judgment and discretion based on patient's best interest and outcomes.[11]

DIETARY INTERVENTIONS FOR LUNG CANCER PATIENT AND SURVIVORS

During the emotional stress of dealing with lung cancer at any stage, patients derive increased quality of life and a sense of control over their lives as the result of receiving supportive advice on diet and lifestyle.[12] Therefore, the use of nutrition intervention can help lung cancer patients maintain body weight and nutrition stores, offering relief from symptoms and improving their quality of life. Whether the goal of lung cancer treatment is cure or palliation, early detection of nutritional problems and prompt intervention is essential.[12]

A general healthful diet is recommended for cancer patients and survivors. It consists of foods low in fat, cholesterol, and sodium and high in fiber. The general healthful diet includes protein sources other than red meat, low-fat or fat-free dairy products, whole grains, and at least five servings per day of fresh fruits and vegetables.

Small, frequent meals, and snacks versus three large daily meals should be considered for those having a hard time with their oral intake. If there is any chewing or swallowing difficulties present, a texture-modified diet is considered to ease chewing or swallowing and maximize intake.

The general healthful diet can be used to achieve and maintain a healthy weight. Addition of medical food supplements or the initiation of enteral or parenteral nutrition (PN) may be considered if oral intake is not adequate to meet estimated needs for preventing undesired weight loss and or loss of muscle mass.

Diet Composition

In the general healthful diet, carbohydrate is equal to 45%−65% of energy, protein is equal to 10%−20% of energy, total fat is equal to 20%−35% of energy, and fiber is equal to 25−30 g per day.

Some cancer patients tolerate liquids better than solids. To help meet estimated energy needs, patients should consider intake of high calorie foods such as whole milk and whole milk products, regular salad dressings, regular mayonnaise, honey, nectar, jam, granola, dried fruits, eggs, egg nog, nuts, nut butters, seeds, seed butters, wheat germ, coconut milk, gravy. Most importantly, patients should eat/drink what they desire, what they find appetizing, and what they are able to tolerate to optimize oral intake. In order to increase calorie and protein intake, oral nutritional supplements may be used.

Intake of vitamins and minerals should not exceed the Dietary Reference Intake (DRI), which is based on age and gender. Higher intake does not provide added benefit and instead may be harmful.

Diet and Inflammation

Lung cancer is associated with chronic inflammation, particularly chronic pulmonary inflammation or persistent lung inflammation such as chronic airway inflammatory conditions. Certain foods can cause inflammation, such as refined carbohydrates (white bread and pastries), margarine, shortening, lard, French fries, other fried foods, sugar, high-fructose corn syrup, soda, other sugar-sweetened beverages, red meat (burgers, steaks), and processed meat (hot dogs, sausage).[13]

The Mediterranean diet may become the preferred diet for reducing chronic inflammation since it has demonstrated antiinflammatory effects when compared with North American and Northern European diets. The Mediterranean diet has a high ratio of monounsaturated (MUFA) to saturated (SFA) fats and omega-3 to omega-6 polyunsaturated fatty acids (PUFAs) plus includes fruits, vegetables, legumes, and grains.[14]

Fat is needed in our body in order for it to function. However, not all fats are produced by our body. Omega-3 polyunsaturated fatty acid is an essential fat that our body cannot create on its own but instead needs to obtain it from the foods we consume. It may help prevent cancer. Before omega-3 supplements are taken, a healthcare provider should be consulted for any possible interaction with current medications.[15]

Omega-3 fatty acids can be found in plant oils, nuts and seeds, such as flaxseed and flaxseed oil, chia seeds, walnuts, canola oil, soybean oil, hemp seeds, navy beans, edamame, kidney beans, herring fish, fish oil, mackerel, salmon, rainbow trout, halibut, cod liver oil, canned tuna, rockfish, shrimp, and catfish. Certain foods, like some eggs, milk, or soy beverages, may have omega-3 added to it. The product food label will indicate if it has been fortified with omega-3.[11]

Nutrition is an important part of cancer treatment and recovery. Eating a healthy diet can promote health and reduce the risk of developing another cancer. The diet should include many types of plant-based foods. Fruits, vegetables, grains, beans, and other plants contain natural health-promoting substances called phytochemicals, which are plant-based chemicals. Some phytochemicals may protect cells from damage that could lead to cancer.[16]

Phytochemicals are antioxidants, which also include vitamin C, vitamin E, and carotenoids. Antioxidants help inhibit cell damage that may play a role in the development of cancer and therefore may aid in cancer prevention.[16]

Since fruits and vegetables contain antioxidants, their consumption may decrease the risk of some types of cancer. Eating a variety of foods rich in antioxidants each day may help cancer survivors in decreasing their risk for second cancers, which are new, different cancers and not the previously diagnosed cancer.[16]

Supplements that contain antioxidants have not been proven to decrease the risk of cancer. Therefore, it is recommended to consume foods instead of supplements containing antioxidants. Supplements may have antioxidants in amounts greater than the indicated DRI.[16]

Taking large doses of antioxidant supplements during chemotherapy or radiation is not recommended by some oncologists because it is believed that the antioxidants may restore the cancer cells damaged during these treatments, making chemotherapy and radiation less potent. To others, the belief that antioxidants repair the damage caused to cancer cells by cancer treatments is only speculation. Instead, they feel like there may be a net benefit in aiding to protect normal cells during cancer treatments.[16]

Currently, there is no science-based guidance whether antioxidant supplements are beneficial or damaging during chemotherapy or radiation treatment. Due to lack of evidence, cancer patients receiving these treatments should avoid supplements unless there is an actual nutrient deficiency indicated by test results, and they should also abstain from supplements that provide greater than 100% of the Daily Value.[16]

Cancer patients should focus on food versus supplements to optimize their nutrition. Meats at some meals should be replaced with legumes (dried beans and peas) weekly. At least five servings of fruits and vegetables, including citrus fruits, dark-green and deep-yellow vegetables, should be consumed daily. High-fiber foods, such as legumes, whole grain breads, and cereals, should be included daily. High-fat foods, particularly those from animal sources, should be limited. Lower-fat milk and dairy products should be considered. Lower-fat cooking methods, such as baking or broiling, should be used. Intake of salt-cured, smoked, and pickled foods should be reduced.

A lung cancer survivor should eat a plant-based diet high in fruits, vegetables, and whole grains. On a daily basis, survivors should consume at least 2.5 cups of fruits and vegetables. They should limit red and processed meats, and avoid cooking these and other high-fat protein sources at high temperatures. Survivors should limit high-fat foods and foods with added sugar. Supplements should only be taken by survivors if they have a nutrient deficiency.

Counseling Strategies

Effective nutrition counseling strategies for cancer patients include setting attainable goals, reducing sugar intake, increasing intake of foods rich in antioxidants, and empowering patients. The clinician should not overwhelm the patient with too much information all at once. Change is a process that takes time and each patient changes at their own pace.

Nutrition goals for cancer patients should follow the SMART criteria (specific, measurable, attainable, realistic, and timely). Goals should be created and agreed to by both patient and practitioner. Collaboration should take place in brainstorming ways to attain all goals and within what timeframe, which should lead to patients being more likely to actually change and reach their goals.

Sugar intake is associated with cancer since glucose is the main source of energy for cancer cells, also known as the Warburg effect. Cancer patients may benefit from a low-sugar diet, primarily added sugars, since it hinders the reproduction of cancer cells. Fruits and vegetables with low glycemic load should be considered over those with a high glycemic load, since it can lead to an increase risk of cancer. A high glycemic load and carbohydrate intake are linked to greater recurrence and mortality for chemotherapy patients.[17]

Intake of antioxidants in foods such as fruits and vegetables has the opposite effect of sugar intake. Individuals who consume the highest amount of vegetables, especially cruciferous vegetables, such as broccoli, cauliflower, cabbage, kale, Brussels sprouts, among others, have a decreased risk of cancer development and recurrence, particularly for lung cancers. Intake of nonstarchy vegetables should be higher than starchy vegetables. Darker-colored vegetables also have a greater nutritional impact.[17]

Empowering cancer patients can be achieved by using a style of counseling known as Motivational Interviewing, where clinicians try to get patients to develop intrinsic motivation to change their own behavior. Motivational Interviewing is defined as a collaborative, goal-oriented style of communication with particular attention to the language of change. Motivational Interviewing is designed to strengthen personal motivation for and commitment to a specific goal by eliciting and exploring the patient's own reasons for change within an atmosphere of acceptance and compassion. Through this strategy, patients are given the opportunity to examine their mixed feelings and contradictory ideas, which results in the patient ultimately coming to the conclusion that their habits need to change. Listening and in letting the patient come to their own decision about what they

need to do with her health is most beneficial. A sense of hope and optimism is linked with improved patient outcomes, including conditions as diverse as cancer recurrence, weight loss, depression reduction, blood pressure reduction, and more. In conclusion, clinicians should balance communicating the effect that lifestyle has on health, without overwhelming patients and contributing to more pressure and fear, since a few steps in the right direction is far better than a sense of overwhelm, paralysis, and inaction.[18]

RESTORATIVE CARE

An estimated 90% of oncology patients in the United States are treated in outpatient cancer settings. Cancer patients receiving out-patient multimodal treatment such as chemoradiation, surgery and, other interventions like immunotherapy are at risk for malnutrition. Treatment can often impair a patient's ability to eat and drink adequately. Most patients receiving out-patient cancer care do not receive routine nutrition referrals, and when they are referred, there are limited standards for out-patient nutrition care across patient populations. Suboptimal oral nutrition intake for a prolonged time can lead to malnutrition, impact treatment outcomes, and increase the risk of poor nutrition quality. Early nutrition screening and interventions can help minimize cancer treatment sequela and may improve overall outcomes. Major indicators for restorative nutrition support in the oncology population include mechanical and functional dysfunctions such as dysphagia, GI obstruction, tumor burdens to the oral cavity, and the inability to digest and absorb adequate foods and liquids.

Oral Nutrition

Once a patient is safe to swallow and can tolerate foods by mouth, oral food intake should be incorporated. Eating by mouth/oral route is of crucial importance to prevent gastrointestinal and mucosal atrophy. The goal of nutrition support of treatment is to meet calorie, protein, and fluid needs. When PO needs are met at > than 75%, enteral nutrition (EN) support may be discontinued.

Enteral Nutrition

The benefit of routine EN as a standard of maintaining proper nutrition in the lung cancer patients is not well documented. There are limited data showing that only ~12% of lung cancer patients receive EN.[19] EN is most often used in lung cancer patients who are receiving multimodal therapy with curative intent, and those experiencing alterations in swallow ability due to mucositis, esophagitis, or dysphagia due to treatment toxicities. Emerging research on the risk factors impacting lung cancer patients at highest risk will dictate if the use of EN will become a standard of nutrition care.

Indications for the Use of Enteral Nutrition Support

Existing malnutrition	Inability to consume adequate nutrients by mouth for greater than 7–14 days	Inability to feed by oral route, intolerance to oral diet	Patients treated with curative intent chemoradiation

Clinical Guidelines of the American Society for Parenteral and Enteral Nutrition (ASPEN).

Parenteral Nutrition

PN, the delivery of nutrition support intravenously, has saved many lives since its inception more than 50 years ago. Considered to be one of the hallmarks of modern medicine, PN remains of clinical significance across patient populations. The clinical debate surrounding the risks and benefits on clinical outcomes remain a hotly debated topic.[20] Historically, evidence-based research on the benefit of parental nutrition in lung cancer patients receiving multimodal treatment that included chemotherapy and radiation revealed mixed results.[21] Randomized controlled trials, undertaken in these early studies, did not show significant impact in outcomes with PN use.[22] Currently, the standard of care is to only use PN in patients without a functional gastrointestinal tract, and in fact PN is not recommended based upon diagnosis or disease state alone.[23] Prior to use of PN, the feasibility of EN is recommended and PN should only be used when adequate EN is not an option or in patients who are malnourished and will not be able to meet near normal and full nutrition needs using the GI tract for a prolonged period of time.

Symptom Management

Nutrition impact symptoms in the lung cancer population have been shown to be more prevalent than in patients with other cancers.[24] There are numerous nutrition-related impact symptoms that can occur in patients undergoing treatment. Common symptoms include loss of appetite, nausea, vomiting, fatigue, dysphagia, esophagitis dysgeusia or changes in taste, parageusia, odynophagia, and early satiety. These symptoms affect the patient's ability to eat and drink adequately and increase the risk of developing malnutrition.[25] Malnutrition prevalence studies show that as

little as two nutrition impact symptoms can cause difficulties in food intake.[26] Nutrition impact symptoms increase risk of malnutrition exponentially in metastatic versus localized lung cancer disease.[27] Interventions provided by the nutrition support team are pertinent and are most efficient when patients are assessed early using a step-wise approach that includes risk stratification. While there is a paucity of research on outcome associated with dietitian-led nutritional counseling and instruction, feasibility of symptom management education is well established.[28] Providing patients with instruction and strategies on how to manage symptoms that compromises appetite and oral intake, for example, has been shown to be most impactful when incorporated with use of oral nutrition supplements rich in branched-chain amino acids and omega-3 fatty acids. Even though omega-3 supplement studies have shown mixed results and larger studies are needed to direct precise interventions, patients appear to appreciate the benefit of calorie rich medical grade drinks to augment their usual food intake when appetite is poor. Nausea and vomiting pose an even greater challenge for lung cancer patients to meet nutrition needs as symptoms can be mild to severe.

Lung rehabilitation strategies for these patients are often dictated by the degree of the nausea and vomiting and require a tailored approach to management. Constipation and diarrhea are similarly troubling and can impact the patient's ability to eat. Constipation can induce early satiety and lead to poor nutritional intake. Diarrhea, defined as more than three loose bowel movements in a 24 h period, that is refractory to medical management and dietary intervention can cause electrolyte imbalance and deficits in hydration that can be detrimental to maintaining proper nutrition before during and after treatment. Dysphagia, the loss of swallowing function, is another significant symptom in lung cancer patients and can develop due to the intensity and proximity of radiotherapy to the organs associated with swallowing. Additionally, a process described as sarcopenic dysphagia has been reportedly observed. Although not well described in the literature, it can have a negative impact on lung cancer patients. A case study illustrating sarcopenic dysphagia described as a loss of swallowing muscle mass and function associated with generalized loss of skeletal muscle mass was observed in a geriatric malnourished patient following surgery, intubation, and diagnosed malnutrition.[29] Rehabilitative nutrition included dysphagia rehabilitation from speech therapy and nutrition support team. Sarcopenia-induced dysphagia should be considered in patients with sarcopenia and dysphagia.

The table below illustrates common real-world nutrition interventions incorporated for nutrition impact symptoms during dietetic supportive care to lung cancer patients.

Nutrition Impact Symptom	Interventions
Loss of appetite/Early satiety	Eat by the clock rather than awaiting hunger cues
Anorexia	Eat smaller more frequent high calorie foods and liquids
Nausea	Eat dry carbohydrate foods versus foods that overwhelm or have extreme odors and temperatures
Vomiting	Consume liquids between meals versus with meals. Limit exposure to foods with extreme odors and smells—Eat cool foods with little odor. Avoid strong smelling lotions and perfumes when in close proximity.
Diarrhea	Encourage a low fat/fiber, modified caffeine diet, use bulking agents such as pectin or soluble fiber foods such as bananas, oats, rice, potatoes to control loose stools
Constipation	Evaluate for medications that may slow gastric emptying for example, opioids, aluminum hydroxide antacids, H2 receptor antagonists, proton pump inhibitors (PPIs)
Dysphagia	Incorporate a modified consistency diet Recommend good posture when eating to help prevent aspiration, avoid distractions and limit talking while eating, encourage double swallow to ensure food clears, Use thickeners in liquids to slow flow and allow safe swallow- refer for speech and language therapist consult
Mucositis/Esophagitis	Inflammation of the mouth or esophagus - a painful irritated throat—described as a lump in the throat. Choose soft textured, low acid foods, practice good oral care

PALLIATIVE AND SUPPORTIVE NUTRITIONAL CARE

Nutrition care and goals for palliative care patients differ depending on whether palliation is concurrent with treatment or if it is initiated later in the disease process. Aggressive nutrition support may not be indicated when goals of care are not curative and the shift is toward end of life or hospice with a focus on comfort measures.[30] In patients with advanced cancer and terminal illness, for example, cancer cachexia is common and there is evidence that suggest that there are opportunities to enhance supportive nutrition care measures. Patients and caregivers convey a feeling of frustration and distress by a lack of response from healthcare teams when it comes to weight loss, weight change, and inability to take oral nutrition.[31] Nutrition by way of solid food or fluid intake is considered basic care across the continuum of cancer care.

In palliative care, the use of artificial nutrition and hydration (ANH) is a dynamic and often controversial topic among patients, caregivers, and healthcare providers. ANH is associated with benefits and burdens, specifically in end of life care. There are many factors that influence acceptance or refusal of ANH. Religious beliefs, culture, whether it is cost prohibitive, and level of care needs dictate the use of ANH. ANH is considered a necessity by some and other consider withdrawing or withholding the appropriate choice.[32] Lack of knowledge about all nutrition options in palliative and end of life care may be an issue in unrealistic expectations of medical interventions. Patients and caregivers perceptions on ANH may conflict with the healthcare team.[33] Patients and family often consider artificial hydration (AH) a way of ensuring a better quality of life, minimizing discomfort, and ensuring a sense of well-being.[34,35] Terminal dehydration is associated with confusion, opioid toxicity, constipation, dry mouth, and thirst. Those opposing AH consider it to cause pain, and promotes vomiting, ascites, edema, and pulmonary congestion.[36] Even though research to explore whether AH improves or worsens symptoms is conflicting,[37,38] the use of AH is not recommended at the end of life.

Contraindications noted are that it causes false hope, and denial of the terminal illness, increases urine output and induces further dehydration, and increases risk or infection. Withholding AH can induce euphoria, decrease agitation, and delirium and offer improvement in sedation in end of life care.

In lung cancer patients with stable, advanced, and terminal disease, the nutrition team can help to provide evidence-based education to patients, caregivers, and the medical team on the benefits and risks of ANH for patients under the care of the palliative medicine team and at end of life.

DIET, NUTRITION, AND PHYSICAL ACTIVITY

Recent systematic reviews suggest that exercise and nutrition interventions are not harmful and may have beneficial effects on unintentional weight loss, physical strength, and functional performance in patients with advanced lung cancer.[39]

Case Study

A 65-year-old gentleman was referred to the radiation oncology clinic after presenting with anterior chest wall pain, a 25 pound unintentional weight loss, and generalized fatigue. Previous inpatient work-up revealed a large 7 cm apical/Pancoast tumor of the right upper lobe with mediastinal adenopathy. He was subsequently diagnosed with a stage IIIB, T4N2M0, NSCLC [adenocarcinoma], and was not deemed a surgical candidate. The treatment consensus was to proceed with concurrent chemo-radiotherapy and adjuvant immunotherapy.[40] At time of initial consultation, this patient was cachectic with a decreased body mass, a thin chest wall, and minimal para-spinal fat seen on cross-sectional imaging (Fig. 12.1). He was reticent and withdrawn, and overwhelmed with cancer diagnosis.

NUTRITION ASSESSMENT

Due to the patient's substantial unintentional weight loss −25 pounds (representing 19% of his usual body weight [UBW]), he was screened by the inpatient nutritionist for further evaluation and management. A nutrition-focused physical examination revealed moderate temple muscle wasting, moderate fat loss in the orbits and cheekbones, moderate fat loss in the triceps,

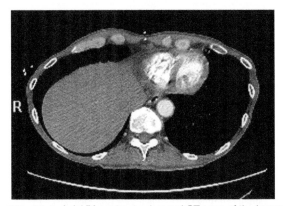

FIG. 12.1 Axial IV-contrast enhanced CT scan of the lower chest and upper abdomen demonstrates an extremely thin chest wall, reduced fat distribution, and reduced muscle bulk in a patient with a newly diagnosed lung cancer, consistent with sarcopenia and malignancy related cachexia.

and protrusion of clavicles. His daily home diet consisted of one large meal nightly without day-time snacks. The nutritionist also noted that the nursing staff frequently removed uneaten meals at patient's bedside. After completion of the comprehensive nutritional assessment, the patient was counseled on the importance of adequate nutrition, and instructed to eat small frequent meals, as well as supplement with caloric nutritional shakes twice daily.

NUTRITION DIAGNOSIS

Acute disease or injury-related malnutrition.

NUTRITION INTERVENTION

The nutritionist followed the patient's progression during the course of his hospitalization, as well as continued with outpatient management upon discharge. They continued to counsel patient weekly on the importance of adequate nutrition and encouraged increased caloric intake. Even though twice daily nutritional shake supplementation was recommended, the patient initially started with only one shake daily due to cost. This led to a revelation of another underlying cause for weight loss—lack of access. The nutrition team subsequently worked with the social work team to provide samples and coupons of nutritional shakes to ensure this barrier was overcome.

CASE DISCUSSION

The established diagnostic criteria for cancer cachexia focused only on weight loss, with 5%−10% being an arbitrary cut off. However, cancer cachexia is a multifactorial syndrome characterized by an ongoing loss of skeletal muscle mass (with or without loss of fat mass) and leads to progressive functional impairment.[41] Cancer cachexia with skeletal muscle depletion is a poor prognostic factor regardless of overall body weight, and is associated with reduced physical function, reduced tolerance to anticancer therapy, and reduced overall survival.[41,42] A full assessment of underlying risk factors, including anorexia, changes in taste and smell, early satiety and nausea, constipation, stomatitis, dyspnea, pain, and socioeconomic stressors, is needed in order to properly establish a treatment regimen. Most worrisome, when patients become malnourished, they are less likely to receive their full oncology treatment and may require treatment breaks, treatment holds, or dose reductions, which may reduce the efficacy of their cancer-directed therapy.

Timely, systematic, and structured nutritional intervention prevented this patient from further weight

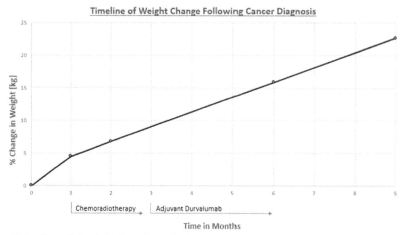

FIG. 12.2 Patient's weight plotted at time of diagnosis, treatment start and during concurrent chemo-radiotherapy, during adjuvant durvalumab, and in follow-up. There was a 22% increase in weight in a 9-month period.

loss and helped him complete his entire 7 week course of concurrent chemo-radiotherapy without interruption (Fig. 12.2). This exemplifies the "parallel pathway," in which routine screening and early intervention starting at the moment a cancer diagnosis is made, and running parallel to the pathway of tumor-directed therapies, improves nutritional outcomes.[43] Perhaps the most significant contributing factor to this patient's weight loss was pain (although decreased appetite and socioeconomic stressors also substantially contributed), which improved dramatically due to therapeutic treatment response. In fact, narcotic pain medication was discontinued half-way through his treatment course due to reduction in the extent of his disease. Having been set up with cancer support services at initial presentation facilitated this patient in completing his entire course of treatment, and illustrates the need for a multidisciplinary treatment approach to cancer care.

CONCLUSION

Experimental and clinical evidence demonstrate cancer cachexia results from profound alterations in nutritional status and metabolic homeostasis.[43] Metabolic disturbances can occur early in the disease course, prior to apparent weight loss. The role of timely nutritional interventions aimed at preventing nutritional decline is becoming increasingly evident. Additional clinical trials are needed in order to evaluate early interventional approaches in at-risk patients, to improve compliance to treatment and ultimately patient outcomes.

REFERENCES

1. Lungcancerresearchfoundation.org. Accessed 10 March 2021.
2. American Cancer Society. *Cancer Facts and Figures 21021*. Atlanta: American Cancer Society; 2020.
3. Dai S, Ming Y, Juan S, Sisi D, Wu J. Impacts of frailty on prognosis in lung cancer patients: a systematic review and meta-analysis. *Front Med.* 2021;8:715513.
4. Gridelli C, Balducci L, Ciardiello F, et al. Treatment of elderly patients with non-small cell lung cancer: results of an international expert panel meeting of the Italian association of thoracic oncology. *Clin Lung Cancer.* 2015;16:325–333.
5. Ethun CG, Bilen MA, Jani AB, Maithel SK, Ogan K, Master VA. Frailty and cancer: implications for oncology surgery, medical oncology, radiation oncology. *CA Cancer J Clin.* 2017;67:362–377.
6. Nakamura R, Inage Y, Tobita R, et al. Sarcopenia in resected NSCLC: effect on post-operative outcomes. *J Thorac Oncol.* 2018;13:895–903.
7. Chen KC, Cheng YJ, Hung MH, et al. Non-intubated thoracoscopic lung resection: a 3 year experience with 285 cases in a single institution. *J Thorac Dis.* 2012;4:347–351.
8. Zijia L, Tan Q, Lijian P, et al. *Anesth Analg.* 2020;131(3):840–849.
9. Sanchez-Lorente D, Navarro-Ripoll R, Guzman R, et al. Pre-habilitation in thoracic surgery. *J Thorac Dis.* 2018;10(Suppl 22):S2593.
10. Polanski J, Jankowska-Polanska B, Uchmanowicz I, et al. Malnutrition and quality of life in patients with non-small cell lung cancer. *Pulm Care Clin Med.* 2017:15–26.
11. Academy of Nutrition and Dietetics. *Nutrition Care Manual.* http://www.nutritioncaremanual.org. Accessed 11 May 2021.

12. Hennekens CH, Buring JE, Manson JE, et al. Lack of effect of long-term supplementation with beta carotene on the incidence of malignant neoplasms and cardiovascular disease. *N Engl J Med.* 1996;334:1145−1149.

13. Kamp DW, Shacter E, Weitzman SA. Chronic inflammation and cancer: the role of the mitochondria. *Oncology.* 2011;25. https://www.cancernetwork.com/view/chronic-inflammation-and-cancer-role-mitochondria.

14. Galland L. Diet and inflammation. *Nutr Clin Pract.* 2010; 25(6):634−640. https://doi.org/10.1177/088453361038 5703. PMID: 21139128.

15. Memorial Sloan Kettering Cancer Center. https://www.mskcc.org. Accessed 29 May 2021.

16. American Cancer Society. http://www.cancer.org. Accessed 14 May 2021.

17. Lyons M. *4 Strategies for Effective Nutrition Counseling for Cancer Patients.* Invitae Cancer Gene Connect; August 24, 2016. https://cagene.com/latest/2016/8/24/4-strategies-for-effective-nutrition-counseling-for-cancer-patients.

18. *MINT Excellence in Motivational Interviewing.* https://motivationalinterviewing.org/understanding-motivational-interviewing. Accessed 21 July 2021.

19. Kiss N, Krishnasamy M, Everett S, et al. Dosimetric factors associated with weight loss during chemo-radiotherapy treatment for lung cancer. *Eur J Clin Nutr.* 2014;68(12): 1309−1314.

20. Mirtallo JM. Parenteral nutrition: can outcomes be improved? *J Parenter Enter Nutr.* 2013;37(2):181−189.

21. Valdivieso M, Frankmann C, Murphy WK, et al. Long-term effects of intravenous hyper alimentation administered during intensive chemotherapy for small cell bronchogenic carcinoma. *Cancer.* 1987;59(2):362−369.

22. McGeer AJ, Detsky AS, O'Rourke K. Parenteral nutrition in cancer patients undergoing chemotherapy: a meta-analysis. *Nutrition.* 1990;6(3):233−240.

23. Worthington P, Balint J, Bechtold M, et al. When is parenteral nutrition appropriate? *J Parenter Enter Nutr.* 2017; 41(3):324−377.

24. Cooley ME. Symptoms in adults with lung cancer: a systematic research review. *J Pain Symptom Manag.* 2000; 19(2):137−153.

25. McCallum P. Nutrition screening and assessment in oncology. In: Elliot L, et al., eds. *The Clinical Guide to Oncology Nutrition.* 2nd ed. Chicago: The American Dietetic Association; 2006:44−53.

26. Segura A, Pardo J, Jara C, et al. An epidemiological evaluation of the prevalence of malnutrition in Spanish patients with locally advanced or metastatic cancer. *Clin Nutr.* 2005;24(5):801−814.

27. Hebuterne X, Lemarie F, Michelle M, et al. Prevalence of malnutrition and current use of nutrition support in patients with cancer. *J Parenter Enter Nutr.* 2014;38(2): 196−204.

28. Naito T, Mitsunaga S, Miura S, et al. Feasibility of early multimodal interventions for elderly patients with advanced pancreatic and non-small-cell lung cancer. *J Cachexia Sarcopenia Muscle.* 2019;10(1):73−83. https://doi.org/10.1002/jcsm.12351.

29. Wakabayashi H, Uwano R. Rehabilitation nutrition for possible sarcopenic dysphagia after lung cancer surgery: a case report. *Am J Phys Med Rehabil.* 2016;95(6):e84−e89. https://doi.org/10.1097/PHM.0000000000000458.

30. Trentham K. Nutrition management of oncology patients in palliative and hospice settings. In: Elliot L, et al., eds. *The Clinical Guide to Oncology Nutrition.* 2nd ed. Chicago: The American Dietetic Association; 2006:44−53.

31. Yamagishi A, Morita T Miyashita M, et al. The care strategy for families of terminally ill cancer patients who become unable to take nourishment orally: recommendations from a nationwide surveyor bereaved family members' experiences. *J Pain Symptom Manag.* 2010;40(5):671−683.

32. Geppert CMA, Andrews MR, Druyan ME. Ethical issues in artificial nutrition and hydration: a review. *J Parenter Enteral Nutr.* 2010;34(1):79−88.

33. Maillet JO, Potter RL, Heller L. Position of the American dietetic association: ethical and legal issues in nutrition , hydration, and feeding. *J Am Diet Assoc.* 2002;102(5): 716−726.

34. Soo L, Grämlich L. Use of parenteral nutrition in patients with advanced cancer. *Appl Physiol Nutr Metabol.* 2008; 33(1):102−106.

35. Cohen MZ, Torres-Vigil I, Burbach BE, de la Rosa A, Bruera E. The meaning of parenteral hydration to family caregivers and patients with advanced cancer receiving hospice care. *J Pain Symptom Manag.* 2012;43(5):855−865.

36. Dev R, Dalal S, Bruera E. Is there a role for parenteral nutrition or hydration at the end of life< Curr Open Support. *Palliat Care.* 2012;6(3):365−370.

37. Good P, Cavenah J, Syrmis W, Jenkins-Marsh S, Stephens J. Medically assisted hydration for adult palliative care patients. *Cochrane Database Syst Rev.* 2008;(2). https://doi.org/10.1002/14651858.CD006274.pub2. Art. no: CD006273.

38. Dalal S, Hui D, Torres-Vigil I, et al. Parenteral hydration (PH) in advanced cancer patients: a multi-center, double-blind, placebo-controlled randomized trial. ASCO 2012 *J Clin Oncol.* 2012;30 (supply;abstr 9025).

39. Payne C, Larkin PJ, McIlfatrick S, Dunwoody L, Gracey JH. *Curr Oncol.* 2013;20(4):e321−e337.

40. Antonia SJ, Villegas A, Daniel D, et al. Overall survival with durvalumab after chemoradiotherapy in stage III NSCLC. *N Engl J Med.* 2018;379:2342−2350. https://doi.org/10.1056/NEJMoa1809697.

41. Fearon K, Strasser F, Anker SD, et al. Definition and classification of cancer cachexia: an international consensus. *Lancet Oncol.* 2011;12:489−495. https://doi.org/10.1016/S1470-2045(10)70218-7.

42. Martin L, Birdsell L, Macdonald N, et al. Cancer cachexia in the age of obesity: skeletal muscle depletion is a powerful prognostic factor, independent of body mass index. *J Clin*

Oncol. 2013;31:1539–1547. https://doi.org/10.1200/JCO.2012.45.2722.

43. Muscaritoli M, Costelli P, Aversa Z, Bonetto A, Baccino FM, Rossi Fanelli F. New strategies to overcome cancer cachexia: from molecular mechanisms to the "Parallel Pathway". *Asia Pac J Clin Nutr.* 2008;17(Suppl 1): 387–390.

FURTHER READING

1. American Lung Association. *State of Lung Cancer.* 2020.
2. Siegel, et al. Cancer statistics, 2021. *CA Cancer J Clin.* 2021; 71:7–33.

CHAPTER 13

Pain Management in Lung Cancer Rehabilitation

AMY K. PARK, DO • CHANEL DAVIDOFF, DO • KIMBERLY BANCROFT, PHD • NAOMI M. KAPLAN, MBBS

INTRODUCTION

Pain Definition

In June 2020, the International Association for the Study of Pain (IASP) revised the definition of pain for the first time since 1979, after 2 years of development.[1] The revised pain definition from the IASP reads as "an unpleasant sensory and emotional experience associated with, or resembling that associated with, actual or potential tissue damage."[1] Six additional notes were added to this revised definition, further describing pain as a personal experience with biopsychosocial factors, as a concept shaped by life experiences, and as distinct from pure nociception.[1] It goes on to emphasize that a patient's pain narrative should be respected, and that verbal communication is not the only way to report pain.[1] Although pain serves as a protective mechanism, it can also seriously impact functional, social, and psychological well-being.[1] The IASP pain definition is widely accepted by international organizations, including the World Health Organization. Patients with lung cancer can have acute pain (<6 months), chronic pain (>6 months), or acute on chronic pain, that can range from mild to severe in intensity, and may be multifactorial in nature, including neuropathic, visceral, and somatic pain components. This will be discussed in depth later in this chapter.

Pain Theories as Related to Cancer

Biopsychosocial Model of Pain. The biopsychosocial model of pain succeeds the biomedical model of pain, which dates back hundreds of years to Descartes, as well as the gate control theory which dates to the 1960s as described by Melzack and Wall.[2,3] The biopsychosocial model described by Turk and Flor posits that biological factors modulate pathophysiological alarms, psychological factors influence the analysis of these internal signals, and that social factors determine the behavioral response to these bodily signs and symptoms.[2,4] This model applies to both acute and chronic pain, is widely accepted within the pain science community, and applies well to cancer pain. The biopsychosocial model focuses on illness instead of disease and proposes that patients can vary in their responses to somatic sensations, based on psychosocial factors.[2] In the biopsychosocial model of pain, the biological, psychological, and social factors can vary in influence at different times within the same patient, as well as vary between patients with the same underlying diagnosis.[2] Ultimately, our understanding of pain has changed throughout the course of human history from a unidimensional construct, to a multidimensional concept which requires an interdisciplinary approach.[2]

Total Pain. Dame Cicely Saunders, founder of the modern hospice movement, with training in nursing, social work, and medicine, introduced the concept of "total pain" to include physical, psychological, social, and spiritual elements, as described in her early writings.[5] Although emphasis is often placed on physical pain, a patient's pain experience may also include any or all components of pain related to their emotional state, loss or change in their societal and familial role, as well existential, religious, and/or spiritual distress. The framework of total pain emphasizes each patient's uniqueness and unique pain experience.

Symptom Clusters. It has been suggested that the symptoms experienced in lung cancer often occur in clusters throughout the course of the disease. In cancer, symptom clusters have been defined as multiple symptoms that exist simultaneously that are related to each other through a common mechanism, although they may not share the same etiology.[6] Hamada and colleagues identified three symptom clusters that predominate in patients with advanced lung cancer: a fatigue/anorexia cluster, a pain cluster, and a numbness

Lung Cancer Rehabilitation. https://doi.org/10.1016/B978-0-323-83404-9.00004-9

cluster.[7] The pain cluster has the strongest influence on an individual's emotions, compounding symptoms of pain, anxiety, and sadness. There is evidence that pain has a positive correlation with fatigue, disrupted sleep, and distress in individuals with lung cancer, suggesting that these symptoms may exist concurrently and intensify overall symptom severity.[8] Symptom clusters affect quality of life (QOL) and functional status to varying degrees. Pain clusters have been shown to interfere with physical, emotional, and social aspects of everyday life.[7] Lin et al. found that the cooccurrence of pain, fatigue, disturbed sleep, and distress negatively correlated with functional status and QOL measures in patients with lung cancer who underwent surgical intervention.[8] Managing pain without considering other cluster symptoms may result in inadequate treatment, persistent symptom burden, and poor QOL. To improve the overall well-being of patients with lung cancer, attention needs to focus on developing comprehensive pain management strategies that address symptom clusters to reduce pain and distress experienced in this population.

PAIN IN LUNG CANCER

Pain in Lung Cancer—Types and Locations

Pain in lung cancer encompasses a broad spectrum of symptomatology and etiology and therefore is often poorly characterized and challenging to treat. One method of classification is by defining whether the patient's pain is directly related to the malignancy or due to the various antineoplastic treatment modalities that are utilized. Pain may also be categorized by location, duration, and/or by its nature.[9]

Somatic or nociceptive pain is defined as "physiological pain due to stimulation of the sensory nociceptors located in tissues." It may occur due to direct damage of local structures, or be referred from visceral organs.[10] **Neuropathic pain**, also called "nerve pain," is caused by an injury or insult to the central or peripheral nervous system, causing the pain centers in the brain, spinal cord, and peripheral nerves to produce abnormal nerve impulses.[11] **Acute pain** usually occurs secondary to a defined injury or insult, with a short duration and predictable course.[12] **Chronic pain** is defined more so by duration. The pain pattern is vaguer, with gradual or ill-defined onset, possibly waxing, and waning severity, and may last the majority of the day. Up to 75% of patients with lung cancer report chronic pain.[13] **Breakthrough pain** is defined as a "transient exacerbation of pain that occurs spontaneously or in relation to a [...] trigger, despite relatively stable [...] background pain."[14]

Chest and back pain are the most common locations of pain in patients with advanced lung cancer.[15] Direct effect of local tumor invasion most commonly causes somatic chest or back pain which is ipsilateral to the site of the malignancy. A Pancoast tumor, located at the apex of the lung, can cause pain in the upper chest and ipsilateral arm as it grows and compresses nearby anatomy causing both somatic and neuropathic pain. Costopleural syndrome, caused by tumor invasion of the pleura, is another direct consequence of the malignancy, most commonly mesothelioma.[16] Metastases to the ribs may cause localized bony pain. If the intercostal nerves are damaged, there is associated neuropathic pain. The main cause of breakthrough pain in lung cancer patients is due to bony metastases. This complex pain pathway is associated with both inflammatory and neuropathic pain at the site of metastasis.[15]

Epidemiology and Prevalence of Pain in Lung Cancer

The incidence of lung cancer continues to be on the rise, accounting for 11.4% of all new cancer cases worldwide.[17] In the United States, there have been notable improvements in survival rates of individuals with lung cancer, owing to tobacco cessation initiatives, early detection, and advancements in treatments for both early and late-stage disease.[18] Yet, lung cancer continues to have the highest mortality rate of all cancer types, accounting for 18% of cancer deaths worldwide.[17] Lung cancer has a high propensity to metastasize or recur locally. In fact, most patients with lung cancer present with advanced stage disease at the time of diagnosis.[19] Recurrence of lung cancer is common within the first 2 years following treatment, with a majority of tumors recurring distally from the primary site.[20,21]

Pain continues to be the most common symptom associated with cancer and, in general, is more prevalent in those with metastatic or terminal disease (66%).[22] As a result, pain is one of the most prevalent symptoms experienced by patients with lung cancer.[9] Improvements in lung cancer survival have impacted the prevalence of pain in this population since more individuals are living with prolonged and persistent symptoms. Unfortunately, management of pain continues to be challenging due to the multifactorial nature of pain associated with lung cancer as well as the overall medical complexity of this patient population. Comprehensive and interdisciplinary assessment is imperative for management of pain in individuals with lung cancer.

Effect of Pain on Quality of Life and Function

Patients with lung cancer experience a variety of symptoms throughout their disease course due to the tumor burden and treatment-related side effects. The most common symptoms reported in this patient population include dyspnea, fatigue, and pain. Compared to other types of cancer, those with lung cancer have higher levels of distress, which can negatively impact overall function and health related QOL.[23,24] In the United States, 32% of patients with advanced stage lung cancer have reported moderate to severe pain.[25] Pain interferes with psychological well-being in patients with lung cancer and has the potential to exacerbate and prolong symptoms of depression, especially if poorly controlled.[26] Identifying and treating symptoms that negatively impact QOL is essential for improving outcomes and overall survival in lung cancer.[27,28] As a result, there has been a paradigm shift toward symptom-focused care in patients with lung cancer which include routine assessment of symptoms and early intervention of supportive services such as rehabilitation and palliative medicine.[29–31]

The Pain Trajectory

Pain from lung cancer and its treatment is present throughout the disease trajectory from the time of diagnosis, through active treatment, and into survivorship or end-of-life care. Knowledge about pain generators throughout the disease continuum is important to improve the management of pain in lung cancer.

Pain at diagnosis. Pain is one of the most common complaints among individuals with lung cancer at the time of diagnosis. Patients diagnosed with primary lung cancer report pain at baseline prior to any treatment or intervention.[32] One reason for this could be that a majority of patients with lung cancer present with late-stage disease at the time of diagnosis[9,24] and, generally, patients with more advanced disease are more likely to experience pain than those with early disease. Lung cancer diagnosed in its early stages (such as incidental pulmonary nodules) is not often associated with pain. It is speculated that a proportion of baseline pain in early-stage lung cancer represents exacerbation of comorbid musculoskeletal pain rather than direct effect of tumor.[32] The leading causes of malignancy-related pain in advanced lung cancer are skeletal metastatic disease, apical Pancoast tumors, and chest wall disease.[33] For individuals with advanced disease at diagnosis, pain can typically occur due to direct, local tumor invasion, malignant pleural effusions, bone metastases, and/or brachial plexopathy.

Thoracic/chest pain is one of the more commonly reported early symptoms at the time of diagnosis and continues to progress throughout the disease course.[34] Chest pain in lung cancer can arise from localized neoplastic spread but also from secondary complications of the disease such as persistent cough, pulmonary embolism, and obstructive pneumonitis.[13] Additionally, pain prior to surgery may be heightened as a result of the emotional and financial stress of being diagnosed with a life-threatening disease in addition to the physical symptoms endured. Studies have recognized that patients with higher preoperative pain are more likely to have persistent pain following surgery.[35] Knowledge about premorbid pain and function can help anticipate complications following interventions and is essential for making informed management decisions.

Pain during treatment. Pain was found to be prevalent in patients with lung cancer at a rate of 39.3% after curative treatment and 55.0% during anticancer treatment.[22] Treatment for lung carcinoma depends on type (nonsmall cell lung cancer vs. small cell lung cancer) and stage of disease (local vs. metastatic).[22] Patients may undergo one or multiple treatment modalities such as surgery, chemotherapy, or radiation therapy. Surgical resection has been shown to improve overall survival in those with operable lung cancer; however, undergoing surgery can result in unexpected complications as well as the development of acute pain syndromes which can further progress to chronic pain if left untreated. Etiologies of pain during treatment are commonly attributed to surgical procedures, chemotherapy, immunotherapy, radiation therapy, or tumor related (see Fig. 13.1).

Acute pain after thoracotomy has been described as the most severe postprocedural pain.[36] This surgery involves manipulation of intrathoracic structures and can result in rib fractures, muscle contusions, stretching of intercostal nerves, and pleural irritation. Management of postoperative pain presents a major challenge to providers due to the complexity of the patient's pain when even the act of taking deep breaths or early mobilization—all important in preventing postsurgical complications—can exacerbate pain. Proper management of postoperative pain is essential as lack of adequate pain control can delay discharge and preclude the patient's ability to participate in rehabilitation which leads to poor outcomes.[37]

Systemic therapy used in lung cancer includes chemotherapy, immunotherapy, or targeted therapy. Patients may receive one or more types of systemic therapy alone or in combination with radiation or surgery. Pain experienced as a result from systemic treatments can be

Diagnosis	Treatment and Post-Operative	Survivorship

Tumor-related
  Chest wall invasion
  Costopleural syndrome
  Pleural effusions
  Malignant brachial
  plexopathy
  Pancoast Tumor
  Metastases:bone, liver,
  brain
 	
Diagnostic procedures
  Lumbar puncture
  Thoracentesis
	Post-Surgical
	  Acute post-thoracotomy pain
	  Chest tube placement
	  Incisional pain
	  Pleuritic chest pain
	
	Systemic Therapy
	  Chemotherapy
	  Painful polyneuropathy
	  (acute)
	
	Radiation Therapy
	  Radiation pneumonitis
		Disease related complications
		  Metastases: bone, liver, brain
		
		  Neuropathy
		  Cervical / Brachial plexopathy
		  Central Pain syndrome (CNS involvement)
		  Post-herpetic Neuralgia
		
		  Paraneoplastic syndromes
		  Hypertrophic osteo-arthropathy
		
		Treatment-related complications
		
		  Chemotherapy induced peripheral
		  neuropathy
		  Radiation Plexopathy
		  Complex Regional Pain Syndrome
		
		Multifactorial
		  Radiation Fibrosis Syndrome
		  Post-thoracotomy pain syndrome

FIG. 13.1 Common causes of pain throughout the lung cancer continuum.

debilitating and negatively impact an individual's function. For example, chemotherapy can induce a painful polyneuropathy in the upper and lower extremities and may result in impairments in gait and activities of daily living. Immune-mediated arthralgias and myalgias have also been reported while taking immune checkpoint inhibitors such as pembrolizumab for nonsmall cell lung cancer.[38]

Pain in survivorship. Many cancer survivors experience physical impairments which may progress to disability if gone undetected or undertreated.[39] Most posttreatment pain syndromes are neuropathic in nature and commonly result from direct nerve injury from prior treatments (surgery, radiation, or chemotherapy) or complications from the cancer itself.[10]

Lung cancer patients can develop chronic pain following thoracotomy also referred to as *post thoracotomy pain syndrome.* It is defined as thoracic pain around the surgical site lasting longer than 2 months following surgery.[40] The exact mechanism is unclear but is hypothesized to have neuropathic and myofascial pain characteristics. Neuropathic pain syndromes can extend into the survivorship stage due to the complexity of symptoms and challenge of mitigating pain related to nerve injury. Moreover, there is a lot of variability between patient symptoms as well as their response to treatment.[41] For cancer survivors in general, it is important to exclude tumor recurrence when presenting with new pain or pain that is persistent and not amenable to treatments.

AN INTERDISCIPLINARY APPROACH TO CANCER PAIN

Team Members in Cancer Pain Management—Providers and Allied Health Professionals

It is not just one specialty's role to provide adequate pain management for patients with cancer. The best way to provide complex pain management is with an interdisciplinary, team approach. Pain is typically a key question on any patient intake form and should be followed up every time. Oncologists, primary care providers, physiatrists, and hospitalists are first-line responders providing *primary* palliative care, which includes pain relief. These providers, although not specialty trained in symptom management, can still provide medications, therapies, and interventions, within their scope, that contribute toward alleviating patients' pain. Palliative medicine specialists, who are subspecialty trained and board certified, are uniquely placed to provide *secondary* or *tertiary* palliative care, which often includes complex pain medication regimens, use of controlled substances, and/or referrals to radiation oncology or even anesthesiology for interventional pain management.

The nonphysician members of the patient care team play an equally integral role in pain management. Social workers and case managers often wear many hats, helping patients with cancer navigate their appointments, providing support for completing the myriad forms needed to ensure care coverage, and depending on their skillset, providing supportive talk therapy that can help patients address the psychosocial components of pain. Talk therapy, in its many forms, can also be provided by clinical psychologists, who are a tremendous asset to oncology programs. Nursing staff is primed to provide patient education about pain medication administration, ensure medication adherence, and answer questions as able. They are also involved in other forms of patient care, such as wound care, which can have a profound impact on pain and discomfort. Physical, occupational, and speech therapists address pain directly through rehabilitation and desensitization techniques, as well as addressing the functional impairments that arise from cancer pain, by means of assistive devices, durable medical equipment, compensatory strategies, and caregiver training. Healthcare chaplaincy can be a great support to both religious and nonaffiliated patients and their families, providing comfort and guidance to alleviate spiritual and existential distress.

Pain Management Locations

Pain management can take place in any patient care location, whether be at home, inpatient admission, or outpatient clinic. Pain management will look different depending on the patient and clinical environment. It's important for them to be consistent and intentional plans for pain control, regardless of the patient location, throughout the continuum of care.

Patients with lung cancer may be at home with oral or subcutaneous pain medications and in-home therapy and nursing services. Hospice and palliative medicine organizations, and some primary care providers, can manage patients' pain via home visits if the patient is homebound and/or is receiving hospice care.

Patients who are still well enough to attend clinic appointments may benefit from intravenous infusions, joint and/or spinal injections, palliative radiation, and medication optimization from outpatient providers. Additionally, outpatient PT, OT, SLP, recreation therapy, social work, and psychology/counseling services can play an important role in outpatient pain management.

Patients with uncontrolled pain symptoms, whose pain is associated with clinical instability, or who have increased morbidity and mortality may be admitted either directly from home, or from the ER, for aggressive inpatient pain management. This typically takes place in a tertiary or quaternary level hospital. For hospice patients with uncontrolled pain, their hospice organization may admit them to a hospice house, nursing home, or medical facility for "general inpatient care." Other specialists that play a role in inpatient pain management include internists, palliative care and pain specialists, anesthesiologists, physiatrists, and radiation oncologists, as well as nurses, therapists, social workers, and chaplains.

PAIN ASSESSMENT

Pain Assessment Strategies

Individuals with cancer experience different pain patterns and characteristics that depend on various pathological, physiological, anatomical, psychological, and social factors.[42] Due the heterogeneity and complexity of pain in cancer, assessment and treatment of pain remains a challenge. Multidimensional pain assessment is a critical first step in providing optimal pain management. In all cancer patients experiencing pain, a comprehensive assessment should be performed which may include the patient's self-report, review of pertinent medical history, a general and focused physical exam, acquirement of essential imaging, psychosocial and functional assessments, and any concerns of financial burden caused by pain. Independent risk factors associated with poor pain control include bone metastases, severe pain, and frequent breakthrough pain. Retrospective analysis of lung cancer patients who reported moderate to severe chronic pain shows that half of the patients had bony metastases. Half of this patient group had neuropathic pain, and a quarter had frequent (>3×/day) breakthrough pain.[15] Factors such as sex, age, tissue pathology, tumor stage, and pain location have not been found to be associated with level of pain control. It was also noted that younger patients are more sensitive and less tolerant to pain.[15]

In addition to pain assessment, psychological assessment should be concurrently evaluated. In a 2014 review, Karen Syrjala and colleagues documented evidence of the interaction between unrelieved pain and emotional distress, depression, anxiety, uncertainty, and hopelessness in patients with cancer.[43] Pain catastrophizing was associated with increased pain severity while pain self-efficacy was associated with lower pain reports. Psychological distress has been shown to both delay and obstruct optimal analgesic management. Poor pain control coupled with psychological distress causes patients to require higher doses of pain medications, leads to polypharmacy with medications from multiple classes, and increases the length of time needed to achieve pain control.[15] Poor pain management can go on to further worsen psychological distress.[44] Physical activity was found to be a protective factor in reducing pain levels in cancer survivors.[43]

Pain and psychological assessment in comprehensive oncology care go hand in hand with clinical work-up. Any new pain or change in pain severity, distribution, or character warrants further investigation for local or distant disease spread. This may include, but is not limited to, lab tests, imaging, and electro diagnostics as appropriate. There is often a role for plain film radiographs, CT, or MRI imaging. At the end of life, symptom management and QOL take priority over work-up for patho-structural changes.

Pain Assessment Tools

There are numerous classification tools and pain scales available to elucidate the nature and severity of pain associated with a patient's malignancy, as well as the patient's unique pain experience.[42] Pain scales provide an objective metric for quantifying pain in a specific domain and are typically unidimensional. Pain scales are often used for screening purposes and evaluation of treatment effectiveness over time. Pain classification tools are more comprehensive and multidimensional including complete evaluation of pain descriptors (intensity, quality, location, duration), physical functioning, emotional functioning, and QOL measures.

Classification tools may be used over pain scales upon initial assessment or when pain is refractory or multifactorial. When selecting a specific assessment tool, providers should take into consideration the specific patient characteristics (cognitive ability and education level) as well as which domain of pain they are looking to investigate.[45]

Currently, there is a lack of validated assessment tools specific for the lung cancer population; however, application of current tools can be used to guide pain management by stratifying patients according to pain characteristics such as nociceptive, neuropathic, as well as breakthrough pain. Situ et al. reviewed the current evidence on classification methodologies and assessment approaches for cancer pain which includes both validated and partially validated classification systems.[42] The review highlights three partially validated classification systems, which includes the Classification of Chronic Pain from the IASP,[46] the Edmonton Classification System for Cancer Pain (ECS-CP),[47] and the Cancer Pain Prognostic Scale (CPPS).[48] These assessment tools, as well as individual pain scales, are listed in Table 13.1, further detailing their clinical applications.

There is currently no universally accepted tool to assess cancer pain, largely because pain characteristics vary between cancer populations as well as between individuals with the same type of cancer. Another issue with assessing cancer pain is that pain is not routinely measured by providers. While a comprehensive assessment is necessary to accurately identify and classify pain syndromes, some tools are too long and cumbersome resulting in less productivity and compliance. The variety of tools and lack of a universal consensus regarding systematic pain assessment adds to the challenges of pain management.

PAIN MANAGEMENT STRATEGIES

WHO Analgesic Ladder

The WHO pain ladder dates to 1986 and was originally developed to address cancer-related pain.[59] Since then there have been no updates, but nonetheless the approach is widely taught, used clinically throughout the world, and has been generalized to include noncancer pain. Patient are escalated sequentially through three steps in the ladder, where medications are classified as nonopioids (such as antiinflammatories), weak opioids (specifically listed as codeine, tramadol, and hydrocodone), and strong opioids (specifically listed as morphine, oxycodone, methadone, hydromorphone, and fentanyl).[59] Each step also includes adjuvant medications, which are not named by the WHO

TABLE 13.1
Pain Scales and Classification Tools Used in Oncology.

PAIN SCALES	
Name	**Domains Assessed**
Numerical Rating Scale (NRS)[49]	Intensity
Verbal Descriptor Scale (VDS)[49]	Intensity
Visual Analog Scale (VAS)[49,50]	Intensity
MD Anderson Symptom Severity Inventory (MDASI)[25]	Intensity
Regional Pain Scale (RPS)[51]	Location
McGill Pain Questionnaire[52]	Intensity, quality, temporal characteristics
Brief Pain Inventory[53]	Intensity, quality, life interference
Leeds Assessment of Neuropathic Signs and Symptoms (LANSS)[54]	Quality, temporal characteristics
EuroQOL-5D questionnaire (EQ-5D)[55]	Function, Quality of life
Pain Management Index (PMI)[56]	Treatment effect
Opioid Escalation Index (OEI)[57]	Treatment effect
Medication Assessment Tool for Cancer Pain Management (MAT-PC)[58]	Treatment effect
CLASSIFICATION TOOLS	
Classification of Chronic Pain of International Association for the Study of Pain (IASP)[46]	Descriptive classification based on location, Intensity, temporal characteristics, onset, duration, medical history
Edmonton Classification system for Cancer Pain (ECS-CP)[47]	Prognostic Classification based on mechanism of pain, incidence, psychological distress, addictive behavior, cognitive function
Cancer Pain Prognostic Scale (CPPS)[48]	Prognostic Classification based on Intensity, emotional well-being, opioid use

but could, for example, include antiepileptics to address nerve pain. Patients may climb the ladder due to medication side effects, drug inefficacy, or increase in pain severity. Other principles laid out by the WHO recommend dosing on a scheduled, rather than as needed basis, and dosing by mouth. This allows for consistent pain relief by the most achievable route of administration. Benefits of the WHO pain ladder include a logical, easy-to-follow approach for clinicians of all specialties to achieve pain control in their patients. Limitations abound though. An obvious critique is that the ladder exclusively focuses on pharmacological pain management, leaving out newer interventional techniques (such as nerve blocks), palliative surgery and radiation, counseling and chaplaincy services, therapy disciplines, and modalities. Furthermore, not every patient may be able to start on the first rung of the ladder, as the second or third step may already be more appropriate, depending on the severity and nature of the pain, especially in the context of cancer pain. Nor does the WHO pain ladder truly integrate the biopsychosocial model of pain, or incorporate the tools needed to manage total pain. Other concepts that the WHO pain ladder fails to address include optimal management of breakthrough pain, as well as the timing and strategy for deescalation of medication (descending the ladder). The reason the WHO pain ladder has endured, namely its simplicity is the same reason it must be considered incomplete, failing to address the complex nature of cancer pain, and pain of all kinds.

A Comprehensive Approach to Pain Management

Comprehensive pain management starts with the WHO analgesic ladder and then goes above and beyond to incorporate the multifactorial needs of the patient as illustrated by the biopsychosocial and total pain models. It takes into account the components of pain—acute, background and breakthrough pain, the pathophysiology of pain—nociceptive, neuropathic, and centralized, as well as the etiology of the pain—cancer related, treatment related, complication related, or psychosocial and existential related. It is delivered by an interdisciplinary team that places the patient and family at the center of a multipronged treatment model, focusing on QOL and timely delivery of holistic patient care.

TYPES OF PAIN MANAGEMENT, IN-DEPTH
Medical Management—Opioids

Opioids are an appropriate and useful tool for managing moderate to severe cancer-related pain, throughout the cancer care continuum, and particularly toward the end of life. Opioids come in short- and long-acting formulations, which are administered orally, sublingually, intravenously, subcutaneously, and transdermally. Subcutaneous administration is possible, but discouraged, as this is a painful route. Opioids act on the mu, kappa, and delta opioid receptors found in the brain, spinal cord, and periphery. They are potent analgesics and a cornerstone to cancer pain management. Common side effects include pruritus, fatigue, constipation, and nausea. All these effects tend to lift in 4–7 days, apart from opioid-induced constipation, to which the GI tract never develops a tolerance. For this reason, opioid prescribers should concurrently prescribe laxatives such as senna glycoside, bisacodyl, or polyethylene glycol, to help patients achieve one soft bowel movement per day.

Short-acting opioids include morphine IR, oxycodone IR, and hydrocodone; the latter is typically incorporated into fixed dose combination products. These can be given to patients orally, q4hrs as needed, for moderate to severe pain. Once it's possible to determine how many morphine equivalents, a patient needs in a 24-h period, the regimen can be adjusted to a scheduled, long-acting opioid with an as needed, short-acting opioid for breakthrough pain. It is helpful to administer sister products together, for example, morphine extended release q12hrs and morphine immediate release q4hrs PRN, as this improves the ease of opioid up- or down-titration.

Transdermal administration of opioids via a patch formulation is appropriate for patients on known, stable doses of opioids, and should only be administered by experienced providers, due to their unique pharmacokinetics. Buprenorphine, a partial opioid agonist, comes as a q96hr patch, and fentanyl, a potent, synthetic mu agonist comes as a q72hr patch.

Patients with lung cancer who are on hospice, and may have limited routes of administration, are well suited to concentrated oral morphine solutions (20 mg/mL) delivered sublingually, or subcutaneous opioid administration via a short- and long-acting daily regimen, or a patient controlled analgesia pump.

Providers who plan to prescribe opioids for cancer-related pain must have the appropriate controlled substance licensing for their region and/or country and are encouraged to pursue continuing medical education in order to be safe and up to date in their prescribing practices.

Medical Management—Adjuvant Medications

The category of adjuvant medications includes drugs that were initially intended for nonpain diagnoses, but are now used for pain, particularly neuropathic pain and/or chronic pain. These include antiepileptic and antidepressant medications. Gabapentin and pregabalin are anticonvulsants which act by inhibiting the alpha 2-delta subunit of voltage-gated calcium channels. These medications can be used for their opioid sparing effects, particularly in cancer-related neuropathies and neuropathic pain, metastatic bone pain, and chronic cancer-related pain. Gabapentinoids can be dosed orally up to 3 times a day, although they have vastly different ceiling doses. Typical side effects may include fatigue, peripheral swelling, gastrointestinal upset, and cognitive fog. It is advised that these medications are discontinued as a taper, as opposed to all at once. In the United States, pregabalin is a schedule V federally controlled substance. At a state, but not federal level, gabapentin is also a schedule V controlled substance in many parts of the United States of America. The schedule V category indicates that the risk for substance use disorder is low, and clinically, the risk is vanishingly rare in the cancer population.

Antidepressants such as duloxetine and venlafaxine can be helpful adjuvant medications, especially for neuropathic pain. They can also have a beneficial effect on mood, which may help in complex pain management. These medications act as serotonin and norepinephrine reuptake inhibitors (SNRIs). SNRIs can be dosed once daily in the evening to avoid the effects of fatigue. Typically, they should not be combined with additional serotonergic agents, to avoid the risk of serotonin syndrome. These medications should be discontinued gradually as opposed to suddenly, to reduce the risk of withdrawal effects which include nightmares.

Tricyclic antidepressants (TCAs), including tertiary amines such as amitriptyline, can also act as an SNRI-type adjuvant medication. Use of these medications is limited by their anticholinergic effects including constipation, urinary retention, dry mouth, and cognitive effects. Non-TCAs, such as those listed above, are more commonly used.

Corticosteroids are an adjuvant pain management tool used frequently by palliative minded physicians that can provide relief from bone pain, neuropathic pain, raised intracranial pressure headaches, and visceral obstructive/inflammatory pain in the setting of lung cancer.[13] Dexamethasone is typically the steroid of choice, with less mineralocorticoid effects.[13] Long-term corticosteroid use has serious ramifications for blood glucose management, bone density, and other hormone-related processes, which must be balanced against the benefits and symptom relief that it provides. Best practice is to use the lowest dose of corticosteroids needed for pain management, for the shortest duration of time, while still optimizing dosing and prioritizing QOL.

Medical Management—Ketamine

Ketamine is a nonopioid medication which has analgesic, amnesic, and anesthetic properties. It is typically used by cancer rehabilitation and palliative providers at lower doses to target pain relief and to avoid amnesia and anesthesia which result from higher doses more commonly used by anesthesiologists. It is a derivative of phencyclidine and acts as an N-methyl-D-aspartate receptor antagonist. It comes as a racemic mixture of S-ketamine and R-ketamine and can be given by all routes available: oral, intravenous, intramuscular, intranasal, subcutaneous, sublingual, and per rectum. Ketamine can play many roles in managing pain in lung cancer. It can be used for cancer pain, neuropathic pain, pain crises, and allow for opioid sparing in the postoperative period. It can also be used for its antidepressant effects to address the mood component of complex cancer pain. It can be applied topically in a compounded cream or a spray for wounds or localized pain. In the United States of America, the use of ketamine in cancer rehabilitation and palliation is entirely off-label, with on-label uses being anesthesia, and FDA-approved intranasal, nonracemic, esketamine which can only be used for treatment-resistant depression through a restricted distribution system. Nonetheless, many palliative and rehabilitation providers may choose to use racemic ketamine for lung cancer pain relief, due to its unique properties and many roles. Adverse events related to ketamine include dizziness, hallucinations, vivid dreams, anxiety, hypertension, tachycardia, and increased salivation. Sialorrhea can be treated with atropine drops or a scopolamine patch; psychosis-related events can be treated with concurrent or PRN dosing of a benzodiazepine. Ketamine is often avoided in patients at risk for raised intracranial pressure, or in patients with untreated psychotic disorders.

Interventional Pain Management

Interventional management of pain in lung cancer may be used as an adjuvant treatment, in conjunction with oral medications. It is typically performed if patients do not achieve sufficient pain relief with oral medications alone, if pain control with oral medications is limited by adverse reactions, or if the goal for treatment is to reduce opioid use. Interventional treatment options are aimed at the anatomic or neurologic cause of pain. It is important to note that injections at or around the tumor site are avoided for several reasons. As tumors grow, they displace and distort the surrounding anatomical structures. This increases the risk of missing the target of the injection. Tumor growth is also associated with vascular neogenesis, which leads to an increased risk of bleeding from injections. As injections consist of introducing a foreign body into the anatomy momentarily, there is a likelihood of seeding cancer cells along the needle track.[60] Interventional modalities include both nondestructive and destructive procedures.[13] The advantages associated with interventional management include targeted treatment with fewer systemic side effects than oral medications, which may facilitate reduction in opioid usage. Interventional procedures should be used as part of the interdisciplinary approach to pain management rather than a stand-alone last resort treatment option.[60]

Interventional Management—Nondestructive Procedures

Nondestructive procedures include peripheral nerve blocks, neuraxial (epidural or intrathecal) blocks, and neuromodulation.

A **nerve block** refers to any procedure in which a needle is used to deposit a local anesthetic within the vicinity of a peripheral nerve thought to be a source of pain. As the agents used for local anesthesia are short-acting, these blocks offer diagnostic information, to guide long-acting or permanent treatment. In patients with lung cancer, the mainstay of treatment for severe pain associated with pathological rib fractures is intercostal blocks.[61] Neurolysis consists of using an ablative solution or radiofrequency with the same technique to achieve localized destruction of the peripheral nerves to diminish the painful sensory stimulus.[60] Proximally, nerve blocks can be performed at the level of the thoracic nerve roots exiting the spine to treat postthoracotomy pain.[62]

Spinal injections are performed to deposit analgesic medication directly at the level of the spinal cord receptors. Intrathecal analgesia should take into account modality selection and patient-related factors such as life expectancy, concurrent treatments, associated comorbidities, and psychosocial factors.[63] Intraspinal neurolysis is performed by injecting neurolytic agents into the epidural or intrathecal space. These procedures are reserved as a last resort option in patients with intractable pain as they cause neurological deficits.[60]

Interventional Management: Destructive Procedures

Destructive procedures are permanent and are another option to impede pain sensation, specifically for severe localized chest wall pain in lung cancer patients.

Anterolateral cordotomy may be performed percutaneously at the level of the spinal cord contralateral to the location of pain to ablate spinothalamic tract fibers. This procedure works to diminish pain sensation, along with temperature sensation as well.[13] Rhizotomy is performed at the level of the nerve root and consists of destruction of the dorsal sensory roots. There are various approaches to rhizotomy, most commonly by surgical resection, chemical neurolysis with phenol, or with radiofrequency ablation.[13]

The Role for Nonpharmacologic Treatments in Cancer Pain Management

It is important to emphasize the interdisciplinary and comprehensive approach to the management of cancer-related pain which may include pharmacological and nonpharmacological treatments. Aside from interventional treatments and medication, other nonpharmacologic options for pain in lung cancer include a rehabilitation program consisting of physical or therapeutic exercise, occupational therapy, and physical modalities.[64] In a seminal review of rehabilitation and exercise recommendations by Stout and colleagues, it was advised that rehabilitation referrals should be based on symptom severity and recommended for individuals with high risk of poor surgical outcomes (Category B guideline).[65]

Therapeutic Exercise and Physical Therapy

Therapeutic exercise and physical therapy are often prescribed as part of a comprehensive rehabilitation program and typically performed under the supervision of a trained rehabilitation specialist (physical therapist, occupational therapist, or exercise physiologist). Both approaches differ slightly in their rehabilitation objectives; however, the outcomes are complimentary. Exercise therapy typically involves aerobic training, resistance training, core/stabilization exercises, and general conditioning with the goal of improving overall physical fitness and optimizing other prescribed exercises. Physical therapy can involve these exercises, although it is more typically prescribed for a specific impairment the patient may be experiencing. For instance, a provider may prescribe physical therapy to improve shoulder mobilization and pain in a patient with adhesive capsulitis from radiation fibrosis syndrome.[66] While it is generally agreed that therapeutic exercise contributes to the improvement of overall function and QOL in cancer patients, there is less consensus over whether it directly reduces pain related to cancer. This may be because cancer pain is multifaceted, making it particularly challenging to ascertain that

therapeutic exercise is effective for alleviating pain. Nonetheless, it is commonly accepted that exercise improves physical fitness, QOL, anxiety, depression, and cancer-related fatigue in cancer survivors and is recommended as standard of care for cancer survivors by the American College of Sports Medicine.[67] The benefit of physical activity on cancer pain is an intuitive concept, but there is limited evidence to support this. What is known is that exercise and physical activity can alleviate symptoms of psychological distress which have a strong association with chronic cancer pain, especially in the setting of lung cancer where symptom burden remains high.[68] In an extensive review by Sommer et al., it was concluded that exercise may be beneficial for exercise capacity and the physical aspect of health-related QOL among patients with NSCLC following lung resection. Although the body of evidence reviewed in this article was not high quality, it was still recommended to consider referring lung cancer patients for exercise interventions following surgery.[69] Preoperative physical conditioning, otherwise referred to as "prehabilitation," is another intervention recommended by the Enhanced Recovery after Surgery Society (ERAS) and the European Society for Thoracic Surgery for lung cancer patients with planning surgical resection to prevent postoperative complications and enhance time to recovery.[70]

Occupational Therapy

Persistent pain can affect an individual's function in day-to-day life. Therefore, rehabilitation for individuals with lung cancer should focus on improving symptom severity, as well as optimizing function. Occupational therapists are integral members of the interdisciplinary cancer team. Their role is to assist in restoring function and preventing disability. Some of their interventions include activity assessments and modifications, equipment prescription, energy conservation techniques, and safety education.[71] For people living with lung cancer, occupational therapy allows patients to improve their mobility and increase their participation in goal-directed therapies. Symptoms in lung cancer can exist in clusters; therefore, reducing dyspnea with energy conservation techniques may subsequently ease overall symptom burden. Working closely with an occupational therapist allows for close monitoring for new or worsening pain symptoms. Functional pain has been found to be a strong predictor of impending pathological fracture[72] and has been identified as a safety consideration for rehabilitation providers.[73] In those with metastatic lung cancer, new functional pain with daily tasks should raise concerns about progression of disease and prompt further investigation. Pain management strategies often assess function to help gauge the severity of impairments in patients, but little is understood about the relationship of pain severity and functional decline in the lung cancer population, and this should be a focus of future research.

Therapeutic Modalities

Modalities that have been accepted as safe for cancer patients include superficial heat, cryotherapy, transcutaneous electrical nerve stimulation (TENS), myofascial release/massage, and desensitization techniques.[74] These modalities are classified as passive rehabilitation contrary to physical and occupational therapy where the patient is an active participant in the program. Therapeutic modalities may be used as an adjunct to conventional pain or rehabilitation strategies and are indicated for pain related to neuromusculoskeletal impairments. Patients who undergo thoracotomy or radiation of the chest wall can benefit from cotreatment with physical modalities to address shoulder joint and scapular dysfunction resulting from muscle and nerve disruption during treatment. Another indication for modalities would be surgical scar and thoracic desensitization which can be a source of persistent postthoracotomy neuropathic pain. It is important to note that these modalities should be used with caution as there are some contraindications that exist in the setting of cancer. For example, it is not advised to apply modalities such as TENS or heat directly to tumor sites.[73] Further, in those with osseous metastatic disease or osteoporosis, precautions should be taken with manual therapies.

Integrative Therapies

Popular mind–body therapies (MBTs) in cancer care include psychological therapies (e.g., cognitive behavior therapy; CBT), relaxation and imagery, hypnosis, yoga, meditation, tai chi and qigong, and art therapies. Existing literature examining MBTs is limited by lack of large sample sizes, active comparison groups, and treatment standardization issues; nevertheless, there is evidence of efficacy for treating many common cancer-related symptoms, including pain, fatigue, nausea and vomiting, mood symptoms, and psychological functioning.[75]

Psychological and Behavioral Interventions. Psychological and behavioral interventions aim to address psychological and social sequelae of cancer, reduce pain severity and functional interference, and improve QOL. From a biopsychosocial approach to pain management, these interventions are considered an essential addition to medical pain management efforts. These treatments can be delivered by trained mental health professionals, such as psychologists, licensed professional counselors, or clinical social workers with professional training and experience working within oncology and/or rehabilitation. Within the field of psychology, there is an emerging specialty of pain psychology with specific competencies in understanding the multidimensional, biopsychosocial nature of pain, assessing, and measuring pain, managing pain, and awareness of how contextual variables affect pain management.[76] Pain psychologists are well poised to join integrated, multimodal, and multidisciplinary pain care teams.

Psychological and behavioral interventions have been shown to have strong and consistent evidence for pain alleviation during procedures and disease treatment across patients with a variety of cancer conditions, including lung cancer. These interventions included education and training with (1) coping skills, which typically include addressing barriers, teaching patients to understand and communicate their pain and medication needs, and self-efficacy enhancement; (2) hypnosis, which typically involves a clinician inviting the patient to focus their awareness and imagination to experience beneficial changes in symptoms and emotional responses; (3) cognitive behavioral approaches targeting depression, anxiety, and QOL related to cancer diagnosis and treatment; and (4) relaxation with imagery, which involves asking a patient to focus on letting go of muscle tension through awareness and suggestions for shifts in perception and interpretation of pain signals.[43] The empirical support of psychological and behavioral interventions in long-term cancer survivors is less robust and the vast majority of data are found within the breast cancer survivorship literature. Physical activity, yoga, and hypnosis demonstrated promising effects for pain reduction in cancer survivors.[43]

In recent years, the application of acceptance-based interventions, such as Acceptance and Commitment Therapy (ACT), has been gaining more attention in both the clinical and research arenas. In contrast to a CBT approach in which patients are taught to identify and change maladaptive thinking patterns in an attempt to reduce pain severity, acceptance-based treatments do not seek to change the experience of pain sensations, per se, but rather to reduce the individual's avoidance of and cognitive fusion to pain by increasing one's psychological flexibility and ability to engage in behaviors consistent with their values despite uncomfortable thoughts, feelings, or sensations. Systematic reviews have demonstrated positive effects on measures of pain acceptance, psychological flexibility, functioning, anxiety and depression within a general chronic pain population[77] and improved emotional state, QOL, and psychological flexibility within an oncological population.[78]

Mindfulness-based interventions have become increasingly employed to address a host of physical illnesses, including cancer. Mindfulness is defined as the awareness that arises by paying attention on purpose, in the present moment and nonjudgmentally.[79] Pioneered by Dr. Jon Kabat-Zinn in the Stress Reduction Clinic at the University of Massachusetts Medical Center in the late 1970s, Mindfulness-Based Stress Reduction (MBSR) is based on systematic training in mindfulness to foster improved physical and psychological health and well-being. MBSR is gaining strong support for its efficacy and effectiveness for stress reduction, symptom management and emotional balance, and positive effects on the brain and immune system.[79] In a recent multicenter, random control trial comparing a group MBSR intervention with 31 patients with lung cancer and their partners to standard of care, patients receiving the mindfulness intervention demonstrated significant less psychological distress, improvements in QOL, mindfulness skills, self-compassion, and less rumination than patients receiving standard care. Further, they found that the level of baseline distress moderated these outcomes, with those experiencing greater distress at baseline benefitting the most.[80]

Pain Neuroscience Education. For cancer survivors whose condition is in remission or "cured", yet who continue to experience persistent, debilitating pain, the effects on day-to-day functioning and lower QOL cannot be understated. Pain education can be an important component to management strategies for patients experiencing chronic postcancer pain.[81] A metaanalysis of 21 trials found that patient-based educational interventions are effective for improving pain severity, knowledge, and self-efficacy for treating cancer-related pain, yet is underused in the field of oncology.[82]

Rather than focusing solely on biomechanical characteristics of pain, pain neuroscience education (PNE) involves teaching patients about the underlying biopsychosocial mechanisms of pain. PNE describes the neurobiology and neurophysiology of pain, and pain processing by the nervous system. This is impacted by pain mechanisms (i.e., nociceptive, neuropathic, central sensitization, mixed pain) as well as by pain perceptions, pain-related fear, fear of movement, maladaptive cognitive patterns (e.g., catastrophizing, perceived injustice, perceived harm, and pain vigilance), pain coping strategies (e.g., avoidance of pain, cognitive fusion with pain), as well as anxiety, depression, and social support. The learning objectives of PNE are to decrease the threat value of pain, increase the patient's knowledge of pain, and reconceptualize pain as an experience produced, constructed, and modulated by the brain that can be partly related to hypersensitivity of the central nervous system.[83] PNE can be delivered by a wide range of healthcare professionals with the prerequisite knowledge, including but not limited to physical therapists, psychotherapists, or nurses.[81]

PNE has already been demonstrated to be well received by patients and effective in changing pain beliefs, improving health status, and pain coping in patients experiencing persistent noncancer pain, including chronic musculoskeletal pain,[84] fibromyalgia,[85] and chronic low back pain.[83] PNE can be an effective first step in pain treatment before more active pain management strategies, such as exercise therapy, stress management, sleep interventions, and nutritional counseling, thereby priming and preparing patients for behavioral changes. PNE interventions can also be useful adjuncts to psychological interventions targeting psychological flexibility, acceptance, and willingness skills. There exists a current need to explore the application, effectiveness, and efficacy of PNE interventions on patient health outcomes and physical and psychological functioning in the field of oncology.

Acupuncture and Acupressure. In light of the ongoing opioid crisis within the United States, there has been a call to move toward nonpharmacological interventions for managing cancer pain, championed by leading organizations within the field, such as the American Society for Clinical Oncology and the National Comprehensive Cancer Network (Swarm, National Comprehensive Cancer Network). Acupuncture is based in traditional Chinese medicine in which specific points on the body are stimulated, most often by inserting thin needles through the skin. In traditional Chinese medicine, acupuncture is explained as a technique for balancing the flow of energy, known as chi or qi, believed to flow through pathways in the body. In contrast, many Western practitioners view acupuncture points as places to stimulate nerves, muscles, and connective tissue. Acupressure is a related practice that involves applying physical pressure to acupressure points using the hand, elbow, or with devices. Acupuncture is considered generally safe, provided the intervention is delivered by trained practitioners using sterile techniques. While research on acupuncture for cancer pain has been growing, findings have been inconsistent.[86] In a 2019 study, researcher Yihan He and colleagues examined the strength of evidence for acupuncture and acupressure on cancer pain through randomized clinical trials (RCTs). Comparison was made with sham acupuncture and analgesic therapy or usual care practices. A total of 17 RCTs (with 1111 patients) were included in the systematic review, and data from 14 RCTs (with 920 patients) were used in the metaanalysis. Results showed association between real acupuncture (vs. sham control) and greater reduction in pain intensity, with a moderate level of certainty. Acupuncture may also be associated with reduced opioid use when added to analgesic therapy. Relatively few adverse events from acupuncture were reported, consisting predominantly of skin and subcutaneous tissue disorder or slight pain at the application site.[87] However, there were notable limitations. Few trials were available for certain types of pain (e.g., neuropathic, osseous metastasis). Further research is needed to investigate the association of acupuncture with specific pain syndromes. Additionally, there existed considerable heterogeneity in the findings, suggesting that outcomes of acupuncture may be variable and thus may not be suitable as a standalone treatment for cancer pain, but rather most appropriate as applied as an adjunctive intervention.[87]

CONCLUSION

In summary, pain is one of the most common symptoms reported by patients with lung cancer. It can have varying degrees of impact on a patient's daily function and health-related QOL throughout the disease course. Members of the cancer rehabilitation team should appreciate the multifactorial nature of pain, including the patient's personal experience of pain. Moving beyond the assessment of pain presentation and etiology to exploring the patient's pain narrative can enhance management strategies and improve care. The complexity and challenge associated with providing effective pain control for patients with lung cancer highlights the importance of multidimensional assessment and comprehensive management. This can be achieved through rehabilitative and palliative approaches, across the disease continuum, from time of diagnosis, through treatment, to survivorship or end of life. Pain management strategies may include pharmacologic agents, interventional procedures, therapeutic exercise, physical and occupational therapy, therapeutic modalities, psychological and behavioral interventions, as well as complementary and alternative medicine therapies as adjuncts to standard care. Therapeutic outcomes in pain management can be enhanced when delivered in a coordinated, interdisciplinary fashion, with the individual patient and their family at the heart of care, with a focus on function and QOL.

REFERENCES

1. Raja SN, Carr DB, Cohen M, et al. The revised International Association for the Study of Pain definition of pain: concepts, challenges, and compromises. *Pain*. 2020;161(9): 1976−1982. https://doi.org/10.1097/j.pain.0000000000 001939.
2. Asmundson GJG, Wright KD. Biopsychosocial Approaches to Pain. In: Hadjistavropoulos T, Craig KD, eds. *Pain: Psychological perspectives Lawrence*. Erlbaum Associates Publishers; 2004. https://psycnet.apa.org/record/2004-00 216-002. Accessed May 27, 2021.
3. Melzack R, Wall PD. Pain mechanisms: a new theory. *Science*. 1965;150(3699):971−979. https://doi.org/ 10.1126/science.150.3699.971.
4. Turk DC, Flor H. Chronic pain: a biobehavioral perspective. In: Gatchel RJ, Turk DC, eds. *Psychosocial Factors in Pain: Critical Perspectives*. The Guilford Press; 1999: 18−34.
5. Clark D. "Total pain", disciplinary power and the body in the work of Cicely Saunders, 1958−1967. *Soc Sci Med*. 1999;49(6):727−736. https://doi.org/10.1016/S0277-9536(99)00098-2.
6. Kim HJ, McGuire DB, Tulman L, Barsevick AM. Symptom clusters: concept analysis and clinical implications for cancer nursing. *Cancer Nurs*. 2005;28(4):270−284. https:// doi.org/10.1097/00002820-200507000-00005.
7. Hamada T, Komatsu H, Rosenzweig M, et al. Impact of symptom clusters on quality of life outcomes in patients from Japan with advanced nonsmall cell lung cancers. *Asia-Pacific J Oncol Nurs*. 2016;3(4):370. https://doi.org/ 10.4103/2347-5625.196489.
8. Lin S, Chen Y, Yang L, Zhou J. Pain, fatigue, disturbed sleep and distress comprised a symptom cluster that related to quality of life and functional status of lung cancer surgery patients. *J Clin Nurs*. 2013;22(9−10):1281−1290. https:// doi.org/10.1111/jocn.12228.
9. Potter J, Higginson IJ. Pain experienced by lung cancer patients: a review of prevalence, causes and pathophysiology. *Lung Cancer*. 2004;43(3):247−257. https://doi.org/10.1016/j.lungcan.2003.08.030.
10. Portenoy RK, Lesage P. Management of cancer pain. *Lancet*. 1999;353(9165):1695−1700. https://doi.org/10.1016/ S0140-6736(99)01310-0.
11. Stute P, Soukup J, Menzel M, Sabatowski R, Grond S. Analysis and treatment of different types of neuropathic cancer pain. *J Pain Symptom Manag*. 2003;26(6):1123−1131. https://doi.org/10.1016/j.jpainsymman.2003.04.002.
12. Carr DB, Goudas LC. Acute pain. *Lancet*. 1999;353(9169): 2051−2058. https://doi.org/10.1016/S0140-6736(99) 03313-9.
13. Simmons CPL, MacLeod N, Laird BJA. Clinical management of pain in advanced lung cancer. *Clin Med Insights Oncol*. 2012;6:331−346. https://doi.org/10.4137/CMO. S8360.
14. Davies AN, Dickman A, Reid C, Stevens AM, Zeppetella G. The management of cancer-related breakthrough pain: recommendations of a Task Group of the Science Committee

of the Association for Palliative Medicine of Great Britain and Ireland. *Eur J Pain*. 2009;13(4):331−338. https://doi.org/10.1016/j.ejpain.2008.06.014.

15. Shi L, Liu Y, He H, Wang C, Li H, Wang N. Characteristics and prognostic factors for pain management in 152 patients with lung cancer. *Patient Prefer Adherence*. 2016;10: 571−577. https://doi.org/10.2147/PPA.S103276.

16. Parker C, Neville E. Lung cancer • 8: management of malignant mesothelioma. *Thorax*. 2003;58(9):809−813. https://doi.org/10.1136/thorax.58.9.809.

17. Sung H, Ferlay J, Siegel RL, et al. Global cancer statistics 2020: GLOBOCAN estimates of incidence and mortality worldwide for 36 cancers in 185 countries. *CA Cancer J Clin*. 2021. https://doi.org/10.3322/caac.21660.

18. Bade BC, Dela Cruz CS. Lung cancer 2020: epidemiology, etiology, and prevention. *Clin Chest Med*. 2019. https://doi.org/10.1016/j.ccm.2019.10.001.

19. Siegel RL, Miller KD, Fuchs HE, Jemal A. Cancer statistics, 2021. *CA Cancer J Clin*. 2021;71(1):7−33. https://doi.org/10.3322/caac.21654.

20. Kenny PM, King MT, Viney RC, et al. Quality of life and survival in the 2 years after surgery for non-small-cell lung cancer. *J Clin Oncol*. 2008;26(2):233−241. https://doi.org/10.1200/JCO.2006.07.7230.

21. Al-Kattan K, Sepsas E, Fountain SW, Townsend ER. Disease recurrence after resection for stage I lung cancer. *Eur J Cardio-thoracic Surg*. 1997;12(3):380−384. https://doi.org/10.1016/S1010-7940(97)00198-X.

22. Van Den Beuken-Van Everdingen MHJ, Hochstenbach LMJ, Joosten EAJ, Tjan-Heijnen VCG, Janssen DJA. Update on prevalence of pain in patients with cancer: systematic review and meta-analysis. *J Pain Symptom Manag*. 2016;51(6):1070−1090.e9. https://doi.org/10.1016/j.jpainsymman.2015.12.340.

23. Akin S, Can G, Aydiner A, Ozdilli K, Durna Z. Quality of life, symptom experience and distress of lung cancer patients undergoing chemotherapy. *Eur J Oncol Nurs*. 2010; 14(5):400−409. https://doi.org/10.1016/j.ejon.2010.01.003.

24. Cooley ME. Symptoms in adults with lung cancer: a systematic research review. *J Pain Symptom Manag*. 2000; 19(2):137−153. https://doi.org/10.1016/S0885-3924(99)00150-5.

25. Mendoza TR, Wang XS, Lu C, et al. Measuring the symptom burden of lung cancer: the validity and utility of the lung cancer module of the M. D. Anderson symptom inventory. *Oncologist*. 2011;16(2):217−227. https://doi.org/10.1634/theoncologist.2010-0193.

26. Andersen BL, Valentine TR, Lo SB, Carbone DP, Presley CJ, Shields PG. Newly diagnosed patients with advanced non-small cell lung cancer: a clinical description of those with moderate to severe depressive symptoms. *Lung Cancer*. 2020;145:195−204. https://doi.org/10.1016/j.lungcan.2019.11.015.

27. Degner LF, Sloan JA. Symptom distress in newly diagnosed ambulatory cancer patients and as a predictor of survival in lung cancer. *J Pain Symptom Manag*. 1995;10(6):423−431. https://doi.org/10.1016/0885-3924(95)00056-5.

28. Pinheiro LC, Reeve BB. Investigating the prognostic ability of health-related quality of life on survival: a prospective cohort study of adults with lung cancer. *Support Care Cancer*. 2018;26(11):3925−3932. https://doi.org/10.1007/s00520-018-4265-3.

29. Ferrell B, Sun V, Hurria A, et al. Interdisciplinary palliative care for patients with lung cancer. *J Pain Symptom Manag*. 2015;50(6):758−767. https://doi.org/10.1016/j.jpainsymman.2015.07.005.

30. Kochovska S, Ferreira DH, Luckett T, Phillips JL, Currow DC. Earlier multidisciplinary palliative care intervention for people with lung cancer: a systematic review and meta-analysis. *Transl Lung Cancer Res*. 2020;9(4): 1699−1709. https://doi.org/10.21037/tlcr.2019.12.18.

31. Shin J, Temel J. Integrating palliative care: when and how? *Curr Opin Pulm Med*. 2013;19(4):344−349. https://doi.org/10.1097/MCP.0b013e3283620e76.

32. Gjeilo KH, Oksholm T, Follestad T, Wahba A, Rustøen T. Trajectories of pain in patients undergoing lung cancer surgery: a longitudinal prospective study. *J Pain Symptom Manag*. 2020;59(4):818−828.e1. https://doi.org/10.1016/j.jpainsymman.2019.11.004.

33. Watson PN, Evans RJ. Intractable pain with lung cancer. *Pain*. 1987;29(2):163−173. https://doi.org/10.1016/0304-3959(87)91033-5.

34. Lövgren M, Levealahti H, Tishelman C, Runesdotter S, Hamberg K, Koyi H. Time spans from first symptom to treatment in patients with lung cancer - the influence of symptoms and demographic characteristics. *Acta Oncol*. 2008;47(3):397−405. https://doi.org/10.1080/02841860701592392.

35. Fagundes CP, Shi Q, Vaporciyan AA, et al. Symptom recovery after thoracic surgery: measuring patient-reported outcomes with the MD Anderson Symptom Inventory. *J Thorac Cardiovasc Surg*. 2015;150(3):613−619.e2. https://doi.org/10.1016/j.jtcvs.2015.05.057.

36. Sparks A, Stewart JR. Review of pain management in thoracic surgery patients. *J Anesthesia Clin Res*. 2018. https://doi.org/10.4172/2155-6148.1000817.

37. Rawal N. Current issues in postoperative pain management. *Eur J Anaesthesiol*. 2016;33(3):160−171. https://doi.org/10.1097/EJA.0000000000000366.

38. Steven NM, Fisher BA. Management of rheumatic complications of immune checkpoint inhibitor therapy − an oncological perspective. *Rheumatology*. 2019; 58(Suppl_7):vii29−vii39. https://doi.org/10.1093/rheumatology/kez536.

39. Silver JK, Baima J, Mayer RS. Impairment-driven cancer rehabilitation: an essential component of quality care and survivorship. *CA Cancer J Clin*. 2013;63(5): 295−317. https://doi.org/10.3322/caac.21186.

40. Arends S, Böhmer AB, Poels M, et al. Post-thoracotomy pain syndrome: seldom severe, often neuropathic, treated unspecific, and insufficient. *Pain Rep*. 2020;5(2):e810. https://doi.org/10.1097/PR9.0000000000000810.

41. Colloca L, Ludman T, Bouhassira D, et al. Neuropathic pain. *Nat Rev Dis Prim*. 2017;3:17002. https://doi.org/10.1038/nrdp.2017.2.

42. Situ D, Wang J, Shao W, Zhu Z-H. Assessment and treatment of cancer pain: from Western to Eastern. *Ann Palliat Med.* 2012;1(1):32−44. https://doi.org/10.3978/j.issn.2224-5820.2011.10.01.

43. Syrjala KL, Jensen MP, Elena Mendoza M, Yi JC, Fisher HM, Keefe FJ. Psychological and behavioral approaches to cancer pain management. *J Clin Oncol.* 2014;32(16):1703−1711. https://doi.org/10.1200/JCO.2013.54.4825.

44. Laird BJA, Scott AC, Colvin LA, et al. Pain, depression, and fatigue as a symptom cluster in advanced cancer. *J Pain Symptom Manag.* 2011;42(1):1−11. https://doi.org/10.1016/j.jpainsymman.2010.10.261.

45. Anderson KO. Assessment tools for the evaluation of pain in the oncology patient. *Curr Pain Headache Rep.* 2007;11(4):259−264. https://doi.org/10.1007/s11916-007-0201-9.

46. Baranowski A, Abrams P, Berger R, et al. *Classification of Chronic Pain* (Revised). 2nd ed. IASP; 2019. https://www.iasp-pain.org/PublicationsNews/Content.aspx?ItemNumber=1673. Accessed May 31, 2021.

47. Nekolaichuk CL, Fainsinger RL, Aass N, et al. The edmonton classification system for cancer pain: comparison of pain classification features and pain intensity across diverse palliative care settings in eight countries. *J Palliat Med.* 2013;16(5):516−523. https://doi.org/10.1089/jpm.2012.0390.

48. Hwang SS, Chang VT, Fairclough DL, Kasimis B. Development of a cancer pain prognostic scale. *J Pain Symptom Manag.* 2003;24(4):366−378. https://doi.org/10.1016/S0885-3924(02)00488-8.

49. Hjermstad MJ, Fayers PM, Haugen DF, et al. Studies comparing numerical rating scales, verbal rating scales, and visual analogue scales for assessment of pain intensity in adults: a systematic literature review. *J Pain Symptom Manag.* 2011;41(6):1073−1093. https://doi.org/10.1016/j.jpainsymman.2010.08.016.

50. Aitken RCB. A growing edge of measurement of feelings [Abridged]: measurement of feelings using visual analogue scales. *J R Soc Med.* 1969;62(10):989−993. https://doi.org/10.1177/003591576906201005.

51. Wolfe F. Pain extent and diagnosis: development and validation of the regional pain scale in 12,799 patients with rheumatic disease. *J Rheumatol.* 2003;30(2):369−378.

52. Melzack R. The McGill pain questionnaire: major properties and scoring methods. *Pain.* 1975;1(3):277−299. https://doi.org/10.1016/0304-3959(75)90044-5.

53. Kumar SP. Utilization of brief pain inventory as an assessment tool for pain in patients with cancer: a focused review. *Indian J Palliat Care.* 2011;17(2):108−115. https://doi.org/10.4103/0973-1075.84531.

54. Bennett M. The LANSS pain scale: the Leeds assessment of neuropathic symptoms and signs. *Pain.* 2001;92(1−2):147−157. https://doi.org/10.1016/S0304-3959(00)00482-6.

55. Koide R, Kikuchi A, Miyajima M, et al. Quality assessment using EQ-5D-5L after lung surgery for non-small cell lung cancer (NSCLC) patients. *Gen Thorac Cardiovasc Surg.*

56. Singh H, Banipal RPS, Singh B. Assessment of adequacy of pain management and analgesic use in patients with advanced cancer using the brief pain inventory and pain management index calculation. *J Glob Oncol.* 2017;3(3):235−241. https://doi.org/10.1200/JGO.2016.004663.

57. Mercadante S, Fulfaro F, Casuccio A, Barresi L. Investigation of an opioid response categorization in advanced cancer patients. *J Pain Symptom Manag.* 1999;18(5):347−352. https://doi.org/10.1016/S0885-3924(99)00099-8.

58. Håkonsen GD, Hudson S, Loennechen T. Design and validation of a medication assessment tool for cancer pain management. *Pharm World Sci.* 2006;28(6):342−351. https://doi.org/10.1007/s11096-006-9060-4.

59. Ventafridda V, Saita L, Ripamonti C, De Conno F. WHO guidelines for the use of analgesics in cancer pain. *Int J Tissue React.* 1985;7(1):93−96.

60. Hochberg U, Elgueta MF, Perez J. Interventional analgesic management of lung cancer pain. *Front Oncol.* 2017;7:17. https://doi.org/10.3389/fonc.2017.00017.

61. Simpson KH. Interventional techniques for pain management in palliative care. *Medicine.* 2011;39(11):645−647. https://doi.org/10.1016/j.mpmed.2011.08.011.

62. Cohen SP, Sireci A, Wu CL, Larkin TM, Williams KA, Hurley RW. Pulsed radiofrequency of the dorsal root ganglia is superior to pharmacotherapy or pulsed radiofrequency of the intercostal nerves in the treatment of chronic postsurgical thoracic pain. *Pain Physician.* 2006;9(3):227−236.

63. Deer TR, Smith HS, Burton A, et al. Comprehensive consensus based guidelines on intrathecal drug delivery systems in the treatment of pain caused by cancer pain. *Pain Physician.* 2011;14(3). https://doi.org/10.36076/ppj.2011/14/e283.

64. Silver JK. Nonpharmacologic pain management in the cancer patient. In: Stubblefield MD, ed. *Cancer Rehabilitation: Principles and Practice.* 2nd ed. Springer Publishing Company; 2018:560−2018. https://doi.org/10.1891/9780826121646.0043.

65. Stout NL, Santa Mina D, Lyons KD, Robb K, Silver JK. A systematic review of rehabilitation and exercise recommendations in oncology guidelines. *CA Cancer J Clin.* 2021;71(2):149−175. https://doi.org/10.3322/caac.21639.

66. Hojan K, Milecki P. Opportunities for rehabilitation of patients with radiation fibrosis syndrome. *Rep Practical Oncol Radiother.* 2014;19(1):1−6. https://doi.org/10.1016/j.rpor.2013.07.007.

67. Campbell KL, Winters-stone KM, Wiskemann J, et al. Exercise guidelines for cancer survivors: consensus statement from international multidisciplinary roundtable exercise guidelines for cancer survivors: consensus statement from international multidisciplinary roundtable special communications. *Med Sci Sports Exerc.* 2019;51(11):2375−2390. https://doi.org/10.1249/MSS.0000000000002116.

68. Zaza C, Baine N. Cancer pain and psychosocial factors: a critical review of the literature. *J Pain Symptom Manag*

2002;24(5):526–542. https://doi.org/10.1016/S0885-3924(02)00497-9.

69. Sommer MS, Staerkind MEB, Christensen J, et al. Effect of postsurgical rehabilitation programmes in patients operated for lung cancer: a systematic review and meta-analysis. *J Rehabil Med.* 2018;50(3):236–245. https://doi.org/10.2340/16501977-2292.

70. Batchelor TJP, Rasburn NJ, Abdelnour-Berchtold E, et al. Guidelines for enhanced recovery after lung surgery: recommendations of the enhanced recovery after surgery (ERAS®) society and the European Society of Thoracic Surgeons (ESTS). *Eur J Cardio-thoracic Surg.* 2019;55(1): 91–115. https://doi.org/10.1093/ejcts/ezy301.

71. White KM. The role of the occupational therapist in the care of people living with lung cancer. *Transl Lung Cancer Res.* 2016;5(3):244–246. https://doi.org/10.21037/tlcr.2016.05.02.

72. Mirels H. Metastatic disease in long bones: a proposed scoring system for diagnosing impending pathologic fractures. 1989. *Clin Orthop Relat Res.* 2003;(415 suppl l). https://doi.org/10.1097/01.blo.0000093045.56370.dd.

73. Maltser S, Cristian A, Silver JK, Stephen Morris G, Stout NL. A focused review of safety considerations in cancer rehabilitation. *PM R.* 2017. https://doi.org/10.1016/j.pmrj.2017.08.403.

74. Cheville AL, Basford JR. Role of rehabilitation medicine and physical agents in the treatment of cancer-associated pain. *J Clin Oncol.* 2014;32(16):1691–1702. https://doi.org/10.1200/JCO.2013.53.6680.

75. Carlson LE, Zelinski E, Toivonen K, et al. Mind-body therapies in cancer: what is the latest evidence? *Curr Oncol Rep.* 2017;19(10). https://doi.org/10.1007/s11912-017-0626-1.

76. Wandner LD, Prasad R, Ramezani A, Malcore SA, Kerns RD. Core competencies for the emerging specialty of pain psychology. *Am Psychol.* 2019;74(4):432–444. https://doi.org/10.1037/amp0000330.

77. Hughes LS, Clark J, Colclough JA, Dale E, McMillan D. Acceptance and commitment therapy (ACT) for chronic pain. *Clin J Pain.* 2017;33(6):552–568. https://doi.org/10.1097/AJP.0000000000000425.

78. González-Fernández S, Fernández-Rodríguez C. Acceptance and commitment therapy in cancer: review of applications and findings. *Behav Med.* 2019;45(3): 255–269. https://doi.org/10.1080/08964289.2018.1452713.

79. Kabat-Zinn J. *Full Catastrophe Living: Using the Wisdom of Your Body and Mind to Face Stress, Pain, and Illness.* 2nd ed. Bantam Books; 2013.

80. Schellekens MPJ, van den Hurk DGM, Prins JB, et al. Mindfulness-based stress reduction added to care as usual for lung cancer patients and/or their partners: a multicentre randomized controlled trial. *Psycho Oncol.* 2017; 26(12):2118–2126. https://doi.org/10.1002/pon.4430.

81. Nijs J, Wijma AJ, Leysen L, et al. Explaining pain following cancer: a practical guide for clinicians. *Braz J Phys Ther.* 2019;23(5):367–377. https://doi.org/10.1016/j.bjpt.2018.12.003.

82. Bennett MI, Bagnall AM, José Closs S. How effective are patient-based educational interventions in the management of cancer pain? Systematic review and meta-analysis. *Pain.* 2009;143(3):192–199. https://doi.org/10.1016/j.pain.2009.01.016.

83. Moseley GL, Butler DS. Fifteen years of explaining pain: the past, present, and future. *J Pain.* 2015;16(9): 807–813. https://doi.org/10.1016/j.jpain.2015.05.005.

84. Louw A, Diener I, Butler DS, Puentedura EJ. The effect of neuroscience education on pain, disability, anxiety, and stress in chronic musculoskeletal pain. *Arch Phys Med Rehabil.* 2011;92(12):2041–2056. https://doi.org/10.1016/j.apmr.2011.07.198.

85. Van Oosterwijck J, Meeus M, Paul L, et al. Pain physiology education improves health status and endogenous pain inhibition in fibromyalgia: a double-blind randomized controlled trial. *Clin J Pain.* 2013;29(10):873–882. https://doi.org/10.1097/AJP.0b013e31827c7a7d.

86. Zia FZ, Olaku O, Bao T, et al. The national cancer institute's conference on acupuncture for symptom management in oncology: state of the science, evidence, and research gaps. *J Natl Cancer Inst Monogr.* 2017;2017(52):68–73. https://doi.org/10.1093/jncimonographs/lgx005.

87. He Y, Guo X, May BH, et al. Clinical evidence for association of acupuncture and acupressure with improved cancer pain: a systematic review and meta-analysis. *JAMA Oncol.* 2020;6(2):271–278. https://doi.org/10.1001/jamaoncol.2019.5233.

CHAPTER 14

Cognitive Impairment in Lung Cancer and Brain Metastases

LINDSAY M. NICCOLAI, PHD • JENNIE L. REXER, PHD

INTRODUCTION

Over the past few decades, advances in cancer treatments have significantly extended survival. With an increase in the number of cancer survivors, there has been a greater appreciation for potential adverse side effects of cancer treatments. Cognitive functioning in cancer patients has increasingly received research attention, particularly with the side effects of chemotherapy on cognition, which are often referred to by patients as "chemo brain" or "chemo fog."[1] Importantly, cognitive complaints are among the most frequently reported side effects from treatments, even in patients with non-central nervous system (non-CNS) cancers. Cognitive impairment can have detrimental impacts on patients' quality of life by affecting their functional abilities, school or occupational performance, social relationships, and participation in leisure activities.[2]

Much of the research on cognition in cancer patients has focused on breast cancer, but several studies have observed cognitive impairments in patients with a variety of other non-CNS cancers including lung cancer. In this chapter, we will focus on cognitive impairment in patients with small cell or non-small cell lung cancer (SCLC and NSCLC, respectively) as well as those lung cancer patients who develop brain metastases. We will summarize the literature on the incidence and pattern of cognitive impairment in lung cancer and brain metastases, the brain-related changes associated with various cancer treatments, and potential approaches to prevent or treat cognitive impairment.

EPIDEMIOLOGY

More than one in three persons will be diagnosed with cancer in their lifetime.[3] Most of these cancers are outside of the central nervous system (CNS). Lung cancer, including both SCLC and NSCLC, is the second most common cancer in men and women. Breast cancer is the most common in women, while prostate cancer is the most common in men. Lung cancer accounts for nearly 25% of all cancer-related deaths,[3] which is the most common cancer-related death in the United States but also in the world.[4] The most common lung cancer type is NSCLC, accounting for approximately 85% of cases, while the often more aggressive SCLC accounts for about 15% of cases.[3] Lung cancer mainly occurs among older adults and the average age at diagnosis is 70. Smoking drastically increases the risk of lung cancer with approximately 85%–90% of cases attributed to smoking.[5] Fortunately, the incidence of lung cancer cases has decreased in recent years due to more people quitting smoking.[3]

Around 20% of cancer patients will develop brain metastases, and lung cancer is the most common primary site for brain metastases across patients irrespective of sex.[6] Lung cancer patients often tend to present with multiple brain metastases, although they may have a solitary lesion if it is detected early.[7] Lung cancer patients with brain metastases can often have a poor prognosis. However, prognosis varies considerably based on molecular markers, such that some patients with brain metastases from NSCLC can have differences in median survival from 12 months to even 4 years.[8] About 20%–40% of NSCLC patients eventually develop brain metastases.[9] Approximately 10% of SCLC patients present with brain metastases at diagnosis, while an additional 40%–50% go on to have brain metastases.[10] At times, the brain metastasis may be discovered before lung cancer is even identified as the primary cancer. Most brain metastases are supratentorial, and they are often discovered at the junction between the gray and white matter and in watershed areas between vascular territories.[6] SCLC has one of the highest incidences of leptomeningeal metastases, a subset of metastases growing in the lining of the brain or spine and/or disseminated in the cerebrospinal spinal fluid, which is associated with a poor prognosis.[6,11]

Cognitive complaints are relatively frequent in patients with both non-CNS cancers along with brain metastases.[2] Up to 70% of adult patients with non-CNS cancers have cognitive complaints during cancer treatments and approximately 30% demonstrate cognitive impairment on formal neuropsychological assessments.[12] Specifically in lung cancer, cognitive dysfunction appears to be common in SCLC with prevalence rates ranging from 15% to 90%.[13] Among patients with NSCLC who had not yet received treatment, prevalence rates range from 23% to 95% having cognitive impairment at baseline. In patients with brain metastases, cognitive impairment is almost ubiquitous with approximately 90% of patients presenting with cognitive impairment prior to receiving any treatments.[14]

In addition to brain metastases, another potential cause of CNS involvement in lung cancer is paraneoplastic neurologic syndromes (PNS). PNS are a heterogeneous group of disorders, which are often caused by an immune response to cancer and not by direct invasion, metastasis, or an effect of cancer treatments.[14a] PNS can affect any part of the nervous system. The immune response is often associated with antineuronal antibodies, and these can serve as biomarkers of the origin of the neurological syndrome and may also reveal the primary cancer. For instance, paraneoplastic limbic encephalitis (PLE) is strongly associated with the antineuronal antibody and anti-Hu, which is often found in SCLC.[15] While PNS can occur with any type of cancer, SCLC is one of the most frequent causes of PNS.[16] SCLC has been found to be associated with a variety of PNS: PLE, Lambert–Eaton myasthenic syndrome, paraneoplastic encephalomyelitis, paraneoplastic sensory neuropathy, and paraneoplastic cerebellar degeneration.[16] Of these disorders, the one that may be most relevant to cognition is paraneoplastic limbic encephalitis (PLE).

PLE is a relatively rare disorder (i.e., approximately 1 in 10,000 of cancer patients;[17] in which 50% are due to SCLC.[18] PLE may occur as a part of a multifocal encephalomyelitis or as an isolated syndrome. Patients with PLE often present with significant cognitive impairments, seizures, and psychiatric symptoms.[19] PLE typically presents as an amnestic syndrome characterized by pronounced memory loss along with deficits in attention, language, visuospatial skills, and executive functioning.[20] Memory loss can be accompanied by confabulations and a lack of insight. The seizures may be generalized or focal. Common psychiatric symptoms may consist of symptoms of depression, anxiety, emotional lability, personality changes, as well as hallucinations and delusions. Overall, the diagnosis of PLE can be difficult to ascertain given the similarity of these symptoms with other cancer-related complications, including brain metastases, toxic and metabolic encephalopathies, viral etiologies such as herpes simplex encephalitis, and the side effects of various cancer treatments.[21] The neurological symptoms of PNS can even precede the detection of the cancer, which can be more difficult to identify it as a paraneoplastic syndrome.

CAUSES AND MECHANISMS
Cognitive Impairment in Lung Cancer
Prior to Treatment

Several studies have demonstrated that patients with a variety of non-CNS cancers may have cognitive impairments prior to cancer treatments.[22] This relationship between cancer and cognitive impairment at baseline may be linked to several factors. Cancer may lead to increased production of proinflammatory cytokines, which may thereby lead to neuroinflammation, which can have untoward effects on cognition.[22] Inflammation also plays a role in "sickness behavior" (e.g., fatigue, sleep disturbance, and decreased appetite).[23]

In addition, genetic variation is another possible mechanism of cancer-related cognitive impairment and may be helpful in identifying individuals who are at increased risk for cognitive impairment following treatments, such as chemotherapy. One of the most frequently studied genes is apolipoprotein ε4 (*APOE4*), which has been extensively studied as a risk factor for the development of Alzheimer's disease as well as poorer outcomes of other neurological conditions such as stroke and head injury.[24] The APOE ε4 allele has been linked increased oxidative stress and inflammation, reduced turnover of neural progenitor cells, and dysfunction of the blood–brain barrier.[25] Since chemotherapy can alter these processes, the influence of *APOE4* may play a key role in cancer-related cognitive impairment. Additionally, DNA damage and DNA repair deficiencies have been associated with an increased risk for both cancer and neurodegenerative disorders, with impaired DNA repair leading to cellular dysfunction, inflammation, and cell senescence.[26,27]

Furthermore, cognitive impairment prior to treatment may be exacerbated by physical symptoms (e.g., fatigue) and psychological distress that are commonly found in individuals diagnosed with cancer.[2] Fatigue is the most commonly reported symptom throughout the disease course in lung cancer patients.[28] Fatigue can negatively impact cognitive efficiency.

Unfortunately, fatigue can often cooccur with other physical symptoms such as sleep disturbance and cancer-related pain. Psychological distress, with symptoms of depression and anxiety, is also highly prevalent in lung cancer patients, and patients with SCLC or those not offered cancer treatments may be at higher risk.[29]

In lung cancer patients,[30] it is shown that patients with SCLC had cognitive impairments in verbal memory and executive functioning as well as reduced motor coordination prior to receiving chemoradiation[31] and found that 97% (29 out of 30) of patients with limited-stage SCLC had cognitive impairment prior to prophylactic cranial irradiation. The most frequent impairments were in verbal memory, executive functioning, and fine motor dexterity. Grosshans et al.[32] also examined patients with SCLC prior to receiving prophylactic cranial irradiation and found that 47% of patients had baseline cognitive impairment. In a review paper of cognitive impairment in patients with SCLC and NSCLC treated with prophylactic cranial irradiation, Zeng and colleagues[33] examined eight different randomized clinical trials and eight observational studies and found that 23%–95% of lung cancer patients had cognitive impairments at baseline. In a study comparing patients with SCLC and NSCLC to healthy controls, both lung cancer groups exhibited a higher rate of cognitive impairments (30%–39%) compared to healthy controls (5%), and there were no significant differences between the lung cancer groups.[34]

In addition, lung cancer patients are often older adults who may be more vulnerable to cognitive decline and have multiple medical comorbidities. Some of these medical comorbidities are directly related to smoking, which is much more frequent among lung cancer patients than in the general population.[35] Smoking has been associated with a higher incidence of respiratory conditions (e.g., chronic obstructive pulmonary disease and obstructive sleep apnea) and vascular conditions (e.g., hypertension and peripheral arterial disease),[35] all of which can lead to cerebrovascular changes and higher rates of cognitive impairment. Also, smoking by itself has been associated with an increased risk of cognitive decline,[36,37] and proposed brain-related mechanisms are increased oxidative stress and inflammation.[36] Other medical conditions can also commonly co-occur in lung cancer patients, which are unrelated to smoking, such as diabetes, which is also a common cerebrovascular risk factor.[35]

Cognitive Impairment Following Lung Cancer Treatments

The impact of cancer treatments for SCLC and NSCLC on cognition is an important consideration when choosing different treatment options, particularly when treatments are not curative.[38] A large portion of lung cancer patients receive platinum-based chemotherapy (e.g., cisplatin and carboplatin) as some part of their treatment regimens, and these therapeutics have been shown to be neurotoxic.[39] Patients with NSCLC may have cognitive impairments soon after chemotherapy.[39] One-month postchemotherapy, 62% of patients showed cognitive declines; however, these cognitive effects were not apparent at 7 months posttreatment. There also appeared to be some cognitive decline in patients with NSCLC receiving either palliative chemotherapy or adjuvant chemotherapy after 2–4 months, with recovery in some cases after 4–6 months.[38] Simó et al.[40] compared patients with SCLC and NSCLC and healthy controls following chemotherapy treatment. The SCLC group performed worse than healthy controls on measures of visuospatial skills and verbal fluency. The NSCLC group performed worse than both healthy controls and SCLC group in verbal memory. In addition to chemotherapies, patients may also receive targeted therapy. One study compared patients with NSCLC treated with targeted therapy versus chemotherapy versus no treatment. About a third (30%–35%) of participants exhibited cognitive impairment in at least one domain in each group regardless of the treatment modality.[41] Slowed psychomotor speed was the most common area of impairment.

Chemotherapy is often administered with thoracic radiation in patients with SCLC.[40] However, SCLC remains difficult to cure and has a propensity to develop distant metastases, in particular, brain metastases. Prophylactic cranial irradiation (PCI) has been used to reduce the incidence of brain metastases and extend overall survival in patients with SCLC. In patients with NSCLC, PCI may increase disease-free survival without an improvement in overall survival.[40] However, PCI can have neurotoxic effects and lead to an increased risk of cognitive decline. PCI may be associated with structural brain changes, such as whole brain volume loss[42] and decreased gray and white matter in multiple areas[40] in patients with SCLC. Decreased gray matter in the hippocampus, insular cortex, and the superior temporal gyrus have been found following PCI.[40] They also found decreased white matter microstructure in the corpus callosum.

Unsurprisingly, cognitive impairments have also been associated with these brain-related structural changes following PCI. Patients with SCLC have demonstrated cognitive declines following PCI in the areas of verbal memory,[42,43] verbal fluency,[40] language skills, and executive functioning.[32] The declines in language skills and executive functioning appeared to be transient, such that they were present at earlier follow-ups but not observed at later time points. In the Radiation Therapy Oncology Group (RTOG) protocols 0212 (limited-disease SCLC) and 0214 (NSCLC), patients in both trials demonstrated verbal memory decline at 6 and 12 months following PCI.[43] Patients treated with PCI also self-reported cognitive decline, although this was not closely correlated with objective cognitive impairment. There are often discrepancies between subjective cognitive complaints and objective impairments on formal neuropsychological testing, which have been demonstrated in various neurological disorders.[44] Self-reported cognitive symptoms may be secondary to emotional distress (e.g., depression and anxiety) as well as fatigue. This emphasizes the need for formal neuropsychological evaluation being used in conjunction with patient-reported symptoms.

Cognitive Impairment in Patients with Brain Metastases
Prior to Treatment
Meyers et al.[14] studied cognitive functioning in patients with various cancers with brain metastases (251 had NSCLC, 75 had breast cancer, and 75 with other cancers) and found about 90% of patients had cognitive impairment at baseline. Performances on cognitive measures of memory retrieval, fine motor speed, and executive functioning were correlated with the total volume of brain metastases. Therefore, cognitive functioning may be more related to tumor volume, or overall brain metastasis burden, rather than the actual number of metastases.[14] Interestingly, Meyers et al.[14] also found that cognitive functioning prior to treatment was a significant predictor of overall survival.

Following Treatments
Treatment approaches of brain metastases consist of surgical resection, stereotactic radiosurgery (SRS), and whole brain radiation treatment (WBRT). Surgical resection is often used with larger tumors that may have mass effect. However, even in the cases of gross total resection, there is about a 50% risk of recurrence at the resection site.[45] Therefore, many patients with brain metastases are often treated with radiotherapy, local radiation in the case of SRS, or widespread radiation in WBRT. SRS is often selected for limited brain metastases arising from most tumor types. The selection of SRS over WBRT is often preferred secondary to concerns of neurotoxicity and subsequent cognitive decline with WBRT without significant benefit to overall survival. When comparing the radiation treatments, patients have demonstrated lower rates of cognitive decline when treated with SRS alone

(cognitive decline in 24% patients) versus patients treated with SRS plus WBRT.[46] WBRT has also been associated with 4- and 6-month decline in verbal learning and memory.[47] Of note, these studies have often excluded patients with SCLC due to concerns of possible rapid neurologic progression. WBRT is still often used in patients with SCLC with a limited number of metastases or even a single brain metastasis.[48] Cordeiro et al.[49] reviewed SCLC patients who were treated with first-line SRS or had prior PCI or WBRT and found no significant difference in overall survival.

Cranial radiation has been associated with diffuse radiographic periventricular white matter changes (i.e., leukoencephalopathy).[50] Leukoencephalopathy has been shown to be far more frequent with WBRT than SRS.[50] To prevent the adverse impacts of WBRT on cognitive functioning, an intensity-modulated radiotherapy technique has been developed to conformally avoid the hippocampus, known as hippocampal avoidance WBRT (HA-WBRT).[51] In patients with brain metastases outside of the hippocampal region, 100 patients (56 of which had lung cancer) were treated with HA-WBRT and compared to a WBRT historical control group.[51] The HA-WBRT showed preservation of memory up to 6-month follow-up. This demonstrated that damage to the hippocampus during WBRT is likely a central mechanism of radiation-induced memory decline.

In addition to HA-WBRT, research has examined the pharmacologic mitigation of cognitive impairment with the use of memantine, an N-methyl-D-aspartate receptor agonist, in patients with brain metastases receiving WBRT primarily in those with lung cancer.[52] Patients treated with memantine had delayed time to cognitive decline versus placebo, specifically in the areas of memory, executive functioning, and processing speed. Memantine was also generally well tolerated by patients. Preservation of cognitive functioning in cases of WBRT remains an active area of research with the hope to maximize the quality of life in patients with brain metastases.

PREVENTION AND INTERVENTION
Understanding the underlying mechanisms of cognitive impairment is key for developing strategies geared toward prevention and intervention. First, early identification of which individuals are at increased risk for cognitive impairment is critical. Risk factors for cognitive decline include higher age, genetic polymorphisms (e.g., APOE ε4), comorbid medical conditions (e.g., hypertension), and smoking. Some of these risk factors are modifiable, for instance, with smoking cessation and maintaining a healthy diet and regular exercise regimen.

Different studies have investigated pharmacological and non-pharmacological approaches to prevent and/or intervene against cognitive impairment in cancer patients. Most of these studies have examined interventions in patients with breast cancer,[53] but this is a burgeoning area of research with extension to other cancer types, including lung cancer.

Pharmacological Interventions

The evidence for effective pharmacological interventions to treat cancer-related cognitive impairment has been limited. Psychostimulants and other medications that are traditionally used to treat attention deficit hyperactivity disorder, as well as narcolepsy, have been studied for their potential improvement of inattention and/or fatigue. In lung cancer patients, methylphenidate improved alertness, increased energy, and global cognitive function.[54] In a study in which the majority were lung cancer patients, modafinil improved psychomotor speed, attention, and processing speed.[55] There were also significant improvements in depression and drowsiness. Similarly, Blackhall and colleagues[56] found that modafinil alleviated fatigue along with improved depression and anxiety symptoms and overall quality of life. In patients with brain metastases, primarily related to lung cancer, patients treated with methylphenidate showed improved alertness and attention.[57] Modafinil may optimize locus coeruleus function and thereby increase binding of dopamine and norepinephrine, thus increasing prefrontal functioning.[58] Although these results in smaller studies have been promising, larger studies with longer follow-ups are needed to establish the efficacy of treating cognitive impairment with stimulants in cancer patients.

Another pharmacologic agent that has received research attention is donepezil, an acetylcholinesterase inhibitor commonly used in Alzheimer's disease. Donepezil initially showed promise in preclinical studies, although phase III studies indicated limited efficacy in treating cancer-related cognitive impairment.[2] In one study of patients with SCLC treated with donepezil and vitamin E, there were no significant differences in cognition when compared to controls following PCI.[58a] There is also no conclusive evidence for *Ginkgo biloba* or erythropoietin, a drug that increases red blood cell production, to treat cancer-related cognitive impairment.[59]

Non-pharmacological Interventions
Cognitive Rehabilitation

The most often studied intervention in cancer patients is cognitive rehabilitation. Different cognitive rehabilitation approaches have been investigated, including cognitive strategy training where the patient learns compensatory strategies, whereas cognitive retraining (otherwise known as computerized training or "brain training") has the patient repeatedly complete exercises focused on particular cognitive domains. Cognitive strategy training with compensatory strategies has shown to be beneficial for cognitive impairments in cancer patients.[60] However, cognitive retraining may demonstrate some objective improvement in specific areas, but may not generalize beyond the skills in the repetitive exercises. Therefore, these programs may lack the fundamental transfer of skills needed for functioning in daily life.

Complementary Interventions

Complementary interventions may be used to target physical and psychological symptoms, which may exacerbate cognitive impairment in cancer patients. Complementary interventions consist of physical activity and relaxation-based strategies including mindfulness-based stress reduction. Physical activity has shown to have beneficial effects on cognitive functioning in healthy cognitively normal adults. The underlying mechanism may be increasing stimulation of neurogenesis in the hippocampus as well as increasing oxygen saturation and cerebral blood flow, as well as reducing oxidative stress and inflammation.[61] Vaquero et al.[62] showed neuroplastic changes in the bilateral hippocampi following a 3-month physical activity program in patients with SCLC and NSCLC. In addition to physical activity, mindfulness-based interventions that target symptoms of depression, anxiety, and stress and may also reduce inflammation and fatigue.[63] Mindfulness-based interventions tend to reduce subjective cognitive complaints; however, they have not been demonstrated to improve objective cognitive functioning.[63] Taken together, additional research is needed to shed light on the effects of complementary interventions on cognition in lung cancer patients.

PATIENT EDUCATION

Health care providers are encouraged to inquire about cognitive difficulties prior to and following cancer treatments. It is important to ask family members and/or other caregivers in addition to the patient since patients with cognitive impairments can often lack insight into their deficits. If patients or their family members do in fact report concerns about cognitive functioning, we would recommend that providers place a referral to a neuropsychologist who can comprehensively evaluate cognitive functioning to determine the etiology of the cognitive changes, such as due to the effects of cancer and cancer treatments or a possible underlying neurodegenerative process. Neuropsychologists can then offer tailored recommendations to educate patients and their families and provide resources in an effort to preserve or improve patients' overall quality of life.

Recommendations to patients and caregivers can vary a great deal depending upon the referral question asked, the nature of the cognitive impairments and underlying etiology, and the goals of the patient and/or caregiver. Lung cancer patients with cognitive changes secondary to chemotherapy may be given education and instructions regarding different compensatory strategies, for instance, utilizing external memory aids and internal memory strategies. Lung cancer patients often have co-occurring physical symptoms that can negatively affect cognition, such as sleep disturbance and fatigue. Therefore, medical providers may offer education regarding strategies for sleep hygiene and energy conservation. Some lung cancer patients experience emotional distress and adjustment issues related to coping with their cancer diagnosis and treatments. These patients may benefit from participating in individual psychotherapy and/or a support group and may also receive psychiatric consultation.

For individuals with more severe cognitive impairment, as in the cases of some patients with brain metastases as well as many of those with neurodegenerative diseases, recommendations are often geared toward ensuring safety and advising that caregivers provide assistance with activities of daily living that could be potentially hazardous, such as driving and managing medications. Caregivers often benefit from receiving caregiving resources through various local and national organizations, which can offer helpful information about cognitive disorders along with supportive services.

CONCLUSION

Many lung cancer patients present with cognitive impairment prior to and following treatments. At baseline, lung cancer patients may have cognitive impairment secondary to multiple factors including increased inflammation, advanced age, medical comorbidities, smoking, and significant fatigue. Lung cancer patients may experience significant cognitive declines following cancer treatments, such as chemotherapy and prophylactic cranial irradiation, which have known neurotoxic effects. As compared to other primary cancers, lung cancer patients may be susceptible to neurological complications of brain metastases and paraneoplastic neurological disorders that have

deleterious impacts on cognitive functioning. Cranial irradiation for brain metastases may also lead to significant brain-related changes and associated cognitive decline. For instance, in WBRT, there are often periventricular white matter changes as well as pronounced memory decline.

Additional research is needed to identify which lung cancer patients are at higher risk for cognitive impairment. Some of these risk factors are likely modifiable, such as promoting smoking cessation and exercising regularly. There are different pharmacological and non-pharmacological approaches aimed at potentially preventing cognitive decline or restoring cognitive functioning in lung cancer patients and those patients who develop brain metastases. In patients with brain metastases treated with whole brain radiation, hippocampal avoidance and memantine may preserve memory functioning. In patients with lung cancer without brain metastases, cognitive rehabilitation and/or complementary interventions may be beneficial for improving cognitive functioning. Some of these non-pharmacological approaches can also demonstrate improvements in patients' mood state and physical functioning. Even mild cognitive problems can affect occupational and social functioning resulting in negative impacts on quality of life; thus, developing effective cognitive interventions is essential. Future prospective studies may further our knowledge of the efficacy of various prevention and intervention strategies to maximize cognitive functioning in lung cancer patients and improve their overall quality of life.

REFERENCES

1. Wefel JS, Lenzi R, Theriault R, Buzdar AU, Cruickshank S, Meyers CA. 'Chemobrain' in breast carcinoma?: a prologue. *Cancer.* 2004;101(3):466–475.
2. Schagen SB, Klein M, Reijneveld JC, et al. Monitoring and optimising cognitive function in cancer patients: present knowledge and future directions. *EJC Suppl.* 2014;12(1): 29–40.
3. American Cancer Society. *Key Statistics in Lung Cancer.* https://www.cancer.org/cancer/lung-cancer/about/key-statistics.html. Retrieved on February 18, 2021.
4. Molina JR, Yang P, Cassivi SD, Schild SE, Adjei AA. Non-small cell lung cancer: epidemiology, risk factors, treatment, and survivorship. *Mayo Clin Proc.* 2008;83(5): 584–594.
5. Samet JM, Avila-Tang E, Boffetta P, et al. Lung cancer in never smokers: clinical epidemiology and environmental risk factors. *Clin Cancer Res.* 2009;15(18):5626–5645.
6. Achrol AS, Rennert RC, Anders C, et al. Brain metastases. *Nat Rev Dis Prim.* 2019;5(1):5.

7. Ali A, Goffin JR, Arnold A, Ellis PM. Survival of patients with non-small-cell lung cancer after a diagnosis of brain metastases. *Curr Oncol.* 2013;20(4):e300−e306.
8. Sperduto PW, Yang TJ, Beal K, et al. Estimating survival in patients with lung cancer and brain metastases: an update of the graded prognostic assessment for lung cancer using molecular markers (Lung-molGPA). *JAMA Oncol.* 2017; 3(6):827−831.
9. Barnholtz-Sloan JS, Sloan AE, Davis FG, Vigneau FD, Lai P, Sawaya RE. Incidence proportions of brain metastases in patients diagnosed (1973 to 2001) in the metropolitan detroit cancer surveillance system. *J Clin Oncol.* 2004; 22(14):2865−2872.
10. Quan AL, Videtic GM, Suh JH. Brain metastases in small cell lung cancer. *Oncology.* 2004;18(8):961−987.
11. Chamberlain MC. Leptomeningeal metastasis. *Curr Opin Neurol.* 2009;22(6):665−674.
12. Chung NC, Walker AK, Dhillon HM, Vardy JL. Mechanisms and treatment for cancer- and chemotherapy-related cognitive impairment in survivors of non-CNS malignancies. *Oncology.* 2018;32(12):591−598.
13. Kanard A, Frytak S, Jatoi A. Cognitive dysfunction in patients with small-cell lung cancer: incidence, causes, and suggestions on management. *J Support Oncol.* 2004;2(2): 127−140.
14. Meyers CA, Smith JA, Bezjak A, et al. Neurocognitive function and progression in patients with brain metastases treated with whole-brain radiation and motexafin gadolinium: results of a randomized phase III trial. *J Clin Oncol.* 2004;22(1):157−165.
14a Dalmau J, Gultekin H, Posner J. Paraneoplastic neurologic syndromes: pathogenesis and physiopathology. *Brain Pathol.* 1999;9(2):275−284.
15. Alamowitch S, Graus F, Uchuya M, Reñé R, Bescansa E, Delattre JY. Limbic encephalitis and small cell lung cancer. Clinical and immunological features. *Brain.* 1997;120(Pt 6):923−928.
16. Gozzard P, Woodhall M, Chapman C, et al. Paraneoplastic neurologic disorders in small cell lung carcinoma: a prospective study. *Neurology.* 2015;85(3):235−239.
17. Lalani N, Haq R. Prognostic effect of early treatment of paraneoplastic limbic encephalitis in a patient with small-cell lung cancer. *Curr Oncol.* 2012;19(5):e353−e357.
18. Ochenduszko S, Wilk B, Dabrowska J, Herman-Sucharska I, Dubis A, Puskulluoglu M. Paraneoplastic limbic encephalitis in a patient with extensive disease small-cell lung cancer. *Mol Clin Oncol.* 2017;6(4): 575−578.
19. Lawn ND, Westmoreland BF, Kiely MJ, Lennon VA, Vernino S. Clinical, magnetic resonance imaging, and electroencephalographic findings in paraneoplastic limbic encephalitis. *Mayo Clin Proc.* 2003;78(11): 1363−1368.
20. Gibson LL, McKeever A, Coutinho E, Finke C, Pollak TA. Cognitive impact of neuronal antibodies: encephalitis and beyond. *Transl Psychiatr.* 2020;10(1):304.
21. Gultekin SH, Rosenfeld MR, Voltz R, Eichen J, Posner JB, Dalmau J. Paraneoplastic limbic encephalitis:

22. Ahles TA, Saykin AJ, McDonald BC, et al. Cognitive function in breast cancer patients prior to adjuvant treatment. *Breast Cancer Res Treat.* 2008;110(1):143−152.
23. Dantzer R, Kelley KW. Twenty years of research on cytokine-induced sickness behavior. *Brain Behav Immun.* 2007;21(2):153−160.
24. McAllister TW, Ahles TA, Saykin AJ, et al. Cognitive effects of cytotoxic cancer chemotherapy: predisposing risk factors and potential treatments. *Curr Psychiatr Rep.* 2004; 6(5):364−371.
25. Fernandez HR, Varma A, Flowers SA, Rebeck GW. Cancer chemotherapy related cognitive impairment and the impact of the alzheimer's disease risk factor APOE. *Cancers.* 2020;12(12):3842.
26. Madabhushi R, Pan L, Tsai LH. DNA damage and its links to neurodegeneration. *Neuron.* 2014;83(2): 266−282.
27. Bagnall-Moreau C, Chaudhry S, Salas-Ramirez K, Ahles T, Hubbard K. Chemotherapy-induced cognitive impairment is associated with increased inflammation and oxidative damage in the Hippocampus. *Mol Neurobiol.* 2019; 56(10):7159−7172.
28. Carnio S, Di Stefano RF, Novello S. Fatigue in lung cancer patients: symptom burden and management of challenges. *Lung Cancer.* 2016;7:73−82.
29. Carlsen K, Jensen AB, Jacobsen E, Krasnik M, Johansen C. Psychosocial aspects of lung cancer. *Lung Cancer.* 2005; 47(3):293−300.
30. Meyers CA, Byrne KS, Komaki R. Cognitive deficits in patients with small cell lung cancer before and after chemotherapy. *Lung Cancer.* 1995;12(3):231−235.
31. Komaki R, Meyers CA, Shin DM, et al. Evaluation of cognitive function in patients with limited small cell lung cancer prior to and shortly following prophylactic cranial irradiation. *Int J Radiat Oncol Biol Phys.* 1995;33(1): 179−182.
32. Grosshans DR, Meyers CA, Allen PK, Davenport SD, Komaki R. Neurocognitive function in patients with small cell lung cancer : effect of prophylactic cranial irradiation. *Cancer.* 2008;112(3):589−595.
33. Zeng H, Hendriks LEL, van Geffen WH, Witlox WJA, Eekers DBP, De Ruysscher DKM. Risk factors for neurocognitive decline in lung cancer patients treated with prophylactic cranial irradiation: a systematic review. *Cancer Treat Rev.* 2020;88:102025.
34. Simó M, Root JC, Vaquero L, et al. Cognitive and brain structural changes in a lung cancer population. *J Thorac Oncol.* 2015;10:38−45.
35. Leduc C, Antoni D, Charloux A, Falcoz PE, Quoix E. Comorbidities in the management of patients with lung cancer. *Eur Respir J.* 2017;49(3):1601721.
36. Anstey KJ, von Sanden C, Salim A, O'Kearney R. Smoking as a risk factor for dementia and cognitive decline: a meta-analysis of prospective studies. *Am J Epidemiol.* 2007; 166(4):367−378.

37. Sabia S, Elbaz A, Dugravot A, et al. Impact of smoking on cognitive decline in early old age: the Whitehall II cohort study. *Arch Gen Psychiatr.* 2012;69(6):627–635.

38. van de Kamp HJ, Molder MT, Schulkes KJG, et al. Impact of lung cancer treatment on cognitive functioning. *Clin Lung Cancer.* 2020;21(2), 114–126.e3.

39. Whitney KA, Lysaker PH, Steiner AR, Hook JN, Estes DD, Hanna NH. Is "chemobrain" a transient state? A prospective pilot study among persons with non-small cell lung cancer. *J Support Oncol.* 2008;6(7):313–321.

40. Simó M, Vaquero L, Ripollés P, et al. Longitudinal brain changes associated with prophylactic cranial irradiation in lung cancer. *J Thorac Oncol.* 2016;11(4):475–486.

41. Kang HL, Chen VC, Hung WL, Hsiao HP, Wang WH. Preliminary comparison of neuropsychological performance in patients with non-small-cell lung cancer treated with chemotherapy or targeted therapy. *Neuropsychiatric Dis Treat.* 2019;15:753–761.

42. Gui C, Chintalapati N, Hales RK, et al. A prospective evaluation of whole brain volume loss and neurocognitive decline following hippocampal-sparing prophylactic cranial irradiation for limited-stage small-cell lung cancer. *J Neuro Oncol.* 2019;144(2):351–358.

43. Gondi V, Paulus R, Bruner DW, et al. Decline in tested and self-reported cognitive functioning after prophylactic cranial irradiation for lung cancer: pooled secondary analysis of Radiation Therapy Oncology Group randomized trials 0212 and 0214. *Int J Radiat Oncol Biol Phys.* 2013;86(4):656–664.

44. Wefel JS, Kesler SR, Noll KR, Schagen SB. Clinical characteristics, pathophysiology, and management of noncentral nervous system cancer-related cognitive impairment in adults. *CA Cancer J Clin.* 2015;65(2):123–138.

45. Patchell RA, Tibbs PA, Walsh JW, et al. A randomized trial of surgery in the treatment of single metastases to the brain. *N Engl J Med.* 1990;322:494–500.

46. Brown PD, Jaeckle K, Ballman KV, et al. Effect of radiosurgery alone vs radiosurgery with whole brain radiation therapy on cognitive function in patients with 1 to 3 brain metastases: a randomized clinical trial [published correction appears in JAMA. 2018 Aug 7;320(5):510]. *JAMA.* 2016;316(4):401–409.

47. Chang EL, Wefel JS, Hess KR, et al. Neurocognition in patients with brain metastases treated with radiosurgery or radiosurgery plus whole-brain irradiation: a randomised controlled trial. *Lancet Oncol.* 2009;10(11):1037–1044.

48. Robin TP, Rusthoven CG. Radiosurgery for small-cell lung cancer brain metastases: a review. *J Thorac Dis.* 2020;12(10):6234–6239.

49. Cordeiro D, Xu Z, Shepard M, et al. Gamma Knife radiosurgery for brain metastases from small-cell lung cancer: institutional experience over more than a decade and review of the literature. *J Radiosurg SBRT.* 2019;6:35–43.

50. Stokes TB, Niranjan A, Kano H, et al. White matter changes in breast cancer brain metastases patients who undergo radiosurgery alone compared to whole brain radiation therapy plus radiosurgery. *J Neuro Oncol.* 2015;121(3):583–590.

51. Gondi V, Pugh SL, Tome WA, et al. Preservation of memory with conformal avoidance of the hippocampal neural stem-cell compartment during whole-brain radiotherapy for brain metastases (RTOG 0933): a phase II multi-institutional trial. *J Clin Oncol.* 2014;32(34):3810–3816.

52. Brown PD, Pugh S, Laack NN, et al. Memantine for the prevention of cognitive dysfunction in patients receiving whole-brain radiotherapy: a randomized, double-blind, placebo-controlled trial. *Neuro Oncol.* 2013;15(10):1429–1437.

53. Vance DE, Frank JS, Bail J, et al. Interventions for cognitive deficits in breast cancer survivors treated with chemotherapy. *Cancer Nursing.* 2017;40(1):E11–E27.

54. Gagnon B, Low G, Schreier G. Methylphenidate hydrochloride improves cognitive function in patients with advanced cancer and hypoactive delirium: a prospective clinical study. *J Psychiatry Neurosci.* 2005;30(2):100–107.

55. Lundorff LE, Jønsson BH, Sjøgren P. Modafinil for attentional and psychomotor dysfunction in advanced cancer: a double-blind, randomised, cross-over trial. *Palliat Med.* 2009;23(8):731–738.

56. Blackhall L, Petroni G, Shu J, Baum L, Farace E. A pilot study evaluating the safety and efficacy of modafinal for cancer-related fatigue. *J Palliat Med.* 2009;12(5):433–439.

57. Bruera E, Miller MJ, Macmillan K, Kuehn N. Neuropsychological effects of methylphenidate in patients receiving a continuous infusion of narcotics for cancer pain. *Pain.* 1992;48(2):163–166.

58. Volkow ND, Fowler JS, Logan J, et al. Effects of modafinil on dopamine and dopamine transporters in the male human brain: clinical implications. *JAMA.* 2009;301(11):1148–1154.

58a Jatoi A, Kahanic S, Frytak S, et al. Donepezil and vitamin E for preventing cognitive dysfunction in small cell lung cancer patients: preliminary results and suggestions for future study designs. *Support Care Cancer.* 2005;13(1):66–69.

59. Karschnia P, Parsons MW, Dietrich J. Pharmacologic management of cognitive impairment induced by cancer therapy. *Lancet Oncol.* 2019;20(2):e92–e102.

60. Fernandes HA, Richard NM, Edelstein K. Cognitive rehabilitation for cancer-related cognitive dysfunction: a systematic review. *Support Care Cancer.* 2019;27(9):3253–3279.

61. Wagner MA, Erickson KI, Bender CM, Conley YP. The influence of physical activity and epigenomics on cognitive function and brain health in breast cancer. *Front Aging Neurosci.* 2020;12:123.

62. Vaquero L, Rodríguez-Fornells A, Pera-Jambrina MÁ, Bruna J, Simó M. Plasticity in bilateral hippocampi after a 3-month physical activity programme in lung cancer patients. *Eur J Neurol.* 2020. https://doi.org/10.1111/ene.14670.

63. Van der Gucht K, Melis M, Ahmadoun S, et al. A mindfulness-based intervention for breast cancer patients with cognitive impairment after chemotherapy: study protocol of a three-group randomized controlled trial. *Trials.* 2020;21(1):290.

CHAPTER 15

Neuropathy in Lung Cancer

CHRISTINA PAUL, MD • CHRISTIAN M. CUSTODIO, MD

INTRODUCTION

There is a wide variety of neuromuscular diseases that impact patients with lung cancer and patients undergoing treatment for lung cancer. Neuropathy is a disease of peripheral nerves, with multiple primary, secondary, and tertiary consequences that can be debilitating for a patient's function and overall quality of life. For the purposes of this chapter, we will review the relationship of the neuropathic disease and function, various etiologies and their standard electrodiagnostic findings, clinical pearls for practical diagnostic evaluation. Finally, we will discuss management and current evidence for both treatment and rehabilitation.

OVERVIEW

The peripheral nervous system includes the spinal roots, brachial or lumbosacral plexus, peripheral axons and/or myelin sheaths, the neuromuscular junction, and the muscle fibers. Anatomically, any level of the peripheral nervous system may be impacted by cancer and its treatment. The variety of mechanisms of injury and broad scope of clinical presentations makes it challenging to estimate the true incidence and prevalence of neuromuscular disorders in cancer patients. However, it is estimated that up to one-third of adult chronic cancer pain patients, across all tumor types and stages, are felt to have cancer-related neuropathic pain.[1]

Cancer can directly affect the peripheral nervous system at any level via numerous mechanisms. Examples inlcude direct nerve compression or infiltration of the cancer itself (such as a Pancoast tumor compressing or infiltrating the brachial plexus or metastatic osseous disease of the spine causing radiculopathy), hematogenous or lymphatic spread, leptomeningeal dissemination, or perineural spread. Indirect effects from cancer include the body's immune response to cancer, such as paraneoplastic syndromes which often manifest with neuromuscular dysfunction (such as Lambert–Eaton Myasthenic Syndrome [LEMS]), or cancer-associated medical complications such as infections, weight loss, or malnutrition. Cancer treatment acquired neuropathies can result from effects of therapies, be it surgery (intercostal nerve injuries during thoracotomies or compressive neuropathies), chemotherapy (inducing peripheral neuropathy), radiation therapy, or immunologic therapy. Finally, patients may also have preexisting neurologic conditions, such as diabetic or hereditary neuropathies, or previous nerve injuries that can make the nerves more susceptible to cancer or its related treatments above.

Neuropathy has a wide variety of symptoms and presentations, ranging from pure sensory to pure motor, and from slight numbness and weakness in patients with chronic axonal neuropathy to significant loss of muscle strength including the respiratory muscles. Early recognition and accurate diagnosis is essential to proper treatment, rehabilitation and reduction of disability.

NEUROPATHY AND FUNCTIONAL CONSEQUENCES

Neuropathy can make one's simple activities of daily living more challenging. An essential aspect of the rehabilitation treatment program for patients affected by lung cancer involves proper identification of the type of disease impairments and understanding of their primary, secondary, and tertiary consequences.

Disease is identified as a disorder of structure or function.

Impairment is a loss of normal function of part of the body.

Disability is when a person is not able to perform an activity in a normal way as a result of an impairment.

Handicap is when there are barriers that prevent a person with a disability from performing a role that is normal for that person. These limitations may be imposed by society, the environment, or by one's own attitude.

Neuropathy can result in different types of impairments depending on the type of nerves of nerves

Lung Cancer Rehabilitation, https://doi.org/10.1016/B978-0-323-83404-9.00007-4

affected by the disease. Examples of this include the following:

Disease of Sensory Nerves: This can cause impairments in sensation, such as with painful paresthesia, dysesthesia, cold sensitivity, tingling, numbness, alteration in vibration and proprioception, or a change in reflexes. Disability occurs, for example, when it impacts an individual's ability to shower, as standing and balancing, and temperature sensation in the shower is significantly impacted. Handicap would occur for example when an individual declines a social activity with friends due to the tremendous amount of effort required for self-hygiene.

Disease of Motor Nerves: This can impair an individual's muscles and motion, such as muscle weakness or decreased coordination fine motor control. Disability can occur for example when it impacts one's ability to walk or when preparing food as opening cans or holding utensils to eat requires much more effort. Handicap would be if an individual were no longer able to perform their task at work due, such as a previously working full time hair dresser declining work due to weakness in her hands and no longer able to cut hair.

Disease of Autonomic Nerves: This affects the autonomic regulation of internal organs and can cause impairments such as with orthostatic hypotension, constipation, urinary retention, irregular heart rate, and sexual dysfunction. Disability occurs, for example, when a patient's standing tolerance is severely impacted. An example of handicap from autonomic neuropathy would potentially be strained relationships due to sexual dysfunction or decreased ability to participate social activities due to limited standing tolerance.

When disease and injury cause an impairment, rehabilitation medicine is an essential aspect of care for the lung cancer patient, as early intervention, including prevention, identification, and treatment, can reduce the occurrence of functional limitations.

NEUROPATHY IN THE CANCER PATIENT

In the field of oncology, the etiology of neuropathy can be broken down into three categories: disease-related, cancer treatment-related, and patient-related. There may be a combination of several processes at once.

Disease Related

Disease related includes direct effects from the cancer itself and secondary paraneoplastic disease.

Radiculopathy

After spinal stenosis and disc disease, tumors involving the spine are the most common cause of radiculopathy and may result in compression or irritation of individual nerve roots via tumor infiltration.[2] The most common primary malignancies that can metastasize to the spine include lung, breast, prostate, colon, thyroid, and kidney.

Any patient with cancer presenting with new onset back or neck pain will need a detailed evaluation. Spinal metastases most commonly affect the thoracic spine (70%), followed by the lumbar (20%) and cervical spine (10%).[3]

Patients can present with an asymmetric array of symptoms resulting from radicular or polyradicular involvement, including focal and radicular pain (commonly described as shooting pain along the dermatomal distribution of a nerve root), areflexia, paresthesias, and lower motor neuron weakness, similar to nonmalignant radiculopathies.

MRI of the spine with and without contrast is the gold-standard diagnostic modality, given its utility with future treatment-related planning. However, electrodiagnostic studies may also be helpful in identifying the primary etiology of symptoms if there are multiple disease processes present (i.e., carpal tunnel syndrome vs. C6 radiculopathy). For radiculopathies, sensory responses should be normal on NCS, as the location of involvement is proximal to the dorsal root ganglion, thereby making the segment of sensory nerve fibers tested metabolically and histologically intact. Motor responses within the affected myotomes may be normal or reduced in amplitude, depending on severity. Needle EMG is the most sensitive electrodiagnostic test for evaluation of a radiculopathy. Neuropathic abnormalities should be recorded in at least two muscles innervated by different peripheral nerves but sharing the same root innervation. Examples of these include increased insertional activity, fibrillation potentials, reduced recruitment, and large, polyphasic motor unit potentials (MUPs). Because paraspinal muscles are innervated by the dorsal primary rami, branching directly off of the nerve root, abnormal neuropathic EMG findings noted in the paraspinals further support the diagnosis of radiculopathy.

Treatment may consist of physical therapy with an emphasis on core and spine extensor strengthening, neuromodulators, radiation therapy, and surgical nerve root decompression.

Leptomeningeal disease

Leptomeningeal disease (LMD)/carcinomatosis, also known as neoplastic meningitis or carcinomatous meningitis, refers to the infiltration of the meninges surrounding the brain, cerebrospinal fluid, and spinal cord by malignant tumor cells. Diagnosis may be particularly challenging as patients can present with a highly variable constellation of symptoms depending on where the tumor has infiltrated the neurologic tissue. Symptoms may include both radicular and focal pain, paresthesias, weakness, areflexia, upper motor neuron signs, and cranial nerve involvement. Patients may also exhibit nausea, vomiting, gait abnormalities, positional headaches, and altered mental status secondary to obstructive hydrocephalus increasing intracranial pressure.[4]

Presently there is currently no standardized diagnostic evaluation with respect to the assessment of leptomeningeal disease, however, evaluation generally consists of three elements: radiographic evaluation of the brain and spinal cord, CSF cytology, and a standardized neurological exam.[5] MRI findings may include enhancing nodules of the leptomeninges and sulcal, linear ependymal, and cranial nerve root enhancement. CSF studies may reveal the presence of tumor cells. Electrodiagnostic studies in LMD can sometimes be consistent with a polyradiculopathy, with preserved sensory nerve action potentials and abnormal paraspinal needle EMG findings. Absent F-waves or prolonged F-wave latencies on NCS are felt to be an early indicator of nerve root involvement but are not specific for either radiculopathy or LMD.

There is no generally accepted standard of care in the treatment of LMD. Treatment is personalized and dependent on disease burden, patient functional status, and associated medical comorbidities.[6] Both radiation therapy and chemotherapy (intrathecal and systemic) can be utilized. However overall prognosis is poor, with a typical median survival of 1–4 months, and treatment often is considered more palliative than curative.[7]

Plexopathy

It has been estimated that neoplastic (tumor) brachial plexopathies occur with a frequency of approximately 0.43% in patients with cancer, most commonly occurring in those with lung (37%) and breast (32%) cancers.[1] Distribution of symptoms is dependent on the anatomic location of the lesion. When there is tumor involvement of the plexus, pain is the most common presenting symptom (75%–98%), followed by the development of weakness and sensory deficits in the distribution of plexus involvement.[1] Metastatic disease can involve any portion of the brachial plexus, but usually involve the lower trunk preferentially, due to its proximity to axillary lymph nodes and the superior sulcus of the lung.

Additionally tumors located in the superior sulcus of the lung, also known as Pancoast Tumors, may invade muscles, upper ribs, thoracic vertebral bodies, subclavian vessels, the inferior portion of the brachial plexus, and sympathetic chain of the autonomic nervous system including the stellate ganglion leading to a unique clinical presentation known as "Pancoast syndrome" that is important to recognize. Clinically, signs and symptoms may include the combination of severe unrelenting shoulder and arm pain along the C8 and T1 root nerve distributions, Horner's syndrome (ptosis, miosis and anhidrosis) and atrophy of hand intrinsics. As with most malignancies, patients with early-stage disease at diagnosis and better performance status are generally indicators of good prognosis. In the context of lung cancer, tumors in this location are rare, accounting for 3–5% of all primary lung cancers.[8] Unfortunately, initial misdiagnosis is not uncommon, as the initial symptoms of painful shoulder and back generally will preclude the more typical pulmonary symptoms concerning for lung cancer (such as cough, hemoptysis, and dyspnea) due to the peripheral location of these tumors and the more advanced stage of disease required to present with pulmonary symptoms. Patients may initially be misdiagnosed as bursitis or osteoarthritis. For this reason, it is especially important for rehabilitation clinicians to recognize and re-evaluate patients that are not responding to treatments for chronic shoulder conditions as expected. The greatest risk factor associated with Pancoast tumors is cigarette smoking, the average age at presentation is the sixth decade of life,[4] and men are affected more frequently than women.[8] It is very important to promptly identify the symptoms and diagnose Pancoast syndrome as they are often stage IIB or higher by the time they are diagnosed.[9]

MRI, CT, and positron emission tomography scans all serve diagnostic purposes, with MRI scans providing the best anatomic detail for potential surgical resection. While tumor plexopathies may involve the whole plexus, electrodiagnostic studies have shown involvement of the lower trunk and medial cord occurring more commonly.[4] Treatment commonly involves local radiation therapy with improvement of pain in approximately 46%–86% of patients.[1] Patients may benefit from early intervention utilizing a multimodal approach including physical and occupational therapy, bracing evaluation, analgesics, and specialized interventional procedures, such as regional nerve blocks.[6]

Mononeuropathy

Focal mononeuropathies related to cancer may occur as a result of direct compression or infiltration from a primary tumor or metastases. Metastases to individual nerves are rare. Clinical presentation is dependent upon the individual nerves being affected. In patients with lung cancers, mononeuropathies more commonly result as an indirect complication from the cancer or treatment, such as rapid weight loss resulting in a peroneal nerve compression neuropathy. NCS and needle EMG should correspond to clinical abnormalities, limited to the distribution of the individual nerve, involving both sensory and motor fibers depending on the composition of the particular nerve involved.

Paraneoplastic syndromes

Although rare, it is important for clinicians to recognize the presentation of neuromuscular paraneoplastic syndromes. These syndromes cause damage to the peripheral nervous system due to remote effects from a malignant neoplasm or its metastases. Almost all tumor types have been associated with paraneoplastic syndromes, and any part of the nervous system can be affected. Clinical neurologic presentations are usually more severe and can be more rapidly progressive than what would normally be expected. Because paraneoplastic syndroms often precede the diagnosis of cancer, early recognition may increase survival. Treatment of the underlying malignancy generally results in improvement of neurologic symptoms.

In some disorders, neuronal antigens expressed by the tumor have been identified. These result in an autoimmune response against both the tumor as well as healthy neural tissue. Identification of these markers can help facilitate the workup of diagnosis a primary tumor.[3] For example, the presence of anti-Hu antibodies has a strong association with small cell lung cancer, neuroblastoma, or prostate cancer. One to 3% of patients with small cell lung cancer develop LEMS associated with anti-VGCC (voltage-gated calcium channel) antibodies.[5] Although some syndromes are associated with identifiable autoantibodies, frequently no such marker is detected.

Paraneoplastic sensory neuronopathy/ganglionopathy can present with either an acute or insidious onset of pain and sensory loss. Clinical findings of sensory ataxia and pseudoathetosis are often present. Clinical and electro diagnostic findings are diffuse and notably are more severe in the upper extremities. Motor dysfunction is usually absent. A pattern of more severe sensory abnormalities on nerve conduction studies in the upper extremities compared to the lower extremities helps distinguish this entity from a length-dependent sensory neuropathy. Needle EMG is usually normal, although poor volitional activation of MUPs may be noted, due to the severity of sensory abnormalities. The most common associated neoplasm is small cell lung cancer.

The diagnosis of a true paraneoplastic distal, symmetric, sensorimotor polyneuropathy in the absence of autoantibodies is difficult to confirm, as there are many more likely known etiologies that can cause this pattern of involvement, including diabetes mellitus, nutritional deficiencies, and chemotherapy-induced polyneuropathy. Sensorimotor polyneuropathy as a paraneoplastic syndrome is often a diagnosis of exclusion. Symptoms and signs can include pain, paresthesias, numbness, and weakness in a stocking-glove distribution, along with hyporeflexia. A more rapidly progressive course may be the only distinguishing factor differentiating a paraneoplastic syndrome from other etiologies. Electrodiagnostic findings are consistent with an axonal process, with reduction in motor and sensory amplitudes on NCS and the presence of fibrillation potentials and large, polyphasic MUPs in distal limb muscles on needle EMG. This syndrome has been associated with small cell lung cancer.

A pattern of clinical and electrophysiologic involvement resembling mononeuritis multiplex may represent a paraneoplastic vasculitic neuropathy. This syndrome has been most commonly reported in association with small cell lung cancer. The anti-Hu antibody has also been associated with this syndrome.

LEMS is probably the best understood paraneoplastic neuromuscular disorder. It is considered the hallmark of presynaptic disorders of neuromuscular transmission. Patients present with fatigue, proximal weakness, hyporeflexia, and autonomic dysfunction. Repeated strength testing may reveal a "warming-up" phenomenon, and patients display an initial increase in strength with repetition followed by eventual fatigue. Bulbar involvement is rare, distinguishing it from myasthenia gravis. While LEMS can occur independently from cancer, up to 40%−60% of cases are associated with small cell lung cancer.[6]

Electrodiagnostic studies, especially repetitive nerve stimulation studies, are invaluable in diagnosing LEMS. Motor responses are reduced in amplitude at baseline. Repetitive stimulation of motor nerves at low frequency (2−3 Hz) demonstrates a further decrement in amplitude. Following brief isometric exercise, facilitation occurs and compound muscle action potential amplitudes show at least a 100% increase. This finding is considered pathognomonic for LEMS. Sensory nerve action potentials and needle EMG findings are usually normal, except for the presence of varying, unstable MUPs. Anti-VGCC antibodies are seen in up to 92% of LEMS patients.[6]

Treatment Related

Chemotherapy induced peripheral neuropathies

Chemotherapy-induced peripheral neuropathy (CIPN) is a common and often disabling toxicity associated with the administration of chemotherapy. Approximately 20–40% of patients with cancer who receive neurotoxic chemotherapy (e.g., taxanes, platinums, vinca alkaloids, bortezomib) will develop painful chemotherapy-induced peripheral neuropathy (CIPN).[11] While CIPN is a well-recognized phenomenon, it is likely underreported. Understanding the epidemiology of CIPN is vital as the onset and progression of symptoms may ultimately require modification or discontinuation of chemotherapeutic protocols.

A wide variation of CIPN prevalence exists, owing mainly to the utilization of numerous different measurement tools and scales such as the National Cancer Institute Common Terminology Criteria for Adverse Events (NCI-CTCAE), CIPN Assessment Tool, Total Neuropathy Scale (TNS), and the Patient Neurotoxicity Questionnaire (PNQ). Despite this wide variability, literature has shown that both prevalence and incidence continue to be high.[6]

While nearly all chemotherapeutic agents have been associated with peripheral neuropathies, there are specific groups that are notorious for expressing neurotoxic effects.

CIPN is classically described as a symmetric, length-dependent, sensory more than motor polyneuropathy. As such, a typical stocking-glove pattern is seen with the majority of agents. Alternatively, a glove-stocking pattern may be seen with platinum compounds in the setting of direct cytotoxic effects causing neurotmesis. Patients describe a wide range of predominantly sensory symptoms including paresthesias, numbness, allodynia, and hypersensitivity to temperature. Loss of proprioception and vibration may also occur, causing difficulty with fine motor tasks and gait. Symptom onset may be acute to subacute during chemotherapy. A phenomenon described as "coasting" has also been observed with vinca alkaloids and platinum-based compounds, in which symptoms either continue to progress despite completion of treatment or patients who were previously asymptomatic start to develop new symptoms.[7] Risk factors include underlying or preexisting peripheral neuropathies, duration of treatment, dosing and frequency of treatment, and co-administration with other neurotoxic agents.[8]

Evaluation should begin with a standard neurologic examination with close attention to sensation, strength, proprioception, vibration, gait, and balance. Clinical history alone may be the most valuable aspect for diagnosis of CIPN. If a patient receiving neurotoxic chemotherapy develops new or worsening numbness, tingling, and/or pain in their hands and/or feet, without any additional possible causes for them to have developed these symptoms, then the diagnosis is made. While neurologic tests, such as electromyography, can be used, they are not essential for making the diagnosis; however, patients with more atypical symptoms may still benefit from electrodiagnostic testing. Atypical features may include asymmetry, nonlength dependence, motor predominance, acute onset, prominent autonomic involvement, severe or rapidly progressive symptoms, or sensory ataxia.

A neuropathy panel may be valuable to evaluate for reversible causes of peripheral neuropathy, including diabetes mellitus, thyroid abnormalities, and nutritional deficiencies, among others, keeping in mind that in the general patient population, idiopathic neuropathy accounts for 40% of all cases.[6]

Unfortunately, there are no standard preventative measures for CIPN. As of 2020, the American Society of Clinical Oncology clinical practice guidelines have not recommended any agents for the prevention of CIPN. The use of acetyl-L-carnitine for the prevention of CIPN in patients with cancer is no longer recommended. Clinicians should assess the appropriateness of dose delaying, dose reduction, substitutions, or stopping chemotherapy in patients who develop intolerable neuropathy and/or functional impairment. Additionally clinicians should assess the risks and benefits of agents known to cause CIPN among patients with underlying neuropathy and with conditions that predispose to neuropathy such as diabetes and/or a family or personal history of hereditary neuropathy.[10] The treatment approach for CIPN is multimodal. Physical and occupational therapy typically includes focus on fine motor skills, desensitization techniques, nerve gliding techniques, strengthening, proprioception, and gait and balance training. Medications may also be used. Currently, duloxetine is the only agent with appropriate evidence to support its use for patients with painful CIPN.[11] Neuromodulators, such as gabapentin and pregabalin, have been used anecdotally; however, supporting studies are limited. These medications may provide relief for positive symptoms (i.e., painful paresthesias, burning, sharp pain); however, they may provide little to no relief for negative symptoms (i.e., numbness).

Radiation induced peripheral neuropathies

Radiation induced brachial plexopathy (RIBP) is a delayed, nontraumatic brachial plexus injury following radiotherapy to adjacent areas including the chest wall, axilla, and neck.[6]

While RIBP is a well-recognized phenomenon, the pathophysiology remains less understood. Radiation may cause direct neurotoxic damage to the mature nerve, including the axon and vasa nervorum, from ionizing radiation with additional secondary and progressive microvascular injury. Nerve trunk fibrosis with components of demyelination and axon loss has been found during surgery and at postmortem evaluation.[12] Risk factors may be either treatment related or patient related. Treatment-related factors include total dose of radiation, dose per fraction, and treatment schedule. Chemotherapy has been suggested to increase the risk as well. Patient-related factors may include advanced age, obesity, and underlying medical conditions such as hypertension, dyslipidemia, diabetes mellitus, and premorbid peripheral neuropathy.[13]

There appears to be a delayed onset of neurological symptoms with median time to onset typically described at 1.5 years, however, ranging from 6 months to 20 years after completion of radiation therapy.[6] Patients classically present with symptoms of paresthesias, which may decrease as numbness develops. Distribution of symptoms depends on the level of injury. Pain is typically less common. Weakness may develop later on, tends to be progressive, and may eventually result in paralysis of the affected upper extremity. Neurologic deficits tend to progressively worsen over the span of several years to the point of significant functional impairment in approximately 2/3rd of patients. Spontaneous neurologic recovery at this point is much less likely.[12]

In patients with cancer, distinguishing brachial plexopathy signs caused from tumor infiltration versus radiation therapy can be challenging. Clinical criteria more commonly associated with radiation injury are painless upper trunk lesions (C5-C6) with lymphedema, while painful lower trunk lesions (C7-8, T1) with Horner syndrome were more commonly associated with tumor infiltration.[17] Electrodiagnostic studies demonstrate myokymia on EMG in approximately 60% of patients.[1] It should be noted that while myokymia by itself is not pathognomonic for radiation-induced injury, it is assumed that this is in fact the etiology when it is present in patients who have received radiotherapy. It

should be noted, however, that the absence of myokymia on electrodiagnostic studies does not rule out the possibility of radiation induced injury. MRI of the brachial plexus remains useful in further evaluation of compressive or infiltrative lesions. In cases of RIBP, brachial plexus MRI may demonstrate linear areas of high signal intensity suggesting fibrosis. More proximal imaging of the cervical spine should also be considered to rule out confounding involvement of the cervical nerve roots.

When developing a treatment plan, expectations should be set given the known clinical trajectory and depending on the patient's individual severity of symptoms. Physical therapy should focus on cervical, shoulder, and scapular range of motion and stretching exercises, chest expansion exercises, shoulder girdle and spine extensor strengthening, and myofascial release. Occupational therapy may also be beneficial for neuromuscular reeducation and fine motor skills. Intermittent bracing may be necessary to prevent development or progression of glenohumeral joint subluxation. If the patient is experiencing pain, neuropathic agents or a short course of prednisone may be considered.

Surgically related neuropathies

Because the nature of surgical procedures for the cancer patient is likely to be more complex, it is thought that the likelihood of neuromuscular complications is greater in oncologic surgeries. The pattern and extent of neurologic involvement following surgery depends on the location of the tumor, patient positioning during surgery, and the patient's overall preoperative status and propensity to nerve injury. Direct nerve injury during surgery occurs in approximately 1% of patients undergoing thoracic surgery.[14] Depending on the specific area of operation, injuries to the recurrent laryngeal nerve, the phrenic nerve, vagus nerve, long thoracic nerve, intercostal nerves, or the sympathetic chain can result.[14]

Perioperative neuropraxic injuries, resulting from either compression or traction of peripheral nerves, are well-recognized phenomena. It is felt that these injuries result from the patient's position during anesthesia and surgery or during the immediate postsurgical recovery period. Common sites of injury and associated surgical procedures include brachial plexus injury during thoracotomy, given the abducted position of the involved upper extremity. Abduction of the upper extremity greater than 90° during surgery can cause inferior subluxation of the humeral head, resulting in compression of the lower part and traction of the upper part of the brachial plexus. Patients upon awakening report varying degrees of pain, weakness, and numbness in both the upper and lower trunk distribution. Complete, spontaneous recovery within weeks is common, even in cases of severe plegia. Ulnar neuropathies at the elbow, resulting from arm boards used to secure intravenous lines, and radial neuropathies at the spiral groove, resulting from prolonged time in the lateral decubitus position, are also noted following thoracic surgery. Findings of focal slowing, temporal dispersion, or conduction block across the level of injury can be demonstrated on motor NCS.[6]

Patient-Related Neuropathies

Cancer treatments may exacerbate preexisting medical conditions which may cause worsening of an underlying peripheral neuropathy. Steroids may exacerbate previously well-controlled diabetes in patients. Endocrine complications of immune checkpoint inhibitors may lead patients to develop endocrinopathies that were previously subclinical. Patients with cancer are often times immunocompromised and as such are at higher risk for secondary infections. Herpes zoster may become reactivated and cause postherpetic neuralgia. Toxic neuropathy may also develop as a result of extended use of antibiotic treatment for infections. Fluoroquinolones, linezolid, metronidazole, and nitrofurantoin, among others, have been shown to cause peripheral neuropathy. Critical illness itself may also cause peripheral neuropathy. Usually presenting as flaccid and symmetric weakness, it has been estimated to occur in 25%−45% of patients admitted to the intensive care unit.[15] Weight loss as a complication of malignancy may also cause focal mononeuropathy as seen in compression neuropathy of the peroneal nerve at the fibular head. Malnutrition, in turn, may cause vitamin B12 deficiency, ultimately causing demyelination of sensory nerve fibers.

Patient education is an important component for management for peripheral neuropathy. It is equally important for clinicians to educate their patients on potential neurologic complications related to their cancer and treatment. Patients should be aware that certain chemotherapeutic agents in lung cancers may cause peripheral neuropathy. Clinicians should be able to manage expectations regarding radiation therapy and educate their patients on potential life-long complications related to radiation-induced injuries. Patients should also be educated on expectations in regards to pain management and early intervention after surgical treatments to minimize postoperative pain and dysfunction. Patient education, management of expectations, and reassurance is a key component of the treatment plan for patients with lung cancer.

General advice for patients is included below:
- Avoiding things that make your peripheral neuropathy worse, such as hot or cold temperatures, or snug clothes or shoes
- Avoiding alcoholic drinks
- Controlling your blood sugar if you have diabetes
- Protecting your hands by wearing gloves when you clean or work outdoors
- Using handrails, a walker, or a cane for support so you do not lose your balance
- Taking care of your feet. Look at them once a day, especially the bottoms, to see if you have any injuries or sores
- Being careful when using knives, scissors, box cutters, or other sharp objects
- Consider physical therapy or occupational therapy

CONCLUSION

As the overall number of cancer survivors continues to increase, most clinicians will manage more of these patients in some manner. New developments in cancer care continue to revolutionize treatment and improve survivorship. It is crucial to have at least a basic understanding of neurologic complications of both cancer and its treatment and its impact on patient functional status and quality of life. There are multiple underlying etiologies for neuropathy in lung cancer including disease related, therapy related, and patient related. Identification is essential for comprehensive rehabilitation and reduction of disability and handicap.

REFERENCES

1. Jaeckle KA. Neurologic manifestations of neoplastic and radiation-induced plexopathies. *Semin Neurol.* 2010; 30(3):254−262.
2. Shelerud RA. Rarer causes of radiculopathy: spinal tumors, infections and other unusual causes. *Phys Med Rehabil Clin.* 2002;13(3):645−696.
3. Sciubba DM, Petteys RJ, Dekutoski MB, et al. Diagnosis and management of metastatic spine disease. A review. *J Neurosurg Spine.* 2010;13(1).
4. Custodio CM. Neuromuscular complications of cancer and cancer treatments. *Phys Med Rehabil Clin.* 2008; 19(1):27−45 (v-vi).
5. Chamberlain M, Junck L, Brandsma D, et al. Leptomeningeal metastases: a RANO proposal for response criteria. *Neuro-Oncology.* 2017;19(4):484−492. https://doi.org/10.1093/neuonc/now183.

6. König F, Custodio C. *Peripheral nervous system involvement in breast and gynecologic cancers. Breast Cancer and Gynecologic Cancer Rehabilitation.* Elsevier; 2021:253–261.

7. Yang JCH, Kim SW, Kim DW, et al. Osimertinib in patients with epidermal growth factor receptor mutation-positive non-small-cell lung cancer and leptomeningeal metastases: the BLOOM study. *J Clin Oncol.* 2020;38(6): 538–547. https://doi.org/10.1200/JCO.19.00457.

8. Panagopoulos N, Leivaditis V, Koletsis E, et al. Pancoast tumors: characteristics and preoperative assessment. *J Thorac Disease.* 2014;6(Suppl 1):S108–S115. https://doi.org/10.3978/j.issn.2072-1439.2013.12.29.

9. Waseda R, Klikovits T, Hoda MA, et al. Trimodality therapy for Pancoast tumors: T4 is not a contraindication to radical surgery. *J Surg Oncol.* 2017 Aug;116(2):227–235.

10. Ko K, Sung DH, Kang MJ, et al. *Ann Rehabil Med.* 2011; 35(6):807–815.

11. Dropcho EJ. Neurologic paraneoplastic syndromes. *Curr Oncol Rep.* 2004;6:26–31.

12. Breinberg HR, Amato AA. Neuromuscular complications of cancer. *Neurol Clin N Am.* 2003;21:141–165.

13. Cavaletti G, Alberti P, Frigeni B, et al. Chemotherapy-induced neuropathy. *Curr Treat Options Neurol.* 2011; 13(2):180–190.

14. Tzatha E, DeAngelis LM. Chemotherapy-induced peripheral neuropathy. *Oncology.* 2016;30(3):240–244.

15. Smith EM, Pang H, Cirrincione C, et al. Effect of duloxetine on pain, function, and quality of life among patients with chemotherapy-induced painful peripheral neuropathy: a randomized clinical trial. *JAMA.* 2013;309(13): 1359–1367. https://doi.org/10.1001/jama.2013.2813.

16. Loprinzi CL, Lacchetti C, Bleeker J, et al. Prevention and management of chemotherapy-induced peripheral neuropathy in survivors of adult cancers: ASCO guideline update. *J Clin Oncol.* 2020;38(28):3325–3348. https://doi.org/10.1200/JCO.20.01399.

17. Dropcho EJ. Neurotoxicity of radiation therapy. *Neurol Clin.* 2010;28(1):217–234.

18. Delanian S, Lefaix JL, Pradat PF. Radiation-induced neuropathy in cancer survivors. *Radiother Oncol.* 2012; 105(3):273–282.

19. Kori S, Foley K, Posner J. Brachial plexus lesions in patients with cancer=100 cases. *Neurology.* 1981;31(1). https://doi.org/10.1212/WNL.31.1.45.

20. Krasna MJ, Forti G. Nerve injury: injury to the recurrent laryngeal, phrenic, vagus, long thoracic, and sympathetic nerves during thoracic surgery. *Thorac Surg Clin.* 2006;16: 267–275.

21. Zhou C, Wu L, Ni F, Ji W, Wu J, Zhang H. Critical illness polyneuropathy and myopathy: a systematic review. *Neural Regen Res.* 2014;9(1):101–110. https://doi.org/10.4103/1673-5374.125337.

CHAPTER 16

Complications and Rehabilitation Challenges of Lung Cancer Surgeries

ADY M. CORREA-MENDOZA, MD • DIANA MOLINARES, MD

SURGICAL TECHNIQUES

Tumor resection is the mainstay treatment of early stages of lung cancer (stage I, II, and some stage III). The first total pneumonectomy reported in the United States was performed in the 1940s by Dr. Evarts Graham, in Saint Louis, Missouri **Graham**. Since then, advances in technology have been developed to decrease morbidity and mortality associated with the procedure. Less invasive surgical techniques with smaller resections have been developed, including wedge resection, segmentation, and lobectomy. The current standard procedure is pulmonary lobectomy or polylobar resection depending on the size and extent of the tumor.[1]

There are three surgical approaches used to perform lung tumor resection.

Open Thoracotomy

The most conventional approach is the open thoracotomy that involves separation of the ribs using a retractor (Fig. 16.1). It consists of an approximately 8 cm incision, performed most commonly through the posterolateral thorax, at the fourth or fifth intercostal space. This approach divides the latissimus dorsi, intercostal muscles, and sometimes the trapezius and rhomboid muscles. An alternate anterior approach could be used, where an axillary incision is performed. The anterior approach involves splitting the serratus anterior and intercostal muscles in order to access the pleural cavity. This procedure allows the surgeon to use the two-handed surgical technique to properly expose and dissect the tumor.

The muscle-sparing thoracotomy is performed using an anterolateral approach, with a vertical skin incision at the midaxillary line, from below the hairline to the ninth intercostal space. The latissimus dorsi muscle is elevated and retracted, and the serratus anterior muscle is detached from its rib insertion. The intercostal muscle is divided anteriorly and posteriorly. Muscles retractors are used to maintain the serratus and pectoralis muscles anteriorly and the latissimus dorsi posteriorly.

Video-Assisted Thoracoscopic Surgery

As a less morbid alternative to the open thoracotomy, the video-assisted thoracoscopic surgery (VATS) is preferred for the early stages of lung cancer. This technique spares rib separation and consists of a skin incision of 4–5 cm through the sixth intercostal space at the anterior axillary line, where the thoracoscope is inserted. Additional 3–5 small incisions of approximately 1–2 cm are used for positioning additional surgical equipment. Intraoperatively, the camera allows only a two-dimensional view of the thoracic cavity, and the surgeon has to perform a sweeping method for visualization. Thus, this limits the VATS to patients with peripherally located tumors of up to 7 cm, without nodal involvement or distant organ metastasis, which do not require access to difficult areas for fine nodal or vascular dissection.[2–4]

Robotic-Assisted Thoracoscopic Surgery

The robotic-assisted thoracoscopic surgery (RATS) requires 8 mm incisions in the posterolateral thorax for ports placement. The surgeon controls the instruments from a console and does not have direct contact with the organs. The RATS has multiple advantages, including an optimal tridimensional view of the surgical field, allowing better access to difficult areas that require fine and controlled dissection, including hilar structures, central tumors, and mediastinal lymph nodes in locally advanced disease. Despite its multiple advantages, the RATS technique is limited by the elevated cost of the equipment and its maintenance and the highly specialized surgical training.[5]

Lung Cancer Rehabilitation. https://doi.org/10.1016/B978-0-323-83404-9.00013-X

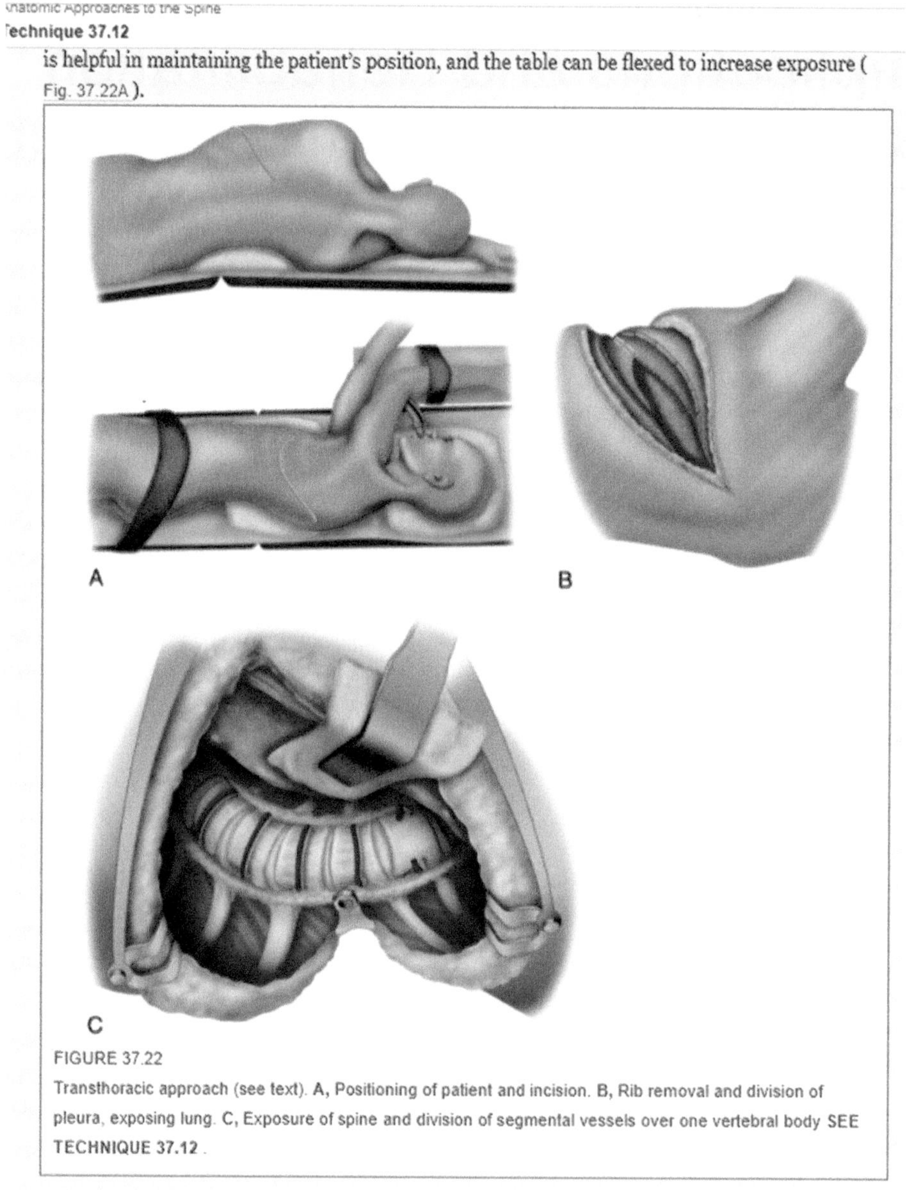
Anatomic Approaches to the Spine
Technique 37.12
is helpful in maintaining the patient's position, and the table can be flexed to increase exposure (Fig. 37.22A).
A
B
C
FIGURE 37.22
Transthoracic approach (see text). A, Positioning of patient and incision. B, Rib removal and division of pleura, exposing lung. C, Exposure of spine and division of segmental vessels over one vertebral body SEE TECHNIQUE 37.12 .

FIG. 16.1 Video-assisted thoracic surgery technique 37.13 (Mack et al).

SURGICAL COMPLICATIONS

Posthoracotomy Pain Syndrome

Posthoracotomy pain refers to persistent or recurrent pain around the surgical incision for more than 2 months postsurgery. Its incidence varies between 30% and 75%, and it is estimated that up to 65% of the patients will develop chronic symptoms. Pain is multifactorial and could be associated with the damage of muscles, fascia, neurovascular structures, joints, and the parietal pleura, but the most common cause reported of postthoracotomy pain syndrome (PTPS) is intercostal neuralgia.

PTPS is often associated with other complications such as atelectasis and pneumonia due to impaired breathing and secretion clearance. Ochroch and colleagues compared postsurgical pain in a group of patients who underwent conventional thoracotomy versus muscle-sparing thoracotomy. In this study, no difference in pain levels was found up to 48 weeks post-surgery. In addition, studies have demonstrated that even with the less invasive video-assisted thoracic surgery technique, postthoracotomy pain is a prevalent comorbidity in this patient population.

Intercostal Neuralgia

Intercostal neuralgia results from an injury to the intercostal nerve, which is located in the subcostal groove at the lower border of the corresponding rib and adjacent to the subcostal artery and vein. The intercostal nerve could be injured intraoperatively while performing the intercostal incision, using rib retractors, or while closing the surgical wound. In addition, postoperatively, the development of adhesions, scarring, or fibrotic tissue can be contributing factors. The pathophysiology of these injuries can be associated with ischemia secondary to nerve compression or an overstretch nerve injury (**Timmermans**).

The patient may report burning pain, allodynia, hyperalgesia, paresthesias, and numbness over the rib cage at rest or with activities such as coughing, deep breathing, or trunk movements. Motor deficits can present with chest wall asymmetry as the intercostalis muscles stabilize the ribs while breathing. Additionally, ipsilateral weakness during bending and contralateral weakness during rotation can be observed if the obliquus externus muscles are affected. In some cases, patients have a positive Schepelmann's sign, manifested as pain in the thoracic cage reproducible with bending toward the affected side. It is essential to perform thorough neurological and musculoskeletal evaluations to rule other possible diagnoses.

Intercostal neuralgia is a clinical diagnosis. Improvement after an intercostal nerve block could aid in the diagnosis and simultaneously provide relief of the symptoms (Fig. 16.2). In some cases, electrophysiologic studies can also help evaluate the intercostal nerves function and rule out other possible nerve injuries. Imaging studies are usually not necessary. However, radiographic studies could be helpful when there are signs suggestive of fractures. Similarly, computed tomography scans and/or magnetic resonance imaging are recommended when recurrent cancer or metastatic disease to the chest wall is suspected. Laboratory workup including inflammatory markers CRP, sedimentation rate, and CBC may help evaluate possible infectious or inflammatory processes. Costosternal syndrome, myofascial pain, or pleuritic pain after thoracic tube placement should be considered as part of the differential diagnoses.

The treatment of intercostal neuralgia starts with preventive measures. Preemptive analgesia refers to the administration of analgesics before the surgical procedure and has been recommended to prevent central sensitization and decrease postoperative pain.[6] Thoracic epidural analgesia is the gold standard of preemptive analgesia for the treatment of postthoracotomy pain (Fig. 16.3). However, there is insufficient evidence that its administration prior to surgery decreases the intensity of acute pain compared to epidural analgesia administered after the surgical procedure.[7] Paravertebral blocks of the intercostal nerves, opioids, acetaminophen, and nonsteroidal antiinflammatories (NSAIDs) are other options used as preemptive analgesics.[6] Intraoperative cryoanalgesia of the intercostal nerves has been studied in patients undergoing VATS technique; however, it has been associated with long-term

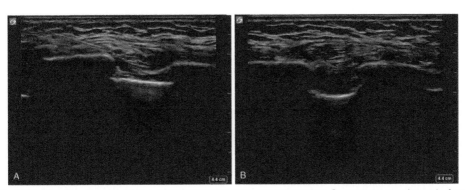

FIG. 16.2 "Dent" in the pleural line after intercostal nerve block injection. Sonograms are shown before **(A)** and after **(B)** injection (approach over rib). (Gray AT, MD, PhD, Chapter 51 *Atlas of Ultrasound-Guided Regional Anesthesia*. 3rd ed. ClinicalKey. Philadelphia, PA: Elsevier:233–238.)

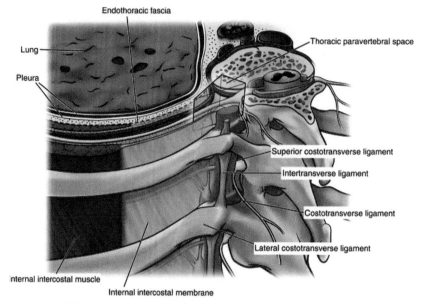

FIG. 16.3 Anatomy of the thoracic paravertebral region showing the various paravertebral ligaments and their anatomical relationship to the thoracic paravertebral space. (Gray A. *Atlas of Ultrasound-Guided Regional Anesthesia, Chapter 61 Thoracic Paravertebral Block*. 3rd ed., ClinicalKey. Philadelphia, PA: Elsevier; 2018: 286–315.)

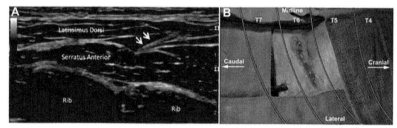

FIG. 16.4 **(A)** Demonstration of ultrasound-guided (in-plane) serratus anterior block. Infiltration of bupivacaine into the fascial plane superficial to the serratus anterior muscle plane. *White arrows* indicate location of the needle. **(B)** Left lateral mini-thoracotomy for entry into left ventricular apex. (Bhatt HV, Montgomery ML, Mittnacht AJC, Shariat A, El-Eshmawi A, Adams DH, Weiner MM. Serratus anterior plane block for transapical off-pump mitral valve repair with neochord implantation. *J Cardiothorac Vasc Anesth.* 2019;33(7):2105–2107. https://doi.org/10.1053/j.jvca.2019.01.051. Epub 2019 Jan 24. PMID: 30876768.)

neuropathic pain.[6] Serratus anterior plane blocks under ultrasound guidance at the levels of T4–T5 have also been suggested, specifically in the perioperative period, as it may decrease the use of opioids in patients who have undergone VATS procedure (Figs. 16.4 and 16.5). Nonetheless, it is also important to control exacerbating factors, such as excessive coughing, which can improve with cough suppressive medication. Postoperative pain can be managed with different medications, depending on the severity of the symptoms. If the pain is mild, NSAIDs are usually recommended, while in cases of moderate to severe pain, patient-controlled

analgesia with narcotics (especially morphine, hydromorphone, and fentanyl) is indicated. Opioid adjuncts such as ketorolac, acetaminophen, gabapentin and pregabalin, tricyclic antidepressants, serotonin–norepinephrine receptor inhibitors, topical lidocaine patches, and ketamine may help to improve symptoms.[8,9]

Ultrasound-guided intercostal nerve blocks have been effective in reducing thoracic neuralgia when compared to fluoroscopic-guided epidural blocks.[10] Immediately after VATS surgery, intercostal nerve blockade with bupivacaine resulted in good analgesia,

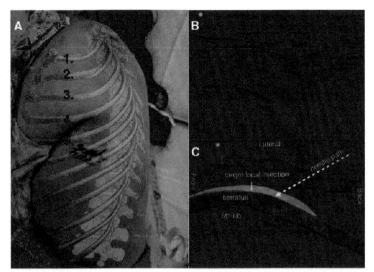

FIG. 16.5 Injection superficial to the anterior serratus muscle. **(A)** The patient in left lateral decubitus position for an in-plane, posterior approach SAPB with approximate location of ribs shown (Henry Gray, Anatomy of the Human Body, 1918). **(B and C)** Ultrasound still image showing the space superficial to the serratus anterior muscle with bolus local anesthetic injection. (Durant E, Dixon B, Luftig J, Mantuani D, Herring A. Ultrasound-guided serratus plane block for ED rib fracture pain control. *Am J Emerg Med*. 2017;35(1):197.e3–197.e6. https://doi.org/10.1016/j.ajem.2016.07.021. Epub 2016 Jul 19. PMID: 27595172.)

reducing morphine requirements in the acute postoperative period.[11] If treatment plan is to target one intercostal nerve, it is recommended to block the cephalad and the caudal nerves. The needle insertion site for this procedure is usually below the lower edge of the rib and medial to the posterior axillary line. Additional potential benefits reported of ultrasound guided intercostal nerve blocks include avoiding pneumothorax and avoidance of potential arterial puncture (**Gray Atlas US**).

Shoulder Pain

Acute postthoracotomy shoulder pain. The occurrence of acute ipsilateral shoulder pain after thoracotomy procedure is very common, with a prevalence between 31% and 97% of patients. Acute pain occurs secondary to visceral and somatic components. The musculoskeletal etiology of pain may include ligament and muscle strains secondary to rib retraction. Additionally, trauma to the latissimus dorsi muscles, glenohumeral, or acromioclavicular joint injury has been related to the patient's position during surgery—lateral decubitus position, with the abduction of the shoulder.[12]

In other cases, the pain is referred to the shoulder from other structures rather than resulting from a direct injury to the musculoskeletal components of the shoulder girdle. Several etiologies of referred shoulder pain have been described after lung cancer surgery, including phrenic nerve damage, transection of a major bronchus, as well as pain from irritation of the mediastinum and diaphragmatic surface. Prolonged surgery duration of more than 2 hours, open thoracotomy versus VATS, and increased body mass index are a risk for the occurrence of shoulder pain after surgery.[13,14]

The patient may present with moderate to severe pain as early as the first postoperative hour. The pain is commonly described as dull and aching, sometimes with neuropathic features including burning, tingling, and numbness. It is mainly reported in the ipsilateral posterior or posterior–lateral shoulder, over the deltoid muscle, or at the distal clavicle and could be present either at rest or with shoulder motion. In most cases, the pain improves or resolves by the fourth postoperative day.[13,15]

On physical examination, the patient may assume a "rounded-shoulder" posture due to pain. Abduction and flexion usually exacerbate the pain, and rest may alleviate the symptoms. In cases of phrenic nerve irritation or damage, the patient could present with decreased sensation on the C4—C5 dermatome distribution. The diagnosis is clinical, but laboratory workup may be indicated if infectious or inflammatory processes are suspected (CBC, CRP, ESR). Shoulder radiographs may help identify joint abnormalities or osseous pathology that could have exacerbated the pain during the surgical procedure as well as the postoperative shoulder alignment. Evaluation for shoulder asymmetries, masses, or effusion may help identify hematomas, collections, or a possible inflammatory process. In the presence of neuropathic symptoms, an abnormal neurologic examination with motor or sensory deficits may indicate peripheral nerve damage, plexopathies, or radiculopathies. Patients with neurological deficits should be evaluated with special imaging (cervical or brachial plexus MRI) and electrodiagnostic studies.[13]

The treatment approach for acute shoulder pain should be multimodal. In most cases, pain management used for postthoracotomy pain syndrome alone does not provide enough pain relief. Perioperative acetaminophen administration for the first 24—48 h or intramuscular NSAIDs in patients with no renal contraindications has been beneficial in preventing postoperative shoulder pain. In addition, periphrenic fat pad injection of ropivacaine has been effective in some studies in reducing the incidence and severity of shoulder pain as well as interscalene blockade or stellate ganglion blocks. The interscalene nerve block under ultrasound guidance is a relatively safe procedure that provides long-lasting analgesia with improved sensory blockade when compared to stimulation-guided techniques (Figs. 16.6 and 16.7).[16,17] It targets the C5—C6 levels, which provide innervation to the glenohumeral joint and cutaneous distribution provided by C3—C4 levels. The stellate ganglion block procedure can be reliably performed under fluoroscopic guidance. However, the use of ultrasound guidance is an ideal tool as it may aid in visualization of vessels, nerve roots, muscles, thyroid gland, and the esophagus, thus potentially decreasing risk of damage to these structures.[18] In addition, it avoids patient exposure to radiation. Unfortunately, in patients with predicted lung functional decline after surgery, these injections are contraindicated.

Once the patient is medically cleared, physical and occupational therapy should be started, as early mobilization is a critical component of the treatment of shoulder pain. Physical and occupational therapy efforts aim to improve the function and mobility of the shoulder,

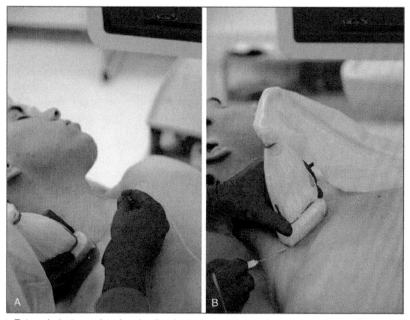

FIG. 16.6 External photographs showing in-plane approaches to interscalene block. The medial to lateral approach **(A)** and the lateral to medial approach **(B)** are shown. (Gray AT, MD, PhD, Chapter 28, Pages 74—83.)

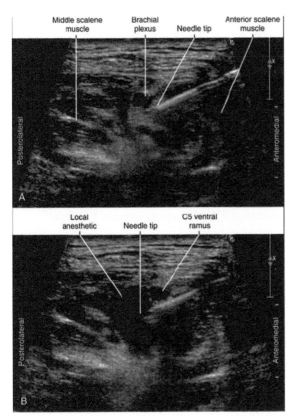

FIG. 16.7 Image sequence showing interscalene block. A medial to lateral in-plane approach is demonstrated where the needle tip is carefully placed adjacent to the components of the plexus **(A and B)**.

focusing on range of motion exercises, in all functional planes, with especial emphasis on flexion and abduction. Early rehabilitation interventions not only help improve shoulder pain, but they are also important in preventing chronic complications such as adhesive capsulitis.[19]

Chronic postthoracotomy shoulder pain. Patients with prolonged shoulder pain and limited range of motion that persists after the perioperative period should raise concern for adhesive capsulitis, commonly known as "frozen shoulder." Adhesive capsulitis results from the accumulation of fibroblasts and chronic inflammatory cells across the glenohumeral joint resulting in increased collagen formation.[20] There are four stages of adhesive capsulitis; In Stage 1 (prefreezing), there is pain associated with limited shoulder motion, Stage 2

(freezing) severe limitation in shoulder motion and pain. In Stage 3 (frozen stage), there is severe stiffness with minimal pain. Finally, in some cases, the shoulder's range of motion may improve with minimal pain in Stage 4. Risk factors for adhesive capsulitis include prolonged immobilization or scar formation during tissue healing after lung surgeries and lung radiation. In addition, age >55−60 years, female sex, and comorbid diagnosis of diabetes mellitus, thyroid disorders, or other systemic diseases increase the risk of developing this pathology. The patients often describe shoulder stiffness, pain, and limited motion that interfere with their daily activities. There is limited active and passive range of motion on physical examination, predominantly with abduction and external rotation. Sometimes, the range of motion limitations may be accompanied by pain over the subacromial, glenohumeral, and bicipital tendon areas. There are no neurological deficits associated. The diagnosis is clinical, but imaging studies may help to rule out other diagnoses. A shoulder X-ray may help evaluate the glenohumeral joint and assess for arthropathy or calcific tendinopathy. In addition, if the adhesive capsulitis is caused by prolonged immobility, the radiograph may reveal osteopenia. Shoulder arthrogram with contrast often shows decreased capsular distension and obliteration of the axillary recess with the early extension of the contrast to the biceps tendon sheath. In addition, the decreased capacity of glenohumeral joint volume less than 10 mL is highly suggestive of adhesive capsulitis, but this study tends to be very painful and is not performed as the standard of care. Static and dynamic ultrasonic guidance for diagnosis of adhesive capsulitis has been accurate and supported in multiple studies (Fig. 16.8). Findings include thickening of the coracohumeral ligament, with proposed cut-off value of 0.7 mm, increased soft tissue in the rotator cuff interval, and there may be increased vascularity in the rotator cuff interval in early stages of the disease along with restricted shoulder external rotation on dynamic evaluation.[21]

The management of adhesive capsulitis has different stages that include operative and nonoperative approaches. In the initial stages of treatment, a combination of physical therapy and NSAIDs is recommended. The therapy program should include modalities, strengthening exercises, and mobilization techniques to improve ROM. Posterior gliding and stretching maneuvers should also be incorporated.[22,23] If the pain and limited mobility persist after completion of the

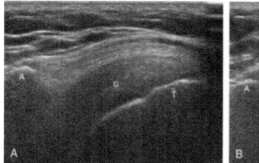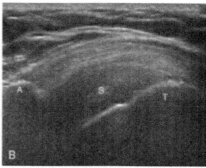

FIG. 16.8 Adhesive Capsulitis. Ultrasound images of the supraspinatus tendon in long axis with arm in neutral position **(A)** and elevated to side **(B)** show that the supraspinatus tendon (S) does not slide beneath the acromion (A), with arm elevation. Note the hypoechoic tendinosis of the supraspinatus tendon. *T*, Greater tuberosity.

therapy program, an intraarticular steroid injection would be recommended as part of the treatment. Though intraarticular hyaluronate injections have been beneficial in some cases, compared to steroid injections, they have not been superior at improving pain and shoulder mobility.[24] Electromyography or ultrasound-guided suprascapular nerve blocks can also be beneficial when the symptoms are refractory to intraarticular injection. If pain persists after 2–3 months of conservative therapies, manipulation under anesthesia with or without arthroscopic release could be considered. Arthroscopic and open capsulotomy are rarely used and are only indicated when manipulation under anesthesia fails.[23]

Rectus abdominis paralysis. The segmental intercostal nerves at the level of T7–T12 are located at the lower border of the corresponding segmental ribs, passing through the subcostal groove with the corresponding artery and vein (Fig. 16.9). These nerves provide innervation to the rectus abdominis muscle and the internal and external oblique muscles. Lower intercostal nerves could be injured after thoracotomy procedure when the surgical incision is performed at the seventh intercostal space or below. Injury of the intercostal nerves can occur during the surgical procedure or could result in late nerve damage secondary to surrounding scar formation.

The patient can present with a "bulging mass" in the ipsilateral abdominal wall, with or without pain. Depending on the severity of the nerve damage, the patient may experience difficulties with expiratory breathing and coughing, with increased risk for postsurgical atelectasis. On inspection of the abdomen, an ipsilateral bulging or distention of the abdomen may be present. However, in obese patients, it could be less evident and only be discovered by palpation while performing Valsalva maneuvers (head elevation while lying supine, coughing, or bilateral leg elevation). The absence of abdominal reflexes could help in excluding a hernia as part of the differential diagnoses. Diagnostic tests include abdominal ultrasound, where an interruption of the posterior rectus sheath suggests a Spigelian hernia. On CT scan under Valsalva, there might be bulging of the abdominal wall and atrophy of the rectus abdominis, internal, and external oblique muscles **Timmermans 3,4**. If abdominal visceral pain and hemodynamic instability are present, imaging studies are imperative to evaluate a possible intraabdominal infectious process or hematoma formation.

Further workup includes electrodiagnostic studies, where denervating potentials in the rectus abdominis muscles can be observed. Neuropathic pain medications (gabapentin, pregabalin, duloxetine, amitriptyline) are indicated in patients with associated neuropathic pain. Rehabilitation interventions focus on core strengthening exercises and neuromuscular reeducation to correct or decrease abdominal weakness and improve patient's discomfort. However, an abdominal binder may be necessary to correct the abdominal defect and improve the quality of life when this result is not achieved.

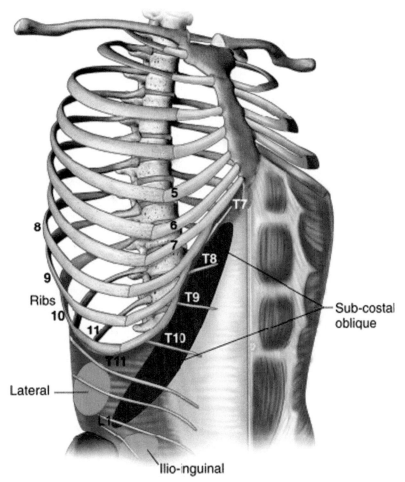

FIG. 16.9 Transversus abdominic pane block zones. (Hebbard P. Chapter 59 *Atlas of Ultrasound-Guided Regional Anesthesia*. 3rd ed., ClinicalKey. Philadelphia, PA: Elsevier: 267–276.)

THE ROLE OF PREREHABILITATION IN LUNG CANCER

Multimodal prerehabilitation program 4–8 weeks prior to lung surgery in patients with COPD and lung cancer has been effective in improving physical fitness, cardiopulmonary function (increased VO2peak and 6MWD), decreased hospital length of stay, and reduced postoperative morbidity.[25–27] Furthermore, in patients with respiratory impairment, smoking history or with high surgical risk, a 4-week prerehabilitation program has shown to improve respiratory function, dyspnea scores and frailty index. The majority of these patients were able to undergo surgery without increased rate of postoperative complications or changes in length of hospital stay.[28,29]

In a metaanalysis performed by[30], preoperative exercise training decreased length of hospital admission by 4.98 days and decreased postsurgical complications when compared to postoperative exercise training alone, but these finding are inconsistent in other studies. However, lack of statistical significance and heterogeneity in some study results have occurred due to lack of randomization, short period of prerehabilitation, patient selection, and small number of patients included. Thus, a multimodal prerehabilitation program that includes aerobic and resistance exercises, respiratory training, nutrition counseling, psychological support, and smoking cessation is a harmless intervention with multiple physiological and psychosocial benefits in lung cancer patients[31] (Tables 16.1 and 16.2).

TABLE 16.1

Rehabilitation Strategies for Musculoskeletal Complications After Lung Cancer Surgeries.

Condition	Symptoms/Signs	Physiotherapy Techniques	Interventional Techniques
Intercostal neuralgia	• Burning over rib cage • Allodynia • Hyperalgesia • Paresthesias • Numbness • Ipsilateral trunk weakness with bending • Contralateral trunk weakness with rotation	• Desensitization techniques • TENS • Cryotherapy • Positioning • Wound support • Breathing exercises • Incentive spirometry • Inspiratory muscle training • Shoulder ROM exercises and gentle scapula mobilization exercises • Leg, trunk, and thoracic mobilization exercises	• US-guided intercostal nerve block • Thoracic epidural analgesia • Paravertebral blocks of the intercostal nerves • Intraoperative cryoanalgesia • Serratus anterior plane blocks
Acute Postthoracotomy Shoulder Pain	• Dull and aching pain • Neuropathic pain over ipsilateral posterior/posterolateral shoulder, deltoid, distal clavicle • Pain with shoulder abduction/flexion • Alleviated by rest • Decreased sensation along C4–C5 dermatomal distribution	• Axillary stretch • Pendulum exercises • Shoulder range of motion exercises • Gentle scapular mobilization exercises • Isometric shoulder exercises in all planes as tolerated • Serratus anterior strengthening in supine • Shoulder shrugs	• Periphrenic fat pad injection • US-guided interscalene nerve block • US-guided stellate ganglion block
Chronic Postthoracotomy Shoulder Pain	• Shoulder stiffness with or without associated pain • Limited active and passive motion, mostly abduction/external rotation	Freezing phase (2–9 months): • Gentle shoulder stretching • Modalities: heat/ice packs Frozen phase (4–12 months): • Stretching exercises • Strengthening exercises: isometrics/statics • Modalities: heat/ice packs Thawing phase (5–26 months): • Stretching exercises • Strengthening exercises: isometrics/static->resistance based	• Intraarticular steroid injections • Intraarticular hyaluronate injections • Suprascapular nerve block • Manipulation under anesthesia • Arthroscopic release • Open capsulotomy
Rectus Abdominis Paralysis	• Bulging mass over ipsilateral abdominal wall worsened with Valsalva • ±Pain • Difficulty with expiratory breathing and coughing • Lack of abdominal reflexes	• Postural training • Breathing exercises • Core strengthening exercises • Strengthening exercises to pelvic floor muscles • Taping or bracing in some cases • Electrical stimulation to rectus abdominis muscles	• US-guided intercostal nerve block • US-guided rectus sheath block • US-guided subcostal transversus abdominis plane block

TABLE 16.2
General Physiotherapy Approach After Lung Cancer Surgeries.

- Wound support
- Positioning: gravity assisted to improve gas exchange and secretion clearance
- Early mobility and ambulation when patient is clinically stable

Hold if:
  - Pulse ≤40/min or ≥140/min
  - Respiratory rate ≤8/min or ≥36
  - Oxygen saturation <85%
  - Systolic blood pressure <80 or >200 mmHg
  - Diastolic blood pressure >110 mmHg
  - Mean arterial pressure 9 MAP <65 mmHg
  - Fever
- Chest expansion techniques:
  - Thoracic expansion
  - Diaphragmatic breathing
  - Sustained maximal inspiration
  - Incentive spirometry
  - Inspiratory muscle training
- Airway clearance
  - Supporting cough
  - Huffing
  - Forced expiration
- Manual chest physiotherapy
- Postural correction/education
- Trunk and thoracic mobilization

REFERENCES

1. Abbas AE. Surgical management of lung cancer: history, evolution, and modern advances. *Curr Oncol Rep.* 2018; 20(12):98. https://doi.org/10.1007/s11912-018-0741-7.
2. Kim HK. Video-assisted thoracic surgery lobectomy. *J Chest Surg.* 2021;54(4):239–245. https://doi.org/10.5090/jcs.21.061.
3. Sihoe ADL. Video-assisted thoracoscopic surgery as the gold standard for lung cancer surgery. *Respirology.* 2020; 25(Suppl 2):49–60. https://doi.org/10.1111/resp.13920.
4. Bendixen M, Jørgensen OD, Kronborg C, Andersen C, Licht PB. Postoperative pain and quality of life after lobectomy via video-assisted thoracoscopic surgery or anterolateral thoracotomy for early stage lung cancer: a randomised controlled trial. *Lancet Oncol.* 2016;17(6):836–844. https://doi.org/10.1016/S1470-2045(16)00173-X.
5. Veronesi G, Novellis P, Voulaz E, Bruschini P. Robotic assisted lung resection for locally advanced lung cancer. *Expet Rev Respir Med.* 2020;14(2):121–124. https://doi.org/10.1080/17476348.2020.1697235.
6. Gharagozloo F, Tempesta B, Meyer M, Gruessner S. *Pain Control Following Robotic Thoracic Surgery.* 2021. https://doi.org/10.1007/978-3-030-53594-0_44

7. Park SK, Yoon S, Kim BR, Choe SH, Bahk JH, Seo JH. Preemptive epidural analgesia for acute and chronic post-thoracotomy pain in adults: a systematic review and meta-analysis. *Reg Anesth Pain Med.* 2020;45(12): 1006–1016. https://doi.org/10.1136/rapm-2020-101708.
8. Imai Y, Imai K, Kimura T, et al. Evaluation of postoperative pregabalin for attenuation of postoperative shoulder pain after thoracotomy in patients with lung cancer, a preliminary result. *Gen Thorac Cardiovasc Surg.* 2015;63(2): 99–104. https://doi.org/10.1007/s11748-014-0466-y.
9. Kelsheimer B, Williams C, Kelsheimer C. New emerging modalities to treat post-thoracotomy pain syndrome: a review. *Mo Med.* 2019;116(1):41–44.
10. Lee HJ, Park HS, Moon HI, Yoon SY. Effect of ultrasound-guided intercostal nerve block versus fluoroscopy-guided epidural nerve block in patients with thoracic herpes zoster: a comparative study. *J Ultrasound Med.* 2019;38(3): 725–731. https://doi.org/10.1002/jum.14758. Epub 2018 Sep 23. PMID: 30244489.
11. Taylor R, Massey S, Stuart-Smith K. Postoperative analgesia in video-assisted thoracoscopy: the role of intercostal blockade. *J Cardiothorac Vasc Anesth.* 2004;18(3):317–321. https://doi.org/10.1053/j.jvca.2004.03.012. PMID: 15232812.
12. Li WW, Lee TW, Yim AP. Shoulder function after thoracic surgery. *Thorac Surg Clin.* 2004;14(3):331–343. https://doi.org/10.1016/S1547-4127(04)00021-0. Review. Pub Med PMID: 15382765.
13. Yousefshahi F, Predescu O, Colizza M, Asenjo JF. Postthoracotomy ipsilateral shoulder pain: a literature review on characteristics and treatment. *Pain Res Manag.* 2016; 2016:3652726. https://doi.org/10.1155/2016/3652726.
14. Bunchungmongkol N, Pipanmekaporn T, Paiboonworachat S, Saeteng S, Tantraworasin A. Incidence and risk factors associated with ipsilateral shoulder pain after thoracic surgery. *J Cardiothorac Vasc Anesth.* 2014;28(4): 979–982. https://doi.org/10.1053/j.jvca.2013.10.008.
15. MacDougall P. Postthoracotomy shoulder pain: diagnosis and management. *Curr Opin Anaesthesiol.* 2008;21(1): 12–15. https://doi.org/10.1097/ACO.0b013e3282f2bb67.
16. Stasiowski MJ, Kolny M, Zuber M, et al. Randomised controlled trial of analgesic effectiveness of three different techniques of single-shot interscalene brachial plexus block using 20 mL of 0.5% ropivacaine for shoulder arthroscopy. *Anaesthesiol Intensive Ther.* 2017;49(3): 215–221. https://doi.org/10.5603/AIT.a2017.0031. Epub 2017 Jul 16. PMID: 28712103.
17. Kapral S, Greher M, Huber G, et al. Ultrasonographic guidance improves the success rate of interscalene brachial plexus blockade. *Reg Anesth Pain Med.* 2008;33(3): 253–258. https://doi.org/10.1016/j.rapm.2007.10.011. PMID: 18433677.
18. Narouze S, Vydyanathan A, Patel N. Ultrasound-guided stellate ganglion block successfully prevented esophageal puncture. *Pain Physician.* 2007;10(6):747–752.
19. Reeve J, Stiller K, Nicol K, et al. A postoperative shoulder exercise program improves function and decreases pain following open thoracotomy: a randomised trial.

J Physiother. 2010;56(4):245–252. https://doi.org/10.1016/s1836-9553(10)70007-2.

20. Gordon JA, Breitbart E, Austin DC, Photopoulos CD, Kelly JD. Adhesive capsulitis: diagnosis, etiology, and treatment Strategies. In: Kelly IVJ, ed. *Elite Techniques in Shoulder Arthroscopy*. Cham: Springer; 2016. https://doi.org/10.1007/978-3-319-25103-5_14.

21. Tandon A, Dewan S, Bhatt S, Jain AK, Kumari R. Sonography in diagnosis of adhesive capsulitis of the shoulder: a case-control study. *J Ultrasound*. 2017;20(3):227–236. https://doi.org/10.1007/s40477-017-0262-5.

22. Bamps M, Dok R, Nuyts S. Low-level laser therapy stimulates proliferation in head and neck squamous cell carcinoma cells. *Front Oncol*. 2018;8:343. https://doi.org/10.3389/fonc.2018.00343.

23. Le HV, Lee SJ, Nazarian A, Rodriguez EK. Adhesive capsulitis of the shoulder: review of pathophysiology and current clinical treatments. *Shoulder Elbow*. 2017;9(2):75–84. https://doi.org/10.1177/1758573216676786.

24. Lee LC, Lieu FK, Lee HL, Tung TH. Effectiveness of hyaluronic acid administration in treating adhesive capsulitis of the shoulder: a systematic review of randomized controlled trials. *Biomed Res Int*. 2015;2015:314120. https://doi.org/10.1155/2015/314120.

25. Jones LW, Peddle CJ, Eves ND, et al. Effects of presurgical exercise training on cardiorespiratory fitness among patients undergoing thoracic surgery for malignant lung lesions. *Cancer*. 2007;110(3):590–598. https://doi.org/10.1002/cncr.22830.

26. Bobbio A, Chetta A, Ampollini L, et al. Preoperative pulmonary rehabilitation in patients undergoing lung resection for non-small cell lung cancer. *Eur J Cardio Thorac Surg*. 2008;33(1):95–98. https://doi.org/10.1016/j.ejcts.2007.10.003.

27. Li T-C, Yang M-C, Tseng H, Lee H. Prehabilitation and rehabilitation for surgically lung cancer patients. *J Cancer Res Prac*. 2017;4. https://doi.org/10.1016/j.jcrpr.2017.06.001.

28. Tarumi S, Yokomise H, Gotoh M, et al. Pulmonary rehabilitation during induction chemoradiotherapy for lung cancer improves pulmonary function. *J Thorac Cardiovasc Surg*. 2015;149(2):569–573. https://doi.org/10.1016/j.jtcvs.2014.09.123.

29. Goldsmith I, Chesterfield-Thomas G, Toghill H. Pretreatment optimization with pulmonary rehabilitation in lung cancer: making the inoperable patients operable. *EClinicalMedicine*. 2021;31:100663. https://doi.org/10.1016/j.eclinm.2020.100663. eCollection 2021 Jan. PubMed PMID: 33554075; PubMed Central PMCID: PMC7846708.

30. Ni HJ, Pudasaini B, Yuan XT, Li HF, Shi L, Yuan P. Exercise training for patients pre- and postsurgically treated for non-small cell lung cancer: a systematic review and meta-analysis. *Integr Cancer Ther*. 2017;16(1):63–73. https://doi.org/10.1177/1534735416645180. Epub 2016 May 5. PMID: 27151583; PMCID: PMC5736064.

31. Sanchez-Lorente D, Navarro-Ripoll R, Guzman R, et al. Prehabilitation in thoracic surgery. *J Thorac Dis*. 2018;10(Suppl 22):S2593–S2600. https://doi.org/10.21037/jtd.2018.08.18.

FURTHER READING

1. Graham EA. The first total pneumonectomy. *Tex Cancer Bull*. 1949;2(1):2–4.

2. Hopkins KG, Rosenzweig M. Post-thoracotomy pain syndrome: assessment and intervention. *Clin J Oncol Nurs*. 2012;16(4):365–370. https://doi.org/10.1188/12.CJON.365-370.

3. Miyazaki T, Sakai T, Tsuchiya T, et al. Assessment and follow-up of intercostal nerve damage after video-assisted thoracic surgery. *Eur J Cardio Thorac Surg*. 2011;39(6):1033–1039. https://doi.org/10.1016/j.ejcts.2010.10.015.

4. Ochroch EA, Gottschalk A. Impact of acute pain and its management for thoracic surgical patients. *Thorac Surg Clin*. 2005;15(1):105–121. https://doi.org/10.1016/j.thorsurg.2004.08.004.

5. Gerner P. Postthoracotomy pain management problems. *Anesthesiol Clin*. 2008;26(2):355–vii. https://doi.org/10.1016/j.anclin.2008.01.007.

6. Timmermans L, Klitsie PJ, Maat AP, de Goede B, Kleinrensink GJ, Lange JF. Abdominal wall bulging after thoracic surgery, an underdiagnosed wound complication. *Hernia*. 2013;17(1):89–94. https://doi.org/10.1007/s10029-012-0971-9.

7. Benedetti F, Amanzio M, Casadio C, et al. Postoperative pain and superficial abdominal reflexes after posterolateral thoracotomy. *Ann Thorac Surg*. 1997;64(1):207–210. https://doi.org/10.1016/s0003-4975(97)82829-9.

8. Ökmen K, Ökmen BM. The efficacy of serratus anterior plane block in analgesia for thoracotomy: a retrospective study. *J Anesth*. 2017;31(4):579–585. https://doi.org/10.1007/s00540-017-2364-9.

9. Erdek MA, Staats PS. Chronic pain and thoracic surgery. *Thorac Surg Clin*. 2005;15(1):123–130. https://doi.org/10.1016/j.thorsurg.2004.10.001.

10. Blichfeldt-Eckhardt MR, Toft P. Treatment of ipsilateral shoulder pain after thoracic surgery-time for comparative studies? *J Thorac Dis*. 2019;11(Suppl 3):S417–S419. https://doi.org/10.21037/jtd.2018.11.91. PubMed PMID: 30997235; PubMed Central PMCID: PMC6424791.

11. Ho J, Richardson JK. Rectus abdominis denervation after subcostal open laparotomy. *Am J Phys Med Rehabil*. 2015;94(5):e43–e44. https://doi.org/10.1097/PHM.0000000000000256.

12. Cho HM, Sim HJ, Kim DH, Lim MH, Lee SK. Paralysis of the rectus abdominis muscle after a video-assisted thoracoscopic surgery. *Ann Thorac Cardiovasc Surg*. 2018;24(1):40–42. https://doi.org/10.5761/atcs.cr.17-00103.

13. Kocher GJ, Mauss K, Carboni GL, et al. Effect of phrenic nerve palsy on early postoperative lung function after pneumonectomy: a prospective study. *Ann Thorac Surg*. 2013;96(6):2015–2020. https://doi.org/10.1016/j.athoracsur.2013.07.006.

14. Han H, Ortoleva JP, Sekhar PM. Ipsilateral shoulder pain after thoracic surgery: chip on our shoulder. *J Cardiothorac Vasc Anesth*. 2021;35(2):563–564. https://doi.org/10.1053/j.jvca.2020.08.062.

15. Welvaart WN, Paul MA, Stienen GJ, et al. Selective diaphragm muscle weakness after contractile inactivity during thoracic surgery. *Ann Surg.* 2011;254(6):1044−1049. https://doi.org/10.1097/SLA.0b013e318232e75b.

16. Chuan A, Scott D. *Regional Anaesthesia : A Pocket Guide.* ProQuest Ebook Central; 2014. https://ebookcentral. proquest.com.

17. Ahmad AM. Essentials of physiotherapy after thoracic surgery: what physiotherapists need to know. A narrative review. *Kor J Thorac Cardiovasc Surg.* 2018;51(5):293−307. https://doi.org/10.5090/kjtcs.2018.51.5.293.

18. Chan HBY, Pua PY, How CH. Physical therapy in the management of frozen shoulder. *Singap Med J.* 2017;58(12): 685−689. https://doi.org/10.11622/smedj.2017107.

19. Uppal V, Sancheti S, Kalagara H. Transversus abdominis plane (TAP) and rectus sheath blocks: a technical description and evidence review. *Curr Anesthesiol Rep.* 2019;9: 479−487. https://doi.org/10.1007/s40140-019-00351-y.

CHAPTER 17

Musculoskeletal and Neurological Complications of Check Point Inhibitors

JESUEL PADRO-GUZMAN, MD • FRANCHESCA KÖNIG, MD

INTRODUCTION

For decades, the standard of care for lung cancer, especially advanced disease, has been chemotherapy. However, the identification of specific genetic mutations and molecular mechanisms by which cancerous cells evade T cell-mediated cytotoxic damage has facilitated the development of immunotherapy.[1] Since 2015, the Food and Drug Administration (FDA) has approved using multiple immunotherapy agents to be used in combination or as monotherapy for lung cancer treatment[2] (see Table 17.1). These agents are antibodies targeting "immune brakes molecules" such as programmed death-1 (PD-1), its ligand PD-L1, and cytotoxic T-lymphocyte associated protein 4 (CTLA-4). Overall, there are known as immune checkpoint inhibitors (ICIs). They work by improving tumor antigen presentation and recognition, thus amplifying antitumor response.[3]

This immune response potentially cause nonspecific activation of the immune system to any organ system. The mechanisms that underlie adverse immune effects (irAE) development are poorly understood but are likely due to increased systemic inflammation caused by ICI, resulting in autoimmune responses and dysregulation of T-cell self-tolerance.[4,5] Musculoskeletal and neurologic adverse effects have been reported up to 30%–40% and 9%–12%, respectively, in multiple clinical trials, where mild symptoms are likely underreported.[6,7] Immunotherapy is now the standard of care for lung cancer patients. Any clinician that takes care of these patients should have a general understanding of the potential complications of immunotherapy and provide adequate care.

This chapter will discuss the adverse effects of ICI on the musculoskeletal and neurologic system and how rehabilitation could play a role in treating the effects of these novel treatments.

Mechanism of Action of Checkpoint Inhibitors

The success of tumor cells depends on their ability to evade the immune system's surveillance and downregulate the T cell response.

TABLE 17.1 FDA approved check point inhibitors for treatment of lung cancers.		
Immune Check Point Inhibitor (ICI)	**Mechanism of Action**	**FDA Approved ICI for Lung Cancer**
Atezolizumab	Antibody blocks programmed death-ligand 1 (PD-L1)	Small cell lung cancer with chemotherapy Squamous NSCLC Nonsquamous NSCLC with platinum chemotherapy
Nivolumab	IgG4 monoclonal antibody blocks programmed death-1 (PD-1)	Small cell lung cancer after platinum chemotherapy Squamous NSCLC
Pembrolizumab	IgG4k monoclonal antibody blocks PD-1	Squamous NSCLC Monotherapy or with platinum chemotherapy Nonsquamous NSCLC with platinum chemotherapy

NSCLC, Nonsmall Cell Lung Cancer.

Lung Cancer Rehabilitation. https://doi.org/10.1016/B978-0-323-83404-9.00002-5

The transmembrane protein PD-1 is present on the surface of B, T, and Natural Kill cells (NK) and is upregulated during the release of proinflammatory cytokines. In normal conditions, once the desired response from the interaction between the antigen-presenting cell (APC) and T cell is no longer needed, the PD-1 receptor on the T cell membrane will interact with the surface ligand on the APC, resulting in the cessation of cytotoxic products release. To escape the immune surveillance, cancer cells produce programmed cell death ligand (PD-L1) on their membrane (see Fig. 17.1).

When PD-1 interacts with the tumor; PD-L1 will downregulate T cells and inhibit apoptosis of the cancer cell. Similarly, the CTLA-4 transmembrane protein expression increases based on inflammatory signals on CD8 and CD4 T cells. When they bind to APC ligands, they reduce the release of cytokines and apoptosis inducing enzymes (see Fig. 17.2). Checkpoint inhibitor treatments are antibodies direct to the PD-1 or CTLA-4 receptors, thus enhancing identification of tumor cells and adequate immune response to eliminate cancer cells.

Musculoskeletal Complications of Immunotherapy

Arthralgias. The incidence of immunotherapy induces arthralgias is approximately 15%.[7] Studies show that the onset of symptoms begins around 5 months of starting therapy. Combination anti-CTLA-4/anti-PD-1 therapy is associated with a greater risk of arthritis than monotherapy.[8] Patients with preexisting autoantibodies and preexisting autoimmune disease are more likely to develop irAEs.[9,10] In a study of 137 with advanced nonsmall cell lung cancer on immunotherapy, those patients positive for any autoantibodies were more likely to develop irAEs than those who were autoantibody negative.[11]

The patient may present with monoarthritis (rare) or, more commonly, oligoarthritis or polyarthritis with or without synovitis. The knee joint has the earliest onset and is frequently underrecognized as an early irAE.[8,12] Examination should include inspection and identification of joint deformity and muscle atrophy since this might suggest an underlying condition. The patient might have active synovitis, reduce range of motion (ROM), and mobility problems.[13] In ICI arthritis, diagnostic evaluation should include serum inflammatory markers (ESR, CRP), evaluation of autoantibodies (ANA, RF, and anti-CCP), and imaging.[12,13] However, in most patients with ICI-induced arthritis are seronegative.[14] On ultrasound, now available in most rehabilitation medicine practices, the presence of effusion, synovial hypertrophy, enthesitis, and enthesophytes and hyperemia are seen in inflammatory arthritis.[15] The majority of patients seen in clinics will have

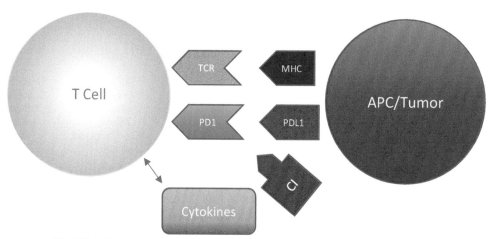

FIG. 17.1 The MCH-TCR interaction leads to the release of cytokines (IFN-gamma, IL-12, granzymes) from T cells. Cancer to T cell binding creates an environment of chronic proinflammatory release that produces PD-1 receptors at the surface of T cell. The tumor PDL1-PD1 connection inhibits apoptosis and inactivation of T cells. CI blocks PD1-PDL1 binding, thus enhancing the recognition of cancer cells. *APC*, antigen-presenting cell; *CI*, checkpoint inhibitor antibody; *MHC*, major histocompatibility complex; *PD1*, programmed cell death-1, Programmed death cell ligand-1; *TCR*, T cell receptor.

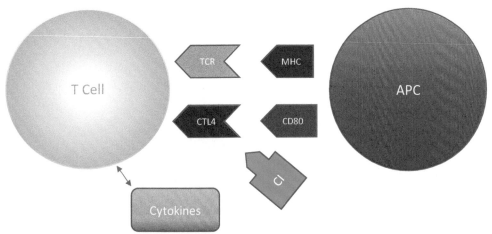

FIG. 17.2 MCH-TCR interaction leads to the release of cytokines (IFN-gamma, IL-12, granzymes) from T cells. Activation of immune cells (CD4 or CD8 T cells) and release of cytokines will lead to upregulation of CTL4 surface receptors. The binding of CTL4 with APC ligands (CD80) reduces the release of cytokines. This inhibitory feedback is considered a "checkpoint" of the immune response. By blocking CTL4, cytokines and other enzymes are released to fight tumor cells. *APC*, antigen-presenting cell; *CD80*, costimulatory receptor; *CI*, checkpoint inhibitor antibody; *CTL4*, cytotoxic T-lymphocyte-associated protein 4; *MHC*, major histocompatibility complex; *TCR*, T cell receptor.

computed tomography (CT) and positron emission tomography (PET) as part of their lung cancer workup and surveillance. It is possible to see findings of muscle or joint inflammation on PET-CT[16](see Fig. 17.3).

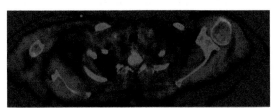

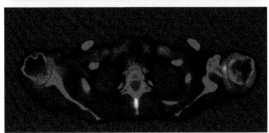

FIG. 17.3 Two cases of nonsmall cell lung cancer patients that presented to our clinic with upper extremity polyarthralgia. They reported symptoms within four to 6 weeks of treatment with check point inhibitors. FDG-PET remarkable for increasing FDG activity at the shoulders, upper back muscles, and around glenohumeral joint. Findings suggestive of inflammation. Follow-up workout reveals high inflammatory markers.

In our practice, many patients present with mild to moderate arthralgias. Initial treatment might include nonsteroidal antiinflammatory drugs or a short course of low-dose steroids. If the patient has single joint involvement, treatment with intraarticular joint injection is preferred to systemic treatment. Patient with seropositive arthritis or severe arthritis consultation with a rheumatologist is recommended.[17] In patients where pharmacotherapy is not indicated, consider the use of modalities such as cryotherapy and transcutaneous electrical nerve stimulation (TENS)[18,19] We recommend joint protection strategies: splinting, compression glove, and adaptive equipment. Therapeutic exercises are often used to restore muscle weakness related to inactivity (see Box 17.1). Muscle strength is

---

BOX 17.1
Rehabilitation Plan for ICI Arthralgia

1. Modalities: Cryotherapy TENS
2. Orthotics: resting splints, compression glove.
3. Therapeutics: joint protections and task modification strategies, endurance, and strengthening exercise including fine motor skills.
4. Range of motion (ROM): Start with active, progress to active assist. Progress base on tolerance and level of pain.
5. Adaptive equipment evaluation.

beneficial for physical function but also for joint stabilization.[20]

Myositis. Myositis is another potential complication of IC treatment. It is considered a rare adverse effect, affecting 1.7–2% of patients.[21,22] It is more common in combination treatment than monotherapy and reported after week 3 of treatment.[23] The patient might present with myalgia or proximal muscle weakness that is often symmetrical. In some cases, ptosis and neck muscle weakness has been reported. It is a diagnostic challenge to the clinician because there are cases of myositis with myasthenia gravis.[24,25] In our experience, patients present with mild to moderate forms of weakness are often sent to rehabilitation medicine with "deconditioning." A thorough musculoskeletal and neurological examination should be performed. At times, the patient with mild symptoms will describe changes in their activities of daily living rather than prominent clinical findings.

When suspected, the Rehabilitation Medicine specialist should communicate diagnostic impressions with the oncology team. If there are concerns for neurological irAE, then the neurology service should be consulted. Differential diagnosis is extensive. In our practice, for mild or moderate cases, we initiate the workout, including creatine phosphokinase (CPK), electromyography test (EMG), inflammatory markers, and basic antiantibodies. If available and to facilitate care, we ask rheumatology and neurology for guidance regarding antibody tests. ICI-induced myositis is usually seronegative and serves to rule out other conditions such as myasthenia gravis.[25,26] The typical workout will show elevated CPK, and a myopathic pattern might be seen in EMG with negative repetitive nerve stimulation. In some cases, the use of magnetic resonance imaging (MRI) is helpful to pick up inflammatory process (see Fig. 17.4) and rule out other types of soft tissue injuries.

The treatment is usually the discontinuation of immunotherapy and steroids. The physiatrist should closely monitor the patient for treatment response and observe for "rebound weakness" associated with steroid therapy. There is no clear rehabilitation protocol for ICI myositis (see Box 17.2). In our practice, we evaluate for adaptive equipment, slow/gentle endurance, and therapeutic exercises. Intensity adjustment depends on reported symptoms. Resistive exercises are well tolerated and safe with active inflammatory myopathy.[27,28] Furthermore, in a patient with inflammatory myopathy, a standardized rehabilitation program that includes strength training, aerobic exercises, transfers, and ROM positively affects function.[29]

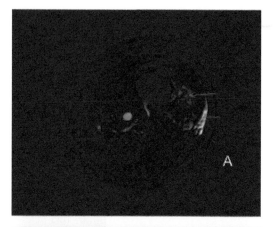

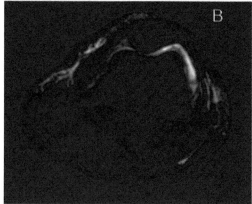

FIG. 17.4 T2 MRI of the thigh. A patient was complaining of leg pain and weakness 4 weeks after initiating treatment with pembrolizumab. **(A)** Image shows edema and enhancement of the vastus lateralis muscle consistent with inflammation. **(B)** There is thickening and enhancement of the knee joint synovium.

BOX 17.2
Rehabilitation Plan for ICI Myositis/Myopathy

1. Therapeutics: gentle aerobic base exercises, strengthening exercise; start with isometric then progress to resistive strength exercises.
2. Sit and stand tolerance activities.
3. ROM: active assist then progresses to passive ROM.
4. Adaptive equipment evaluation.
5. Posture correction.
6. Orthotics: neck collar (for neck extensor weakness) spine brace (posture correction)
7. Caregiver's education and home program.

In neck extensors weakness, neck collar, figure eight, or other spine orthosis have been used with some success. Once the patient completes the rehabilitation program, we recommend close follow-up and physician-guided/monitor home exercises. If the patient resumes treatment, constant communication with the oncology, neurology, and rheumatology team is key to monitoring and treating new symptoms.

Neurologic Complications of Immunotherapy

Compared to the frequency of other irAEs, including gastrointestinal, dermatologic, and hepatic toxicities, neurological irAEs are relatively rare. The overall incidence of such neurological complications is 3.8% with anti-CTLA4, 6.1% with anti-PD1 antibodies, and approximately 12% for combination therapy.[6] The true incidence, however, may be higher due to underreporting of symptoms.

The general scope of clinical syndromes is quite broad, essentially spanning across the entirety of the central and peripheral nervous system. Overall, peripheral nervous system involvement, including peripheral neuropathies and neuromuscular junction, accounts for approximately 70% of neurological irAEs, followed by encephalitis (approximately 20%), meningitis, and vasculitis (approximately 8%–10%), and other inflammatory CNS disorders.[30] Interestingly, clinical manifestations appear to differ among different cancer types; for example, myasthenic syndromes and noninfectious encephalitis/encephalopathy seem to be more common in lung cancer than melanomas.[31] It is important to note, as well, that treatment with immunotherapy may exacerbate preexisting neurological autoimmunity, such as Lambert Eaton syndrome in squamous cell lung carcinoma, with 75% of patients experiencing an exacerbation in one systematic review.[9] The onset of neurologic irAEs most commonly occur within the first 3 months of immunotherapy treatment,[32] although there may be a delayed onset, even possibly months after discontinuation of immunotherapy.

Peripheral neuropathies. As with all neurologic complications of immunotherapies, peripheral neuropathies are highly heterogeneous. Cranial neuropathies appear to occur most commonly, manifested most frequently as the involvement of facial and vestibular nerves.[33] Polyradiculoneuropathies, acute or chronic, such as Guillain–Barre syndrome and axonal or demyelinating sensorimotor polyneuropathies, seem to occur with increased frequency as well.[30] Other manifestations may include mononeuropathies, autonomic neuropathies, and Parsonage–Turner syndrome.

Diagnostic workup is similar to non-ICI-associated peripheral neuropathies. Evaluations should be individualized and tailored to a patient's symptoms, beginning with a thorough neurological examination testing cranial nerves, sensation, strength, proprioception, reflexes, gait, and balance. Reversible causes for neuropathy should also be ruled out, including other medications, vitamin deficiencies, diabetes mellitus, and thyroid dysfunction. Electrodiagnostic studies may help delineate which part of the peripheral nervous system is affected and, ultimately, the severity of the insult for prognostic purposes. CSF analysis for suspected ICI-related Guillain–Barre syndrome should be obtained. However, it may not demonstrate albuminocytologic dissociation. Spinal imaging may also be of use to rule out a compressive lesion.

Depending on the severity of the neurologic symptoms, current guidelines suggest holding immunotherapy and treating with corticosteroids, with high-dose intravenous corticosteroids reserved for more severe cases.[34] Moderate to severe Guillain–Barre syndrome may require ICU-level monitoring and the addition of intravenous immunoglobulins or plasmapheresis in addition to intravenous corticosteroids. Neuromodulators, such as gabapentinoids and duloxetine, may be used for neuropathic pain. Physical and occupational therapy may also be warranted depending on the severity of functional or quality of life deficits. Multidisciplinary inpatient rehabilitation has shown improvement in patient's functional activities.[35] It is ultimately recommended to discontinue immunotherapy for any severity of Guillain–Barre syndrome permanently.

Neuromuscular junction disorders. Neuromuscular junction disorders, such as myasthenic syndromes, have also been described during immunotherapy treatment. While these most commonly present de novo, preexisting neuromuscular junction disorders may also become exacerbated. There are a handful of case reports of Lambert-Eaton myasthenic syndrome after ICI treatment for squamous cell carcinoma, making it difficult to distinguish this as a neurological irAE versus a paraneoplastic neurological syndrome related to cancer itself.[36]

Myasthenic syndromes are more frequently observed with anti-PD-1 antibodies, although they can also occur with anti-CTLA4 treatment. In ICI-related cases, antibodies to the acetylcholine receptor may be negative. The average onset of symptoms has been shown to be within 6 weeks of treatment initiation.[37] It is important to be aware that myasthenic syndromes related to immunotherapy treatment may also present with myocarditis and myositis.[38] Clinically, patients may present with classic signs and symptoms, including ptosis, diplopia, weakness of large muscle groups, dysphagia, and dyspnea. Patients with immunotherapy-related myasthenia gravis frequently present with more clinically severe and life-threatening symptoms at diagnosis, which progress rapidly and ultimately confer a poor prognosis.[39] A complete neurologic evaluation is warranted with any suspicion of myasthenic syndrome. Diagnostic workup with EMG including repetitive stimulation and craniospinal imaging may be necessary. For moderate cases, immunotherapy is recommended to be held, and treatment with pyridostigmine and prednisone is often necessary. For more severe cases, guidelines recommend permanent discontinuation of immunotherapy along with acute neurologic monitoring, high-dose intravenous corticosteroids and plasmapheresis, or intravenous immunoglobulins if no improvement.[34] Immobility might be an issue while the patient is completing medical workup and treatment. Rehabilitation specialists should initiate early mobility programs, energy conservation techniques, and early breathing exercises.

Immunotherapy-related adverse effects involving the central nervous system. Aseptic meningitis in the setting of immunotherapy remains a poorly characterized phenomenon. It has primarily been described in patients treated with anti-CTLA-4, specifically ipilimumab, occurring in approximately 0.1%–0.2% of patients.[40] Clinical presentation may include neck stiffness, headache, and fever. Hypophysitis (inflammation of the pituitary gland), is also associated with ipilimumab and should be considered on the differential. Diagnostic workup should include cerebrospinal fluid analysis, MRI brain with pituitary protocol, and AM cortisol to rule out adrenal insufficiency. Inpatient neurologic monitoring is required in most cases with supportive treatment. Once infectious etiology is ruled out, steroids may be used for treatment. Guidelines recommend consideration of immunotherapy rechallenge in mild to moderate symptoms once these have entirely resolved. In severe cases, immunotherapy should be permanently discontinued.[34]

Encephalopathy related to checkpoint inhibitors may be difficult to diagnose given the broad differential in patients with cancer. Common symptoms include altered mental status, headache, fever, weakness, seizures, and ataxia. In one retrospective study analyzing

immunotherapy-related encephalitis in patients with nonsmall cell lung cancer, the most frequent neurologic sign at diagnosis was confusion in 78% of patients, followed by fever in 45% and cerebellar ataxia in 33%. Symptoms appeared after a median of five infusions.[41] A complete neurologic workup is warranted, including MRI brain, lumbar puncture (including a paraneoplastic panel), and EEG to evaluate subclinical seizures. Further workup to rule out infectious disease, metabolic alterations, and cancer recurrence or progression is also necessary. Treatment with corticosteroids, intravenous immunoglobulins, and plasmapheresis may be required. If paraneoplastic antibodies are found, treatment with rituximab can be considered.[34] In our experience, these patients have a broad spectrum of functional dysfunction. We recommend early interventions including cognitive and balance training. These patients should be followed closely for functional impairments both during admission and upon discharge. Outpatient follow up to promote compensatory techniques, fall prevention, and family training is recommended.

REFERENCES

1. Seebacher NA, Stacy AE, Porter GM, et al. Clinical development of targeted and immune based anti- cancer therapies. *J Exp Clin Cancer Res.* 2019;38(1):156. https://doi.org/10.1186/s13046-019-1094-2. PMID: 30975211; PMCID: PMC6460662.
2. Raju VK, Prakash M, et al. Review of indications of FDA-approved immune checkpoints inhibitors per NCCN guidelines with the level of evidence. *Cancers.* 2020;12:738.
3. Jain P, Jain C, Velcheti V. Role of immune-checkpoint inhibitors in lung cancer. *Ther Adv Respir Dis.* 2018;12:1–13.
4. Moseley KF, Naidoo J, Bingham CO, et al. Immune-related adverse events with immune checkpoint inhibitors affecting the skeleton. *J Immunother Cancer.* 2018;6(1):104. https://doi.org/10.1186/s40425-018-0417-8. PMID: 30305172; PMCID: PMC6180387.
5. Puzanov I, Diab D, Abdallah C. Managing toxicities associated with immune checkpoint inhibitors : consensus recommendations from the Society for Immunotherapy of Cancer Toxicity Management Group. *J. Immunother Cancer.* 2017;5:95. https://doi.org/10.1186/s40425-017-0300-z.
6. Cuzzubbo S, Javeri F, Tissier M, et al. Neurological adverse events associated with immune checkpoint inhibitors: review of the literature. *Eur J Cancer.* 2017;73:1–8. https://doi.org/10.1016/j.ejca.2016.12.001. Epub 2017 Jan 5. PMID: 28064139.
7. Suarez-Almazor ME, Kim ST, Abdel-Wahab N, et al. Review: immune-related adverse events with use of checkpoint inhibitors for immunotherapy of cancer. *Arthritis Rheumatol.* 2017;69:687–699.

8. Cappelli LC, Naidoo J, Bingham III CO, et al. Inflammatory arthritis due to immune checkpoint inhibitors: challenges in diagnosis and treatment. *Immunotherapy*. 2017;9:5−8.

9. Abdel-Wahab N, Shah M, Lopez-Olivo MA, Suarez-Almazor ME. Use of immune checkpoint inhibitors in the treatment of patients with cancer and preexisting autoimmune disease: a systematic review. *Ann Intern Med*. 2018;168:121−130.

10. Belkhir R, Burel SL, Dunogeant L, et al. Rheumatoid arthritis and polymyalgia rheumatica occurring after immune checkpoint inhibitor treatment. *Ann Rheum Dis*. 2017;76:1747−1750.

11. Toi Y, Sugawara S, Sugisaka J, et al. Profiling preexisting antibodies in patients treated with anti-PD-1 therapy for advanced non-small cell lung cancer. *JAMA Oncol*. 2019;5:376−383.

12. Lidar M, Giat E, Garelick D, et al. Rheumatic manifestations among cancer patients treated with immune checkpoint inhibitors. *Autoimmun Rev*. 2018;17:284−289.

13. Cappelli LC, Bingham CO. Immune-related adverse events with check point inhibitors: Arthritis. In: Suarez-Almazor ME, ed. *RheumaticDiseasesand Syndromes Induced by Cancer Immunotherapy*. Switzerland: Springer ;Nature; 2021.

14. Zhong H, Zhou J, Xu D, Zeng X. Rheumatic immune-related adverse events induced by immune checkpoint inhibitors. *Asia Pac J Clin Oncol*. 2021;17:178−185.

15. Albayda J, Dein E, Shah AA, Bingham 3rd CO, Cappelli L. Sonographic findings in inflammatory arthritis secondary to immune checkpoint inhibition: a case series. *ACR Open Rheumatol*. 2019;1(5):303−307.

16. Leipe J, Christ LA, Arnoldi AP, et al. Characteristics and treatment of new-onset arthritis after checkpoint inhibitor therapy. *RMD Open*. 2018;4:e000714.

17. Brahmer JR, Lacchetti C, Schneider BJ, et al. Management of immune-related events in patients treated with immune checkpoint inhibitors therapy: American Society of Clinical Oncology Clinical Practice Guideline. *Clin Oncol*. 2018;36:1714−1768.

18. Abelson K, Langley GB, Sheppeard H, Vlieg M, Wigley RD. Transcutaneous electrical nerve stimulation in rheumatoid arthritis. *N Z Med J*. 1983;96(727):156−158.

19. Fredrikus GJ, Oosterveld FG, Rasker J. Treating arthritis with locally applied heat or cold. *Semin Arthritis Rheum*. 1994;24:82−90.

20. Van den Ende CH, Vliet Vlieland TP, Munneke M, Hazes JM. Dynamic exercise therapy in rheumatoid arthritis: a systematic review. *Br J Rheumatol*. 1998;37(6):677−687.

21. Brahmer J, Reckamp KL, Baas P, et al. Nivolumab versus docetaxel in advanced squamous-cell non-small-cell lung cancer. *N Engl J Med*. 2015;373:123−135.

22. Robert C, Schachter J, Long GV, et al. Pembrolizumab versus ipili- mumab in advanced melanoma. *N Engl J Med*. 2015;372:2521−2532.

23. Touat M, Maisonobe T, Knauss S, et al. Immune checkpoint inhibitor- related myositis and myocarditis in patients with cancer. *Neurology*. 2018;91:e985−e994.

24. Benfaremo D, Manfredi L, Luchetti MM, Gabrielli A. Musculoskeletal and rheumatic diseases induced by immune checkpoint inhibitors: a review of the literature. *Curr Drug Saf*. 2018;13:150−164.

25. Steven NM, Fisher BA. Management of rheumatic complications of immune checkpoint inhibitor therapy-an oncological perspective. *Rheumatology*. 2019;58:vii29−vii39.

26. Liewluck T, Kao JC, Mauermann ML. PD-1 inhibitor- associated myopathies: emerging immune-mediated myopathies. *J Immunother*. 2018;41:208−211.

27. Alexanderson H, Dastmalchi M, Esbjörnsson-Liljedahl M, Opava CH, Lundberg IE. Benefits of intensive resistance training in patients with chronic polymyositis or dermatomyositis. *Arthritis Rheum*. 2007;57:768−777.

28. Alexanderson H, Munters LA, Dastmalchi M, et al. Resistive home exercise in patients with recent-onset polymyositis and dermatomyositis-a randomized controlled single-blinded study. *J Rheumatol*. 2014;41:1124−1132.

29. Vincent T, Francois R, Francois K, et al. Postrehabilitation Functional Improvement in patients with inflammatory myopathies: the results of randomized controlled trial. *Arch Phys Med Rehabil*. 2017;98:227−234.

30. Sechi E, Zekeridou A. Neurologic complications of immune checkpoint inhibitors in thoracic malignancies. *J Thorac Oncol*. 2021;16(3):381−394. https://doi.org/10.1016/j.jtho.2020.11.005. Epub 2020 Nov 11. PMID: 33188910.

31. Johnson DB, Manouchehri A, Haugh AM, et al. Neurologic toxicity associated with immune checkpoint inhibitors: a pharmacovigilance study. *J Immunother Cancer*. 2019;7(1):134. https://doi.org/10.1186/s40425-019-0617-x.

32. Sechi E, Markovic SN, McKeon A, et al. Neurologic autoimmunity and immune checkpoint inhibitors: autoantibody profiles and outcomes. *Neurology*. 2020;95:e2442−e2452.

33. Zivelonghi C, Zekeridou A. Neurological complications of immune checkpoint inhibitor cancer immunotherapy. *J Neurol Sci*. 2021;424:117424. https://doi.org/10.1016/j.jns.2021.117424. Epub 2021 Mar 27. PMID: 33812689.

34. Thompson JA, Schneider BJ, Brahmer J, et al. Management of immunotherapy-related toxicities, version 1.2019. *J Natl Compr Cancer Netw*. 2019 3 1;17(3):255−289 [PubMed: 30865922].

35. Novak P, Šmid S, Vidmar, Gaja b,c. Rehabilitation of Guillain-Barré syndrome patients: an observational study. *Int J Rehabil Res*. 2017;40(2):158−163.

36. Nakatani Y, Tanaka N, Enami T, Minami S, Okazaki T, Komuta K. Lambert- Eaton Myasthenic syndrome caused by Nivolumab in a patient with squamous cell lung Cancer. *Case Rep Neurol*. 2018;10(3):346−352.

37. Makarious D, Horwood K, Coward JIG. Myasthenia gravis: an emerging toxicity of immune checkpoint inhibitors. *Eur J Cancer*. 2017;82:128−136. https://doi.org/10.1016/j.ejca.2017.05.041. Epub 2017 Jun 27. PMID: 28666240.

38. Safa H, Johnson DH, Trinh VA, et al. Immune checkpoint inhibitor related myasthenia gravis: single center experience and systematic review of the literature. *J Immunother Cancer*. 2019 11 21;7(1):319 [PubMed: 31753014].

39. Haugh AM, Probasco JC, Johnson DB. Neurologic complications of immune checkpoint inhibitors. *Expet Opin Drug Saf*. 2020;19(4):479−488. https://doi.org/10.1080/14740338.2020.1738382. Epub 2020 Mar 11. PMID: 32126176; PMCID: PMC7192781.

40. Astaras C, de Micheli R, Moura B, et al. Neurological adverse events associated with immune checkpoint inhibitors: diagnosis and management. *Curr Neurol Neurosci Rep*. 2018;18(1):3 [PubMed: 29392441].

41. Sanchis-Borja M, Ricordel C, Chiappa AM, et al. Encephalitis related to immunotherapy for lung cancer: analysis of a multicenter cohort. *Lung Cancer*. 2020;143:36−39. https://doi.org/10.1016/j.lungcan.2020.03.006. Epub 2020 Mar 17. PMID: 32200139.

CHAPTER 18

Functional Outcomes in Lung Cancer Rehabilitation

ALEXANDRA I. GUNDERSEN, MD • SASHA E. KNOWLTON, MD

INTRODUCTION

While lung cancer is the third most common cancer in males and females (behind breast and prostate cancer), it is the leading cause of cancer related death in the United States.[1,2] The 2-year survival rate ranges from 15% to 42% depending on the type of lung cancer.[2] Risk factors for developing lung cancer include age >50 years, tobacco smoke exposure, and male gender.[2] Smoking cessation can therefore considerably reduce the risk of developing lung cancer along with adequate lung cancer screening for high-risk patients. While small cell lung cancer is associated with cigarette smoking, the most common type of lung cancer is nonsmall cell lung cancer, specifically adenocarcinoma, large cell carcinoma, and squamous cell carcinoma.[1,2]

Treatment for lung cancer depends on the type and stage of the cancer at the time of diagnosis. Surgical intervention includes tumor resection or lobectomy (removal of the affected lobe). Radiation therapy is utilized for regional spread of the cancer and can be used both curatively and palliatively. Common chemotherapy regimens often include a combination of platinum agents (carboplatin), taxols (docetaxel), and/or antimetabolites (pemetrexed, gemcitabine).[3] While chemotherapy directly targets rapidly dividing cells, newer immune checkpoint inhibitors (ICPIs) such as pembrolizumab work to stimulate an immune response against tumor cells.[4]

With improvements in treatment (especially the addition of ICPIs) and tobacco control efforts, the overall mortality of lung cancer has decreased for both the male and female populations.[1,4] Patients are therefore living longer and experiencing a plethora of side effects from the cancer itself and its treatments. These side effects include but are not limited to chemotherapy-induced neuropathy (CIN), radiation fibrosis/myopathy/myelopathy, ICPI-induced neuromuscular disorders, fatigue, chronic pain, cognitive dysfunction, and breathing problems. Early targeted and multidisciplinary treatment of conditions can significantly improve a patient's quality of life and overall health and function.

Cancer rehabilitation as a specialty is focused on anticipating and then addressing these oncologic factors through longitudinal monitoring of cancer patients. Depending on the timing and nature of the side effects, cancer rehabilitation efforts can be broken down into preventative, restorative, supportive, and palliative rehabilitation.[5] Preventative rehabilitation (prehabilitation) focuses on early identification of functional deficits in an effort to prevent or delay complications of cancer therapies.[5] Restorative rehabilitation involves comprehensive therapy for cancer patients who have the potential to return to their functional baseline.[5] Supportive rehabilitation is for patients with more severe and potentially permanent deficits in an effort to maintain as much functional independence as possible.[5] Lastly, palliative rehabilitation focuses on maximizing comfort for patients with advanced disease or treatment refractory cancer and support for their families.[5] For all of these rehabilitation efforts, it is essential to establish the functional baseline of lung cancer patients and accurately monitor any changes in functional level before, during, and after cancer treatment.

ESTABLISHING FUNCTIONAL OUTCOMES

In order to establish this functional baseline for lung cancer patients, a thorough medical and rehabilitation assessment must be completed. The medical assessment includes discussion of any relevant comorbidities (especially pulmonary, cardiac, neuromuscular conditions), family medical history, and a focused physical exam (including heart, lung, neurologic, cognitive, musculoskeletal). The rehabilitation evaluation involves a detailed social history including home and community supports, tobacco/alcohol/drug use, current and previous occupations (for known exposures), and most importantly, the current overall functional level of the patient. There are both subjective and objective assessments to evaluate a patient's function. The short- and long-term goals for the patient are heavily based on their current functional level, the stage of the lung cancer and the prognosis at diagnosis, the treatment plan (chemotherapy, radiation, surgery), and the patient's overall priorities—including quality of life.

Subjective evaluations of function are centered on physical, mental, and social health. Examples of subjective evaluations that can be used in the lung cancer population are described below. The Patient-Reported Outcomes Measurement Information System (PROMIS) is a questionnaire that can focus on emotions (anger, anxiety, depression), pain, physical function, and overall life satisfaction. The Short Form (SF) 36 questionnaire evaluates how a patient's health limits his or her day to day physical activities (walking, climbing, bending). EuroQol 5 Dimensions addresses concerns or problems with mobility, self-care/usual activities, pain/discomfort, and anxiety/depression. The Visual Analogue Scales is a very commonly used psychometric response scale utilizing facial expressions and numbers to evaluate the level of a patient's pain and/or fatigue. The Brief Pain Inventory assesses the severity of pain and its impact on a patient's activity, mobility, sleep, mood, and interactions with others. Similarly, the Piper Fatigue Scale and the Functional Assessment of Chronic Illness Therapy Fatigue Scale evaluate the severity of fatigue and its impact on a patient's emotions and ability to engage in activities.

Objective evaluation of function can be divided into physical and cognitive function assessments. The Functional Independence Measure (FIM) is a common tool used in inpatient rehabilitation facilities that evaluates a patient's independence with mobility, activities of daily living, and cognition; patients can be scored as fully independent to total assist on each measure. The Timed up and Go test is an assessment of mobility over 10 feet which demonstrates an increased risk of falling if a patient requires >12 s to complete. The Berg Balance Scale is a performance-based metric to further define a patient's balance impairment by rating the ability to perform a number of specific exercises. The 2/6/10-min walk tests (2/6/10 MWTs) evaluate a patient's self-paced walking distance as a reflection of functional capacity with age-specific normative data. The sit to stand test calculates functional lower extremity strength and exercise capacity with age-specific normative data while assessment of grip strength focuses on upper body strength and force. For cognitive

evaluation, the Montreal Cognitive Assessment (MoCA), Rowland Universal Dementia Assessment Scale (RUDAS), and Addenbrooke's Cognitive Examination Revised (ACE-R) can detect early cognitive impairment and evaluate the severity of this impairment. The Mini-Mental State Examination (MMSE) is a more concentrated evaluation for cognitive impairment but is similar to the MoCA. The Frontal Assessment Battery is a cognitive test that specifically helps to differentiate between frontotemporal dementia and other types of dementia.

While many subjective and objective functional assessments are generalized for all patients, there are specific functional metrics for cancer patients utilized by medical and surgical oncologists. The Functional Assessment of Cancer Therapy - General (FACT-G) subjectively measures a patient's well-being and quality of life throughout four main domains (physical, social, emotional, and functional); there are also specific FACT domains for certain disease processes. The Eastern Oncology Group (ECOG) and Karnofsky performance scales (KPS) are more objective and are used to assess how a patient's cancer and treatment are tolerated though assessment of impact on activities of daily living, needs, and overall performance status. While both the KPS and ECOG are used interchangeably and often together, some studies have suggested that the ECOG may have a better predictive validity to establish functional status for patients with lung cancer with different prognoses.[6] The goal of these scales is to determine the appropriate medical treatment and overall prognosis for a patient based on current functional status and likely tolerance of treatment. All of these evaluations are being used more frequently to further understand patients' goals and to monitor any changes in emotional, physical, and cognitive function throughout their cancer journey.

FUNCTIONAL OUTCOMES DATA FOR LUNG CANCER PATIENTS

While the data on functional outcomes for lung cancer are limited, the data that are available have been utilized to illustrate the efficacy of lung cancer treatments. Monitoring the functional status of lung cancer patients before, during, and after treatment is important to determine appropriate treatment protocols while enabling maximal functional independence. Establishing a functional baseline prior to initiation of treatment is important to enable monitoring during treatment to assess tolerance, with frequent monitoring of functional status to identify any need for intervention such as treatment reduction or cessation at appropriate intervals. Baka et al., for example, looked at the change in KPS along with symptom palliation throughout two different treatment schedules for gemcitabine.[7] This frequent monitoring can help guide treatment options and ensure adequate attention to function and symptom management. The Karnofsky scale has also been used to indicate better overall survival for patients with lung cancer. Kasmann et al. showed that KPS of >70 was significantly associated with better survival for elderly patients with small cell lung cancer.[8] Performance status as a strong independent factor can help guide prognostication discussions and patient expectations.

Studies are often focused on surgical outcomes and risk factors that affect functional outcomes. Lei et al. found that preoperatively ambulatory status, ECOG performance status, number of involved vertebrae, visceral metastases, and time to development of motor deficit had significant impact on survival for patients with lung cancer with metastatic spinal cord compression.[9] Because the functional outcome (in this study, rated as the ability to walk postoperatively) was noted to be worse after decompression for patients who were prognosticated to have an overall shorter survival, the study recommended these patients instead be treated with radiotherapy and supportive care.[9] Postoperatively, however, 51.5% of previously nonambulatory patients regained the ability to walk. As a result, this study demonstrated that discussion of quality of life is essential as patients with shorter projected survival time may still prioritize a chance for improvement in their walking ability.[9] Rather than using the ability to ambulate as the primary functional outcome, in a similar study Park et al. noted improvement in the ECOG-PS by at least one grade in 66% of cases postoperatively from decompression for metastatic nonsmall cell lung cancer to the spine.[10] The postoperative ECOG-PS was also noted to be an independent factor for overall survival time.[10]

Exercise during cancer treatment has been shown to be safe and associated with strong and consistent improvement in cardiorespiratory fitness, reduced fatigue, enhanced physical, and functional activity as well as emotional well-being in a mixed cancer population. Combined aerobic and muscle strength exercises after lung cancer surgery have shown benefits regarding physical capacity, relief of dyspnea, fatigue, and shoulder pain. For patients undergoing lung cancer surgery (defined as radical lung tumor resection), Brocki et al. found statistical improvement in the bodily domain portion of the SF36 for those who were involved with

supervised exercise training 4 months after surgery versus unsupervised exercise training.[11] Garcia et al. noted that preoperative exercise-based training improves pulmonary function before surgery and reduces in-hospital length of stay and postoperative complications after lung resection surgery for lung cancer.[12]

When examining the functional outcomes for different kinds of lung cancer surgery (video-assisted thoracic surgery (VATS) vs. open lobectomy), Handy et al. showed that patients that underwent VATS had the same or better scores in all SF36 categories at 6 months postoperatively compared to those who underwent open lobectomy.[13] The open lobectomy group had significantly worse SF36 scores in the categories of physical functioning and role functioning at 6 months postoperatively.[13]

With regards to functional status and its correlation with overall survival prediction for patients with lung cancer, multiple tools have been suggested. Saotome et al. specifically looked at the role of inpatient rehabilitation on functional outcomes for patients with a variety of cancer diagnoses, though not specifically for lung cancer diagnoses.[14] Functional gains were noted for total FIM, motor FIM, and KPS following an inpatient rehabilitation stay. Higher total FIM scores (>80) were associated with significantly longer survival.[14] Motor FIM, FIM efficiency, KPS scores, return to home (as opposed to skilled nursing facility), ability to ambulate, and in-home medical/therapy services were also associated with improved survival.[14] Mohajer et al. compared the ECOG to the palliative performance scale and the lung cancer symptom scale (LCSS) to see which tool most accurately predicted survival for patients with advanced NSCLC.[15] The study showed that the LCSS was the best at predicting prognosis.[15] Ganz et al. illustrated that while there was a good correlation between a patient's Karnofsky Performance Status and the Functional Living Index-Cancer (FLIC), the FLIC was overall very difficult for patients to complete and had issues with quality control and data collection.[16] While the KPS and ECOG have both been utilized for prognostication, it can be beneficial to incorporate patient reported quality of life measures for more complete patient assessments. However, quality of life has been exceedingly difficult to quantify using a tool or scale.[16] Utilization of a quality of life measuring tool would prevent providers from relying so heavily on a low KPS score (e.g., KPS <50%) to predict a shortened survival before consulting palliative care and considering hospice.[17] Many patients and their families would benefit from palliative care involvement prior to such a low KPS score. Overall, while studies have been completed to evaluate functional outcome data for lung cancer patients, there are still unknowns that prevent reliable prognostication and symptom management based solely on function.

INTEGRATIVE CANCER CLINIC FOR LUNG CANCER PATIENTS

In order to further monitor functional outcomes for lung cancer patients and how those outcomes correlate with treatment decisions and survival, patients should ideally be seen at an integrative, multidisciplinary cancer clinic. The design of the multidisciplinary clinic would involve a variety of providers from different specialties that would meet the patient at the time of diagnosis and then continually see and treat the patient throughout their cancer journey. The providers would then be able to not only monitor the cancer progression but also diagnose and address any other symptoms or medical issues that come up along the way.

The group of providers would include but is not limited to the primary oncology team (including medical oncology, radiation oncology, surgical oncology), nurse navigators, pharmacy specialist, dietician/nutritionist, social worker, psychologist, cancer rehabilitation physician, and therapy staff (including a physical therapist, occupational therapist, and speech language pathologist as needed). This vast array of providers would ensure that every symptom and concern would be addressed appropriately, whether it was focal limb weakness requiring PT and bracing or pain control requiring specific medications. This design can also facilitate a patient's admission to acute care hospitals, inpatient rehabilitation hospitals, and hospice as appropriate.

Prehabilitation, defined as rehabilitation interventions that are implemented to address impairments identified between the official cancer diagnosis and the onset of treatment, is an important aspect of cancer rehabilitation and an ideal part of an integrative clinic; increasingly, prehabilitation has been well studied for a variety of cancer diagnoses.[18] The goal of prehabilitation is to identify and address physical and psychosocial issues prior to the initiation of treatment with the hopes of a better treatment outcome and less side effects. Prehabilitation interventions can include general conditioning, targeted exercise, nutritional interventions, smoking cessation, psychological well-being, etc.[18] All of these aspects of prehabilitation can be addressed through the multidisciplinary cancer clinic. Unfortunately, there are more limited data specifically for the lung cancer patient population and the effects of prehabilitation on preventing pulmonary complications and improving long-term quality of life.[19]

Lung cancer prehabilitation would ideally include cardiopulmonary exercise testing along with monitoring of forced expiratory volume and peak oxygen consumption (VO2) to be used as predictors for better surgical outcomes along with improving overall muscular strengthening.[20] It is well known that exercise improves cardiorespiratory fitness, muscular strength, and pulmonary function parameters.[21] Exercise as a part of a prehabilitation program prior to lung cancer surgery would reduce the likelihood of postoperative complications and hospital length of stay.[21] This prehabilitation, however, would need to be implemented in a way to not delay surgical intervention. Overall, the general understanding of the benefits of prehabilitation has been established but not how these benefits specifically pertain to the lung cancer population. An integrative cancer clinic would be able to more accurately observe the functional progress of lung cancer patients from the prehabilitation stage through treatment and even through the posttreatment phase.

CONCLUSION

There is evidence to suggest that improvements in functional (monitored by KPS, FIM, ECOG, etc.) are associated with improved quality of life and prolonged survival for cancer patients. Engagement in cancer rehabilitation ideally via an integrative cancer clinic can both monitor and encourage these improvements in function. There remains a lack of data specifically for lung cancer patients regarding functional outcomes throughout their cancer journeys. Efforts are required for streamline rehabilitation programs for these patients to allow for more robust and accurate data collection. Implementing rehabilitation in the lung cancer population starts with the education of both patients and their providers on the importance and role of cancer rehabilitation along with the observation of a patient's function throughout the treatment process. Regular monitoring and intervention will lead to a higher likelihood of all symptoms and medical issues being addressed and for a clearer understanding of a patient's cancer trajectory, potential treatment options, and overall survival.

REFERENCES

1. Wender R, Fontham ETH, Barrera E, et al. American Cancer Society lung cancer screening guidelines. *CA Cancer J Clin.* 2013;63(2):106−117. https://doi.org/10.3322/caac.21172.

2. Siegel RL, Miller KD, Fuchs HE, Jemal A. Cancer statistics, 2021. *CA Cancer J Clin.* 2021;71(1):7–33. https://doi.org/10.3322/caac.21654.

3. Wang S, Wong ML, Hamilton N, Davoren JB, Jahan TM, Walter LC. Impact of age and comorbidity on non - small-cell lung cancer treatment in older veterans. *J Clin Oncol.* 2012;30(13):1447–1455. https://doi.org/10.1200/JCO.2011.39.5269.

4. Matas-García A, Milisenda JC, Selva-O'Callaghan A, et al. Emerging PD-1 and PD-1L inhibitors-associated myopathy with a characteristic histopathological pattern. *Autoimmun Rev.* 2020;19(2):102455. https://doi.org/10.1016/j.autrev.2019.102455.

5. Chowdhury RA, Brennan FP, Gardiner MD. Cancer rehabilitation and palliative care—exploring the synergies. *J Pain Symptom Manag.* 2020;60(6):1239–1252. https://doi.org/10.1016/j.jpainsymman.2020.07.030.

6. Buccheri G, Ferrigno D, Tamburini M. Karnofsky and ECOG performance status scoring in lung cancer: a prospective, longitudinal study of 536 patients from a single institution. *Eur J Cancer A.* 1996;32(7):1135–1141. https://doi.org/10.1016/0959-8049(95)00664-8.

7. Baka S, Ashcroft L, Anderson H, et al. Randomized phase II study of two gemcitabine schedules for patients with impaired performance status (Karnofsky performance status ≤ 70) and advanced non-small-cell lung cancer. *J Clin Oncol.* 2005;23(10):2136–2144. https://doi.org/10.1200/JCO.2005.01.003.

8. Käsmann L, Janssen S, Rades D. Karnofsky performance score, radiation dose and nodal status predict survival of elderly patients irradiated for limited-disease small-cell lung cancer. *Anticancer Res.* 2016;36(8):4177–4180.

9. Lei M, Liu Y, Yan L, Tang C, Yang S, Liu S. A validated preoperative score predicting survival and functional outcome in lung cancer patients operated with posterior decompression and stabilization for metastatic spinal cord compression. *Eur Spine J.* 2016;25(12):3971–3978. https://doi.org/10.1007/s00586-015-4290-6.

10. Park SJ, Lee CS, Chung SS. Surgical results of metastatic spinal cord compression (MSCC) from non-small cell lung cancer (NSCLC): analysis of functional outcome, survival time, and complication. *Spine J.* 2016;16(3):322–328. https://doi.org/10.1016/j.spinee.2015.11.005.

11. Brocki BC, Andreasen J, Nielsen LR, Nekrasas V, Gorst-Rasmussen A, Westerdahl E. Short and long-term effects of supervised versus unsupervised exercise training on health-related quality of life and functional outcomes following lung cancer surgery - a randomized controlled trial. *Lung Cancer.* 2014;83(1):102–108. https://doi.org/10.1016/j.lungcan.2013.10.015.

12. Sebio Garcia R, Yáñez Brage MI, Giménez Moolhuyzen E, Granger CL, Denehy L. Functional and postoperative outcomes after preoperative exercise training in patients with lung cancer: a systematic review and meta-analysis. *Interact Cardiovasc Thorac Surg.* 2016;23(3):486–497. https://doi.org/10.1093/icvts/ivw152.

13. Handy JR, Asaph JW, Douville EC, Ott GY, Grunkemeier GL, Wu YX. Does video-assisted thoracoscopic lobectomy for lung cancer provide improved functional outcomes compared with open lobectomy? *Eur J Cardio-Thorac Surg.* 2010;37(2):451–455. https://doi.org/10.1016/j.ejcts.2009.07.037.

14. Saotome T, Klein L, Faux S. Cancer rehabilitation: a barometer for survival? *Support Care Cancer.* 2015;23(10):3033–3041. https://doi.org/10.1007/s00520-015-2673-1.

15. Mohajer R, Nathan S, Wells K, et al. Survival prediction in ambulatory stage III/IV non small cell lung cancer patients using the palliative performance scale, ecog and lung cancer symptom scale. *Ann Oncol.* 2012;23(September):ix467. https://doi.org/10.1016/s0923-7534(20)33989-2.

16. Ganz PA, Haskell CM, Figlin RA, Soto La N, Siau J. Estimating the quality of life in a clinical trial of patients with metastatic lung cancer using the Karnofsky performance status and the functional living index—cancer. *Cancer.* 1988;61(4):849–856. https://doi.org/10.1002/1097-0142(19880215)61:4<849::AID-CNCR2820610435>3.0.CO;2-B.

17. Chang VT, Scott CB, Gonzalez ML, Einhorn J, Yan H, Kasimis BS. Patient-reported outcomes for determining prognostic groups in veterans with advanced cancer. *J Pain Symptom Manag.* 2015;50(3):313–320. https://doi.org/10.1016/j.jpainsymman.2015.03.016.

18. Santa Mina D, Brahmbhatt P, Lopez C, et al. The case for prehabilitation prior to breast cancer treatment. *PM R.* 2017;9(9):S305–S316. https://doi.org/10.1016/j.pmrj.2017.08.402.

19. Mahendran K, Naidu B. Prehabilitation in lung cancer resection-are we any closer to the ideal program? *J Thorac Dis.* 2020;12(4):1628–1631. https://doi.org/10.21037/jtd.2020.02.15.

20. Gravier FE, Bonnevie T, Boujibar F, et al. Effect of prehabilitation on ventilatory efficiency in non–small cell lung cancer patients: a cohort study. *J Thorac Cardiovasc Surg.* 2019;157(6):2504–2512.e1. https://doi.org/10.1016/j.jtcvs.2019.02.016.

21. Avancini A, Cavallo A, Trestini I, et al. Exercise prehabilitation in lung cancer: getting stronger to recover faster. *Eur J Surg Oncol.* 2021. https://doi.org/10.1016/j.ejso.2021.03.231.

CHAPTER 19

Telemedicine in Lung Cancer Rehabilitation

CHANEL DAVIDOFF, DO • ADRIAN CRISTIAN, MD, MHCM • GENEVIEVE MARSHALL, DO • SUSAN MALTSER, DO

Telemedicine refers to the use of telecommunication technologies to deliver healthcare services at a distance.[1] The concept of telehealth refers to the broader scope of healthcare services, including nonclinical services. In contrast, telemedicine, a subset of telehealth, refers to the delivery of clinical services by a practicing healthcare provider (physician, nurse practitioner, or physician assistant).[2] Throughout this chapter, the terms telehealth and telemedicine will be used synonymously. Telemedicine uses various technology-based applications with the overall goal of enhancing communication between patients and providers, increasing continuity of care, decreasing travel burden, and overcoming workforce shortages in areas lacking specific providers. The rapid growth of telemedicine has extended into various medical disciplines, including oncology and, most recently, physical medicine and rehabilitation. "Teleoncology" and "telerehabilitation" are used to describe the use of telemedicine within these specialties, respectfully. This chapter provides a general overview of cancer telerehabilitation and discusses the practical applications of telerehabilitation, focusing on individuals with lung cancer.

TELEMEDICINE IN CANCER

The growth of telemedicine in oncology began with the goal of redistributing the workforce to rural areas that lack oncologic-specific programs or specialists.[3] In recent years, further adaptations of telemedicine in oncology have given rise to interventions such as remote symptom monitoring, chemotherapy supervision, remote office visits, and home-based rehabilitation programs.[3] Yet, despite the potential benefits of these established programs, integration of telemedicine remained a challenge because of various clinical and administrative barriers including fear of losing interpersonal relationships, need for trained personnel, provider resistance to change, and lack of adequate reimbursement.[4] The use of telemedicine accelerated during the height of the novel, highly virulent, Sars-Cov2 (COVID-19) outbreak in 2020 after clinics and services was closed due to government-mandated physical distancing orders to minimize viral spread and lessen the burden on the healthcare system. There was a dramatic rise in telemedicine services (almost 4000%) in April 2020, mainly due to adaptations by patients and changes in licensing policies and reimbursements by third-party organizations.[5] In oncology, the use of telemedicine during this public health crisis lessened the incidence of viral transmission while simultaneously minimizing disruption of care for cancer patients through improved access to care and timeliness of treatments. Experts are optimistic about the use of telemedicine beyond the COVID-19 pandemic period, given the numerous benefits and implications in cancer care, including improvements in patient–provider communication, participation in multidisciplinary collaboration, symptom monitoring, and participation in cancer clinical trials.

OVERCOMING BARRIERS TO CANCER REHABILITATION WITH TELEMEDICINE

Cancer survivors experience a variety of complex physical and functional impairments as a result of tumor-related or treatment-related adverse effects. Despite robust evidence supporting cancer rehabilitation efforts, cancer patients continue to have unmet rehabilitative needs.[6] The underutilization of cancer rehabilitation services by the patient and referring physicians results from a lack of knowledge that such services exist, lack of access to specialists or programs, or difficulty with adherence due to physical or financial inconveniences.[7] These

Lung Cancer Rehabilitation. https://doi.org/10.1016/B978-0-323-83404-9.00008-6

barriers highlight the importance of integrating cancer rehabilitation into standard cancer care to identify cancer-related impairments early on and prevent functional decline. Over the years, several rehabilitation models have been proposed including prospective surveillance models, triggered rehabilitation referrals, hospitalized-based care delivery pathways, and center-based programs. Implementing these delivery models in clinical settings across the nation has been challenging due to the lack of reimbursement mechanisms and infrastructure.[8,9] Advancements in communication technology can offer cost-effective strategies to effectively integrate rehabilitation in cancer care. Historically, telerehabilitation has focused on neurological rehabilitation in which remote therapies are offered to stroke patients and their progress is monitored.[10] Randomized clinical trials have shown telerehabilitation is an equally effective way of improving patient outcomes after stroke compared to in-clinic care.[11] However, the use of telerehabilitation services in cancer care remains limited. The primary reason for this is that exercise-based rehabilitation programs are not yet part of the standard of care for cancer patients, and therefore, cancer rehabilitation is not regularly recommended by oncologists.[12] There may also be hesitancy to refer a patient to virtual rehabilitation programs versus supervised face-to-face programs due to the perceived fragility and medical complexity of this population. Nevertheless, there is emerging evidence to support the use of telemedicine in cancer rehabilitation as an effective, accessible, feasible, and cost-effective alternative to traditional care.

Lung Cancer Telerehabilitation

Multidisciplinary rehabilitative assessments and interventions are important for individuals living with lung cancer to mitigate symptoms, optimize their physical health, prevent falls, and improve quality of life. This section discusses the role of telerehabilitation to address common rehabilitation needs of lung cancer patients and their symptom management.

PAIN

Pain is one of the most prevalent and complex symptoms in patients diagnosed with lung cancer and can stem from local invasion of chest structures or metastatic disease affecting bones, nerves, or other anatomical structures or as a consequence of treatments. Patients with unrelieved pain also can experience physical symptoms such as insomnia, anorexia, profound fatigue, reduced cognition, and overall reduced vital capacity. Persistent pain can cause existential and spiritual

suffering, limiting the patient's coping skills. This underscores the importance of frequent pain assessments to ensure adequate pain control. The ease of access using telemedicine has allowed for more frequent symptom monitoring through a variety of technological interfaces (video, phone call, web-based messaging, etc.). An NCI-funded clinical trial found that a 6-month physical rehabilitation program delivered by telephone modestly reduced pain and improved function for people with advanced cancer. The telerehabilitation program also reduced the time patients spent in hospitals and long-term care facilities such as nursing homes.[13]

Managing pain through telerehabilitation has many challenges despite advancements in technology such as videoconferencing. Limitations include interpreting nonverbal cues, rapport building, and performing an in-depth physical exam—all of which are necessary parts of pain management visit. With a focused pain history, physical exam, and mental health assessment, a rehab physician's knowledge of pain physiology can assist in identifying the pain generator and assist in designing a therapeutic blueprint.[14] The clinical history not only localizes the pain but distinguishes whether the pain is somatic, visceral, neuropathic, or mixed in etiology. The history provides information about what measures were previously attempted to alleviate pain and can guide future therapies. In addressing pain through telemedicine conferencing, providers may use typical pain scales to aid in assessments such as the numeric rating scale (NRS), verbal rating scale (VRS), and visual analog scale (VAS). It is also possible to use multiple dimension instruments to assess pain such as the McGill Pain Questionnaire and the Brief Pain Inventory (BPI), which incorporates the impact of chronic pain on day-to-day functioning as well as a mental health screening tool as the Patients Health Questionnaire-9 or General Anxiety Disorder-7. Generally, the physical exam follows a standard in-person exam with exceptions made for palpation, range of motion, and special testing, for which the patient or a family member can be guided through to approximate.

DECONDITIONING AND DYSPNEA

Physical activity has also shown to be effective in lessening cardiorespiratory decline associated with cancer and its treatments.[15] In particular, pulmonary rehabilitation programs are designed to increase exercise tolerance. Despite demonstrated benefits in improving muscle strength, endurance, and quality of life, up to half of referred patients never attend or fail to complete an exercise program.[16] Travel and transportation barriers, lack of support from family members, and perception of minimal benefit from participants are some of the barriers to patients obtaining pulmonary rehabilitation.[17] Given the challenges inherent in managing treatments while patients may also be working and managing their home responsibilities, the optimal exercise program for lung cancer patients is flexible, convenient, and promotes self-management of exercise.

For these reasons, telerehabilitation may better meet patient needs. Although telerehabilitation trials for lung cancer remain limited, several studies have evaluated the benefits of home exercise using telerehabilitation in patients with moderate to severe chronic obstructive pulmonary disease. Findings revealed improvements in physical function, participants were able to master use of the technology with minimal difficulty, and no adverse events were reported.[18] The ability to exercise at home with intermittent clinician supervision might help establish behaviors that promote long-term adherence to exercise versus the direct supervision model.

FRAILTY

A position statement from the American Medical Association defined the term "frailty" as characterizing "the group of patients that presents the most complex and challenging problems to the physician and all health care professionals," because these are the individuals who have a higher susceptibility to adverse outcomes, such as institutionalization or mortality.[19] Fried and colleagues identified five frailty markers: nutrition, mobility, strength, energy, and physical activity and reported that older persons with at least three of the five frailty markers are at significantly increased risk of having adverse outcomes such as falls, decreased mobility, disability, hospitalization, and death within 3 years.[20] Collaborative telerehabilitation—such as remote monitoring and web-based exercises—helps minimize functional regression and improve overall functional capacity in cancer patients. Further, the functional improvements gained from remote therapies are maintained months after completion of a program.[10,21] A secondary advantage of telemedicine is the ability to observe the home environment. By doing so, rehabilitation specialists can better assess fall risk, equipment, and caregiver needs as well as barriers to ADLs.

GAIT AND BALANCE DYSFUNCTION

Gait and balance training is recommended for all patients experiencing loss of balance or who are assessed to be at high risk for falls. Chemotherapy-induced

peripheral neuropathy (CIPN) is one of the most frequent side effects caused by antineoplastic agents and is characterized as a primarily sensory neuropathy that may be accompanied by motor and autonomic changes of varying intensity and duration. It is imperative to have ongoing rehabilitation assessments in patients with lung cancer diagnosed with CIPN to ensure mitigation of symptoms and risk as well as improvement of symptoms. Rehabilitation providers and therapists can use video interface applications for surveillance of CIPN throughout and beyond treatment. An example would be to assess for falls by monitoring ambulation in the home setting. In addition, a rehabilitation clinician can provide real-time safety cues relevant to their home environment. It is important to take precautions when using telemedicine to evaluate a patient with gait impairments due to risk of falls. Therefore, it is advised to perform telemedicine assessments under direct supervision of a caregiver or family member who is physically capable of providing hands-on assistance if needed.

Practical Applications of Telemedicine in Lung Cancer Rehabilitation

Referral to cancer rehabilitation specialists from oncologists via telemedicine can help facilitate the initiation of pulmonary rehabilitation for individuals with lung cancer. This section discusses the practical applications of telemedicine in lung cancer rehabilitation, covering the approach to telerehabilitation consultation, ideal patient selection for remote telerehabilitation programs, delivery of remote exercise programs, utilizing telemedicine for prehabilitation, and safety considerations prior to initiating remote therapy.

THE LUNG CANCER TELEREHABILITATION CONSULTATION

In patients with cancer, early identification and intervention for physical, cognitive, and psychological needs are imperative for optimal functional recovery. This is especially true for individuals with lung cancer due to the high symptom burden present throughout the disease continuum. Yet, evidence suggests that in individuals with lung cancer, referral to rehabilitation services usually occurs when patients enter the palliative phase of their illness or following treatment and are less likely to be referred at the early stages of the disease.[22] Individuals with lung cancer could benefit from a cancer rehabilitation consultation even at the time of diagnosis to aid in symptom management and provide baseline functional status that may influence best course of treatment. Using telemedicine to provide ease of access to cancer rehabilitation services will allow for early rehabilitative assessments and interventions. While there is currently no standardized referral process across institutions, multiple cancer rehabilitation referral models have been developed, as mentioned earlier in this chapter. Ideally, following initial diagnosis, the primary oncologist could refer the patient for a cancer rehabilitation consultation via telemedicine for a baseline functional assessment and evaluation for rehabilitative needs as well as other objectives shown in Fig. 19.1.

Another advantage of conducting a remote cancer telerehabilitation consultation is determining the need for a more in-depth, in-person evaluation before starting an exercise or rehabilitation program. The American College of Sports Medicine Exercise is Medicine in Oncology initiative has proposed a clinical pathway for clinicians to assess, advise, and refer cancer patients to either home-based or community-based exercise programs.[23]

There are several things to consider before, during, and after the cancer telerehabilitation consultation. Before the visit, a medical chart review is helpful to determine if the patient is a good candidate for this type of consultation versus an in-person visit.

Office staff can also determine if the person has an adequate video platform and is comfortable using this platform for the telecancer rehabilitation visit. If the person has difficulty using video platform technology for the visit, a family member or close friend should be available to assist with the use of the video platform. The office staff can also instruct the patient on what to expect during the telemedicine consultation and can also collect information from the patient that may be useful in the assessment and for the treatment plan (i.e., self-reported functional outcomes assessing the physical function and fatigue levels of the patient). A medical assistant can provide general instructions to the patient for the consultation. Specifically, he/she should be seated comfortably in a well-lit room, wearing comfortable clothing with easy access to inspect the arms and legs. The patient should be instructed not to drive or engage in other activities that could contribute to an accident during the consultation.

During the actual consultation, it is helpful to have the patient's medical record available whether in written or electronic format to access information during the interview. Accessories for the clinician such as a head set with microphone and video camera holder can make it easier to perform the consultation. It is important for the clinician to be dressed professionally, with a professional background setting and to be on time for the appointment.

The patient's identification should be double checked and patient should be instructed on the limitations in performing a physical examination via telemedicine. The chief complaint, history of present illness, past medical history, past surgical history, allergies, medications, and review of systems are often comparable to those typically performed in an office visit. With respect to the physical examination, some important general elements include observing if the patient

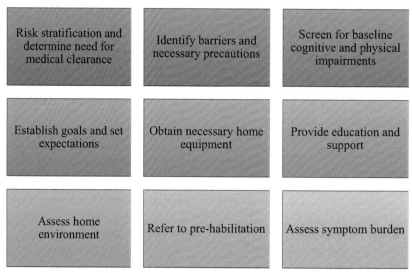

FIG. 19.1 Objectives for initial cancer telerehabilitation consultation.

appears to be cachectic or frail in appearance, short of breath, or demonstrating signs of cognitive impairment. Is he/she able to sit up from chair? walk around his/her home independently, or with the use of an assistive device?

An evaluation of the nervous and musculoskeletal systems can be performed, however, somewhat limited compared to an in-person office visit. The clinician should inspect the upper and lower extremities for atrophy, deformities, or erythema. Range of motion for the upper and lower extremities can be determined with the patient seated by asking him/her to raise arms overhead, flex, and extend elbows, flex and extend wrists, open/close fists, flex hips, flex and extend knees, dorsiflex, and plantar flex ankles. The patient can then be asked to self-palpate the arms and legs and to notify clinician of any sensory deficits or tender points. Gait can be assessed by asking the patient to walk around their home with/without assisted device and checking for presence of foot drop, knee buckling or genu recurvatum or impaired balance. This should only be attempted if clinician deems it to be safe for the patient to do so based on prior medical record review and with input from the patient and family member. While the patient is walking around their home, the clinician can also obtain information about the living environment with respect to potential safety risks such as falls.

Once the physical evaluation has been completed, it is important to discuss the general findings and the problems identified as well as recommended treatment plan. If the clinician has access to the electronic medical record of the patient and can enter orders, then referrals for rehabilitative therapies, and other consultations, medications, and orders for durable medical equipment can be entered. The patient can also be educated on a simple home exercise program if time permits, and information mailed or e-mailed to the patient and his family after the visit has been completed by the medical assistant.

Telerehabilitation follow-up visits can be very beneficial to the patient, regardless if the initial visit was via telemedicine or in-person. However, ideally if the initial visit was via telemedicine, at least the follow-up visit should be in person to complete a more thorough evaluation. An important point is that if the clinician believes that the initial telemedicine or follow-up visit cannot provide adequate information to make an assessment and plan or if the patient requires more immediate attention for a medical problem, then he/she can recommend an in-person evaluation instead of telemedicine visit.

EXERCISE AND PHYSICAL ACTIVITY FOR LUNG CANCER VIA TELEMEDICINE

Based on the recommendations from the 2018 ACSM International Multidisciplinary Roundtable on Exercise and Cancer Prevention and Control, physical fitness assessments are not required prior to starting a standardized, community-based exercise program for most survivors.[24] However, the prevalence of cardiovascular and pulmonary comorbidities in lung cancer has been frequently reported, adding to the medical complexity of their condition.[25] As a result, patients may have poor exercise tolerance at baseline before receiving potentially cardiotoxic chemotherapy agents. Based on the 2021 NCCN Guidelines on survivorship, medical clearance with further evaluation is indicated in patients with medical comorbidities and those with significant disease or treatment-related impairments.[26] A telemedicine consultation by a rehabilitation or exercise professional could be helpful in this situation. Table 19.1 summarizes the medical evaluation and exercise supervision recommendations in lung cancer survivors using telerehabilitation, adapting the triage approach from the NCCN Survivorship guidelines.

TABLE 19.1

Adapted NCCN Triage Approach to Exercise for Lung Cancer Survivors Using Telerehabilitation.[26]

No Comorbidities	No further evaluation necessary Follow general exercise recommendations
Peripheral neuropathy Arthritis/ musculoskeletal issues Osteopenia/ osteoporosis Symptom clusters	Consider in-person preexercise evaluation Consider exercise supervision by trained personnel Provide exercise modifications to general recommendations Referral to telerehabilitation or remote exercise program
Cardiopulmonary disease Lung surgery Bone mets Extreme fatigue Severe nutritional deficiencies Functional decline	In-person preexercise medical evaluation recommended Medical clearance prior to exercise by a physician Supervision by trained personnel with a transition to a home exercise program

Despite the limited supportive evidence, there is still a strong rationale behind recommending exercise to lung cancer survivors to improve cardiovascular fitness and activity tolerance.[15] Compliance and adherence to physical activity and exercise is a known challenge. Therefore, the optimal regimen for this population is one that promotes compliance. The ease of access with telerehabilitation can promote participation and improve adherence to exercise programs. For example, remote monitoring via sensors, mobile applications, or telephone inquiry can address any barriers to participation, such as uncontrolled symptoms or poor tolerability to the current physical activity regimen. Knowing these interferences early on can prompt program modifications or referral for medical evaluation if necessary.

Exercise and rehabilitation programs via telemedicine should ideally follow similar guidelines to in-person programs. A multicomponent rehabilitation program that consists of aerobic, strength, range of motion, and balance training is recommended for cancer survivors. In those with lung cancer, the addition of chest physiotherapy and pulmonary rehabilitation is also beneficial due to their inherent risk to develop pulmonary complications.

Aerobic Exercise — Patients with lung cancer have impaired cardiorespiratory fitness due to various factors that may negatively impact cardiopulmonary reserve.[27,28] The underlying mechanism of aerobic training can lead to favorable improvements in oxygen utilization.[28] Aerobic exercise can mitigate and potentially improve these adverse effects and improve quality of life. Aerobic training modalities can be supervised (through real-time video interface) or unsupervised (biking or walking). For patients requiring additional supervision and guidance, a remote, home-based incremental walking program demonstrated good feasibility and safety in individuals with advanced lung cancer.[13] Preliminary results from a home-based telerehabilitation program that included real-time supervised aerobic activity for lung cancer patients undergoing chemotherapy demonstrated good feasibility and adherence, with no adverse events reported.[29]

Strengthening exercise — Strengthening exercise is important in patients with lung cancer as many sustain generalized weakness due to chemotherapeutic agents, metabolic derangements, physical inactivity, and poor nutrition. Patients may even progress to exhibit cachexia and sarcopenia which are associated with poor outcomes.[30] Progressive resistance training can counteract skeletal muscle dysfunction and potentially attenuate cancer cachexia and improve outcomes by preventing further breakdown of muscles. Resistance training performed remotely can be done using body weight exercises, dumbbells, or Thera-Bands. For rehabilitative strengthening, programs focus on functional exercises utilizing the home environment such as climbing stairs or getting up from a chair. Examples of home-based programs included 2−3 sessions of resistance training per week, two sets of 4−5 upper, and lower body exercises for 8−12 reps.[13,31,32]

Range of motion and flexibility — Range of motion restrictions, particularly of the upper extremity and thoracic cage, is common in individuals with lung cancer throughout the disease trajectory. In those with active disease, etiology of shoulder pain and restrictions can be attributed to metastatic lesions or Pancoast tumors invading structures of the shoulder girdle. There is evidence to support the feasibility of telerehabilitation for range of motion exercises in cancer patients; however, more studies are needed for the lung cancer population. Telerehabilitation exercises to improve shoulder range of motion can include moving fingers up the wall, performing shoulder rolls, or pendulum swings with a light weight can of food.[33]

Coordination and balance — Telerehabilitation considerations for gait and balance training should include adequate supervision (by caregiver) and use of any assisted devices nearby in order to prevent potential falls. Through video interface, therapists can remotely monitor progression of gait as well as instruct the patient and caregiver through various balance exercises.

Chest Physiotherapy — Chest physiotherapy, a component of pulmonary rehabilitation, is commonly recommended for patients undergoing thoracic surgeries and encompasses exercises that promote chest expansion, secretion mobilization, postural correction, and respiratory muscle training.[34] With telerehabilitation, therapists can provide patients and their care givers with skills and techniques that can help optimize pulmonary function and overall endurance to perform daily tasks. For example, therapists may instruct the patient through deep breathing exercises and coughing techniques. Remote therapy programs may also incorporate inspiratory muscle training (IMT), a form of respiratory resistance training that uses a specifically designed device to strengthen muscles involved in breathing. IMT in the postoperative period has been shown to improve oxygenation in high-risk patients following lung cancer surgery and reduce complications (Brocki 2016). IMT devices can be provided to the patient by qualified therapists who can be available remotely to monitor compliance with exercises.

PULMONARY TELEREHABILITATION

Pulmonary rehabilitation is a comprehensive intervention that aims to improve the physical and psychological consequences of chronic respiratory conditions to decrease symptom burden, improve functional capacity, and enhance health-related quality of life.[35] The factors that influence referral to pulmonary rehabilitation by health care providers depend on clinical resources and financial support available within individual healthcare systems. Barriers at the hospital system level included lack of standardized protocols, lack of knowledge of services, staff limitations, and perceived low prioritization of medical services at the time of diagnosis.[36] Additionally, lung cancer patients face personal barriers that impede participation in traditional pulmonary rehabilitation, including low motivation, fear of exercising, poor adherence, uncontrolled symptoms, and other environmental and social barriers (lack of transportation, caregiver burden, etc.).[36] Utilizing telehealth technologies can potentially overcome these barriers by remotely delivering the essential components of pulmonary rehabilitation under the supervision of essential rehabilitation professionals. Examples of remote pulmonary rehabilitation services may include symptom monitoring, pain management, home exercise programs, as well as prehabilitation self-management and education.

LUNG CANCER PRETELEREHABILITATION

Cancer prehabilitation refers to rehabilitation interventions after diagnosis and prior to receiving acute treatment. A prehabilitation program for lung cancer is a multimodal approach that often includes a baseline functional assessment, physical therapy exercises, pulmonary rehabilitation, psychological support, mindfulness strategies, medical management for symptom control, and smoking cessation education.[37,38] The concept of cancer prehabilitation for lung cancer is to optimize patients for anticipated stressors of treatments or surgical interventions. Telerehabilitation provides an opportunity for timely preoperative intervention by allowing for immediate intervention and preventing delay in treatments. Future studies demonstrating the feasibility and validity of such programs are warranted to successfully standardize programs into clinical practice.

PRECAUTIONS AND SAFETY CONSIDERATIONS IN LUNG CANCER TELEREHABILITATION

During or following treatment with chemotherapy or radiation, clinicians overseeing exercise or rehabilitation should take caution in patients who develop neurotoxicity, cardiotoxicity, or hematologic derangements. In these cases, in-person assessment and medical clearance including routine labs may be warranted. Although there is a robust body of evidence to support that exercise in the setting of cancer is safe, precaution is still needed in select populations. As we have learned, lung cancer patients are uniquely complex largely due to due to high disease burden and greater symptom distress throughout the disease trajectory.[39,40]

In all lung cancer patients, throughout their care, it is important to bear in mind potential "red-flag conditions" noted in Table 19.2. These medical conditions may necessitate in person rehabilitation evaluation and medical clearance from necessary providers prior to initiating therapies.

TABLE 19.2
Virtual Safety Considerations and Precautions for Rehabilitation in Lung Cancer.[a]

Red Flags	Concern	Telerehabilitation Precautions and Follow-up Plan
All	Physical impairment, gait dysfunction, fall risk, progression of disease	- In person assessment is warranted - Medical clearance is recommended - Optimize home environment to prevent falls - Prescribe durable medical equipment (DME) as needed - Consider in-person supervision of therapies with vital sign monitoring with transition to home exercise program - Home supervision by care giver is warranted

Continued

TABLE 19.2

Virtual Safety Considerations and Precautions for Rehabilitation in Lung Cancer.[a]—cont'd

Red Flags	Concern	Telerehabilitation Precautions and Follow-up Plan
Dyspnea	Cardiopulmonary toxicity, pulmonary embolism, metastatic disease, progression of tumor, underlying COPD exacerbation, anemia	- Consider referral for pulmonary or cardiac evaluation prior to therapies - Provide portable pulse ox monitor for home therapies - Monitor for worsening lower extremity edema - Educate on self-report tolerance to exercise using RPE scale
Uncontrolled pain	Undertreated visceral, musculoskeletal, or neuropathic pain	- Referral for imaging - Consider medications or refer to pain management for therapeutic interventions
Postoperative (i.e., thoracotomy)	Postthoracotomy pain, wound infection, pneumothorax	- Avoid ROM and stretching of upper limb until removal of any intercostal catheters. - Avoid upper extremity resistance exercises during wound healing (<6 weeks postop)
New neurologic deficits	Tumor recurrence (brain or spinal cord), infiltrative disease, compression neuropathy/plexopathy, chemotherapy-induced peripheral neuropathy (CIPN), paraneoplastic	- Consider advanced imaging to rule out new tumor recurrence - Referral for neurological evaluation (e.g. NCS/EMG) and surgery as indicated - Rehab: Compensatory strategies, PT/OT prescription, bracing, and equipment as needed
Cognitive impairment or altered mental status	Metastatic disease (if symptoms are new), chemotherapy induced, infection, metabolic derangements	- Advanced imaging and labs as indicated - Ensure adequate home supervision - Referral to neuropsychology, compensatory strategies, medications when appropriate
Frailty	Malnutrition, fall risk	- Referral to nutritionist, fall risk assessment, and prevention
Bone metastases	Pathological fracture	- Orthopedic assessment is recommended - Assess risk of pathological fracture - Monitor functional pain (best predictor of pathological fracture) (mirels 1989) - May offload effected limb with assisted device (e.g., Platform walker for upper extremity bony metastasis) - Avoid progressive resistance exercises in affected limb
Cytopenias (anemia, thrombocytopenia, leukopenia/neutropenia)	Infection, bleeding complications	- Fall assessment and prevention, symptom monitoring, review transfusion status

TABLE 19.2
Virtual Safety Considerations and Precautions for Rehabilitation in Lung Cancer.[a]—cont'd

Red Flags	Concern	Telerehabilitation Precautions and Follow-up Plan
		- Platelets <20,000: light activities of daily living - Hgb <8: monitor perceived exertion, energy conservation, short exercise intervals with periods of rest - WBC <1.5109/L (neutropenia): neutropenic precautions per facility guidelines

[a] Referenced from Maltser et al. and Granger et al.[39,40]

CONCLUSION

In summary, individuals with lung cancer endure several functional impairments that warrant rehabilitation interventions. The integration of telemedicine in lung cancer rehabilitation offers a unique opportunity to enhance the way supportive cancer services are delivered and provides solutions to the current barriers that preclude integration of exercise and rehabilitation in supportive lung cancer care. Objectives of telerehabilitation in lung cancer may include functional assessments, fall prevention, medical clearance evaluation, screening for functional impairments, symptom monitoring, caregiver support and education, remote exercise programs, smoking cessation, nutrition counseling, pulmonary rehabilitation, and evaluation for durable medical equipment. Improving access to these services can ease care-giver burden, enhance patient–provider satisfaction, improve communication among patients and providers, and prevent further disability in a population at risk for functional decline.

REFERENCES

1. Manocchia A. Telehealth: enhancing care through technology. *R I Med J*. 2020;103(1):18–20.
2. World Health Organization. *Opportunities and Developments in Member States. Report on the Second Global Survey on EHealth*. Vol. 2. Global Observatory for EHealth Series; 2010.
3. Sirintrapun SJ, Lopez AM. Telemedicine in cancer care. *Am Soc Clin Oncol Educ B*. 2018. https://doi.org/10.1200/edbk_200141.
4. Gogia SB, Maeder A, Mars M, Hartvigsen G, Basu A, Abbott P. Unintended consequences of tele health and their possible solutions. Contribution of the IMIA working group on telehealth. *Yearb Med Inform*. 2016;1:41–46. https://doi.org/10.15265/iy-2016-012.
5. Whaley CM, Pera MF, Cantor J, et al. Changes in health services use among commercially insured US populations during the COVID-19 pandemic. *JAMA Netw Open*. 2020;3(11):e2024984. https://doi.org/10.1001/jamanetworkopen.2020.24984.
6. Thorsen L, Gjerset GM, Loge JH, et al. Cancer patients' needs for rehabilitation services. *Acta Oncol*. 2011;50(2):212–222. https://doi.org/10.3109/0284186X.2010.531050.
7. Stubblefield MD. The underutilization of rehabilitation to treat physical impairments in breast cancer survivors. *PM R*. 2017. https://doi.org/10.1016/j.pmrj.2017.05.010.
8. Cheville AL, Mustian K, Winters-Stone K, Zucker DS, Gamble GL, Alfano CM. Cancer rehabilitation: an overview of current need, delivery models, and levels of care. *Phys Med Rehabil Clin N Am*. 2017;28(1):1–17. https://doi.org/10.1016/j.pmr.2016.08.001.
9. Stout NL, Binkley JM, Schmitz KH, et al. A prospective surveillance model for rehabilitation for women with breast cancer. *Cancer*. 2012;118(Suppl 8):2191–2200. https://doi.org/10.1002/cncr.27476.
10. Peretti A, Amenta F, Tayebati SK, Nittari G, Mahdi SS. Telerehabilitation: review of the state-of-the-art and areas of application. *JMIR Rehabil Assist Technol*. 2017. https://doi.org/10.2196/rehab.7511.
11. Cramer SC, Dodakian L, Le V, et al. Efficacy of home-based telerehabilitation vs in-clinic therapy for adults after stroke: a randomized clinical trial. *JAMA Neurol*. 2019. https://doi.org/10.1001/jamaneurol.2019.1604.
12. Silver JK, Stout NL, Fu JB, et al. *The State of Cancer Rehabilitation in the United States HHS Public Access*. Vol. 1. 2018.
13. Cheville AL, Moynihan T, Herrin J, Loprinzi C, Kroenke K. Effect of collaborative telerehabilitation on functional impairment and pain among patients with advanced-stage cancer: a randomized clinical trial. *JAMA Oncol*. 2019;5(5):644–652. https://doi.org/10.1001/jamaoncol.2019.0011.

14. Nanda U, Luo J, Wonders Q, Pangarkar S. Telerehabilitation for pain management. *Phys Med Rehabil Clin N Am.* 2021;32(2):355–372. https://doi.org/10.1016/j.pmr.2021.01.002.

15. Scott JM, Zabor EC, Schwitzer E, et al. Efficacy of exercise therapy on cardiorespiratory fitness in patients with cancer: a systematic review and meta-analysis. *J Clin Oncol.* 2018;36(22):2297–2304. https://doi.org/10.1200/JCO.2017.77.5809.

16. Rochester CL, Fairburn C, Crouch RH. Pulmonary rehabilitation for respiratory disorders other than chronic obstructive pulmonary disease. *Clin Chest Med.* 2014;35(2):369–389. https://doi.org/10.1016/j.ccm.2014.02.016.

17. Jones AW, Taylor A, Gowler H, O'Kelly N, Ghosh S, Bridle C. Systematic review of interventions to improve patient uptake and completion of pulmonary rehabilitation in COPD. *ERS Monogr.* 2017;3(1). https://doi.org/10.1183/23120541.00089-2016.

18. Choi J, Hergenroeder AL, Burke L, et al. Delivering an in-home exercise program via telerehabilitation: a pilot study of lung transplant go (LTGO). *Int J Telerehabilitation.* 2016;8(2):15–26. https://doi.org/10.5195/ijt.2016.6201.

19. Hendee WR. American medical association white paper on elderly health. Report of the council on scientific affairs. *Arch Intern Med.* 1990;150(12):2459–2472. https://doi.org/10.1001/archinte.150.12.2459.

20. Fried LP, Tangen CM, Walston J, et al. Frailty in older adults: evidence for a phenotype. *J Gerontol Ser A Biol Sci Med Sci.* 2001;56(3). https://doi.org/10.1093/gerona/56.3.m146.

21. Irwin ML, Crumley D, McTiernan A, et al. Physical activity levels before and after a diagnosis of breast carcinoma: the health, eating, activity, and lifestyle (HEAL) study. *Cancer.* 2003;97(7):1746–1757. https://doi.org/10.1002/cncr.11227.

22. Nwosu AC, Bayly JL, Gaunt KE, Mayland CR. Lung cancer and rehabilitation - what are the barriers? Results of a questionnaire survey and the development of regional lung cancer rehabilitation standards and guidelines. *Support Care Cancer.* 2012;20(12):3247–3254. https://doi.org/10.1007/s00520-012-1472-1.

23. Schmitz KH, Campbell AM, Stuiver MM, et al. Exercise is medicine in oncology: engaging clinicians to help patients move through cancer. *CA Cancer J Clin.* 2019;69(6):468–484. https://doi.org/10.3322/caac.21579.

24. Campbell KL, Winters-stone KM, Wiskemann J, et al. Exercise guidelines for cancer survivors: consensus statement from international multidisciplinary roundtable exercise guidelines for cancer survivors: consensus statement from international multidisciplinary roundtable special communications. *Med Sci Sports Exerc.* 2019;51(11):2375–2390. https://doi.org/10.1249/MSS.0000000000002116.

25. Ambrogi V, Pompeo E, Elia S, Pistolese GR, Mineo TC. The impact of cardiovascular comorbidity on the outcome of surgery for stage I and II non-small-cell lung cancer. *Eur J Cardio Thorac Surg.* 2003;23:811–817. https://doi.org/10.1016/S1010-7940(03)00093-9.

26. National Comprehensive Cancer Network. *NCCN Clinical Practice Guidelines in Oncology (NCCN Guidelines). Adult Cancer Pain.* https://www.nccn.org/guidelines. Accessed 23 May 2021.

27. Avancini A, Sartori G, Gkountakos A, et al. Physical activity and exercise in lung cancer care: will promises Be fulfilled? *Oncologist.* 2020;25(3):e555. https://doi.org/10.1634/theoncologist.2019-0463.

28. Lakoski SG, Eves ND, Douglas PS, Jones LW. Exercise rehabilitation in patients with cancer. *Nat Rev Clin Oncol.* 2012;9(5):288–296. https://doi.org/10.1038/nrclinonc.2012.27.

29. Coats V, Moffet H, Simard S, et al. Home-based telerehabilitation program using real-time monitoring and interactive exercise for patient with lung cancer: a feasibility study. *Eur Respir J.* 2015;46:OA3283. https://doi.org/10.1183/13993003.congress-2015.oa3283.

30. Nattenmüller J, Wochner R, Muley T, et al. Prognostic impact of CT-quantified muscle and fat distribution before and after first-line-chemotherapy in lung cancer patients. *PLoS One.* 2017;12(1):e0169136. https://doi.org/10.1371/journal.pone.0169136.

31. Cheville AL, Kollasch J, Vandenberg J, et al. A home-based exercise program to improve function, fatigue, and sleep quality in patients with stage iv lung and colorectal cancer: a randomized controlled trial. *J Pain Symptom Manag.* 2013;45(5):811–821. https://doi.org/10.1016/j.jpainsymman.2012.05.006.

32. Ariza-Garcia A, Arroyo-Morales M, Lozano-Lozano M, Galiano-Castillo N, Postigo-Martin P, Cantarero-Villanueva I. A web-based exercise system (e-cuidatechemo) to counter the side effects of chemotherapy in patients with breast cancer: randomized controlled trial. *J Med Internet Res.* 2019. https://doi.org/10.2196/14418.

33. de Rezende LF, Francisco VE, Franco RL. Telerehabilitation for patients with breast cancer through the COVID-19 pandemic. *Breast Cancer Res Treat.* 2021;185(1):257–259. https://doi.org/10.1007/s10549-020-05926-6.

34. Kendall F, Abreu P, Pinho P, Oliveira J, Bastos P. The role of physiotherapy in patients undergoing pulmonary surgery for lung cancer. A literature review. *Rev Port Pneumol.* 2017;23(6):343–351. https://doi.org/10.1016/j.rppnen.2017.05.003.

35. Spruit MA, Singh SJ, Garvey C, et al. An official American thoracic society/European respiratory society statement: key concepts and advances in pulmonary rehabilitation. *Am J Respir Crit Care Med.* 2013;188(8). https://doi.org/10.1164/rccm.201309-1634ST.

36. Granger C, Denehy L, Remedios L, Parry S. Barriers to implementation of the physical activity guidelines in lung cancer. *Eur Respir J.* 2016;48:PA1900. https://doi.org/10.1183/13993003.congress-2016.pa1900.

37. Silver JK, Baima J. Cancer prehabilitation: an opportunity to decrease treatment-related morbidity, increase cancer treatment options, and improve physical and

psychological health outcomes. *Am J Phys Med Rehabil.* 2013. https://doi.org/10.1097/PHM.0b013e31829b4afe.

38. Sell NM, Silver JK, Rando S, Draviam AC, Mina DS, Qadan M. Prehabilitation telemedicine in neoadjuvant surgical oncology patients during the novel COVID-19 coronavirus pandemic. *Ann Surg.* 2020;272(2):e81–e83. https://doi.org/10.1097/SLA.0000000000004002.

39. Maltser S, Cristian A, Silver JK, Stephen Morris G, Stout NL. A focused review of safety considerations in cancer rehabilitation.PM R doi:10.1016/j.pmrj.2017.08.403.

40. Granger CL. Physiotherapy management of lung cancer. *J Physiother.* 2016;62(2):60–67. https://doi.org/10.1016/j.jphys.2016.02.010.

Index

Note: Page numbers followed by "f" indicate figures, "t" indicate tables and "b" indicate boxes.

CPI Antony Rowe
Eastbourne, UK
April 27, 2022

Contributors

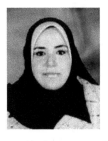

Rania Ahmed Abul-Seoud earned her BSc in communications and electronics engineering from Fayoum University, Fayoum, Egypt, in 1998, her MS in artificial intelligence from the Faculty of Computer Engineering at Fayoum University in 2005, and her PhD in biomedical engineering, artificial intelligence, and its applications to biomedical informatics from Fayoum University in 2008. She is the author of several research papers published in highly reputable journals and conference proceedings. Her current research interests are artificial intelligence and its different applications, biomedical informatics, and routing and security protocols for wireless sensor networks.

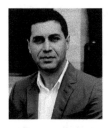

Ozgur B. Akan earned his PhD in electrical and computer engineering from the Broadband and Wireless Networking Laboratory, School of Electrical and Computer Engineering, Georgia Institute of Technology, Atlanta, Georgia, in 2004. He is currently a full professor with the Department of Electrical and Electronics Engineering, Koc University, Istanbul, Turkey, and the director of the Next-Generation and Wireless Communications Laboratory. His current research interests are wireless communications, nanoscale and molecular communications, and information theory. He is an associate editor of the *IEEE Transactions on Communications*, the *IEEE Transactions on Vehicular Technology*, the *International Journal of Communication Systems* (Wiley), the *Nano Communication Networks* journal (Elsevier), and the *European Transactions on Technology*.

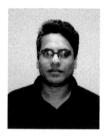

Muhammad Mahbub Alam earned his BS in applied physics and electronics and his MS in computer science in 1998 and 2000, respectively, from the University of Dhaka, Dhaka, Bangladesh. He earned his PhD from the Department of Computer Engineering, Kyung Hee University, South Korea, in 2008. Currently, Dr. Alam is working as a professor in the Department of Computer Science and Engineering at the Islamic University of Technology, Gazipur, Bangladesh. His research interests include wireless and mobile networking and performance modeling and analysis of networking systems.

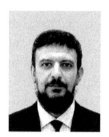

Raghied Mohammed Atta earned his BSc in electronics and communications engineering from the Faculty of Engineering, Cairo University, Cairo, Egypt, his MSc in signal processing from the Faculty of Electronic Engineering, Menoufia University, Menouf, Egypt, in 1992, and his PhD from the Department of Engineering, University of Cambridge, Cambridge, UK. Currently, he is an associate professor in the Electrical Engineering Department, Engineering College, Taibah University, Madinah, Kingdom of Saudi Arabia.

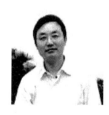

Guilin Chen earned his BS in mathematics from Anhui Normal University, Wuhu, China, in 1985, and MS in computer applications from Hefei University of Technology, Hefei, China, in 2007. Dr. Chen is currently a professor in the School of Computer and Information Engineering at Chuzhou University, Chuzhou, China. His main research interests include cloud computing, the Internet of Things, and big data.

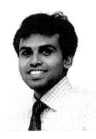

Md. Abdul Hamid earned his BE in computer and information engineering in 2001 from the International Islamic University Malaysia (IIUM), Seoul, Yongin, South Korea. In 2002, he became a lecturer at the Computer Science and Engineering Department, Asian University of Bangladesh, Dhaka, Bangladesh. He earned his PhD from the Computer Engineering Department at Kyung Hee University, Suwon, South Korea, in August 2009. In September 2009, he became an assistant professor in the Department of Information and Communications Engineering at Hankuk University of Foreign Studies, Yongin, South Korea. He then joined Green University of Bangladesh and worked as an assistant professor in the Department of Computer Science and Engineering from September 2012 to May 2013. Dr. Hamid is currently serving as a faculty member in the Department of Computer Engineering, Taibah University, Madinah, Kingdom of Saudi Arabia. His research interests include wireless sensor, mesh, ad hoc, and opportunistic networks with particular emphasis on network security, reliability, fairness, and quality-of-service issues.

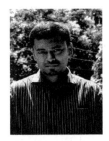

Abu Raihan Mostofa Kamal is currently serving as a faculty member in the Department of Computer Science and Engineering at the Islamic University of Technology, Gazipur, Bangladesh. He worked in the area of embedded networked systems, specifically wireless sensor networks, at the School of Computer Science and Informatics, University College Dublin, Dublin, Ireland. His PhD work focused on enhanced reliability in wireless sensor networks. He completed his PhD research under the supervision of Dr. Chris Bleakley in 2013. The core area of Dr. Kamal's research includes data and network fault detection in sensor networks. He completed his MSc in information and communication security at the Royal Institute of Technology, Stockholm, Sweden, in 2004. Dr. Kamal also worked as a postdoctoral researcher at the Nimbus Centre, Cork Institute of Technology, Cork, Ireland, between May 2013 and May 2014.

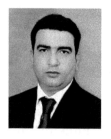

Nour El-Deen Mahmoud Khalifa earned his MS and PhD in 2009 and 2013, respectively, both from the Faculty of Computers and Information, Information Technology Department, Cairo University, Cairo, Egypt. Currently, he is a research doctor at the Faculty of Computers and Information at Cairo University. Dr. Khalifa's academic and research specialties are information technology, multimedia, wireless sensor networks, communication protocols in WMSNs, cryptography, wireless communication security, network security, multimedia security, and NS2.

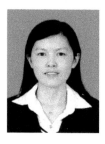

Xiaolan Liu earned her MS in information and communication engineering from Dalian Maritime University, Dalian, China, in 2009. Since 2009, she has been with the School of Computer and Information Engineering at Chuzhou University, Chuzhou, China. Her research interests include wireless camera sensor networks and barrier coverage.

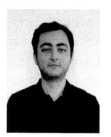

Mustafa Ozger earned his BSc in electrical and electronics engineering from Middle East Technical University, Ankara, Turkey, in 2011, and MSc in electrical and electronics engineering from Koc University, Istanbul, Turkey, in 2013. He is currently a research assistant in the Next-Generation and Wireless Communication Laboratory and pursuing his PhD at the Electrical and Electronics Engineering Department, Koc University, Istanbul, Turkey. His current research interests include cognitive radio networks and cognitive radio sensor networks.

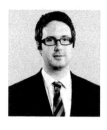

Ecehan B. Pehlivanoglu earned his BSc in electrical and electronics engineering from Middle East Technical University, Ankara, Turkey, in 2011. He is currently a research assistant at the Next-Generation Wireless and Communication Laboratory while pursuing his PhD at the Electrical and Electronics

Engineering Department, Koc University, Istanbul, Turkey. His research interests include cognitive radio, cognitive radio sensor networks, and nanoscale communications.

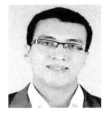

Ahmed Hussein Abbas Salem earned his BSc in communications and electronics engineering from Fayoum University, Fayoum, Egypt, in 2014. He is the author of several research papers published in a number of conference proceedings. His current research interests are network communications and routing, security protocols, and applications for wireless sensor networks.

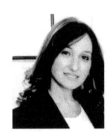

Pinar Sarisaray-Boluk earned her BS and MS in computer engineering from Karadeniz Technical University, Trabzon, Turkey. She earned her PhD in the Computer Engineering Department at Istanbul Technical University, Istanbul, Turkey. In 2013, she did postdoctoral training at the Computer Science Department of Southern Illinois University, Carbondale, Illinois. Currently, she is serving as an assistant professor in the Software Engineering Department at Bahcesehir University, Istanbul, Turkey. Her research interests are wireless sensor networks, network security, and software development, analysis, and design.

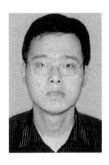

Bin Yang earned his BS and MS in computer science from Shihezi University, Shihezi, China, in 2004, and from the China University of Petroleum, Beijing, China, in 2007, respectively. He is currently a PhD candidate at the School of Systems Information Science, Future University Hakodate, Hakodate, Japan, and is also a faculty member at the School of Computer and Information Engineering, Chuzhou University, Chuzhou, China. His research interests include performance modeling and evaluation, stochastic optimization, and control in wireless networks, LTE-A, and 5G networks.

Introduction

Wireless Sensor Multimedia Networks

Wireless sensor networks (WSNs) are a special class of ad hoc networks in which network nodes are tiny sensors with limited processing power, memory, and battery power. These sensors cooperate to convey messages from each node to the sink node or gateway node.

Wireless sensor multimedia networks (WSMNs) are a special category of WSNs in which sensor nodes are small cameras and microphones, as shown in Figure I.1.

WSMNs differ greatly from WSNs. In WSNs, network nodes cooperate to convey scalar data such as temperature, pressure, humidity, and light to the sink node. In WSMNs, the data being sent are multimedia data such as voice, image, or video. However, scalar data can also be handled by a WSMN node, by adding the required sensors.

WSMNs have appeared as a result of intensive research in various areas such as VLSI, MEMS, digital signal processing, communications, and networks. The availability of inexpensive CMOS cameras and microphones accelerated the use of WSMNs in the market. Currently, WSMNs are attracting a great amount of attention from academia and industry due to the variety of applications where they can be deployed. Moreover, WSMNs have many challenges in their design and deployment.

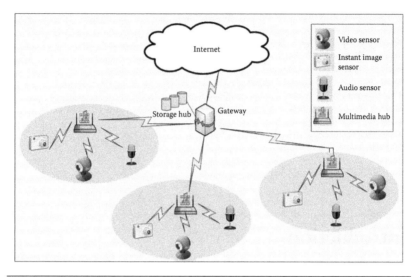

Figure I.1   WMSN architecture.

Benefits of WSMNs

WSMNs have the ability and flexibility to fuse and store multimedia content originating from different camera sources. Deploying multiple visual sensors as cameras has several benefits despite increasing the coverage and enlarging the field of view (FOV), but it also increases redundancy and reliability, as well. WSMNs offer the following benefits:

- Better enhanced FOV: This can be accomplished by using several cameras. When the FOV is dark, using a combination of cameras is beneficial to show the infrared and visible spectrum in the targeted scene.
- Larger FOV: Using several cameras enables a larger FOV. The main idea is to use several low-resolution cameras to trigger the few high-resolution cameras. These advanced cameras can then target the required event, using their pan–tilt–zoom functionality. This technique will provide the necessary quality at a lower cost.
- Adding several points of view: When an area such as a street needs to be monitored, one camera will not suffice, so several cameras are added to provide flexibility and several viewpoints.

These benefits have led to deploying WSMNs in a variety of applications:

- Surveillance, monitoring, and object protection applications: WSMNs help greatly in monitoring streets, public areas, and, more importantly, museums and borders.
- Storing footage of unusual events: WSMNs are able to record accidents, robberies, and traffic violations.
- Traffic congestion avoidance: Traffic in large cities can be monitored, which will help greatly, especially during rush hours.
- Health-care applications: In addition to sensing scalar data relevant to the patient—such as blood pressure, ECG, and heart rate—remote monitoring could be achieved by using motion sensors in conjunction with video and audio sensors. Recording the behavior of elderly people could be useful for research in the medical and health-care areas.
- Environmental applications: WSMNs can be used to monitor the environment and help warn of dangers such as global warming. For example, the polar ice caps could be monitored to predict the effects of global warming on the Earth's water levels.
- Habitat monitoring: Monitoring animals in certain areas will help in understanding the habits of wild animals and animals that prefer quiet settings.
- Localization services: Processing captured images and video may lead to locating missing objects or children and wanted criminals.

One of the challenging problems in WSMNs is routing the data collected from several cameras, especially if high resolution is required. Although providing better quality for images and videos is necessary, it shortens the network lifetime because the batteries will drain quickly. Therefore, minimizing energy consumption and developing energy-efficient protocols have become a must in WSMN.

WSMN Structure

A WSMN may have a simple structure, such as one or more nodes communicating directly to the base station through single-hop communication, which is known as star topology. Such a topology will not succeed in sizable applications. Therefore, it is essential to dissect WSMN operation. By dissecting the operation and the nodes to levels of hierarchy, energy consumption can be decreased and the network will be much more manageable and organized. WSMNs can have four main components:

1. Wireless multimedia nodes (WMNs): WMNs are the end points of the network. These nodes have a camera and a microphone. The WMN is mostly battery powered.
2. Wireless cluster head (WCH): The WCH receives data from several WMNs; it also removes scenes and events that are from the same FOV.
3. Wireless network node (WNN): A WNN acts as a relay node, delivering data from the network to the base station. Its main purpose is to decrease the distance between the network and the base station in order to decrease energy consumption.
4. The base station (BS): It collects the data on the PC for further processing and research applications.

The main goal of such a structure is decreasing energy consumption as much as possible.

The WSMN Node

The WSMN node is designed to be small in size with low power consumption and low cost. All WSMN nodes consist of the following four components:

1. The *communication unit* contains the transceiver, which is usually based on the ZigBee [1] (IEEE* 802.15.4) standard or 6LoWPAN (IPv6 over Low Power Wireless Personal Area Networks) [2]. These standards target low power consumption during transmission and reception processes. The simple difference between both standards is that 6LoWPAN supports relaying the sensor data to the Internet.
2. The *processing unit* will differ significantly from the processors used in normal WSNs, as the WSMN may contain a processor combined with a processor specific for image or

---

* IEEE, Institute of Electrical and Electronics Engineers.

video applications. Microcontrollers, DSPs, and application-specific processors are usually used in such nodes.

3. The *sensing unit* is the main difference between WSNs and WSMNs; WSMNs will have visual sensors like a camera and audio sensors such as a microphone.

4. The *power unit* is usually required to be portable, such as batteries.

WSMN Suppliers

In this section, we would like to point out one of the WSN suppliers, namely, Libelium [3]. Libelium is one of the high-end companies that succeeded in building a completely compatible, unique WSMN node. Libelium delivers a powerful, modular, easy-to-program open-source sensor platform for the Internet-of-Things enabling system. One of these products is the Waspmote. Waspmote is Libelium's advanced mote for WSNs; it can be integrated with different boards, such as the video camera board shown in Figure I.2.

Book Organization

Chapter 1: Multichannel, Multipath-Enabled, Quality-of-Service-Aware Routing for Wireless Multimedia Sensor Networks

This chapter presents a novel quality-of-service-aware routing proto-col to support a high data rate in wireless multimedia sensor networks.

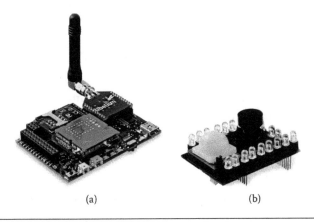

(a)   (b)

Figure I.2   (a) Libelium Waspmote and (b) a video camera board.

*Chapter 2: Adaptation Techniques for Multimedia Communication
in Wireless Sensor Networks*

This chapter first surveys different factors affecting the design of communication protocols and multimedia application algorithms for efficient multimedia communication in sensor networks. It also presents different protocols and algorithms used in the transport, network, and MAC layers of WSMNs. It evaluates them in terms of multimedia transmission. Finally, some multimedia adaptation techniques are presented for each protocol to give an optimistic perspective for future deployment.

*Chapter 3: Multimedia Communication in Cognitive Radio
Ad Hoc and Sensor Networks*

This chapter introduces the use of cognitive radio capability in sensor networks to increase the efficiency of overall spectrum utilization and to decrease the probability of collision and contention. This chapter also presents different factors influencing multimedia communications in cognitive radio ad hoc and sensor networks and demonstrates open research problems at different communication layers.

Chapter 4: Multimedia Streaming in Wireless Multimedia Sensor Networks

This chapter presents different multimedia streaming optimization techniques and highlights the differences between WSN and WSMN requirements for multimedia streaming.

Chapter 5: Coverage Problems for Wireless Multimedia Sensor Networks

This chapter describes the state of the art in influencing factors, deployment mechanisms, sensor selection, and performance metrics for WMSN node coverage. The authors present different types of coverage and state representative solution algorithms. Finally, they discuss existing problems and new research trends in some key realms.

*Chapter 6: A Security Scheme for Video Streaming
in Wireless Multimedia Sensor Networks*

This chapter surveys different attacks on WSMNs. It also proposes a new security scheme that is appropriate for real-time video streaming.

The performance of the proposed scheme is verified by simulation. Open research problems in this area are also presented.

Chapter 7: Power Management for Wireless Multimedia Sensor Networks

This chapter presents several ways of optimizing the power consumption of existing WSMNs. It also identifies various unconventional sources of energy harvesting based on the available techniques and compares their advantages.

Mohamed Mostafa A. Azim
Cairo University, Giza

Xiaohong Jiang
Future University, Hakodate

References

1. IEEE 802.15 WPAN Task Group 4. http://www.ieee802.org/15/pub/TG4.html
2. Kushalnagar, N. et al. IPv6 over Low-Power Wireless Personal Area Networks (6LoWPANs): Overview, assumptions, problem statement, and goals, *IETF RFC 4919*, Aug 2007. http://www.rfceditor.org/rfc/pdfrfc/rfc4919.txt.pdf
3. Libelium. http://www.libelium.com/

Multichannel, Multipath-Enabled, Quality-of-Service-Aware Routing for Wireless Multimedia Sensor Networks

MD. ABDUL HAMID, ABU RAIHAN MOSTOFA KAMAL, AND MUHAMMAD MAHBUB ALAM

Contents

The majority of sensor network routing protocols consider energy efficiency as the main objective and assume data traffic with unconstrained delivery requirements. However, the introduction of image and video sensors demands a certain quality of service (QoS) from the routing protocols and underlying networks. Managing such real-time data requires both energy efficiency and QoS assurances to ensure efficient usage of sensor resources and accuracy of the collected information. In this chapter, we discuss this issue and present a novel QoS-aware routing protocol to support a high data rate for wireless multimedia sensor networks (WMSNs). With multichannel, multipath technology, routing decisions are made according to dynamic adjustment of the required bandwidth and path-length-based proportional delay differentiation (PPDD) for real-time data. To justify QoS requirements and to offer differentiated service, we classified and prioritized the sensor data. Finally, we evaluated the protocol performance through rigorous simulation under different scenarios. The simulation results demonstrate significant improvement in performance in terms of average end-to-end delay, average lifetime, network throughput, packet drop ratio (PDR), and delivery ratio. In particular, we delve into a performance evaluation of single-sink and multiple-sink schemes.

1.1 Introduction

Wireless sensor networks (WSNs) have unique characteristics, such as self-configuration, low cost, easy deployment, and distributed sensing capacity. As a result, the field of WSNs has enjoyed tremendous research attention over the past decade. Traditional WSNs are often deployed in hard-to-reach areas for prolonged durations to report various real-time scalar data such as temperature, humidity, and light intensity. Usually such networks are operated for a long time without any human intervention. Successful WSN deployment [1–3] has gained a new and promising dimension among the research community with the introduction of multimedia data such as image and video. As a result, applications can get high-dimensional data with increased accuracy both in event detection and periodic monitoring. Furthermore, for cost–benefit analysis, recent trends indicate that multiple applications with varied QoS requirements can be efficiently deployed in a single network [4,5]. Consequently, WMSNs have received a great deal of research attention in recent years. Traditional protocols for WSN cannot cope with MWSN gracefully because they were designed to handle scalar data from a single application. In this chapter, we present a novel QoS-aware packet delivery technique to support high data rates and delay bound requirements for WMSNs. The promising pace of technological growth has led to the design of sensor nodes with the capability of sensing the environment and producing multimedia data. However, because multimedia traffic contains images, video, audio, and scalar data, each merits a different metric. To accommodate a high data rate, designing an efficient routing protocol is of primary interest. The significance of such a protocol becomes clear with a few challenging and motivating facts. First, research challenges found in Ref. [6] state that existing data rates of about 40 and 250 kbit/s supported by the MICA2 and MICAz [7] motes are not geared to support multimedia traffic. Instead of improving the hardware and thus increasing cost, an alternate approach is to more efficiently utilize the available bandwidth. By using multiple channels in a spatially overlapped manner, the existing bandwidth can be leveraged to support multimedia applications. Second, the use of multipath technology has two clear advantages: (1) the load may be balanced so as not to overwhelm the limited buffers at the intermediate sensor nodes and (2) one path condition may not permit a high data rate for the entire duration of the event being monitored. By allowing multiple paths, the effective data rate of each path gets reduced and the application can be supported. This chapter presents a protocol that targets the application of WMSNs where sensors produce multimedia content from the deployed area to deal with both critical and general data. Applications may include critical condition monitoring and security surveillance tasks such as monitoring a volcano explosion, toxic gases, or a forest fire; military applications such as sniper or enemy detection; and civil applications such as the location of survivors for rescue services. Once a node detects an important event, fast and reliable delivery is required; late or failed delivery may cause disaster. In a real-time application such as multimedia streaming, delivered data can become useless in only a few milliseconds.

Though most currently deployed sensor networks use the same channel to communicate information among nodes, a significant number of current sensor node prototypes use radio modules capable of transmission on multiple channels. For example, the radio capabilities of the MICAz mote allow communication on multiple frequencies as specified in IEEE* standard 802.15.4. The idea of using multiple channels in wireless networks is not new. One study [8] has shown how the capacity of a static multichannel network scales as the number of nodes in the network increases. The authors show that it may be possible to build capacity optimal multichannel networks with as few as one interface per node. The authors of [9] present a multichannel defense mechanism against jamming attacks in WSNs by automatically and efficiently assigning nodes to different channels in the jammed area to defeat an attacker. The work presented in Ref. [10] introduces a control-theoretic approach for maximizing throughput in multichannel sensor networks by choosing node communication frequencies such that the total network throughput is maximized.

Classical multipath routing has been explored for two reasons. The first is load balancing (where traffic is split across multiple disjoint paths) and the second is to increase the likelihood of reliable data delivery (multiple copies of data are sent along different paths). Although a plethora of techniques have been developed for sensor networks, all protocols featured either multipath or multichannel technology. In fact, QoS provisioning is a challenging task for multimedia sensor networks because link capacity and delay vary continuously and may be bursty in nature [6]. Creating a QoS provisioning routing protocol with the efficient use of both multipath and multichannel technology to support the high data rate requirement for WMSNs has not been addressed. In this chapter, we present a mechanism for packet delivery over a multipath, multichannel-provisioned WMSN in which multimedia sensors ubiquitously retrieve multimedia contents from the environment. The initial version of this work can be found in Ref. [11]. Our main goal is to support a high data rate while maintaining the attainable delay so that packets can be delivered to the destination

---

* IEEE, Institute of Electrical and Electronics Engineers.

with their bandwidth and delay requirements. The main contributions of the chapter can be summarized as follows:

- We designed a QoS-aware routing protocol for WMSNs. More specifically, our design is based on multipath, multichannel technology, which influences how routing decisions for real-time and non-real-time multimedia traffic are made, using dynamic bandwidth adjustment and PPDD. To meet bandwidth requirements, the proposed technique provides network-wide dynamic bandwidth-adjustment options for the nodes in a distributed manner. To meet delay requirements, the proposed technique provides PPDD options, extending the idea of the PDD mechanism in Ref. [12].
- In order to define QoS in WMSNs, we classified data traffic, which facilitates the prioritization of different data packets.
- Rigorous simulation was carried out to evaluate the performance of the proposed design. The results show the advantages of our approach over the existing approach in terms of throughput, end-to-end delay, lifetime, PDR, and network-wise delivery ratio (NDR). Improvement was also noticed in multiple-sink scenarios, which is a natural solution for a very large network.

The rest of this chapter is organized as follows. Section 1.2 describes an overview of existing background works. Section 1.3 provides the network model and assumptions. Section 1.4 presents the proposed QoS-aware routing protocol in detail. Section 1.5 presents performance evaluation through simulation. Finally, Section 1.6 concludes this work with a summary and some future research challenges.

1.2 Background

A large number of studies have been carried out in this area since data collection became the most important aspect of WSNs. The findings of research challenges and the current status of the literature on multimedia communication in WSNs are presented in Refs. [6,13,14]. More specifically, factors influencing multimedia delivery over WSNs and currently proposed solutions for application, transport, and network layers are pointed out along with their shortcomings and open research issues. Cucchiara [15] gives a short overview of the hot topics in multimedia surveillance systems and introduces some research activities currently underway worldwide. For example, a multiflow real-time transport protocol described in Ref. [16] does not specifically address energy efficiency considerations in WMSNs, but is suited for real-time streaming of multimedia content by splitting packets over different flows. In Ref. [17], a wakeup scheme is proposed that tries to balance energy and delay constraints. In Ref. [18], the proposed protocol has an interesting feature: to establish multiple paths (optimal and suboptimal) with different energy metrics and assigned probabilities. Hence, it is inherently a multipath protocol with QoS measurements and a good fit for routing of multimedia streams in WSNs.

Recently, Hamid and Bashir [19] proposed a cross-layer QoS protocol for WMSNs. The protocol provides interaction between energy-based admission control, delay- and interference-aware routing, and dynamic duty cycle assignment in the MAC layer. Kim and Sung [20] proposed a scheme for efficiently and reliably delivering real-time multimedia streams in WSNs. To specify the property of streams, a multimedia stream is modeled as an (m,k)-firm stream that is known to have the characteristics of a weakly hard real-time system. A cross-layer framework is proposed in Ref. [21] to support QoS in WMSNs to enhance the number of video sources, given that the QoS constraint of each individual source is also preserved. Their goal is achieved by implementing Wyner–Ziv lossy distributed source coding at the sensor node with variable group of pictures size, exploiting multipath routing for real-time delivery and link adaptation to enhance the bandwidth under the given bit error rate. Touil et al. [22] analyzed energy consumption and evaluated the performance of the 802.11e enhanced distributed channel access (EDCA) with and without the contention-free burst (CFB) mechanism, compared with IEEE 802.11 DCF. They showed that the use of EDCA CFB gives better performance and offers a very good relationship between energy consumption and traffic performance, which is recommended in WMSNs.

A QoS provisioning multipath and multi-SPEED routing protocol (MMSPEED) was proposed [23]; MMSPEED spans the network layer and medium access control layer to provide QoS differentiation in timeliness and reliability. To support both best-effort and real-time traffic at the same time, a class-based queuing model was employed in Ref. [24]. The queuing model allows service sharing for real-time and non-real-time traffic. The bandwidth ratio r is defined as an initial value set by the gateway and represents the amount of bandwidth to be dedicated both to the real-time and non-real-time traffic on a particular outgoing link in case of congestion. As a consequence, the throughput for normal data does not decrease, provided that this r value is properly adjusted. However, the same r value is initially set for all nodes; the selection is done in such a way that it will satisfy the delay requirement for the least hop node, which does not allow flexible adjustment of bandwidth sharing for different links. Moreover, the average delay increases with a higher real-time data rate. The protocol was extended in Ref. [25] by assigning a different r value for each node to achieve better utilization of the links. In addition, the average delay per packet does not increase overly much with an increase in the real-time data rate. However, finding the r values and sending these to a particular node not only requires overhead but is energy consuming as well, because the r values have to be unicasted to every single node. Moreover, when a route changes, a set of new r values has to be calculated for all the nodes in the new route and transmitted to the nodes. In our protocol, each node locally adjusts the bandwidth and delay requirement based on the path-length and incoming traffic.

1.3 Network Model

WMSNs have several additional features and challenges compared with traditional WSNs. We considered a static wireless network containing multimedia sensor nodes capable of performing all possible application tasks (e.g., capable of sensing video, audio, scalar data). The following definitions describe a network scenario where the proposed routing protocol fits well.

- Multimedia node (M node): A sensor node capable of generating multimedia data (such as video and image) in real-time interaction with the environment is termed an M node. M nodes are often equipped with additional storage capacity to store their local data.
- Scalar node (S node): S nodes are limited to scalar data such as temperature, humidity, and light intensity.

- Sink: A node with higher computational and storage capacity is regarded as the data collection point for the network. For a single sink scheme, the network inherits a many-to-one traffic pattern; all data packets are routed to the sink node.
- Relay node (R node): Due to the limitations of short-range radio connectivity, a network often requires additional nodes to simply relay incoming packets to its next nodes toward the sink.
- Processing hub (PH): Essentially, PH nodes are a subset of R nodes whose main task is some in-network processing (i.e., data aggregation, discard of redundant data) in a distributed fashion in the network. Some PHs are called multimedia processing hubs (MPHs) because of their higher capabilities to process multimedia sensor data.
- Target area: The core purpose of WMSNs is to observe a specified area and report the status in real time. We term this area the *target area*, or *monitored area*.
- Network size: A network is said to have a network size N if there exist a total of N nodes, with the implicit assumption that nodes are uniformly distributed.

Figure 1.1 demonstrates the above components in a single network setup. Both the M nodes and MPH are equipped with a single radio

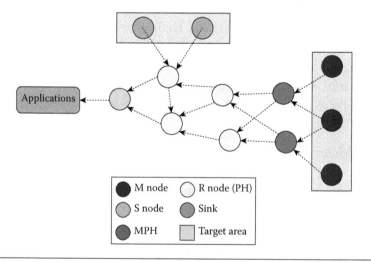

Figure 1.1   Network model: wireless multimedia sensor network.

interface and multiple channels, and the radio interface is capable of transmitting or receiving data on one channel at a given time. The task of the multimedia nodes is to dynamically serve the need of multimedia data to travel from the target area to the sink.

1.4 QoS-Aware Routing Protocol

A QoS-aware routing protocol is presented in this section. In the following, first a multipath, multichannel-provisioned network topology is constructed and, second, a packet-scheduling technique is presented to meet the QoS requirements.

1.4.1 Multipath, Multichannel Network Topology Construction

To realize the network with multipath, multichannel provisions, we used techniques based on a multipath construction mechanism [26] and multichannel assignment technique [9]. The outcome of these techniques was to assign each network node with the knowledge of available paths and channels to transmit and receive data packets. Figure 1.2 shows one possible multipath construction scheme, which has been described [26] as multiple localized, disjoined paths that use localized information alone and do not rely on global topology. As shown in Figure 1.2a, some path request packets have initially been flooded throughout the network by the source nodes. The sink then has some empirical information about which of its neighbors can provide it with the highest quality data (lowest loss or lowest delay).

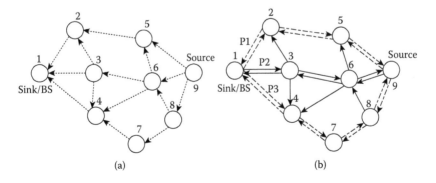

Figure 1.2 Multipath construction: (a) multipath dissemination using flooding (single source to single sink is shown) and (b) three alternative paths P1, P2, and P3 shown with double arrow lines.

To this preferred neighbor, it sends out a primary-path (P3) reinforcement, as shown in Figure 1.2b. As with the basic directed diffusion scheme, that neighbor then locally determines its most preferred neighbor in the direction of the source, and so on. Accordingly, alternative paths P1 and P2 are constructed [26].

The next task is to assign each node its transmission activities to efficiently utilize the bandwidth using multiple frequencies (channels). Mutually orthogonal Latin square (MOLS) based scheduling is applied to assign transmission and reception activities, presented in Ref. [9], as described below.

Definition 1: A $p \times q$ rectangular array formed by the symbols 1, 2, ..., k, where $k \geq p$ and $k \geq q$, is called a Latin rectangle if every symbol from the symbol set appears at most once in each column and once in each row.

Definition 2: A Latin square A of order p is a $p \times p$ matrix with entries from a set of p distinct symbols such that each row and column contains every element exactly once. The symbol in the ith row and the jth column is written as $a_{i,j}$.

Definition 3: Two distinct $p \times p$ Latin squares A and B, where $a_{i,j}$ and $b_{i,j} \in 1, 2, ..., p$, are said to be orthogonal if the p^2 ordered pairs $\langle ..., (a_{i,j}, b_{i,j}) ... \rangle$ are all different.

The square matrices S and R as shown in Figure 1.3 are examples of Latin squares of order 7. In Latin square–based scheduling, channels correspond to the rows and time slots correspond to the columns [27]. According to Definition 3, the two 7×7 Latin squares S and R are orthogonal.

Lemma 1: If two nodes are assigned two symbols from two different orthogonal Latin squares, then there is at most one collision for these two nodes in every time frame (proof is given in Ref. [27]).

$$S = \begin{bmatrix} 0 & 1 & 2 & 3 & 4 & 5 & 6 \\ 1 & 2 & 3 & 4 & 5 & 6 & 0 \\ 2 & 3 & 4 & 5 & 6 & 0 & 1 \\ 3 & 4 & 5 & 6 & 0 & 1 & 2 \\ 4 & 5 & 6 & 0 & 1 & 2 & 3 \\ 5 & 6 & 0 & 1 & 2 & 3 & 4 \\ 6 & 0 & 1 & 2 & 3 & 4 & 5 \end{bmatrix} \quad R = \begin{bmatrix} 1 & 2 & 3 & 4 & 5 & 0 & 6 \\ 2 & 3 & 4 & 5 & 6 & 1 & 0 \\ 3 & 4 & 5 & 6 & 0 & 2 & 1 \\ 4 & 5 & 6 & 0 & 1 & 3 & 2 \\ 5 & 6 & 0 & 1 & 2 & 4 & 3 \\ 6 & 0 & 1 & 2 & 3 & 5 & 4 \\ 0 & 1 & 2 & 3 & 4 & 6 & 5 \end{bmatrix}$$

Figure 1.3 Example of two Latin squares of order 7.

During the network initialization phase, a distributed distance-2 vertex coloring algorithm [28] is performed. This approach requires only local information from immediate neighbors to assign the vertex color to the network node. The algorithm outputs different vertex colors to all nodes within interference range of each other (the two-hop distance is a good approximation of the carrier sensing range in ad hoc networks, and node activation scheduling usually requires all neighbors of a node within two hops to be silent when the node transmits [9]). Therefore, the problem of assigning square symbols to network nodes can be modeled as a distance-2 graph coloring problem such that each node can directly use its assigned vertex color as its square symbol. In addition to vertex coloring, MOLS matrices are generated during the network initialization phase.

The orthogonality of the squares corresponds to there being exactly one time/channel assignment for every pair of nodes in different squares. In this way, a node can decide to be a sender or a receiver by picking the appropriate square. For example, let the entries in the square labeled S represent the set of sender nodes and the entries in square R represent the set of receiving nodes. Combining the two squares together will result in a unique time/channel assignment for each pair of senders/receivers, as shown in Figure 1.4. The uniqueness of each pair assignment is guaranteed by the orthogonality of the two squares.

As shown in Figure 1.5, suppose nine nodes numbered from one to nine get seven different colors numbered from zero to six. Any pair of communicating nodes may select appropriate symbols according to their vertex colors to be a sender/receiver pair for a collision-free transmission/reception. With these multipath multichannel provisions,

$$SR = \begin{bmatrix} (0,1) & (1,2) & (2,3) & (3,4) & (4,5) & (5,0) \\ (1,2) & (2,3) & (3,4) & (4,5) & (5,6) & (6,1) \\ (2,3) & (3,4) & (4,5) & (5,6) & (6,0) & (0,2) \\ (3,4) & (4,5) & (5,6) & (6,0) & (0,1) & (1,3) \\ (4,5) & (5,6) & (6,0) & (0,1) & (1,3) & (2,4) \\ (5,6) & (6,0) & (0,1) & (1,2) & (2,3) & (3,5) \\ (6,0) & (0,1) & (1,2) & (2,3) & (3,4) & (4,6) \end{bmatrix}$$

Figure 1.4   Example of SR matrix.

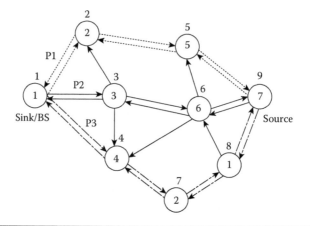

Figure 1.5 Vertex coloring to assign Latin square symbols to nodes. Each circle represents a network node, and assigned colors are numbered inside the circle.

nodes in the network may decide to forward packets to the appropriate path/channel depending on the desired QoS requirements (i.e., required bandwidth and delay as described later).

1.4.2 QoS-Aware Packet Scheduling

In this section, we describe different types of multimedia traffic and queuing models, how to provide QoS assurance, and how to route the traffic toward the destination.

1.4.2.1 Traffic Classification and Queuing Model Sensor data may originate from various types of events that have different levels of importance, as depicted in Table 1.1. Hence, packet-scheduling policy should consider different priorities (importance) for different types of traffic classes. Time-critical (delay bound) packets are assigned a high priority compared to non-time-critical packets to meet the deadlines. Because local packet drop policy is aware of the type of packet it receives, we rationalize it by expanding the length L of each queue q_i a function of its p value. More specifically,

$$L(q_i) = \frac{1}{p\,\text{value}(q_i)} \times \alpha \qquad (1.1)$$

where α is a network-dependent constant.

Table 1.1   Multimedia Traffic Classification for Wireless Multimedia Sensor Networks

TRAFFIC CLASS	NAME/EXAMPLE	DELAY	LOSS	BANDWIDTH
Class I ($p = 1$)	Real-time/ video–audio streams	Bounded	Tolerant	High
Class II ($p = 2$)	Real-time/ monitoring processes	Bounded	Intolerant	Low to moderate
Class III ($p = 3$)	Non-real-time/ video–audio stream	Unbounded	Tolerant	High
Class IV ($p = 4$)	Non-real-time/ scalar, snapshot	Unbounded	Tolerant	Low

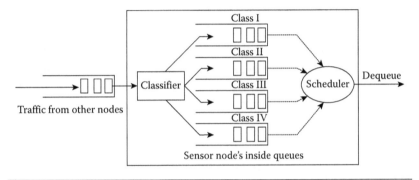

Figure 1.6   Queuing model on a multimedia sensor node.

Figure 1.6 shows the queuing model for a sensor node considering the different traffic classes described in Table 1.1. On each node, there is a classifier to check the type of the incoming packet and to send it to an appropriate queue. Finally, there is a scheduler that schedules the packets according to the delay bound and bandwidth requirements. Note that Equation 1.1 ensures that a high priority packet is assigned to a longer queue and vice versa.

1.4.2.2 QoS Assurance   To meet the QoS requirements for a packet from source to destination along a path, let us derive a path-specific condition. Suppose a packet p_i on path P originated at the source node at time t_i and has to reach the destination by $t_i + T_i$, where T_i is the deadline of packet p_i. The arrival time of the packet at hop

j denotes the time it is inserted into the queue at that node. The departure time of p_i from hop j denotes the time the transmission of p_i is completed. The arrival time of p_i at hop $j + 1$ is equal to its departure time from j plus propagation delay. Let the time this packet p_i spends at hop j be d_j, which is the interval between its arrival time and departure time at hop j; let s_j denote the switching delay from one channel to another at each hop. So, the packet p_i will reach the destination while preserving the delay bound if

$$\sum_{j=1}^{H} d_j + \rho_j + s_j \leq T_i \tag{1.2}$$

where ρ_j is the propagation delay for each hop j and H is the total number of hops a packet travels. The propagation delay in Equation 1.2 can be neglected, since packet propagation occurs at the speed of light and is therefore much faster than transmission and queuing delays. Considering the delay for a specific path, the sink (network designer) may determine the required bandwidth consumed by different traffic classes. We denote B as the required bandwidth. Initially, the sink will determine the value of B based on the observed delay for a time-critical traffic class and will broadcast this value. After receiving the value, all nodes will dynamically calculate their own value for B considering the distance of the nodes from the sink for a particular path. Then a PPDD model will determine the delay encountered by each packet in a particular queue along the path. Finally, the waiting time priority (WTP) algorithm [12] will be exploited to dequeue packets from the queues according to the service class and waiting time.

Dynamic Bandwidth Adjustment As both real-time and non-real-time traffic coexist, bandwidth should be used effectively, so that not only are the QoS requirements of real-time traffic met but service to the non-real-time traffic is also maximized. As mentioned earlier, a parameter B is used to control the bandwidth used by real-time and non-real-time traffic. As shown in Figure 1.7, Node 4 has more traffic than Node 3, 2, or 1; accordingly, Node 4 should allocate more bandwidth. We assume that the rate of real-time data is almost inversely proportional to the hop count of the node from the sink.

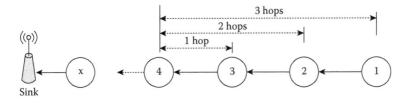

Figure 1.7 Dynamic bandwidth adjustment and path-length-based proportional delay differentiation calculation.

As stated earlier, if the sink broadcasts a value for B based on the observed delay for time-critical traffic, then each node adjusts its own B value according to the following equation:

$$B_H = \frac{B}{H + \alpha} \tag{1.3}$$

Here, H is the hop count of the node from the sink; α is the adjusting factor and the node will set this value based on the incoming traffic. When the sink observes that the end-to-end delay is increasing, it increases the value of B to allocate more bandwidth to real-time traffic, and vice versa. In addition, the sink tries to make the value of B as low as possible without violating the QoS requirement to maximize the bandwidth use of non-real-time traffic.

PPDD: The PPDD is a differentiated services based proposal that is an extension of PDD [12], defined for wired networks. The PPDD scheduler services packets in classes and realizes proportional average per-hop queuing delays among them locally at each node along the path. At node k, packets from class i experience smaller delay than class j for all $i > j$, $i, j \in S_{b,k}$, where $S_{b,k}$ is the set of backlogged classes at node k. Usually, the end-to-end delay of a packet is proportional to the number of hops. For example, for a path, a packet that is H hops away from the sink experiences a smaller end-to-end delay than a packet that is more than H hops away from the sink. As shown in Figure 1.5, a packet from Node 1 will experience more end-to-end delay than a packet from Node 4. The spacing between delays is tuned by the sink based on observed delay of the real-time packet with a set of class differentiation parameters. As its name suggests, the model not only holds at each node it also holds across all nodes in a path. The PPDD service model is defined as follows.

Let $1 = \partial_1 > \partial_2 > \ldots > \partial_H > 0$ be delay differentiation parameters that define that a packet of a node smaller hops away from the sink may allow higher delay than a packet that arrives from a node more hops away. Let d_H^k denote the average queuing delay of a packet at node k that is H hops away from the sink. Then, the PPDD requirement is given according to the following equation:

$$\frac{d_H^k}{d_{H+1}^k} = \frac{\partial_H}{\partial_{H+1}} \tag{1.4}$$

Then, with WTP, each class is serviced with a separate first-in-first-out queue. The head-of-line packet of a class is assigned a WTP based on the service class and waiting time of the packet. The scheduler always schedules the highest priority head-of-line packet for transmission.

1.4.2.3 Routing Single Sink The packets are routed through the nodes along the path from the source to the destination; nodes choose the paths/channels that meet the bandwidth and delay requirements. Each node knows the available path options and collision-free channel assignment among its two-hop neighbors and adjusts bandwidth and delay according to Equations 1.2 and 1.3, respectively, to relay traffic along the path. Packets that do not meet the deadline (i.e., QoS requirements) are discarded. Best-effort traffic is routed through the alternative paths to balance the distribution of the remaining traffic. Redundant data are aggregated by the PHs to reduce the network traffic.

Multiple Sinks Initially, we considered deployment of WMSNs based on a many-to-one communication paradigm, where a single sink collects data from a number of data sources. Because our protocol deals with real-time and non-real-time data, we may exploit scenarios with multiple sinks to further balance the distribution of traffic. With the resulting many-to-many communication paradigm, each node might adjust the bandwidth, delay, and path length of different sinks to route the packets. For example, real-time data may be routed to the nearest sink (i.e., with a path length smaller than that of other available sinks), and less sensitive non-real-time data may be routed to the longest route, because the delay requirement is flexible for such data.

1.5 Performance Evaluation

The effectiveness of the proposed QoS routing approach was evaluated through simulation in ns-2 [29] under various situations. Initially, we considered a network of size 100 (N = 100) uniformly placed in a 1000 × 1000 meter area. Nodes were positioned as a 10 × 10 square grid. Nodes within one and two hops were marked as R nodes. The sink was placed at the center (0,0). Other nodes were operated as either M nodes or N nodes. Table 1.2 shows the simulation parameters in more detail. Some parameters of the table were taken from Ref. [25]. To evaluate the performance of the proposed routing approach, we used the following performance metrics, which apply to the entire evaluation section:

- EDP (end-to-end delay per packet): The EDP is measured as the time difference between sensing the data and receiving it by the sink.
- PDR: The PDR indicates the number of packets dropped per time unit due to congestion or local buffer overflow.
- NDR: The NDR is computed as the ratio of the total number of successfully delivered packets to the total number of packets sent by all source nodes in the network [30].
- Network throughput: The network throughput is measured as the total number of data packets received at the sink divided by the entire simulation time.

Table 1.2   Simulation Parameters

PARAMETERS	VALUE
Network size (N)	100
Radio model*	Free space
Packet generation rate (non-real-time)*	1 packet/s
Packet generation rate (real-time)*	8 packet/s
Maximum data packet length*	10 kbit
Maximum control packet length*	2 kbit
Total number of channels	7
Channel switching delay	250 ms
Number of M nodes	15 (15% of N)
Number of S nodes	15 (15% of N)
Simulation duration	100 s
Number of iterations	10

1.5.1 Effects on End-to-End Delay

First, we consider the impact of the real-time data rate on the average delay per packet for both real- and non-real-time data. The average delay per packet is defined as the average time a packet takes to travel from a sensor node to the sink. We observed that both multiple-r and single-r mechanisms had a higher average delay compared to our proposed protocol, as shown in Figure 1.8a. The multiple-r mechanism performed better than the single-r mechanism, as expected; every particular node adjusts its r value based on the resources available. This method is more efficient than the single-r mechanism, in which a unique r value is imposed by the sink for all the nodes. Intuitively, the average delay per packet for the proposed protocol is less than for the single-r mechanism. The reason is that forwarding nodes locally adjust the bandwidth (value of B) proportional to the expected load instead of assigning a single value of r for all forwarding nodes. Moreover, even though the value of B is not set exactly like the multiple-r mechanism, the average delay is less for the multiple-r mechanism. The rationale behind this system is that the multiple-r mechanism uses unicast transmission to deliver the individual value to the nodes; our protocol requires smaller control packets (because a single B value is sent to all nodes), which in turn increases the forwarding rate of the data packets.

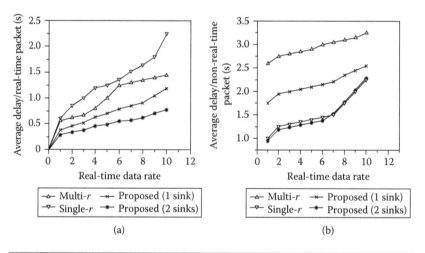

(a)   (b)

Figure 1.8   Impact of the real-time data generation rate on the (a) average delay per real-time packet and (b) average delay per non-real-time packet.

Figure 1.8b shows the effect of the real-time data rate on the average delay per non-real-time packet. The delay increases with the rate, because packets incur more queuing delay and share the same amount of bandwidth. Note that the average delay for non-real-time packets using the multiple-r mechanism is greater than for the single-r mechanism. With the multiple-r mechanism, the increase in the throughput of non-real-time packets causes an extra queuing delay on the nodes, leading non-real-time packets to experience end-to-end delay [25]. Our protocol has less average delay compared to the multiple-r protocol, because the nodes can schedule non-real-time packets and exploit multiple paths.

1.5.2 Scalability Assessment

To evaluate the scalability of the proposed routing scheme, we repeated the simulation with different settings for the network size (N). In this case, we varied N from 25 to 200. Note that the end-to-end delay with a smaller network ($N \leq 50$) was not significantly different for either the previous or proposed schemes (Figure 1.9). However, with a larger network, the improvement was remarkable; for instance, a network with $N = 200$ using our proposed routing scheme (with one source) experienced an average of 47.8% less delay compared with that of the previous method using the single-r mechanism. Apart from this advantage, the presented methods showed a linear increase in their end-to-end delay parameters with respect to network size. Therefore, the routing mechanism presented herein can be efficiently deployed for a larger network.

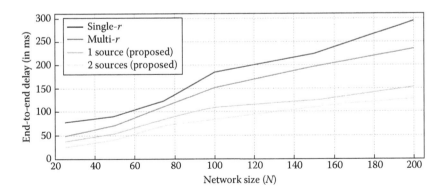

Figure 1.9   End-to-end delay for a large network.

1.5.3 Effects on Network Throughput

Next, we consider network throughput, which is measured as the total number of data packets received at the sink divided by the simulation time. Figure 1.10a shows the non-real-time data throughput. Our protocol outperforms existing protocols due to efficient utilization of the wireless spectrum. When the number of real-time packets increases, it gets more difficult to satisfy the increasing need for QoS paths, leading to rejection of paths or packet drops for non-real-time data and causing throughput for such data to decrease. Figure 1.10b shows the average lifetime of the nodes, illustrating that our model consumes less energy compared to both the other models. The reason is that our model does not require multiple unicast transmission of the r value, unlike the multiple-r mechanism. Moreover, the PHs perform in-network data aggregation and channel assignment, which results in fewer collisions.

1.5.4 Packet Drop Ratio

One of the major motivations for this work stems from the fact that, in multi-application WSN setups, it is not wise to treat every data packet equally, as most routing protocols do [30]. In this section, we analyzed the trace from the simulation to assess the effects of PDR on each type of traffic (Classes I to IV). Figure 1.11 depicts the findings. It shows that

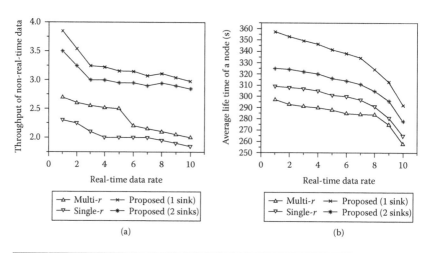

Figure 1.10 Impact of the real-time data generation rate on (a) the throughput of non-real-time data and (b) the average lifetime of a node.

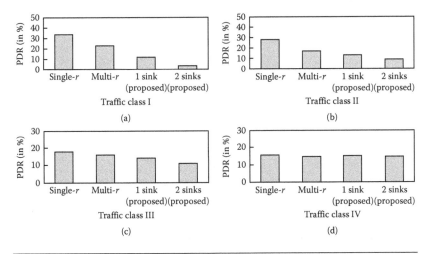

Figure 1.11 Packet drop ratio: a comparative study with different classes of data traffic.

for traffic of Classes I, II, and III, the traditional methods (multiple-r and single-r mechanisms) incurred a higher PDR compared with our proposal. This higher rate is a result of the prioritization of each packet. High priority packets are assigned to longer queues, which ensures lower probability of being dropped because of local buffer overflow. Furthermore, they are transmitted in a multipath fashion to attain higher network reliability. In the case of low priority packets (Class IV), the achievement is not noticeable, because these packets are the primary targets to be dropped. We occasionally obtained a higher PDR using our proposal (data not shown; only the averaged value is plotted in Figure 1.11).

1.5.5 Network-Wise Delivery Ratio

The primary goal of this work is to ensure higher reliability in delivering sensor information for MWSNs. We assessed the NDR to justify the network-wise overall improvement. We varied the network size N from 25 to 200. The findings are graphed in Figure 1.12. For smaller networks, the NDR was almost 100% for all schemes. With multiple-r and single-r schemes, the NDR dropped rapidly when N became larger than 50: the average NDRs recorded were 81.67% and 83.78% for the single-r and multiple-r schemes, respectively. Using our proposed schemes, the average NDRs were 92.7% and 95.167% for one- and two-sink networks, respectively. These figures suggest that our proposed scheme ensures a high degree of reliability in terms of NDR even for a very large network.

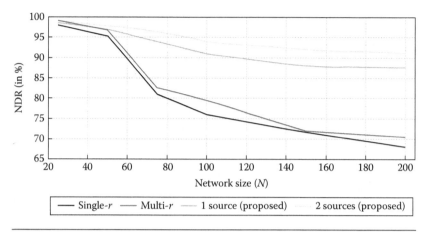

Figure 1.12   Network-wise delivery ratio: a comparative study.

1.6 Conclusions

In this chapter, we described and presented a QoS-aware routing mechanism to meet the challenges posed by WMSNs. We considered many-to-one and many-to-many communication scenarios to evaluate the performance of the scheme using a single sink and multiple sinks (two sinks). In all cases, the sensor nodes were considered to be static. We showed that the proposed QoS-aware routing mechanism provides a significant performance improvement in terms of average delay, average lifetime, network throughput, PDR, and NDR. In particular, we showed that, with more than one sink, data gathering can be further improved with the proper routing technique. In future works, it would be interesting to experiment with performance issues for the mobile sink and at the same time to implement this protocol in a test-bed to measure its efficiency with commercial sensors.

References

1. Szewczyk, R., Mainwaring, A., Polastre, J., Anderson, J., Culler, D. An analysis of a large scale habitat monitoring application. In: *Proceedings of the 2nd International Conference on Embedded Networked Sensor Systems, SenSys '04*, pp. 214–226. ACM, New York, NY, 2004. DOI: 10.1145/1031495.1031521.
2. Tolle, G., Polastre, J., Szewczyk, R., Culler, D., Turner, N., Tu, K., Burgess, S. et al. A macroscope in the redwoods. In: *Proceedings of the 3rd International Conference on Embedded Networked Sensor Systems, SenSys '05*, pp. 51–63, ACM, New York, NY, 2005. DOI: 10.1145/1098918.1098925.

3. Ingelrest, F., Barrenetxea, G., Schaefer, G., Vetterli, M., Couach, O., Parlange, M. Sensorscope: Application-specific sensor network for environmental monitoring. *ACM Transactions on Sensor Networks* 6, 1–32, 2010. DOI: 10.1145/1689239.1689247.

4. Tavakoli, A., Kansal, A., Nath, S. On-line sensing task optimization for shared sensors. In: *Proceedings of the 9th ACM/IEEE International Conference on Information Processing in Sensor Networks, IPSN '10*, pp. 47–57. ACM, New York, NY, 2010. DOI: 10.1145/1791212.1791219.

5. Bhattacharya, S., Saifullah, A., Lu, C., Roman, G.C. Multi-application deployment in shared sensor networks based on quality of monitoring. In: *Proceedings of the 2010 16th IEEE Real-Time and Embedded Technology and Applications Symposium, RTAS '10*, pp. 259–268, IEEE Computer Society, Washington, DC, 2010. DOI: 10.1109/RTAS.2010.20.

6. Akyildiz, I.F., Melodia, T., Chowdhury, K.R. A survey on wireless multimedia sensor networks. *Computer Networks* 51(4), 921–960, 2007. DOI: 10.1016/j.comnet.2006.10.002.

7. Data Sheet for Micaz Mote. http://www.xbow.com/Products/wCatalogs.aspx, 2010.

8. Kyasanur, P., Vaidya, N.H. Capacity of multi-channel wireless networks: Impact of number of channels and interfaces. In: *Proceedings of ACM International Conference on Mobile Computing and Networking (MobiCom)*, pp. 43–57, Cologne, Germany, 2005.

9. Alnifie, G., Simon, R. A multi-channel defense against jamming attacks in wireless sensor networks. In: *Proceedings of the 3rd ACM Workshop on QoS and Security for Wireless and Mobile Networks Chania*, pp. 95–104, Crete Island, Greece, 2007.

10. Le, H.K., Henriksson, D., Abdelzaher, T. A control theory approach to throughput optimization in multi-channel collection sensor networks. In: *Information Processing in Sensor Networks, 2007. IPSN 2007. 6th International Symposium*, pp. 31–40, ACM: New York, NY, 2007. DOI: 10.1109/IPSN.2007.4379662.

11. Hamid, M.A., Alam, M.M., Hong, C.S. Design of a QoS-aware routing mechanism for wireless multimedia sensor networks. In: *IEEE Global Communications Conference (GLOBECOM)*, pp. 800–805, 2008.

12. Dovrolis, C., Stiliadis, D., Ramanathan, P. Proportional differentiated services: Delay differentiation and packet scheduling. *IEEE/ACM Transactions on Networking* 10(1), 12–26, 2002.

13. Gurses, E., Akan, O.B. Multimedia communication in wireless sensor networks. *Annales des Telecommunications* 60(7–8), 872–900, 2005.

14. Ehsan, S., Hamdaoui, B. A survey on energy-efficient routing techniques with QoS assurances for wireless multimedia sensor networks. *IEEE Communications Surveys Tutorials* 14(2), 265–278, 2012.

15. Cucchiara, R. Multimedia surveillance systems. In: *VSSN '05: Proceedings of the Third ACM International Workshop on Video Surveillance & Sensor Networks*, pp. 3–10, ACM, New York, NY, 2005. DOI: 10.1145/1099396.1099399.

16. Mao, S., Bushmitch, D., Narayanan, S., Panwar, S. MRTP: A multiflow real-time transport protocol for ad hoc networks. *IEEE Transactions on Multimedia* 8(2), 356–369, 2006.

17. Yang, X., Vaidya, N.H. A wakeup scheme for sensor networks: Achieving balance between energy saving and end-to-end delay. In: *Proceedings of IEEE RTAS*, 10th IEEE, pp. 19–26, 2004. DOI: 10.1109/RTTAS.2004.1317245.

18. Shah, R., Rabaey, J. Energy aware routing for low energy ad hoc sensor networks. 2002. citeseer.ist.psu.edu/shah02energy.html

19. Hamid, Z., Bashir, F. XL-WMSN: Cross-layer quality of service protocol for wireless multimedia sensor networks. *EURASIP Journal on Wireless Communications and Networking* 2013(1), 1–16, 2013.

20. Kim, K.I., Sung, T.E. Modeling and routing scheme for (m, k)-firm streams in wireless multimedia sensor networks. *Wireless Communications and Mobile Computing* 15(3), 475–483, 2013.

21. Shah, G., Liang, W., Akan, O. Cross-layer framework for QoS support in wireless multimedia sensor networks. *IEEE Transactions on Multimedia* 14(5), 1442–1455, 2012.

22. Touil, H., Fakhri, Y., Benattou, M. Energy-efficient MAC protocol based on IEEE 802.11e for wireless multimedia sensor networks. In: *2012 International Conference on Multimedia Computing and Systems (ICMCS)*, pp. 53–58, 2012.

23. Felemban, E., Lee, C.G., Ekici, E. MMSPEED: Multipath multi-speed protocol for QoS guarantee of reliability and timeliness in wireless sensor networks. *IEEE Transactions on Mobile Computing* 5(6), 738–754, 2006.

24. Akkaya, K., Younis, M. An energy-aware QoS routing protocol for wireless sensor networks. In: *Proceedings of the MWN*, pp. 710–715, 2003. DOI: 10.1109/ICDCSW.2003.1203636.

25. Akkaya, K., Younis, M. Energy and QoS aware routing in wireless sensor networks. *Cluster Computing* 8(2–3), 179–188, 2005. DOI: 10.1007/s10586-005-6183-7.

26. Ganesan, D., Govindan, R., Shenker, S., Estrin, D. Highly-resilient, energy-efficient multipath routing in wireless sensor networks. SIGMOBILE Mob, *Comput. Commun. Rev.* 5(4), 11–25, 2002.

27. Ju, J., Li, V.O.K. TDMA scheduling design of multihop packet radio networks based on Latin square. *IEEE Journal on Selected Areas in Communications* 17(8), 3499–3504, 1999.

28. Kubale, M., Kuszner, L. A better practical algorithm for distributed graph coloring. In: *PARELEC '02: Proceedings of the International Conference on Parallel Computing in Electrical Engineering*, p. 72. IEEE Computer Society, Washington, DC, 2002.

29. The Network Simulator—ns-2. http://www.isi.edu/nsnam/ns/index.html, 2010.

30. Puccinelli, D., Haenggi, M. Reliable data delivery in large-scale low power sensor networks. *ACM Transactions on Sensor Networks* 6, 28:1–28:41, 2010. DOI: 10.1145/1777406.1777407.

Adaptation Techniques for Multimedia Communication in Wireless Sensor Networks

PINAR SARISARAY-BOLUK

Contents

2.1 Introduction

New advances in (complementary metal-oxide semiconductor) CMOS technology have led to an increase in the availability of cameras and microphones. Wireless multimedia sensor networks (WMSNs) have gained attention after integration of this multimedia-enabled low-cost hardware into traditional sensors [6,12,31]. WMSNs are the next-generation WSNs; they are specially designed to retrieve and transmit multimedia data from wireless environments. They support various multimedia applications including multimedia surveillance networks, target classification, disaster prevention and environmental monitoring, and many more. A comprehensive survey of multimedia communication over WMSNs is presented in Refs. [5,36]. Real-time data transmission over the wireless medium has rigid quality-of-service (QoS) needs; several requirements based on multimedia applications are also given in Refs. [7,25]. Traditional sensor nodes are not suitable for multimedia applications due to their exhaustive requirements. Instead, various improved series of wireless sensor nodes such as Imote2 [26], TelosB motes [28], and MICAz [Crossbow technology, California, www.xbow.com] may be utilized for multimedia applications.

Figure 2.1 shows several new imaging platforms for sensor motes, specifically the CMUcam3 [Carneige Mellon University, Pittsburgh] [31], Cyclops [Agilent Laboratories and the Center for Embedded Network Sensing at UCLA, Los Angeles] [29], and Stargate board [Crossbow technology, California] with webcam [15]. The Crossbow Stargate platform provides a processing platform that can plug into a webcam for medium-resolution imaging. It is utilized as a video sensor node in WMSNs. The Cyclops may be connected to a sensor node such as Crossbow's Mica2 or MICAz [44] that provides low-resolution imaging. It also contains several special image processing libraries. The CMUcam3 is a recent series of embedded cameras that can plug into the TMote Sky. It is composed of the OmniVision CMOS camera sensor module and open-source libraries.

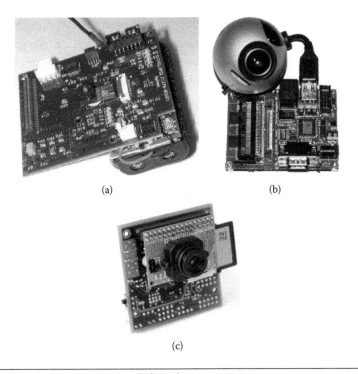

(a)   (b)

(c)

Figure 2.1   Several recent imaging platforms for sensor motes.

These libraries include several image processing algorithms such as frame differentiae, JPEG compression, histogramming, and edge detection, as presented in Figure 2.1.

Construction of a WSN for a specific application is affected by various considerations such as scalability, operating environment, network topology, production costs, hardware constraints, transmission media, and energy consumption [4]. There are several additional factors that affect the performance of WMSNs, for example, multimedia coding techniques, high bandwidth demand, and application-specific QoS requirements. Because sensor nodes have limited power resources, storage, computation, and communication capability, it is challenging to fulfill the application layer QoS requirements for multimedia communication over lossy wireless links. To transmit multimedia data effectively, these factors should be considered in the design of WMSN protocols [16,33].

They are explained in more detail as follows:

- Application-specific QoS requirements: Due to the nature of the wireless medium, multimedia traffic is exposed to losses during transmission, which leads to perceptual quality degradation for viewers at the sink. Furthermore, applications generally require that transmission of multimedia data be completed in a certain time period, referred to as a *delay bound*. This time period is composed of processing time and communication latency. Hence, protocols should be designed to fulfill the reliability and delay requirements of multimedia transmission.

- High bandwidth demand: Most multimedia applications require a certain bandwidth to provide the perceptual quality and delay bound required by the application layer. Otherwise, the application layer QoS requirements cannot be satisfied by the network. Hence, solutions for meeting high bandwidth requirements should be considered in the design of WMSN protocols [7,25,37].

- Error control: To decrease the effects of data loss on multimedia data, error-mitigating techniques are utilized in coded video [1]. However, the perceptual quality of multimedia data is still very sensitive to losses due to the lossy environment and sensor node failures. Hence, error mitigation techniques should be analyzed and designed for WMSNs so as to decrease quality degradation during communication [8].

- Packet prioritization: Multimedia data may be composed of valuable parts and parts that contain less information. Losses of the valuable parts of multimedia data lead to more perceptual quality degradation at the end-user. In order to protect the more valuable parts during transmission, multimedia packets should be prioritized with respect to their significance [10].

There are only a few studies related to satisfying multimedia requirements in WMSN. Many of the proposed protocols do not consider the real-time requirements of applications or only try to meet the deadlines as fast as possible [3,14,17]. Few studies take into account the nature of the multimedia data during communication in WMSNs [19,34]. They generally ignore the transmitted data content, which plays a big role in meeting requirements of the application. Due to this lack of awareness, WMSNs cannot employ the most appropriate transmission techniques to present the needed quality for the application layer. It is vital for QoS-based WMSN applications to provide accurate interaction between the content of the multimedia data and communication protocols. In this chapter, detailed information is provided about well-known existing communication protocols from the media access control (MAC) layer to the transport layer for WSNs. However, these communication protocols were not designed for real-time multimedia communication; therefore, each underlying communication protocol must be adapted to fulfill the requirements of the applications. To satisfy QoS-based WMSN applications, the characteristics of the multimedia data are integrated with the communication architecture of the sensor networks. To remedy this situation, we describe the weaknesses of the existing protocols. We then provide some adaptation techniques to make them suitable for multimedia communication.

The rest of this chapter explains WSN protocols and algorithms and evaluates them in terms of multimedia transmission. Some multimedia adaptation techniques are described for each protocol to provide a better perspective for future deployment. Section 2.2 presents transport layer protocols. Section 2.3 provides network layer protocols that are essential to sensor network applications. Section 2.4 illustrates MAC layer protocols. Finally, Section 2.5 contains our conclusions.

2.2 Transport Layer Protocols

Transport protocols are a means of dealing with reliability and congestion, supporting fair bandwidth sharing, and assuring end-to-end (E2E) reliability. Although these objectives are still absolute for multimedia applications, additional vital issues must be addressed in these protocols. Transport layer protocols should meet real-time requirements such as delay, jitter, bandwidth, etc. In this section, we consider several transport protocols for WSN and check their suitability for WMSN applications. Additionally, several solutions are given to increase the suitability of these protocols for multimedia applications.

2.2.1 Event-to-Sink Reliable Transport Protocol

The event-to-sink reliable transport (ESRT) algorithm [2,39] maintains reliable event detection without intermediate caching requirements. The most important characteristics of ESRT are its self-configuring ability, energy attentiveness, and congestion control. ESRT utilizes both the observed reliability, which is the number of packets that are passed from the event to the sink, and the required reliability, which is the desired number of such packets for the event to be successfully tracked to adjust reporting frequency. If the observed reliability of the event is less than the requirement, then ESRT increases the reporting frequency. On the contrary, if the required reliability degree has been transcended, ESRT reduces the reporting frequency to preserve energy. The frequency at which sensors must send their reports is conveyed to them through broadcasts from the sink, after appropriate calculations, so that the necessary reliability is achieved. Congestion control is performed by controlling buffer levels at forwarding sensors. In this protocol, a sensor node does not require a sensor ID because it uses the event ID for the communication. The advantage of ESRT algorithms is that the protocol is mainly executed in the sink with a plentiful energy. Minimal functions of the protocol run on resource-constrained sensor nodes. This protocol has some limitations in supporting multimedia data.

Limitations:

- E2E QoS [11]: Multimedia applications have different QoS requirements so as to provide user-level satisfaction in WMSNs. Hence, the QoS parameters traditionally used may not be adequate for these applications. Several new QoS metrics are needed for effective evaluation of the transmission of real-time data.

  The QoS requirements of WMSN multimedia applications may vary, and traditional E2E QoS parameters may not be sufficient to portray WMSN application-specific QoS requirements. Consequently, new QoS parameters are required for measuring the delivery of multimedia data in an efficient and effective way [9].

- Inability to cope with bursty multimedia traffic: ESRT mainly considers reliability and energy conservation, without paying enough attention to congestion. Transmission of especially large amounts of multimedia data may lead to congestion over the network. Congestion consumes the limited energy as a result of a large number of retransmissions and packet losses. It precludes event discovery reliability [41].

- Weak algorithm for high bandwidth applications [25]: Multimedia data represent a high volume of data. Hence, it is necessary to fragment the data into smaller packets.
- Rate control: ESRT presents reliability on an application level. However, it does not afford real-time data-dependent source rate managing.

Solutions:

- Because ESRT protocol is based on events, many sensors may be involved in transmitting high-volume multimedia traffic. An event report may be divided into smaller packets coming from the source. Thus, it requires a redefinition of the observed reliability to examine the number of obtained reports taken by the sink instead of the packets. Before transmission of this traffic, a filter may be required to reduce the amount of data to be sent. Additionally, a smarter algorithm regulating the data rate of the source is needed to handle congestion and jitter because of the nature and size of multimedia traffic. The algorithm should control the reporting frequency adaptively.

2.2.2 Pump Slowly, Fetch Quickly: A Reliable Transport Protocol for Sensor Networks

The reliable event-to-sink communication necessary for the delivery of data from the sink to sensors contains retransmission of the packets as well as an acknowledgment procedure, which drains sensor network resources. Hop-by-hop retransmission and Negative Acknowledgment (NACK) mechanisms are generally superior to acknowledgment (ACK) mechanisms and E2E retransmissions in providing energy efficiency. The sink, with abundant energy, storage, and processing and communication resources, takes a greater share of responsibility in the sink-to-sensor communication on the reverse path by using a powerful antenna. Hence, data communication along this path may be subject to less congestion than the forward path, which is based on multihop communication.

Less congestion leads to decreased usage of the congestion-control mechanisms on the reverse path in WSN. Pump slowly, fetch quickly (PSFQ) [38] is a reliable, robust, scalable, and customizable transport protocol. It consists of three operations: message relaying (pump), error recovery (fetch), and selective status reporting (report). The pump function delivers data to the sensor nodes while controlling flow; it localizes loss by guaranteeing buffering of data packets at intermediate nodes. Thus, the errors on one link are rectified locally without propagating them down the entire path. Intermediate sensor nodes send the packet by considering loose delay bounds. Whenever a receiver discerns gaps in the received sequence numbers, a loss is denoted, and it goes into fetching mode. PSFQ deduces that data loss results from unsatisfactory link conditions rather than traffic congestion. It uses a link-based error correction scheme, which causes overhead because it requires intermediate nodes to become aware of a forwarded packet. It requests missing packets to be sent from neighboring nodes. An attempt is made to aggregate losses—that is, several message losses are batched into a single fetch operation, which is especially appropriate for burst losses. PSFQ performs a reporting operation to assure feedback on packet transmission status to the source. The farthest target sensor initiates its report on the reverse path of data, and all intermediate nodes append their reports to the same report. Hence, PSFQ guarantees that data segments are delivered to all necessary receivers in a scalable and reliable manner, even in environments with poor channel conditions.

Limitations:

- Congestion is unaccounted for: This protocol attempts to restrict congestion by injecting packets more slowly. However, the delivery of multimedia data to the network may lead to congestion. The huge volume of multimedia data quickly drains sensor resources as well as network bandwidth. It results in severe packet losses and node failures. Although PSFQ lacks the ability to differentiate the reason for packet losses, it presumes that the packet losses occur due to channel problems without considering congestion. As a result, there is no operation to handle congestion problems in this protocol.
- Slow pump operation and buffering cause large delays: As slow pumping causes a delay at intermediate hops,

the WMSN suffers from high latency. However, the transmission of the multimedia data should be completed in a certain time period. This time period includes the processing time and communication latency.

• Hop-by-hop error correction (recovery) with cache requires more buffers: When the receiver realizes that there is a missing packet, it caches received packets until the lost one is taken. This operation introduces overhead at the receiver node, which has limited buffer storage.

Solutions:

• This algorithm does not function adequately, because all losses are reported as channel losses. This misclassification decreases the performance of PSFQ over wireless channels for multimedia transmission. A new algorithm that includes loss differentiation and source rate adjustment should be implemented to differentiate channel and congestion status.

2.2.3 CODA: Congestion Detection and Avoidance in Sensor Networks

CODA's [40] goal is to provide no protocol overhead throughout normal network conditions. However, it should react quickly to alleviate congestion around hotspots, whenever congestion is noted. Congestion detection, open-loop hop-by-hop back pressure, and closed-loop E2E multisource regulation are three functions included in the protocol. In CODA, congestion is determined by monitoring channel and buffer usage. If buffer and channel load are greater than a predefined value, it indicates congestion. In case of congestion, upstream nodes are alerted to lessen their transmission rate by way of open-loop hop-by-hop back pressure. By means of this mechanism, upstream nodes reduce their transmission rate. These nodes may then propagate the back-pressure upstream depending on the local congestion status. CODA can also adjust the multisource rate using a closed-loop E2E approach. With this approach, when the sensor rate is greater than the theoretical throughput, the sensor sets a regulation bit in an event packet. If the sink receives an event packet with a regulation bit, it transmits an ACK message to the other sensors to reduce their rate. When the congestion is cleared, another ACK message is delivered to the nodes to notify them to increase their rate. CODA has some limitations such as

Limitations:

- Design avoids reliability: This algorithm considers not reliability but congestion control. It tries to prevent congestion, which leads to an increase in the performance of network. However, it does not consider reliability.
- Very low link utilization: Wireless channels may not allow a high data rate during monitoring of the event.
- Resource wastage problem: The suppression messages and ACK mechanism cause waste of resources such as energy and bandwidth.
- Experienced delay: The reaction time for closed-loop multi-source regulation increases with excessive congestion because there is a high probability of loss for the ACK coming from the sink.
- Weak algorithm for Real Time (RT) and high bandwidth applications: CODA cannot cope with bursty multimedia traffic at intermediate nodes due to queue lengths.

Solutions:

- A new multipath algorithm should be implemented for reliability purposes. It should also cope with congestion problems by splitting a large data burst into smaller ones.

2.2.4 Sensor Transmission Control Protocol

Sensor Transmission Control Protocol (STCP) is a reliable and robust transport layer protocol whose functions are generally performed by the sink. It provides regulated reliability and congestion detection-avoidance mechanisms for multiple network applications. In this protocol, first the sensor nodes send a session initiation packet to notify the sink of the number of flows coming from the transmitter, transmission rate, type of data flow, and needed reliability [21]. After receiving the session initiation packet, the sink records all of the information, adjusts timers for each flow, and sends an acknowledgment.

Whenever sensor nodes receive the ACK, they begin to transport packets to the sink. The session initiation packet is used to organize multiple streams. If the sensor node has multiple sensing devices and needs to transmit data obtained from more than one device, it sends a session initiation packet for all flows. Because the transmission attributes may be mismatched, the source node independently transmits packets belonging to each flow.

In continuous flows, the sink can calculate the expected arrival of the next packet by utilizing the transmission rate. If the sink does not receive a packet within the expected window of time, it then sends an NACK to sensor nodes, notifying them to retransmit the packet.

To resend the lost packets, the transmitted packets are held in the buffer of the sensors. A buffer timer is used to avoid buffer overflow. Here, the size of the buffer is monitored; if it reaches the threshold, the buffer is cleared. The sink cannot measure arrival times of data packets in event-driven flows. Whenever the sink receives a packet, it transmits an ACK to the sender to provide reliability. Provided that the sender does not obtain an ACK in a predetermined time, it resends the packet. Until an ACK is received, the sender will keep the transmitted packets in its buffer.

The session initiation packet is used to indicate the needed reliability for each flow. A running average of the reliability is measured by the sink through the fraction of the packets successfully received for a continuous flow. As long as current reliability fulfills the needed reliability in the session initiation packet, a NACK packet will not send for a lost packet in the flow. For event-driven flows, reliability is defined as the ratio of packets obtained to the maximum sequence numbered packet taken. Before transmitting the packet, a sensor node checks the reliability of transmission by assuming that the packet will get lost. If the obtained reliability satisfies the needed reliability, the node will not buffer the packet, leading to saved memory usage. In STCP, congestion is detected by the intermediate nodes based on queue length. To indicate congestion, a congestion notification bit is set in the header of the STCP packet. Upon getting an STCP packet in a congested network flow, the sink alerts the source to the congestion by setting a bit in the ACK packet. When the source receives this ACK packet, it may change its paths or reduce its transmission rate.

In data-centric applications, because the number of sources may be immense, acknowledgment for reliability will be an extremely resource-consuming task in terms of network resources and energy. Hence, STCP does not employ any ACK-based schemes. It assumes that data from different sensors are redundant, hence, events can be transmitted to the sink in a reliable manner.

Limitations:

- E2E and not scalable: STCP includes E2E congestion-control techniques. Hence, delivering congestion information in a WSN, which includes a huge number of sensor nodes, is a time-consuming process. This process leads to delay in the network.
- Inability to cope with bursty multimedia traffic: Multimedia traffic causes high data rates and thus congestion in the network. Acknowledgment (ACK and NACK) is also a time- and energy-consuming process. The algorithm is weak for high bandwidth applications.

Solutions:

- A smarter algorithm integrating Random Early Detection (RED) and an E2E approach could be tailored to STPC. Multimedia traffic should be differentiated depending on the content of the data. A proactive scheme along with this prioritization scheme could be employed to transmit the packets by taking advantage of the multistreaming scheme of the protocol. Packet loss could be handled separately depending on the reasons of it (congestion or link failure). The techniques for reliability should include a hop-by-hop approach depending on the importance of the packets and reasons for the losses.

2.3 Network Layer Protocols

The network layer employs a routing protocol to find paths between the source and destination [27]. Due to transmission distortions induced by channel problems, energy restrictions, and software or hardware malfunctions, the routing performance may not be acceptable for QoS-based WMSN applications. Thus, the routing protocol is a prominent issue to meet the application layer QoS requirements for transmitting multimedia data. In this section, we discuss several routing protocols and their weaknesses in terms of multimedia transmission. Furthermore, we recommend various solutions to increase the suitability of network protocols for multimedia applications.

2.3.1 Sensor Protocols for Information via Negotiation

The routing protocol, referred to as sensor protocols for information via negotiation (SPIN), is proposed in Ref. [22]. Source adjustment and negotiation mechanisms used by SPIN cover the deficiencies of flooding. Negotiation decreases overlap and implosion problems, while a threshold-based resource-aware algorithm provides the improvement of network lifetime. SPIN employs three different types of messages: Advertisement (ADV), Request (REQ), DATA. A sensor node broadcasts an ADV including metadata, describing the actual data with fewer bytes. Provided that a neighbor decides to receive the data, it transmits a REQ message to the source; in turn, the data are disseminated through the source over the network. In SPIN, each sensor requires knowledge about only its single hop neighbors, hence topological changes are not necessary to handle in the communication process.

Limitations:

- Limited scalability: The SPIN protocol does not adapt well to a WSN size increase. Its performance may decrease dramatically for a larger number of hops.
- Inability to guarantee data delivery: The data may not be transmitted due to uninterested nodes on the path between sender and receiver. As a result, this protocol is not good for applications that need reliability.
- Algorithm overhead: Control messages cause overhead in terms of energy and delay. Generating metadata is also an impractical function for resource-limited nodes in terms of processing, energy, and storage.
- Unbalanced energy consumption: The nodes around the sink could exhaust their energy if there are too many events to be interested by the sink.

Solutions:

- A new algorithm for reliability could be implemented to guarantee data delivery while decreasing message overhead for a small WMSN. By means of the control messages, the algorithm should differentiate multimedia packets depending on importance. Relay nodes receiving data info could apply the same adaptive methods to transmit high priority packets to the destination.

2.3.2 Directed Diffusion

Directed diffusion protocol [20] is convenient in scenarios where the sensor nodes deliver queries for information captured by other nodes, rather than the queries originating only from a sink. By utilizing interest gradients, directed diffusion protocol improves on data diffusion. Wireless sensor nodes identify information amidst the attributes, while the other nodes decide their interest based on these attributes. As long as the sink requires the data to be reported to it, it repeatedly messages its interest. The data are transmitted on the reverse path of the interest diffusion. A gradient built at the time of interest propagation is used for attribution for each path. Negative gradients restrain the distribution of data on a particular path, and positive gradients support data flow along the path.

The advantage of this scheme is that it results in multiple paths from source to sink with different gradients. During transmission, nodes cache or locally transform (aggregate) data in the diffusion model, increasing the scalability of communication and also decreasing the number of message transmissions needed. A reinforcement process is utilized if the sink needs more periodic updates from the sensors, which have discovered an event. Then, the sink broadcasts its interest in a higher data rate requirement. By contrast, if the sink requires only a few updates, it employs negative reinforcement by lowering required data rates. In network processing, the data can be fused into directed diffusion, so that each node actively aggregates queries conveying the same interest and reports including correlated data.

Limitations:

- High complexity: A high degree of complexity results in high latency and extensive usage of computational power and storage.

- High overhead: In-network processing is a drawback for multimedia transport. It requires significant processing power, leading to death of the sensor nodes in the network. As a result, the topology of the network may change and even cause network disruption.
- Weak algorithm for RT and high bandwidth applications: Because directed diffusion is not designed for QoS applications, it does not provide QoS guarantees.

Solutions:

- A new algorithm should be created to utilize multipath technology and leverage in-network processing. A multipath scheme could be used to balance network load and to differentiate packets depending on their importance. When deciding paths, QoS metrics should be considered.

2.3.3 Low-Energy Adaptive Clustering Hierarchy

Low-energy adaptive clustering hierarchy (LEACH) is a well-known hierarchical routing protocol for WSNs. It forms clusters based on signal strength and selects cluster heads (CHs) randomly from the sensor nodes [18]. By means of the rotating CH roles among the sensors, the energy load is distributed to the sensor nodes. The CH nodes aggregate data coming from the sensor nodes in the cluster and then transmit the combined data to the sink. This method decreases the number of messages transported to the sink. MACs based on time division multiple access Time division multiple access (TDMA) and CDMA are utilized to lessen collisions, which may occur inside or outside of the clusters. Data gathering is carried out periodically or on demand in a centralized manner. LEACH is composed of two phases: the setup phase and the steady-state phase. The setup phase includes forming the clusters and electing the CH nodes. In the steady-state phase, data communication travels from the sensors to the sink. In the setup phase, a certain ratio of the nodes (p) is determined as CHs. In this process, a sensor node produces a random number (r). If this number (r) is greater than a predefined value, $T(n)$, the node wins the current round. It is then assigned as a CH.

All chosen CHs transmit an advertisement message to all the non-CH nodes in the WSN. Based on the signal strength of this message, all non-CH nodes determine which clusters they belong to. All non-CH nodes transport a packet to the appropriate CH node so as to join the related cluster. A CH allocates a time slot for each node belonging to it; the nodes in that cluster can only transmit their data to the CH. All nodes are informed of their defined time slot.

The sensors can start sensing and sending data to the CHs in the steady-state phase. The CH node, after receiving all the data, combines it before transporting it to the sink. After a predetermined time, the network triggers the setup phase again and new CHs are selected at the end of this phase. Different CDMA codes are used to decrease interference incoming from the other nodes owned by the other clusters.

Limitations:

- In-network processing issue: In-network processing is a drawback for multimedia transport. It leads to energy consumption by the sensors.
- Higher resource cost: The dynamic nature of the protocol—the CH changes, messaging, etc.—causes additional overhead, which increases energy consumption of the protocol. Additionally, in this protocol, data gathering is performed periodically, which is unsuitable and one of the causes of energy waste for event-based WMSN applications.
- Lack of scalability: LEACH presumes that all nodes have enough power to reach the sink and always have data to transmit. Additionally, it assumes all sensors start with an equal amount of energy in each selection round. Therefore, it may not be appropriate for large networks.

Solutions:

- A new algorithm adjusting channel status and communication load could be implemented with a consideration given to scalability. LEACH should also be improved to account for nonuniform energy nodes.

2.3.4 Power-Efficient Gathering for Sensor Information Systems

Power-efficient gathering for sensor information systems (PEGASIS) [24] is a data-collecting protocol. It is assumed that the topology information is available to all nodes and a leader node can reach the sink in one hop. PEGASIS aims to minimize the distance over which each node sends transmissions, the number of packets that need to be transmitted to the sink, and broadcasting overhead; it also aims to distribute the energy consumption equally across all nodes. Sensor nodes, starting with the node furthest from the sink, build a chain by using a greedy algorithm. The nearest unvisited neighbor is added to the chain at each step. Before beginning data transmission, the chain is established *a priori*; when nodes die out, it is reconstructed. Data fusion or aggregation is performed at every node, so that only one message is forwarded from one node to the next. A node entitled as the leader lastly transports the message to the sink. Leadership is assigned to the next one in a sequential manner and a token is passed on in the chain to transmit the data.

Limitations:

- Delay: Until all of the messages are captured, the leader does not start to communicate with the sink. This situation leads to too much delay for distant nodes in the chain.
- High overhead: PEGASIS has high overhead in terms of delay, computational power, and storage. Aggregation at each hop is a drawback for multimedia transport and may cause erroneous information.
- Lack of scalability: Single-leader concept used in this protocol may be a bottleneck in the network.

Solutions:

- A new scalable algorithm is needed that considers both energy efficiency and delay sensitivity in WMSNs. A smart aggregation algorithm could be performed to decrease the amount of data to be transmitted. This algorithm should decide if aggregation is required or not for the data held in a given sensor node. At this point, sensor nodes can combine their data with the incoming message and then transmit or only behave as relay nodes.

2.3.5 Minimum Energy Communication Network and Small MECN

Location awareness provides an increase in the performance of a network in terms of delay and energy consumption [13]. Minimum energy communication network (MECN) utilizes the location information to make effective routing decisions. It uses a GPS to build and sustain a MECN for a WSN. MECN tries to find a subnetwork with a lower number of nodes where the energy conservation between any two nodes is provided. Global minimum power paths can be found by using a localized search for individual sensor nodes in their transmission region. MECN protocol includes two phases as follows: (1) a sparse graph (enclosure graph) based on two-dimensional positions is constructed. The graph is composed of all the enclosures of each transmitting node. The construction of the graph requires local computations at the nodes. (2) The algorithm finds optimal links in terms of energy waste on the enclosure graph. The distributed Bellman–Ford shortest path algorithm is utilized with energy consumption as the cost metric. Due to MECN self-configuration topology, both node failures and new sensor deployment can be easily handled. Additionally, MECN modifies the minimum cost links adaptively for topological changes.

The small MECN (SMECN) [23] is a modified version of the MECN protocol. MECN assumes that every node can always transport to other sensors, whereas SMECN considers the possible barriers between any two nodes due to availability. MECN and SMECN are categorized into proactive routing protocols, which keep the recent routing information. SMECN is superior to MECN [23] in terms of energy usage and maintenance cost of the links, at the expense of escalated overhead in the algorithm.

Limitations:

- Weak algorithm for RT and high bandwidth applications: Because of its proactive behavior, topological changes cause high delay.
- High overhead: Building a subnetwork with a smaller number of edges leads to overhead.

Solutions:

- A new algorithm should be designed to account for delay factors, leveraging proactive and reactive style. Other QoS parameters as well as energy can be integrated into the MECN during subnetwork building.

2.3.6 *Sequential Assignment Routing*

The sequential assignment routing (SAR) [35] algorithm is a table-driven multipath protocol that provides QoS-based routing in WSNs. It aims to find optimal routes between the sink and the source in terms of energy usage and reliability. In this protocol, a weighted QoS metric is computed and then minimized so as to multiply the lifetime of the network. SAR uses three considerations: priority levels of the packets, QoS on each path, and energy resources. A multipath routing approach and path restoration techniques are utilized to obviate path failure. A tree is created to obtain multiple paths from the sink to the sensors. During the final part of this procedure, each sensor node is included in more than one path. Node failures because of energy constraints or the wireless environment result in topology changes, hence the path is rebuilt. The sink also recomputes the paths periodically to cope with the changing topology.

Limitations:

- Lack of testing: Performance testing is needed for multimedia transmission.
- Lack of scalability: As the number of nodes in the network is increased, SAR suffers from processing time overhead for handling the tables and status data for each of the sensor nodes.

Solutions:

- SAR does not consider the nature of multimedia data during communication. A new scalable algorithm can be designed to give priority to the multimedia packets in terms of bandwidth utilization and reliability.

2.3.7 *A Stateless Protocol for Real-Time Communication (SPEED)*

SPEED [17] is a well-known QoS-based routing algorithm that provides real-time anycast for data transmission. Because SPEED is based on hop-by-hop data transmission, it does not need a routing table, which causes minimal control packet overhead. A special packet-naming periodic beacon is used between neighboring nodes. To adapt network condition alterations, two different kinds of beacon packets are used for congestion detection and delay assessment. Using topographic information, data packets are transmitted specifically to the nodes that are nearer to the sink. Among the suitable nodes, the nodes with the minimum estimated delay are selected as intermediate nodes. In the absence of a sensor node to satisfy the delay restraint, the packet is dropped. Although SPEED does not have packet priorities, it provides real-time data communication over WSNs by supplying assurance on the maximal delay.

The Multipath Multi-SPEED Protocol (MMSPEED) protocol [14], which is an enhanced version of the SPEED protocol, supports service differentiation and a probabilistic QoS guarantee. Global network state information and E2E path setup are not required for all functions in MMSPEED. Hence, the protocol is scalable and adaptable to network dynamics. In MMSPEED, different packet transportation speeds are given for different traffic types as stated in their E2E deadlines. The reliability required by the application is provided with a probabilistic multipath forwarding technique that regulates the number of delivery routes in the communication.

Limitations:

- Channel throughput problem: Due to a certain parameter naming the maximum delivery speed, SPEED does not transmit packets at an increased speed, even if the network can present higher rates.
- Trade-off between energy and delay: SPEED and MMSPEED do not consider the energy–delay trade-off. There is no delay guarantee in a dynamically changing network.
- No consideration of Aggregation issues: No network layer aggregation scheme is employed in these protocols. Additionally, MMSPEED does not account for the number of hops between source and destination in making route decisions.
- No consideration of energy issues: SPEED and MMSPEED do not take into account further energy metrics.
- Resource requirement: MMSPEED needs to buffer the reliable forwarding probabilities of the neighboring nodes, which require several updates.

Solutions:

- A modified algorithm should be adopted using a probabilistic approach based on energy constraints. The algorithm could deal with a mapping process from application layer quality to network parameters. It could also be integrated with a localization algorithm to obtain high scalability.

2.3.8 An Energy-Aware QoS Routing Protocol for WSNs

The energy-aware QoS routing protocol for WSNs given in Ref. [3] locates the least costly path by considering energy efficiency and specific E2E delay constraints. The cost of the link is calculated using several transmission metrics such as the energy reserve of the node, energy consumed by transmission, error rate, and so forth. In this protocol, best-effort and real-time traffic are supported by means of a class-based queuing model. The protocol also provides resource distribution for real-time and non-real-time traffic. In case of congestion, a bandwidth ratio r shows the amount of both types of bandwidth-adjusted traffic on certain outgoing links. A number of less costly paths are located and a path is chosen from among those that satisfy the E2E delay requirement. This protocol consistently performs well in terms of QoS and energy parameters. However, an equal r value is utilized for all nodes in the network.

Limitations:

- No prioritization for real-time traffic: The protocol does not contain a function to provide different priorities for multimedia traffic.
- Lack of scalability: Because it calculates multiple paths, for each node the algorithm needs complete information about the network topology.
- Bandwidth sharing issue: The protocol does not support adaptive assigning of bandwidth sharing for different links.

Solution:

- A modified algorithm with scalability could be adopted based on packet-level priority. It should support adaptive bandwidth sharing for different links.

2.4 MAC Layer Protocols

MAC protocols are responsible for channel adjustment and error control–recovery techniques to provide robust, error-free data transfer between the nodes with minimal energy consumption. The quality of wireless links changes dramatically over time for various reasons such as scattering, diffraction, and many more. This dynamic nature of wireless links causes packet losses and also the degradation of perceptual quality of a multimedia application. Hence, new robust transmission mechanisms are required to provide QoS for multimedia [32]. There are two additional QoS metrics that should be considered for multimedia transmission [8,25]: packet latency and multiple priorities for varying services. Due to the high volume of data involved, energy consumption is still an issue for efficient multimedia data transmission for MAC layer protocols.

2.4.1 Sensor MAC Protocol

Sensor MAC (SMAC) focuses on energy efficiency and self-configuration issues to ensure the sustainability of the WSN. SMAC focuses on energy and self-configuration issues to ensure the sustainability of the WSN. It identifies control packet overhead, overhearing, collision, and idle listening as major sources of energy wastage in WSNs. Hence, SMAC utilizes several techniques to decrease energy consumption. To this end, the low duty cycle technique is used for multihop WSNs. To decrease control overhead and to allow traffic-adaptive wake-up, sensor nodes create virtual clusters depending on their sleep periods. The other technique used is channel signaling, which provides a way for nodes to stop overhearing uninteresting traffic. Ultimately, message passing is used to lower contention latency for those WSN applications needing data aggregation. Because of sleep schedules, the energy consumption for idle listening is decreased. The announcements for sleep schedules lead to reducing time synchronization overhead.

Limitations:

- Increased collision probability results from broadcast data packets without RTS/CTS.

- Trade-off between energy and delay/throughput: This protocol preserves energy at the expense of degraded throughput and latency.
- Schedule exchange between neighbors can cause high overhead for video/audio traffic.
- SMAC may not be able to handle synchronization and coordination of the nodes when sensor nodes have a dynamic duty cycle.
- Sudden buffer overflow may occur at the receiver.
- Because sleep and listen periods are predefined, there may be a reduction in the performance of the algorithm for different traffic loads.

Solution:

- An energy-efficient algorithm should be implemented that preserves E2E delay and throughput concerns.

2.4.2 Traffic-Adaptive MAC Protocol

Traffic-adaptive MAC protocol (TRAMA) [30] aims to increase the usage of traditional TDMA in an energy-efficient and collision-free approach. Two techniques are used to reduce energy consumption: (1) assuring unicast and broadcast transmission without collision and (2) assuring that sensor nodes that are not communicating are allowed to enter a low power and idle state. TRAMA partitions time into a series of random-access signaling periods and scheduled-access (transmission) periods. TRAMA chooses one transmitter within each two-hop neighborhood for each time slot. This selection operation dispenses with the hidden terminal problem, and hence the nodes within one hop of the neighborhood of the transmitter are not exposed to collision. TRAMA exhibits higher percentages of sleep time and lower collision probability compared to Carrier sense multiple access (CSMA)-based protocols. Moreover, intended receivers are indicated in a bitmap; less communication overhead occurs for multicast and broadcast traffic compared to other protocols [42].

Limitations:

- High overhead: TRAMA includes a complex election algorithm and data structure and explicit schedule propagation.
- Delay: TRAMA produces a higher queuing delay.

Solution:

- A resource-efficient algorithm could be implemented to prevent delay.

2.4.3 Diff-MAC

Diff-MAC [43] provides differentiated services and hybrid prioritization for WSN applications. It proposes to increase channel utilization with service differentiation and to provide fair and fast distribution of data. Diff-MAC is used for QoS-based WMSN applications, which generally transmit heterogeneous traffic. Several techniques are utilized to provide QoS in WSNs. Video data are fragmented into tiny packets and then transported as a burst that enables a decrease in retransmission cost in case of link failures. The congestion window size is adjusted depending on the data QoS requirements, leading to reduced packet delays and fewer collisions. The protocol adjusts the duty cycle of the sensor nodes by taking into consideration the current traffic class and attempts to balance latency and energy consumption. Finally, fair data distribution among wireless nodes and all traffic classes is provided by intranode and intraqueue prioritization. Diff-MAC is also easily adapted to varying network conditions.

Limitations:

- Due to its network statistics and dynamic adaptation, it has a high complexity. Additionally, Diff-MAC has several complex and overwhelming functions such as monitoring networks statistics and dynamic adaptation.
- Packet latency: Diff-MAC has packet delays due to early sleeping. However, the absence of sleep–listen synchronization among nearby sensor nodes does enhance the scalability of the protocol.

Solutions:

- An energy-delay efficient algorithm should be integrated with this protocol. The algorithm can minimize E2E delay by limiting packet latency. In addition, the complex techniques used in this protocol should be energy-aware.

2.5 Conclusion

WMSN applications have several QoS requirements such as perceptual quality and timeliness. Unstable wireless links and the tight resource constraints of sensor nodes lead to QoS degradation during multimedia communication. Hence, some new approaches are imperative to ensure that the QoS requirements of applications are met. These approaches need to observe the current status of the network and to take action in an adaptive manner to sustain an acceptable level of quality for multimedia transmissions. In this context, providing accurate mapping from application layer perceptual quality requirements to lower layer system parameters is essential. Because application layer requirements depend heavily on the transmitted multimedia data, the characteristics of the data are associated with the communication architecture of WMSNs. To satisfy the QoS-based WMSN applications, the nature of the multimedia data should be integrated with the communication architecture of the sensor networks. In this chapter, we have presented an overview of well-known communication layer protocols from the transport layer to the MAC layer for WSNs. We have highlighted design constraints and open research issues to suggest further avenues of research in the field of QoS provision in WMSNs at the transport, routing, and MAC layers. We believe that this work will lead to reuse of well-known WSN protocols by adapting them for multimedia transmission in WMSNs.

References

1. Aaron, A., Rane, S., Setton, E., Girod, B. Transform-domain Wyner–Ziv codec for video. In: *Proceedings of SPIE Visual Communications and Image Processing*, volume 5308, pp. 520–528. Citeseer, San Jose, CA, 2004.
2. Akan, O.B., Akyildiz, I.F. Event-to-sink reliable transport in wireless sensor networks. *IEEE/ACM Transactions on Networking,* Maryland University, Baltimore, MD, 13(5), 1003–1016, 2005.
3. Akkaya, K., Younis, M. An energy-aware QoS routing protocol for wireless sensor networks. In: *Proceedings, 23rd International Conference on Distributed Computing Systems Workshops, 2003*, pp. 710–715. IEEE, 2003.
4. Akyildiz, I.F., Su, W., Sankarasubramaniam, Y., Cayirci, E. Wireless sensor networks: A survey. *Computer Networks* 38(4), 393–422, 2002.

5. Akyildiz, I.F., Melodia, T., Chowdhury, K.R. A survey on wireless multimedia sensor networks. *Computer Networks* 51(4), 921–960, 2007.

6. Akyildiz, I.F., Melodia, T., Chowdhury, K.R. Wireless multimedia sensor networks: Applications and testbeds. *Proceedings of the IEEE* 96(10), 1588–1605, 2008.

7. Akyildiz, I.F., Melodia, T., Chowdury, K.R. Wireless multimedia sensor networks: A survey. *IEEE Wireless Communications* 14(6), 32–39, 2007.

8. Boluk, P., Baydere, S., Harmanci, A. Robust image transmission over wireless sensor networks. *Mobile Networks and Applications* 16, 149–170, 2011. DOI: 10.1007/s1 1036-010-0282-2.

9. Boluk, P.S., Baydere, S., Harmanci, A.E. Perceptual quality-based image communication service framework for wireless sensor networks. *Wireless Communications and Mobile Computing* 14(1), 1–18, 2011.

10. Boluk, P.S., Baydere, S., Harmanci, A.E. Perceptual quality-based image communication service framework for wireless sensor networks. *Wireless Communications and Mobile Computing* 14(1), 1–18, 2014.

11. Chen, D., Varshney, P.K. QoS support in wireless sensor networks: A survey. In *International Conference on Wireless Networks,* volume 13244, pp. 227–233. Citeseer, Las Vegas, Nevada, 2004.

12. Culurciello, E., Andreou, A.G. CMOS image sensors for sensor networks. *Analog Integrated Circuits and Signal Processing* 49(1), 39–51, 2006.

13. Ehsan, S., Hamdaoui, B. A survey on energy-efficient routing techniques with QoS assurances for wireless multimedia sensor networks. *Communications Surveys & Tutorials, IEEE* 14(2), 265–278, 2012.

14. Felemban, E., Lee, C.G., Ekici, E. MMSPEED: Multipath multi-speed protocol for QoS guarantee of reliability and timeliness in wireless sensor networks. *IEEE Transactions on Mobile Computing* 5(6), 738–754, 2006.

15. Feng, W., Kaiser, E., Feng, W.C., Baillif, M.L. Panoptes: Scalable low-power video sensor networking technologies. *ACM Transactions on Multimedia Computing, Communications, and Applications (TOMCCAP)* 1(2), 151–167, 2005.

16. Hao, J., Kim, S.H., Ay, S.A., Zimmermann, R. Energy-efficient mobile video management using smartphones. In: *Proceedings of the 2nd Annual ACM Conference on Multimedia Systems,* pp. 11–22. ACM, Santa Clara, CA, 2011.

17. He, T., Stankovic, J.A., Lu, C., Abdelzaher, T. SPEED: A stateless protocol for real-time communication in sensor networks. *International Conference on Distributed Computing Systems,* 0, 46, 2003.

18. Heinzelman, W.R., Chandrakasan, A., Balakrishnan, H. Energy-efficient communication protocol for wireless microsensor networks. In: *Proceedings of the 33rd Annual Hawaii International Conference on System Sciences, 2000,* pp. 10, IEEE, Island of Maui, 2000.

19. Hyung, S.L., Hee, Y.Y., Jung, H. Context-aware cross-layered multimedia streaming based on variable packet size transmission. In: *Proceedings of the International Conference on Computer Science and Its Applications (ICCSA 2006)*, pp. 691–700. Glasgow, UK, 2006.
20. Intanagonwiwat, C., Govindan, R., Estrin, D. Directed diffusion: A scalable and robust communication paradigm for sensor networks. In: *Proceedings of the 6th Annual International Conference on Mobile Computing and Networking*, pp. 56–67. ACM, Boston, MA, 2000.
21. Iyer, Y.G., Gandham, S., Venkatesan, S. STCP: A generic transport layer protocol for wireless sensor networks. In: *Proceedings, 14th International Conference on Computer Communications and Networks, 2005. ICCCN 2005*, pp. 449–454. IEEE, San Diego, California, 2005.
22. Kulik, J., Heinzelman, W., Balakrishnan, H. Negotiation-based protocols for disseminating information in wireless sensor networks. *Wireless Networks* 8(2), 169–185, 2002.
23. Li, L., Halpern, J.Y. Minimum-energy mobile wireless networks revisited. In: *IEEE International Conference on Communications, 2001. ICC 2001*, volume 1, pp. 278–283. IEEE, Helsinki, Finland, 2001.
24. Lindsey, S., Raghavendra, C.S. PEGASIS: Power-efficient gathering in sensor information systems. In: *IEEE Aerospace Conference Proceedings, 2002*, volume 3, pp. 3–1125. IEEE, Big Sky, Montana, 2002.
25. Misra, S., Reisslein, M., Xue, G. A survey of multimedia streaming in wireless sensor networks. *IEEE Communications Surveys & Tutorials* 10(4), 18–39, 2008.
26. Nachman, L., Huang, J., Shahabdeen, J., Adler, R., Kling, R. Imote2: Serious computation at the edge. In: *International Wireless Communications and Mobile Computing Conference, 2008. IWCMC'08*, pp. 1118–1123. IEEE, Crete Island, Greece, 2008.
27. Pantazis, N.A., Nikolidakis, S.A., Vergados, D.D. Energy-efficient routing protocols in wireless sensor networks: A survey. *Communications Surveys & Tutorials, IEEE* 15(2), 551–591, 2013.
28. Polastre, J., Szewczyk, R., Culler, D. Telos: Enabling ultra-low power wireless research. In: *4th International Symposium on Information Processing in Sensor Networks, 2005. IPSN 2005*, pp. 364–369. IEEE, UCLA, Los Angeles, California, 2005.
29. Rahimi, M., Baer, R., Iroezi, O.I., Garcia, J.C., Warrior, J., Estrin, D., Srivastava, M. Cyclops: In situ image sensing and interpretation in wireless sensor networks. In: *Proceedings of the 3rd International Conference on Embedded Networked Sensor Systems*, p. 204. ACM, San Diego, CA, 2005.
30. Rajendran, V., Obraczka, K., Garcia-Luna-Aceves, J.J. Energy-efficient, collision-free medium access control for wireless sensor networks. *Wireless Networks* 12(1), 63–78, 2006.
31. Rowe, A., Goode, A., Goel, D., Nourbakhsh, I. CMUcam3: an open programmable embedded vision sensor. Technical Report CMU-RI-TR-07-13, Robotics Institute, Carnegie Mellon University, Pittsburgh, PA, 2007.

32. Sarisaray-Boluk, P. Performance comparisons of the image quality evaluation techniques in wireless multimedia sensor networks. *Wireless Networks* 19(4), 443–460, 2013.

33. Sen, J., Bhattacharya, S. A survey on cross-layer design frameworks for multimedia applications over wireless networks. *International Journal of Computer Science and Information Technology (IJCSIT)* 1(1), 29–42, 2010.

34. Shu, L., Zhang, Y., Yu, Z., Yang, L.T., Hauswirth, M., Xiong, N. Context-aware cross-layer optimized video streaming in wireless multimedia sensor networks. *The Journal of Supercomputing* 54(1), 94–121, 2010.

35. Sohrabi, K., Gao, J., Ailawadhi, V., Pottie, G.J. Protocols for self-organization of a wireless sensor network. *IEEE Personal Communications* 7(5), 16–27, 2000.

36. Soro, S., Heinzelman, W. A survey of visual sensor networks. *Advances in Multimedia*, 1–21, 2009.

37. Su, W., Cayirci, E., Akan, O. Overview of communication protocols for sensor networks. In: *Handbook of Sensor Networks: Compact Wireless and Wired Sensing Systems* (Eds. M. Ilyas, I. Mahgoub), pp. 374–392, Boca Raton, FL, USA, CRC Press, p. 374, 2004.

38. Wan, C.Y., Campbell, A.T., Krishnamurthy, L. PSFQ: A reliable transport protocol for wireless sensor networks. In: *Proceedings of the 1st ACM International Workshop on Wireless Sensor Networks and Applications*, pp. 1–11. ACM, Atlanta, GA, 2002.

39. Wan, C.Y., Campbell, A.T., Krishnamurthy, L. Reliable transport for sensor networks. In: *Wireless Sensor Networks* (Eds. C.S. Raghavendra, K.M. Sivalingam, and T. Znati), pp. 153–182. Springer, Berlin, Germany, 2004.

40. Wan, C.Y., Eisenman, S.B., Campbell, A.T. CODA: Congestion detection and avoidance in sensor networks. In: *Proceedings of the 1st International Conference on Embedded Networked Sensor Systems*, pp. 266–279. ACM, Los Angeles, CA, 2003.

41. Wang, C., Sohraby, K., Lawrence, V., Li, B., Hu, Y. Priority-based congestion control in wireless sensor networks. In: *IEEE International Conference on Sensor Networks, Ubiquitous, and Trustworthy Computing, 2006*, volume 1, pp. 8. IEEE, Newport Beach, CA, 2006.

42. Yahya, B., Ben-Othman, J. Towards a classification of energy aware MAC protocols for wireless sensor networks. *Wireless Communications and Mobile Computing* 9(12), 1572–1607, 2009.

43. Yigitel, M.A., Incel, O.D., Ersoy, C. QoS-aware MAC protocols for wireless sensor networks: A survey. *Computer Networks* 55(8), 1982–2004, 2011.

44. Zacharias, S., Newe, T. Technologies and architectures for multimedia-support in wireless sensor network. In: *Smart Wireless Sensor Networks*, (Ed. Y. K. Tan) InTech, Rijeka, Croatia, pp. 18–25, 2010.

3

MULTIMEDIA COMMUNICATION IN COGNITIVE RADIO AD HOC AND SENSOR NETWORKS

MUSTAFA OZGER, ECEHAN B. PEHLIVANOGLU, AND OZGUR B. AKAN

Contents

3.1 Introduction

Small and low-cost sensor nodes are available, thanks to developments in micro-electro-mechanical systems (MEMS) technology. These sensor nodes have irreplaceable batteries and they are deployed in specific regions of interest. The deployment of these sensor nodes forms wireless ad hoc networks, namely wireless sensor networks (WSNs). The application areas of these networks are environmental or habitat monitoring, military surveillance, medical applications, multimedia applications, and so forth. The sensor nodes sense the environment—heat, pressure, sound, light, or motion depending on the application—and form packets related to the observations. The sensor nodes collaborate with each other to convey these packets in a multihop manner to a base station or sink [1].

Reliable and timely delivery of data packets is a vital requirement for multimedia communication. The inherent demands of multimedia communication are limited delay, large bandwidth, jitter control, no abrupt changes of transmission rate, and loose reliability [2]. Hence, a new networking paradigm—wireless multimedia sensor networks (WMSNs)—has been proposed to realize multimedia communication in WSNs. Multimedia communication demands more resources than mainstream data-sensing applications. Event features in sensor networks and the packets generated by source nodes in ad hoc networks contain large byte streams, because they are in the form of multimedia, for example, video, audio, and still images. Hence, the main challenges posed by multimedia communication are high bandwidth demand and strict time constraints [3].

Ever-increasing demand in wireless communication has led to the spectrum scarcity problem. Furthermore, the electromagnetic spectrum is not utilized efficiently due to the fixed frequency assignment approach. Cognitive radio (CR) technology has become the solution to the problems of spectrum scarcity and inefficient utilization. Communication between wireless nodes becomes spectrum-aware by cognitive cycle operations, namely spectrum sensing, spectrum decision, and spectrum handoff [4]. The inherent features of CR have increased electromagnetic spectrum efficiency and have overcome the spectrum scarcity challenge. The main CR application areas are ad hoc networks and sensor networks [5].

A typical CR ad hoc network consists of two types of users: primary users (PUs) and secondary users (SUs). PUs are the legacy users of the licensed spectrum. SUs are the CRs, and they utilize the licensed bands opportunistically [6]. The CR capability of wireless nodes makes them adaptable to environmental changes in the network. A CR node can find vacant spectrum bands by spectrum sensing and can make use of them through the spectrum decision process. If a channel that is being utilized becomes occupied by a PU, the communication continues on another vacant channel through the spectrum handoff function. Hence, CR can change its operating parameters to enable seamless communication.

WSNs are characterized by a fixed frequency assignment policy; hence, they also suffer from the spectrum scarcity challenge [5]. The event-driven nature of WSN communications causes bursty traffic. The injection of event packets leads to packet collisions and excessive contention delay due to high traffic and high node density in the network. Furthermore, sensor nodes have inherent limitations in power, communication, processing, and memory resources. Hence, the CR sensor network (CRSN) has been proposed by integrating CR capability into sensor networks. Providing sensor nodes with CR capability increases the efficiency of overall spectrum utilization and decreases the probability of collision and contention by utilizing multiple channels opportunistically. Adaptability to the existing spectrum meets the unique requirements of WSNs. To this end, CRSNs benefit from the potential advantages of the salient features of dynamic spectrum access, such as adaptability to environmental changes to decrease collision and to reduce power consumption and accessing multiple channels to provide flexibility in spectrum usage.

Sensor nodes in CRSNs sense the environment as well as the spectrum. The event readings of the sensor nodes in the event region are collaboratively conveyed in a multihop manner through vacant channels. A typical CRSN architecture for multimedia communication is shown in Figure 3.1. In this architecture, multimedia CRSN nodes and PUs coexist and there is a sink with CR capability. Base stations serve as PUs, and CRSN nodes communicate without interfering with PUs. The CR-capable sink can receive multiple data with its CR-capable transceivers. Furthermore, a typical CRSN topology can be ad hoc, clustered, hierarchical, and mobile, depending on the application.

A wide range of potential applications for CRSNs exists in the literature. These applications include indoor sensing applications, multiclass heterogeneous sensing applications, and real-time surveillance

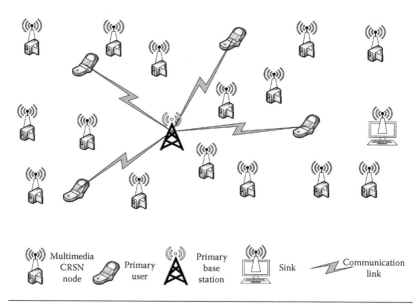

Figure 3.1   A typical cognitive radio sensor network architecture.

applications [5]. Furthermore, one of the most significant areas of application is multimedia communication [3].

Multimedia communication has been investigated in a wireless sensor and ad hoc network context extensively [2,3,7]. However, there is no research on multimedia communication in CR ad hoc and sensor networks. The dynamic radio environment poses distinctive challenges in multimedia communication. Multimedia communication requires seamless communication, bounded delay, and a certain level of quality of service (QoS). However, with CR capability, communication may be interrupted by the arrival of PUs, resulting in delay, route changes, and variation in QoS. Hence, multimedia communication in a CR network (CRN) regime intensifies existing challenges. In this chapter, we survey the approaches proposed for each network layer in WSNs, CRNs, and WMSNs; we examine the challenges and potential approaches to overcome them.

We survey existing studies and present research opportunities on multimedia communication from the perspective of network layers in CR ad hoc and sensor networks. We examine the state-of-the-art approaches related to WMSN communication and how these methods can be applied to multimedia communication in CR ad hoc and sensor networks. We clearly indicate the challenges posed by CR and sensor networks for multimedia communication and investigate how the union of sensor networks and CR in multimedia communication poses new challenges.

Multimedia streams must be conveyed in a timely manner. However, CR introduces some delays due to cognitive cycle operations and coordination activities, such as the need for communicating parties to tune to the same channel. Hence, these are the specific challenges caused by enabling wireless nodes with CR capability. Furthermore, multimedia applications require limited delay and mandate the transport of packets in a timely manner. In the light of the above-mentioned challenges and limitations, we investigate the existing protocols and open issues. In the application layer, we investigate multimedia encoding techniques and present open issues for CR sensor and ad hoc networks. We examined the existing transport layer approaches for multimedia communication in WSNs, CRNs, and CRSNs, and we present the potential approaches for CR and ad hoc networks according to reliability of the transport and congestion control. We investigated routing issues in the network layer by examining the previous works on WSNs, CRNs, and CRSNs. We present potential approaches in the medium access control (MAC) layer for medium access control protocols for CR ad hoc and sensor networks. We outline the open research issues in each layer to facilitate multimedia communication in CR ad hoc and sensor networks.

3.2 Factors Influencing Multimedia Communication in Cognitive Radio Ad Hoc and Sensor Networks

Designing protocols for CR ad hoc and sensor networks imposes limitations such as constrained energy and memory capability, decentralized architecture, node failures, dynamic radio environment, and so on. Energy and memory limitations are inherited from the WSN paradigm; opportunistic spectrum access is inherited from the CR capability. These challenges are amplified by the union of the sensor network paradigm and CR. On the other hand, multimedia communication has unique requirements—high bandwidth demand, application-specific QoS requirements, and delay bound [3]. These requirements must be revisited from the perspective of the dynamic radio environment. Satisfying these requirements is the main motivation to facilitate multimedia communication. These requirements are also the main factors influencing the quality of multimedia communication. These factors are explained as follows.

- High bandwidth demand: Multimedia traffic contains large packets and they must be transported to the destination within a certain delay. Hence, high bandwidth is a vital requirement for real-time multimedia communication. However, the dynamic radio environment poses a significant challenge here because of PU activities. The channel conditions change with the arrival of PUs and spectrum handoff.
- QoS requirements and limited delay: Either processing time or communication latency in WMSN may cause delay [3]. Furthermore, channel access delay should be taken into account for the delay in CR ad hoc and sensor networks. Low delay and high throughput are the main QoS requirements in multimedia communication. In addition, jitter degrades the performance of

continuous media such as audio and video. It can be avoided by replay buffering at the receiver side.

- Dynamic radio environment: The cognitive capability of nodes offers flexibility in utilizing communication channels. However, they pose significant challenges. For example, the coordination of communication is a difficult task, since the communication between cognitive nodes requires tuning to the same channel for communication.
- Power consumption: Nodes have irreplaceable batteries; hence, energy efficiency is a vital requirement. Collision, unnecessary packet transmission, extensive overhead due to communication coordination, and high duty cycle operation are the most important factors in power consumption.

3.3 The Application Layer in Multimedia Communication for Cognitive Radio Ad Hoc and Sensor Networks

The application layer is perhaps the most important platform in multimedia communication, since it governs the communication quality of the end user. In a WSN or CRSN, the application layer needs to compress the field data efficiently and obtain a proper representation to it, such that data are transported via wireless links in multihop manner.

The application layer is responsible for

- Managing traffic based on application requirements
- Performing source coding via a suitable approach based on the resource constraints of the sensor nodes

Both of these challenging tasks were previously investigated in the context of WSNs. However, intermittent communications in the CR concept and its additional operational requirements necessitate revisiting these tasks and assessing their applicability to CRSNs.

3.3.1 Challenges and Requirements

The challenges faced by the application layer in WMSNs and multimedia communication in CRSNs are mostly driven by the high bandwidth multimedia nature of the data to be communicated. We invite users interested in general challenges on application layer of traditional WSN to read Ref. [1], an excellent survey of WSNs and their challenges. Refs. [2,3,7] are excellent sources for a general overview on the challenges and requirements of the application layer for WMSNs. Based on the tasks of managing traffic with respect to the application requirements and source coding, the challenges of the application layer in WMSNs and CRSNs will be investigated along different dimensions, as shown in Figure 3.2.

- QoS is an important metric to be considered in sensor networks, even more in multimedia sensor networks. In that sense, based on application requirements, sensor nodes may need to differentiate different types of traffic. Therefore, existing measures in this respect and their applicability to CRSNs are worthy of consideration.

- Multimedia applications demand high bandwidth, which is scarce in the industrial, scientific, and medical bands populated by WSNs. Although CRSNs can offer a remedy to the bandwidth problem, efficient source coding techniques are needed to carry out source-to-sink multimedia relaying in an energy-efficient manner. Depending on the network and application, distributed source coding (DSC) or individual source coding may be used in WMSNs [2]. Moreover, different compression techniques exhibit differences in resilience to errors, energy efficiency, and adaptability to network conditions, among other properties. Communication is intermittent in CRSNs, with constant adaptation of communication parameters and additional tasks regarding cognitive cycle bringing additional challenges in communications and energy expenditure. Therefore, compression techniques need to be revisited for multimedia communications in CRSNs.

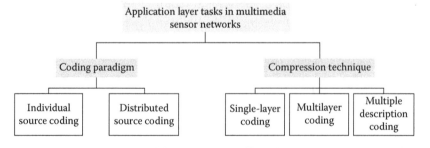

Figure 3.2 Application layer tasks in a multimedia sensor network.

3.3.2 *Existing Application Layer Solutions*

3.3.2.1 WMSNs In traffic management, application layer responsibility in a WMSN depends on whether the application is delay-tolerant and is concerned about a multimedia stream or a specific data. In real-time applications, tolerance for delay is very low, which in turn requires CR nodes (for CRSNs) to carry out the cognitive cycle in a quicker manner, with the shortest possible spectrum-sensing duration and acceptable false alarm and false detection levels. In real-time applications, greedy forwarding and nearest neighbor forwarding should be assessed to determine which would cause less delay, and action should be taken, which in turn requires cross-layer coordination. In a delay-tolerant setting, CRSN nodes can periodically turn on and off their transceivers, field-sensing units, or both. To date, no study has considered a sleeping schedule for transceivers and field-sensing units of CRSN nodes at the same time, which would be governed by the traffic-management task of the application layer.

In terms of the coding paradigm, with individual source coding, each node codes its own field readings independently [2]. Simplicity is an advantage of individual source coding because it does not require communication and/or coordination between nodes for coding purposes. Such individual coding has been shown to be suboptimal, especially if the spatiotemporal correlation of the sensed field is significant [8]. Accordingly, in a WMSN, it is possible to choose a representative number of nodes M for an event and adjust their reporting frequency f such that significant power savings can be achieved while conforming to a maximum distortion at the sink, that is, $D(f, M) < D_{max}$.

The video compression technology H.264 possesses excellent rate-distortion performance with its advanced compression techniques [9]. The newly proposed H.265 [10] will even surpass it in terms of compression efficiency. Nevertheless, such predictive coding schemes bring processing complexity and require excessive energy consumption for compression. In addition, predictive coding schemes require complex encoders and decoders. It is not feasible for resource-constrained sensor nodes to use these complex encoders. To solve these problems, DSC has been proposed as the paradigm to balance communication needs and processing cost with a good rate-distortion performance.

Slepian and Wolf [11] first proved that, for lossless compression of two correlated signals, separate simple encoding and joint decoding is as efficient as joint decoding. Considering X and Y as two correlated random variables, from Shannon's source coding theorem, a rate $R \geq H(X, Y)$ is sufficient. This may be obtained by a rate $R_Y \geq H(Y)$ and $R_X \geq H(X \mid Y)$, which in turn produces a total rate of $R_X + R_Y \geq H(X \mid Y) + H(Y) = H(X, Y)$. Slepian and Wolf stated that $R \geq H(X, Y)$ is sufficient for the separate encoding of correlated X and Y, which translates to $R_X \geq H(X \mid Y)$ being achievable without knowing the explicit Y at the encoder but knowing the joint statistics of X and YY only. Wyner–Ziv coding was proposed as an extension to Slepian and Wolf, where correlated discrete signals are coded in a lossy manner this time, with respect to a fidelity criterion. Wyner–Ziv is challenged, though, by the fact that obtaining explicit joint probability density functions to compress the sources (nodes) in a distributed manner is difficult [12]. Exploitation of spatial correlation among sources is the key to overcoming this challenge. This is natural, given the fact that video sources are usually anisotropic. From a CRSN perspective, leveraging spatial correlation via DSC is still more challenging, since DSC would require synchronization between two nodes to be jointly decoded at the sink. Due to temporal variation of licensed user traffic, even neighboring nodes might not be able to communicate for proper synchronization, especially in delay-intolerant applications.

DSC via the Wyner–Ziv paradigm (simple encoder at nodes, complex decoder at sink) is a very attractive technique for exploiting the temporal correlation of each source's readings within itself. DSC is indeed one of the hot topics in research, with various studies conducted to find a balance between computation and communication efficiency in sensor networks [13,14,15,16]. On exploitation of temporal correlation of each node, routing schemes may need to be revisited particularly in the case of CRSNs, where routes to the sink may lose connectivity, even permanently, depending on the PU behavior.

On the compression technique side, single layer and multi-layer coding techniques have been nicely summarized in Ref. [2].

Accordingly, in single layer coding, a reference layer and only consecutive differences between frames are transmitted until the next reference frame. This type of coding does not provide error resilience. Nevertheless, in underlay cognitive networks, besides bad channel conditions for SUs, a frame is to be retransmitted (potentially through another channel) regardless once it is interrupted via licensed user traffic. However, for CRNs using underlay spectrum sharing, transmission can still continue until the tolerable threshold limit on licensed users has been crossed by the SUs. In that sense, it is more suitable to employ multilayer coding, which allows for joint source and channel coding, and hence error resilience, in underlay CRSNs.

3.3.2.2 Cognitive Radio and Sensor Networks   There are far fewer studies regarding multimedia communications in CRNs and CRSNs than in WSNs, given that they are relatively new paradigms.

Ref. [17] is a related work in the context of CRNs, where QoS is optimized by varying the intra-refreshing rate together with the access strategy and spectrum sensing of CR nodes. The idea with the intra-refreshing rate is that an intra-coded macroblock does not depend on previous blocks, which might have been corrupted by errors in previous transmission, thus limiting error propagation and lowering of QoS. Nevertheless, because the study focuses on CRNs, the assumed multimedia model is based on advanced compression techniques of H.264 and alike, which are not suitable for the low complexity nodes of CRSNs.

Dastpak et al. [18] also study multimedia communications in CRN. A streaming optimization problem is set and is solved based on the bandwidth budget available to CR nodes. The results reveal that group-of-picture (GoP)-based optimization is less computationally expensive, but it also has slightly less QoS compared to frame-based optimization. Again, the work is based on the H.264 scalable video codec and is not directly applicable to resource-constrained CRSNs.

Ref. [19] is an interesting work in CRSNs regarding the optimal allocation of power to two sensing tasks, namely field sensing and spectrum sensing. Although the results are insightful, the network model needs to be extended to a multihop network, which is usually the case in CRSNs.

3.3.3 Open Research Issues for the Application Layer

Several open issues exist in CRSN regarding the application layer, as follows:

- For traffic management, an application layer protocol that decides upon sleep and wake-up schedules of the transceivers and field sensor of CRSN nodes is needed for enhanced network lifetime.
- An energy-efficient, cross-layer scheme for source and channel coding in CRSN is needed to ensure reliable monitoring.
- Routing schemes need to be revisited in the CRSN aspect, to make sure that Wyner–Ziv coding that is targeted to leverage node-based temporal correlation makes each packet arrive at the sink, given that connectivity in CRSNs is intermittent among many nodes.

3.4 The Transport Layer in Multimedia Communication for Cognitive Radio Ad Hoc and Sensor Networks

The transport layer provides end-to-end reliability for data transfer and congestion and flow control in traditional computer networking. Transport layer protocols regulate data flows, control congestion, decrease packet loss, and guarantee a certain level of end-to-end reliability in WSNs [20]. However, due to the inherent features of WSNs, such as network topology, traffic characteristics, and their application-dependent nature, the traditional transport layer protocols such as transmission control protocol (TCP) and user datagram protocol (UDP) do not suit WSN.

Transport layer solutions are vital for the realization of multimedia communication in CR ad hoc and sensor networks. Reliable data delivery of event features and the amount of traffic injection upon event detection are the main issues of the transport layer. The existing challenges for CR and sensor networks need to be reconsidered for the realization of the multimedia communication in CR ad hoc and sensor networks. Apart from the WSN paradigm, CR ad hoc and sensor networks impose new challenges for transport layer functionalities. To achieve efficient transport layer solutions, the unique characteristics of CR ad hoc and sensor networks paradigm and the distinctive requirements of multimedia communications must be analyzed in detail to develop transport layer solutions.

3.4.1 Challenges and Requirements

The main duties of the transport layer are reliability and congestion control. Multimedia communication in wireless networks is delay-sensitive data communication. Hence, timely delivery of data packets is more important for performance than reliability. Delay bound and strict QoS demands impose significant challenges on communication. The multimedia packets have a higher size than conventional data packets. Hence, the potential delays cause buffer overflows and the loss of data packets.

In sensor networks, event readings are injected to the network, and this injection creates high and bursty traffic. This situation requires a certain level of congestion control and end-to-end reliability to preserve the limited resources of the nodes. The end-to-end reliability is achieved by the arrival of a sufficient number of event packets at the sink. Congestion control is enabling the event traffic toward the sink to not exceed the capacity of ad hoc or sensor networks. These functionalities of the transport layer are used to provide energy efficiency and to prevent the waste of communication resources [5].

CR has unique features that should be carefully considered to propose efficient solutions. The inherent features of CR give rise to unique challenges, which can be itemized as follows.

- Spectrum sensing: Spectrum sensing is a vital cognitive cycle operation that provides information about spectrum availability. During spectrum sensing, the transmission function is paused, since they cannot be performed simultaneously. The operating channels can be changed after channel sensing. The channel characteristics may change or it may even become occupied by a PU. Furthermore, the channel-sensing period may be changed due to spectrum efficiency and interference avoidance [21]. The scheduling of sensing duration must be organized to decrease collision probability. Different sensing periods of nodes results in variation of packet latency, that is, jitter. Transport layer functionality rate control must consider this heterogeneity in the spectrum-sensing duration that causes the degradation of transport layer performance.

- Interference by the PU: The main spectrum-sensing technique is energy detection. This technique may cause faulty detection; thus, the transmission continues despite the existence of a legacy user on that communication band. Furthermore, a packet transmitted by a CR source node may be received erroneously. The precious resources of wireless nodes are wasted. The probability of successful packet transmission decreases with PU activities.

- Spectrum handoff: During communication between event and sink in CRSNs, and between source and destination in cognitive radio ad hoc networks (CRAHNs), changes in licensed user activity are observable. These changes may degrade the performance of the secondary network. Upon detection of a licensed user in the communication channel, spectrum handoff is performed. The communication is stopped until a new vacant channel can be found. In addition, the delay characteristics and the loss rate change on the communication link, which affects the communication performance.

- Dynamic spectrum access: If a CR does not find a vacant band, then it has to wait for a spectrum opportunity. This waiting time causes extra time delay for packet transmission. In sensor networks, the data packet may become obsolete due to the delay.

- Spectrum mobility: The CR capability of CR ad hoc and sensor nodes provides a change of operating parameters in case of spectrum handoff. The channel and delay characteristics, and also the level of noise change due to the variations in the operating channel parameters.

- Spectrum coordination: The dynamic spectrum environment requires spectrum coordination. The exchange of control packets for channel selection and sensing duration are the main functionalities of spectrum coordination. Spectrum coordination is highly necessary to perform cognitive cycle operations such as spectrum decision and spectrum handoff.

The challenges posed by the CR ad hoc and sensor network paradigm are amplified by the unique requirements of multimedia communication. The dynamic spectrum access scheme provides gain by opportunistic channel access; however, licensed user activities may deteriorate multimedia communication. Furthermore, energy efficiency is an important challenge for resource-constrained wireless nodes. Hence, dynamic spectrum access (DSA) and licensed user activities should be carefully examined to avoid unnecessary power consumption due to collision, interference, and loss through buffer overflow.

3.4.2 Existing Transport Layer Solutions

3.4.2.1 *WSNs* The main duties of transport protocols are to mitigate congestion and packet losses and to fairly allocate limited bandwidth between the wireless nodes. Hence, we propose a number of WSN transport protocols, according to energy efficiency, reliability, and fairness metrics.

Different techniques can be combined to control and mitigate congestion in WSNs. In Ref. [22], three techniques—hop-by-hop flow control, a source rate limiting scheme, and a prioritized MAC layer that gives priority to backlogged nodes—are combined to mitigate and control congestion. Congestion is detected when the fraction of space of the output queue is less than a certain threshold [22]. To mitigate congestion, hop-by-hop rate adjustment is performed. By contrast, Wan et al. [23] detect congestion in WSNs by also observing the state of the channel for a certain period of time. If channel utilization surpasses a certain threshold, the congestion bit in the outgoing packet is set to one. Congestion mitigation is performed by hop-by-hop back pressure to locally change congestion policy or end-to-end source rate regulation.

Congestion can be detected in several ways in WSN. For example, in Ref. [24], the authors look at packet service time to find congestion. On the other hand, Ref. [20] uses interarrival times of the packets in addition to the service time of the packet to detect congestion. Furthermore, congestion is mitigated by hop-by-hop rate adjustment in Refs. [20,24]. Table 3.1 outlines congestion detection and mitigation techniques used in the literature.

Table 3.1 Existing Congestion Control Protocols in Wireless Sensor Networks

PROTOCOL	CONGESTION DETECTION	CONGESTION MITIGATION
Fusion [22]	Observing output queues	Hop-by-hop rate adjustment
CODA [23]	Observing state of channel	Hop-by-hop rate backpressure
Congestion Control & Fairness Protocol [24]	Observing service time of packets	Hop-by-hop rate adjustment
PCCP [20]	Observing inter-arrival time of packets and service time	Hop-by-hop rate adjustment

Multimedia communication in CR ad hoc and sensor networks requires efficient congestion detection and mitigation mechanisms, because congestion strongly affects real-time communication. Large packet size, the dynamic radio environment, and limited capabilities of sensor nodes necessitate novel schemes by considering the challenges posed by the CRSN paradigm.

Apart from congestion detection and mitigation techniques, reliability is another important functionality of the transport layer in WSNs. Reliable multi-segment transport (RMST) [25] provides end-to-end reliability for all the packets in WSN and does not take into account the correlated nature of the event packets. Packet reliability is provided by requesting data by NACK from the source or the cache nodes. Multi-path and multi-SPEED (MMSPEED) [26] provides reliability at different QoS levels, in addition to timeliness. It utilizes multipath method to increase the delivery probability of packets and to propose a dynamic compensation scheme such that inaccurate decisions made by a node in the path can be compensated for along the route to the sink. Pump slowly fetch quickly (PSFQ) [27] injects or pumps messages slowly to the network. Furthermore, the intermediate nodes cache data for local loss recovery. If there is a gap in the received file fragments, a NACK is sent in the reverse path to recover the lost packets. However, packet loss due to congestion is not addressed in PSFQ.

The transport layer requires end-to-end reliability in wireless ad hoc networks. However, sensor observations are correlated in sensor networks [8]. Hence, end-to-end reliability is not a strict requirement. A sufficient number of sensor observations must be collected by the sink to extract event features with a certain estimation distortion. This reliability model is known as *event reliability* [28]. TCP protocols, which require retransmission of lost packets, are not efficient for the WSN paradigm because retransmission consumes the scarce resources of sensor nodes.

End-to-end reliability is provided at the sink or source nodes. In Ref. [28], the application-dependent reliability level is satisfied at the sink according to the reporting rate of source nodes in the event region. If the packets received according to sensor reports satisfy the reliability level, the reporting rate is decreased. Otherwise, the reporting rate is increased to achieve the desired level of event reliability. With this adaptive feature of event-to-sink reliable transport (ESRT), the event is extracted as a result of the correlated nature of sensor observations.

Rate-controlled reliable transport (RCRT) [29] is a reliable transport protocol for applications that are not tolerant to packet losses. It utilizes end-to-end loss recovery. Furthermore, congestion detection and rate adaptation are done at the sink. It implements a NACK-based end-to-end loss recovery scheme to guarantee reliability. It also utilizes cumulative ACK to remove the packets at the source node that are received by the sink.

Wireless sensor and actor networks are heterogeneous networks where sensor nodes and actors coexist. Sensors observe the environment and actors perform actions according to the sensor observations. $(RT)^2$ [30] proposes real-time reliable transport for sensor–actor and actor–actor communication. It considers event reliability as in ESRT [28].

In CR ad hoc and sensor networks, reliable delivery of all multimedia communication data packets is not necessary due to the correlated nature of sensor observations. Hence, the protocols must consider event reliability and offer a certain level of QoS. Table 3.2 outlines reliable transport protocols in WSNs and their advantages and disadvantages for multimedia communications.

3.4.2.2 Cognitive Radio Ad Hoc and Sensor Networks The unique constraints encountered at the transport layer in WSNs are amplified by the CR capability in CRAHNs. Cognitive cycle operations affect the transport layer protocol design. For example, transport layer functionality is disrupted by spectrum sensing and, if a timeout occurs, the source rate is decreased without congestion. The delay between two nodes increases by spectrum switching due to PU arrival on the communication channel. In Ref. [31], the optimal balance is achieved between the spectrum-sensing duration and the throughput

Table 3.2 Reliability of Transport Protocols in Wireless Sensor Networks

PROTOCOL	MULTIMEDIA COMMUNICATION ISSUES
RMST [25]	– End-to-end reliability for all packets
	– No consideration of correlation between packets
	– NACK-based retransmission
MMSPEED [26]	+ Reliability at different quality of service levels and timeliness
	+ Multipath support
	+ Dynamic compensation against inaccurate decisions
PSFQ [27]	+ Caches data for loss recovery
	– NACK-based retransmission
	– No congestion loss consideration
ESRT [28]	+ Event reliability
	+ Reporting rate adjustment
RCRT [29]	+ Real-time support
	– End-to-end loss recovery by NACK
$(RT)^2$ [30]	+ Event reliability
	+ Real-time reliable transport

Note: Advantages and disadvantages are indicated by + and –, respectively.

of the CRN. It is known that if sensing duration increases, end-to-end throughput decreases [32]. Spectrum switching due to PU activities causes changes in channel characteristics. These changes result in variation of the bandwidth and hence the TCP congestion window is adaptively modified [31]. Consequently, classical TCP is adapted to a dynamic radio environment. In an earlier work, transport protocol for cognitive radio ad hoc networks (TP-CRAHN) [33] was proposed for establishing a spectrum-aware window-based transport layer protocol.

Cross-layer design is also used to improve the performance of the transport layer in CRNs. In Ref. [34], the cognitive cycle operations, physical layer coding and modulation scheme, and data-link layer frame size are concurrently optimized to maximize TCP throughput in CRNs. Furthermore, the effects of varying link capacity and PU detection errors on TCP throughput were studied in a dynamic spectrum access network with a centralized base station [32]. However, this study did not consider the ad hoc nature of the communications.

For CRAHNs, existing works mainly regard the adaptation of TCP to the dynamic radio environment by considering cognitive cycle operations. The transport layer has also been investigated in CRSNs.

In Ref. [35], it was pointed out that existing WSN transport layer solutions are not suitable for CRSNs, because they do not consider the additional delay caused by spectrum sensing and spectrum mobility. These were indicated as open research issues for the CRSN transport layer. It was concluded that to propose novel transport layer solutions, packet losses and delays due to the cognitive cycle must be considered together with the energy constraints of CRSN nodes.

3.4.2.3 WMSNs Multimedia communication in WSN requires the transportation of a great volume of data with high transmission rate and bounded delay. The high volume of data produced by multimedia applications results in buffer overflow and congestion. Queue-based Congestion Control Protocol with Priority Support (QCCP-PS) [36] was proposed for fair and reliable transport in WMSNs. In this protocol, queue length is used as a measure of congestion degree, and rate assignment to a traffic source is done according to its priority index and congestion degree. The priority index is used to ascertain the priority of the traffic sources in WMSNs. However, this approach does not consider spectrum-aware communication and hence it cannot be directly applied to CR ad hoc and sensor networks.

3.4.3 Open Research Issues for the Transport Layer

In preceding subsections, we investigated the challenges for multimedia communication in CR ad hoc and sensor networks. Furthermore, we surveyed the important existing transport layer solutions in WSNs, CRAHNs, CRSNs, and WMSNs.

Transport layer protocols for WSNs cannot be applied to CR and ad hoc networks due to lack of support for DSA functionalities. CRAHN and CRSN solutions do not satisfy the unique requirements of multimedia communication such as bounded delay, jitter control, and smooth variation of throughput. WMSN transport layer solutions satisfy multimedia communication requirements; however, they do not consider spectrum awareness. Hence, the open research issues can be itemized as follows:

- In light of the above discussions, it is necessary to develop novel transport layer algorithms to satisfy the requirements of multimedia communication and DSA functionalities.

The proposed transport protocol should be adaptive to licensed user activities and cognitive cycle operations to deliver multimedia data in an energy-efficient and timely manner.

- Varying network capacity is detrimental for multimedia communication. Spectrum handoff results in a change of operating channel parameters, and link capacity changes accordingly. Hence, licensed user behavior can be estimated to prevent frequent spectrum handoff and deterioration of multimedia communication.

- A novel congestion detection mechanism should be developed that considers the extra delay caused by cognitive cycle operations such as spectrum sensing and spectrum handoff.

- A novel rate control mechanism should be designed to decrease buffer overflow and retransmission. Rate control in CR ad hoc and sensor networks should consider the varying licensed user activity, spectrum-sensing duration, and spectrum handoff delay.

- In addition to reliable transport protocols for multimedia communication, they should support real-time communication to satisfy multimedia application deadlines.

- Due to energy constraints, the limited capabilities of sensor nodes, and the dynamic spectrum environment and DSA capability, cross-layer communication protocols should be investigated to support energy-efficient and reliable multimedia communication in CRSNs.

3.5 The Network Layer in Multimedia Communication for Cognitive Radio Ad Hoc and Sensor Networks

The network layer provides the connection between the transport layer and the MAC layer. It mainly provides routes from the source to destination that satisfy certain QoS requirements such as energy efficiency and delay. In wireless ad hoc networks, multihop communication is utilized to save energy and to maintain high-quality communication links. Hence, efficient network layer solutions are imperative for establishing energy-efficient routes and providing information to the transport layer.

3.5.1 Limitations and Challenges

Multimedia communication in CR sensor and ad hoc networks has some inherent limitations. Furthermore, spectrum awareness of wireless nodes poses extra challenges in the network layer.

Multimedia communication has stringent delay requirements and requires high bandwidth. Furthermore, there are limitations on multimedia communication in WSNs as stated in Ref. [3], which are summarized as follows. Multimedia communication has a query-driven or event-driven data delivery model. Continuous data delivery drains the energy of wireless nodes. Source aggregation and in-network processing are not efficient methods for multimedia communication due to the anisotropic nature of video signals. Furthermore, the cost due to the multimedia information gathering and processing in local communication should be limited. Multimedia communication should also satisfy a certain level of QoS. This limitation could be overcome by utilizing multipath communication.

The limitations of multimedia communication are amplified by the unique features of CR. For example, data delivery models must be revisited for the spectrum sensing and spectrum hand-off mechanisms. In addition, the dynamic radio environment poses challenges for multipath communication, because multipath routes between an event and the sink may be disrupted by the activities of PUs. Predetermined routes may break due to dynamic channel conditions.

3.5.2 Existing Network Layer Solutions

3.5.2.1 WSNs Wireless sensor nodes have energy and processing constraints, hence energy efficiency is the main consideration of routing protocols in WSNs. The route is established and maintained at the network layer to maximize the lifetime of the WSN. Furthermore, an excessive number of sensor nodes is deployed in sensor networks; classical IP addressing would be an overhead for energy-constrained WSN regimes. Hence, attribute addressing is used such that the node having the attributed data communicates to the sink over multiple hops.

Routing protocols in WSNs are classified into three categories— flat, hierarchical, and location-based [37]. In flat network routing, all the nodes in the network have the same role and collaboratively send observation data to the sink. Hierarchical network routing employs clustering; cluster heads behave as source aggregation nodes and decrease message content to provide energy efficiency. In geographical network routing, each node in the network knows its position by triangulation and localization techniques. The source packets are routed toward the sink with the location information.

Sensor protocols for information via negotiation (SPIN) [38] is a flat network routing protocol where every node sends an advertisement (ADV) message to announce its data packet. The node needing this packet sends a request (REQ) message to the node, and the node with the data sends it with a DATA message. This protocol is not suitable for multimedia communication in CR ad hoc and sensor networks because it does not guarantee the delivery of data packets, which degrades the performance of the multimedia communication. Furthermore, Directed Diffusion [39] is a query-based data-centric routing protocol where the sink sends an interest signal to request information from the source nodes. Source nodes set up gradients toward the sink and the sink reinforces some paths according to QoS requirements. Source nodes send the information from reinforced paths. This process requires end-to-end control data transfer, hence the routing discovery process may increase delay bound. By contrast, the multipath support satisfies the multipath limitation of multimedia communication. A variant of Directed Diffusion, Rumor Routing [40], which decreases energy consumption by avoiding flooding the queries, does not provide multipath support; therefore, it is not suitable for multimedia communication.

Hierarchical routing for multimedia communication has some drawbacks because of the communication and processing burden of multimedia data at the cluster head and poor channel quality between cluster heads, which is the result of a high communication range between the cluster heads. In Low-Energy Adaptive Clustering Hierarchy (LEACH) [41], the data collected by the cluster members are gathered at the cluster head, and an aggregation technique is applied. LEACH proposes a routing architecture such that the aggregated data at each cluster head are conveyed collaboratively by all cluster heads. It offers scalability, lifetime improvement, and energy efficiency. Due to the aggregation limitations of multimedia data and the poor quality of the communication link between cluster heads, this architecture is not suitable for multimedia communication.

On-the-fly event-driven clustering was proposed in Ref. [42], where it is called "Event-to-Sink Directed Clustering" (ESDC). Upon detection of an event, a routing corridor is established between the event and the sink. The data packets are routed by the cluster heads. Multimedia packets are large packets and their processing, that is, aggregation, requires a large memory size, which is not suited to the limited capabilities of sensor nodes. Hence, this approach has a disadvantage for multimedia communication.

Clustering-based routing is very promising for WSNs; however, if the network is homogenous, the multimedia applications cannot use the benefits of hierarchical routing. By contrast, if the cluster heads are more powerful nodes that are capable of processing multimedia data, hierarchical routing becomes an efficient means for providing network layer solutions in multimedia applications.

In another approach, the event packets are propagated directly towards the sink, if the direction of the base station is known. First, the node broadcasts its packet to its one-hop neighbors; the node with the least cost to the base station continues the data flow. In this approach, known as the "Minimum Cost Forwarding Algorithm" (MCFA) [43], each node knows the cost to reach the base station through messages sent by the base station. This protocol is convenient for multimedia communication, since the multimedia data are forwarded to the base stations upon the detection of an event without any delay for setting up routes.

In location-based networks, routing is performed according to the location information. For example, in Geographical and Energy Aware Routing (GEAR) [44], location-aware and energy-aware nodes utilize a heuristic approach for selecting a neighbor to route the packets toward the sink. In Ref. [45], energy minimization is achieved through location information and relay region determination accordingly. Minimum energy paths are established beforehand; hence, the topology changes and reconfiguration of WSNs may lead to inefficiency of the routing protocol. However, location-based networks set up routes with smaller delay and reduced energy consumption. Hence, it is more appropriate for multimedia communication.

Routing protocols can also be divided into five categories, according to protocol operation: negotiation-based, multipath, query-based, QoS-based, and coherence-based protocols [37]. In negotiation-based protocols, negotiation is performed between nodes to prevent duplication and redundancy before data communication. In multipath communication, the same data are sent along different paths to increase reliability and bandwidth. Query-based protocols start data transmission and set up routes upon queries sent by the sink. QoS-based routing protocols establish routes to satisfy certain parameters such as delay, throughput, jitter, and so on. In coherence-based routing protocols, the raw data are processed at the nodes. According to this characterization, multipath and QoS routing protocols are suitable for multimedia communication because it requires reliability, high throughput, and low delay bound and jitter.

QoS-based protocols set up and maintain the routes according to certain metrics such as link delay, bandwidth, energy efficiency, residual energy, or a weighted combination of some of these. In Ref. [46], an energy-aware QoS routing protocol is proposed. It considers the end-to-end delay to establish QoS routes for real-time data delivery. According to a cost function—which is evaluated by transmission energy, error rate, and residual energy—the least-cost path is selected with delay constraint. Real-Time Power-Aware Routing (RPAR) [47] addresses the challenge of energy-efficient communication with a certain QoS requirement—specifically, delay. RPAR is achieved by adapting the transmission power of the nodes and routing decisions dynamically, based on packet deadlines. It supports real-time communication in WSNs. This type of protocol is very promising for multimedia communication in CR ad hoc and sensor networks because it satisfies a certain QoS requirement—delay, with energy-efficiency constraints. However, such protocols do not support CR functionality. Hence, they need to be modified to adapt to spectral changes.

Table 3.3 outlines routing protocols in WSNs and their advantages and disadvantages for realizing multimedia communication in CR ad hoc and sensor networks.

3.5.2.2 Cognitive Radio Ad Hoc and Sensor Networks The dynamic spectral environment and cognitive cycle operations of wireless nodes make routing a very challenging task in CRNs. The flexibility

Table 3.3 Routing Protocols in Wireless Sensor Networks

PROTOCOL	MULTIMEDIA COMMUNICATION ISSUES
SPIN [38]	− Flat network routing
	− No guarantee of data delivery
Directed Diffusion [39]	+ Query-based data-centric routing
	+ Multipath support
	− Delay due to end-to-end control data
Rumor Routing [40]	+ A variant of directed diffusion [39]
	+ No flooding of queries
	− No multipath support
LEACH [41]	+ Scalability and lifetime improvement
	− Poor link quality between cluster heads
ESDC [42]	+ On-the-fly event-driven clustering
	+ Routing corridor between event and sink
GEAR [44]	+ Route selection according to energy and location
[45]	+ Relay region determination through location information
MCFA [43]	+ Routing toward the sink
	+ No delay to set up routes to the sink
[46]	+ Energy-aware QoS-based routing
	+ QoS routes for real-time data delivery
RPAR [47]	+ Energy-efficient routing with low delay
	+ Routing decisions according to packet deadline

Note: Advantages and disadvantages are indicated by + and −, respectively.

in spectrum access brings about complexity in the protocol design. The main challenges of the routing multihop CRN are spectrum awareness, setup of quality routes, and route maintenance/repair [48]. Furthermore, routing protocols in CRNs depend on either full-spectrum knowledge or local-spectrum knowledge.

With full-spectrum knowledge in CRNs, optimal routes can be set up. In practical networks, full knowledge may not be achievable; however, optimal routes can be used as a benchmark for the routing protocols. In the routing process, avoidance of interference with PUs is a requirement; hence, routing protocols establish routes to not interfere with licensed users. In Ref. [49], spectrum information is known *a priori* and mixed integer linear programming is used to provide fair routing for different traffic demands by considering spectrum sharing and flow routing with interference considerations.

Spectrum-Aware Opportunistic Routing [50] was proposed to employ multipath transmissions and QoS guaranteed throughput with decreased delay. SAOR creates a spectrum map from local sensing observations and opportunistic routing. Furthermore, opportunistic cognitive routing was proposed in Ref. [51]. CRs select the relay node based on the location information and channel usage statistics. A new metric, cognitive transport throughput, is defined to assess the potential relay gain.

Link scheduling is important for CRNs to decrease interference. The routing problem in multihop CRNs has been studied with link scheduling [52]. Scheduling and routing are performed alongside the unpredictable activities of PUs. They try to perform opportunistic spectrum access, scheduling, and multipath multihop routing in CRNs by minimizing network resource usage. The spectrum vacancy of a licensed band is modeled as a random variable to estimate the channel availability. Ref. [52] is an important study for realizing multimedia communication in CR ad hoc and sensor networks.

Spectrum-Aware On-Demand Routing protocol is a reactive protocol that balances channel switching and spectrum sharing through routing and frequency band selection [53]. Routes are selected according to their effectiveness in terms of spectrum switching delay and back-off delay. Ma et al. [54] also propose an on-demand routing and channel assignment protocol that does not utilize a common control channel (CCC). The protocol also decreases back-off delay and the overhead due to channel switching and tries to avoid the deafness problem due to channel switching. Reactive protocols are more advantageous than proactive protocols because the dynamic nature of the environment renders obsolete the routes established beforehand. Hence, on-demand (reactive) routing protocols are more applicable to CR ad hoc and sensor networks.

Enabling multimedia communication of WMSNs over CRSNs poses challenges due to the distributed nature of CRSNs and the dynamics of network and spectrum usage. Hence, routing protocols should provide rate adaptation with opportunistic bandwidth, as well as delay and jitter control [55]. Spectrum-Aware Clustering Protocol for Energy Efficient Routing (SCEEM) [55] was proposed such that clustering manages dynamic spectrum access and QoS routing for multimedia communication in CRSNs. The contributions of

Table 3.4   Routing Protocols in Cognitive Radio Networks

PROTOCOL	MULTIMEDIA COMMUNICATION ISSUES
Joint Spectrum and Fair Routing Protocol [49]	+ Can be considered a benchmark
	+ Fair routing for different traffic demands
	− Spectrum information known *a priori*
SAOR [50]	+ Multipath opportunistic routing
	+ QoS guaranteed throughput with decreased delay
	+ Local spectrum sensing
Opportunistic Cognitive Routing (OCR) [51]	+ Relay node selection based on location information and channel usage statistics
Joint Routing and Link Scheduling Protocol [52]	+ Joint routing and scheduling
Spectrum-aware On-Demand Routing Protocol [53]	+ Balances spectrum sharing and channel switching
	+ Considers spectrum switching and back-off delay
Multi-hop single transceiver CRN Routing Protocol [54]	+ Route selection according to energy and location
SCEEM [55]	+ Smooth delivery of multimedia data
	+ Clustered QoS routing

Note: Advantages and disadvantages are indicated by + and −, respectively.

SCEEM are smooth multimedia data delivery by the isolation of time and frequency variability of the spectrum and energy efficiency with QoS-aware routing.

Table 3.4 outlines several routing protocols in CRNs and CRSNs and their advantages for multimedia communication in CR ad hoc and sensor networks.

CRN routing protocols consider delay, throughput, and licensed user activities; however, they do not deal with the challenge of energy efficiency. Delay and throughput considerations are compatible with the requirements of multimedia communication. By contrast, these protocols need appropriate modifications such as energy efficiency to be utilized in CR ad hoc and sensor networks.

3.5.2.3 WMSNs   New routing solutions have been proposed to satisfy the unique requirements of multimedia communication in WMSNs. Readers may refer to the comprehensive survey about routing protocols in WMSN presented by Abazeed et al. [56]. In this section, we present some of the recent proposals for routing in WMSNs.

Li et al. [57] extend directed diffusion to reinforce multiple paths with a high quality of links and low latency. This protocol offers better throughput with lower delay than directed diffusion. Furthermore, Ref. [58] proposes a multichannel, multipath routing protocol in which routes are determined by adjusting the required bandwidth dynamically and by the differentiation of delay that is proportional to the path length for real-time data. Ref. [59] provides the necessary bandwidth for multimedia applications by establishing disjoint routes and avoiding intersession and intrasession interference. One path is built for each session; if there is congestion or lack of bandwidth, additional paths are established. Interfering nodes are forced to be passive to decrease interference and unnecessary energy consumption.

A routing protocol has also been proposed for multimedia streaming, which requires delay bound and high bandwidth demand [60]. This protocol is an online multipath routing protocol for WMSNs. Route decisions are made at each hop using location information. Two schemes are used to achieve energy efficiency and load balancing: a smart greedy forwarding scheme that selects the most appropriate node and a walk-back scheme to bypass network holes.

Table 3.5 outlines the state-of-the-art routing protocols and their advantages for realizing multimedia communication in CR ad hoc and sensor networks. In general, the proposed routing solutions in the literature employ location-based and multipath routing. They support traffic demanding high bandwidth and low delay. However, the proposed solutions do not consider the dynamic radio environment, which is a missing issue for multimedia communication in CR ad hoc and sensor networks.

Table 3.5   Routing Protocols in Wireless Multimedia Sensor Networks

PROTOCOL	MULTIMEDIA COMMUNICATION ISSUES
Delay Constrained High Throughput Protocol [57]	+ Reinforces multiple paths with high quality links with low latency
QoS Routing Protocol [58]	+ Multichannel multipath routing
	+ Real-time data delivery
Maximally radio-disjoint multipath routing Protocol [59]	+ Disjoint route establishment
	+ Additional paths in case of congestion and lack of bandwidth

Note: Advantages and disadvantages are indicated by + and −, respectively.

3.5.3 Open Research Issues for the Network Layer

Numerous efforts focus on network layer solutions in WSNs, CRNs, and WMSNs. These efforts mainly concentrate on routing protocols. Multimedia communication requirements are satisfied by WMSN routing solutions. However, they must also overcome the challenges of CR and sensor networks. Open research issues in the network layer can be itemized as follows.

- Back-off delay and channel-switching delay must be taken into account to provide delay-bounded path establishment. Additional delay occurs due to licensed user activities in CR ad hoc and sensor networks.
- The dynamic radio environment causes changes in spectrum opportunities; hence, reactive protocols would be more appropriate for multimedia communication in CR ad hoc and sensor networks. This type of protocol should be designed.
- Due to the dynamic spectral environment, established paths can become obsolete. Hence, multipath protocols are appropriate for multimedia communication, and there is no existing study of multipath protocols in CR ad hoc and sensor networks.

3.6 The MAC Layer in Multimedia Communication for Cognitive Radio Ad Hoc and Sensor Networks

The MAC layer is mainly responsible for the channel access mechanism, scheduling, buffer management, and error control mechanisms in wireless networks. The channel access mechanism affects the delay and reliability of the packet; scheduling is used to schedule packet transmission in the medium to decrease collision probability. The bursty nature of multimedia communication requires efficient buffer management policies to decrease buffer overflows. If the received packet has errors, the transmitter simply resends the packet in ARQ scheme. However, in FEC scheme, the receiver can detect and recover the errors in the packet without any retransmission. Due to the real-time data delivery requirement of multimedia communication, the ARQ scheme may not be used, because it requires retransmission of the packet.

Energy-aware MAC layer solutions are necessary to satisfy the unique requirements of the sensor network paradigm as well as the requirements of multimedia communication. Novel techniques are required for adaptation to the dynamic spectral environment in CR ad hoc and sensor networks. Access to the medium, error control, and packet transmission reliability are highly influenced by the requirements of multimedia communication, sensor networks, and CR. In this section, we survey MAC layer solutions in the literature and how they can be extended to multimedia communication in CR ad hoc and sensor networks.

3.6.1 Challenges and Requirements

The major requirements of MAC protocols in sensor networks are real-time or QoS requirements, decentralized operation, power awareness, and flexibility to different kinds of applications [61]. The main requirement of multimedia communication in the MAC layer is packet transmission with minimal error, delay, and collision. Contention in the medium access may result in collision and, hence, delay and energy consumption. Latency, delay, and jitter are the vital QoS parameters for multimedia communication.

The most important challenge for multimedia communication in CR ad hoc and sensor networks is intermittent communication due to cognitive cycle functions. These fundamental operations result in delay and channel quality degradation and, hence, a decrease in communication quality for multimedia communication. In CR communication, there is a nonzero probability of colliding with the packets of PUs, as well as with the packets of SUs. Furthermore, there are many more parameters that need to be taken into account to realize multimedia communication in CR ad hoc and sensor networks.

3.6.2 Existing MAC Layer Solutions

There have been some surveys on the MAC layer in WSNs [62] and CRNs [63,64]; however, they do not explain how to enable efficient multimedia communication in dynamic radio environments. In this section, in addition to explaining the state-of-the-art solutions for the MAC layer, we emphasize the changes necessary to realize multimedia communication in CR ad hoc and sensor networks.

3.6.2.1 WSNs Many MAC layer protocols have been proposed with different objectives for WSNs. However, they do not satisfy the requirements of multimedia communication and the challenges posed by CR and sensor networks. In sensor networks, the primary concerns are energy efficiency and scalability; however, throughput and latency attributes are secondary concerns [62]. They must all be treated as primary concerns for multimedia communication.

MAC protocols can be divided into two categories: contention-free protocols and contention protocols. The contention-free protocols are time division multiple access (TDMA), frequency division multiple access (FDMA), and code division multiple access (CDMA). By contrast, contention protocols do not reserve resources; they are allocated to network users on demand. The carrier sense multiple access (CSMA) protocol and its variants are used for medium access control in sensor networks as contention protocols.

The main attributes of MAC protocols are energy efficiency, scalability and adaptivity, channel utilization, latency, throughput, and fairness [65]. In contention-free protocols, scheduling is organized by time, frequency, or code domain to eliminate interference and collisions. TDMA protocols [66] support low duty cycle operation, which decrease idle listening; however, TDMA protocols have scalability issues and do not support distributed functionality. Furthermore, TDMA protocols require global synchronization, which is a burden for sensor networks. The clustering approach has been proposed to resolve the scalability issue and scheduling. LEACH [41] proposes TDMA scheduling for its cluster and cluster members. Furthermore, the protocol in Ref. [67] uses different subchannels by frequency division and code division and, hence, utilize FDMA and CDMA. Reservation of network resources decreases collision, delay, and jitter; increases throughput; and provides real-time guarantees, which are fundamental requirements of multimedia communication [2]. However, the centralized control and the complexity of the protocols are the disadvantages.

The contention-based protocols use carrier-sensing and collision avoidance mechanisms [61]. The challenge of contention-based protocols is collision due to insufficient coordination. For example, two disparate nodes may send packets to the same receiver and there may be collision at the receiver node. Such an event is termed a *hidden node terminal problem*. Multiple access with collision avoidance (MACA) [68] eliminates this problem with extra control signals, request to send (RTS) and clear to send (CTS). It uses three-way handshaking to coordinate communication. The control signals may collide; however, the collision probability is low due to the small control packet size. Variants of this approach exist, such as multiple access with collision avoidance for wireless (MACAW) [69] and MACA with piggybacked reservation (MACA/PR) [70].

Institute of Electrical and Electronics Engineers (IEEE) 802.11 [71] is a standardized protocol for wireless LAN. It combines the features of CSMA/CA, MACA, and MACAW. The IEEE 802.11 distributed coordination function is designed for ad hoc networks. It utilizes the CSMA/CA and RTS/CTS handshaking mechanism. If the medium is idle for a predefined interval, the node is allowed to transmit. If the channel is sensed to be busy, a random back-off interval is been chosen uniformly from the contention window interval. Furthermore, ACK and virtual carrier sensing by network allocation vector are used. The main disadvantage of this protocol is the listening to the channel during the back-off period, which is energy-consuming.

Hybrid schemes combine the contention-based period with the contention-free period. Nodes in a neighborhood first contend for reservation of the medium. After the reservation period, the reserved communication resources are used by the nodes. CSMA approaches do not require clock synchronization or global knowledge about the network. However, contention-free protocols are not tolerant to sensor node failures, and clock synchronization and a central controller are necessary. Dynamic topology changes in sensor networks may be costly due to the global rearrangement of schedules. Low contention in sensor networks causes lower channel utilization and higher delay than CSMA, since the node must wait for its TDMA schedule to communicate; by contrast, in CSMA the node communicates when the channel is sensed to be idle [72]. Hence, Rhee et al. proposes Z-MAC, a hybrid MAC protocol that combines the strengths of CSMA and TDMA while decreasing their inefficiencies. The main advantage of Z-MAC is the adaptability of network contention level. With low contention it becomes TDMA; with high contention it becomes TDMA.

From the perspective of multimedia communications, collision-free protocols can provide real-time guarantees, as well as tolerable delay

Table 3.6 MAC Protocols in Wireless Sensor Networks

PROTOCOL	TYPE	TECHNIQUE	DISADVANTAGE
Low Power TDMA [66]	Contention-free	TDMA	Global synchronization
LEACH [41]	Contention-free	TDMA	Clustered structure
Self Organization Protocol [67]	Contention-free	CDMA-FDMA	Lack of scalability
Real time communication and coordination protocol [61]	Contention	Carrier sensing	Coordination
MACA [68]	Contention	Carrier sensing	Collision
IEEE 802.11 [71]	Contention	CSMA/CA	Idle listening
Z-MAC [72]	Hybrid	CSMA-TDMA	—

bounds and desirable throughput by organizing the communication schedule. On the other hand, this type of protocol is not scalable, and they do not adapt to the dynamic environment of sensor networks. Contention-based protocols cannot provide real-time guarantees due to collisions. Hybrid protocols can be used for multimedia communication, since the disadvantages of contention-based and contention-free protocols are minimized by combining them. Hybrid mechanisms are more resilient to scalability, energy consumption, and collisions.

Table 3.6 outlines MAC protocols, their types, techniques used, and disadvantages for multimedia communication in CR ad hoc and sensor networks.

3.6.2.2 Cognitive Radio Networks   One of the most fundamental challenges for designing MAC protocols in CRNs is spectrum management. Medium access is highly affected by spectrum-sensing results, and communication between nodes is interrupted by spectrum handoff and spectrum sensing. Resource allocation is performed to eliminate collision between CRs and to avoid harmful interference with PUs.

MAC protocols can be split into two categories: Direct Access Based (DAB) and DSA [64]. In DAB protocols, every node optimizes its own goals and resource allocation is performed by sender–receiver handshake. DSA protocols try to achieve global network optimization.

Coordination among the nodes is a difficult challenge in CRNs. Two nodes within the communication region of each other communicate if they have a common channel. Agreement on communication channel can be reached on an in-band or out-of-band channel. In-band channel negotiation utilizes data channels; by contrast, out-of-band channel negotiation utilizes a different channel for negotiation and sharing of the spectrum-sensing results. Generally, the out-of-band approach is used in MAC protocols. The out-of-band approach can be divided into CCC and split phase (SP). CCC uses a common control channel for signaling [73], and SP allows the transceiver on each node to switch between control phase and data phase in a time frame [74]. CCC needs two transceivers and handles synchronization problems; SP is cost-efficient but reduces network utilization due to the separate control phase. The CCC approach is much more convenient than the SP approach, because it overcomes the problem of synchronization and system inefficiency. However, it is not practical to place two transceivers on one sensor node. Multimedia QoS requirements can be satisfied in a more robust way by the CCC approach. Nevertheless, it should be noted that it is not feasible to guarantee CCC among the network members due to the dynamic nature of the spectral environment in CRNs. By contrast, the Frequency Hopping Sequence (FHS) approach utilizes in-band control channel, and sensing interruptions do not affect system performance by hopping the frequency to enable communication [75]. FHS generally satisfies the throughput and QoS requirements of multimedia communication.

Contention in CRNs can be avoided by centralized or distributed algorithms. As classified in Ref. [63], there are three kinds of CR MAC protocols: random access, time-slotted, and hybrid. In random access MAC protocols, CRs utilize CSMA/CA as architecture for accessing the medium for control and data packets. A centralized carrier-sensing CSMA-based mechanism has been proposed for CRNs coexisting with a primary system. It utilizes in-band signaling, and CR nodes have single transceivers. In time-slotted MAC protocols, time is synchronized and slots for data and control channels are reserved. In cognitive MAC (C-MAC) [76], time is divided into superframes which contain slots for beacon period and data transmission period. It uses multiple transceivers to enable high throughput and resilience to the dynamic spectrum environment. A rendezvous channel is used for node coordination. A back-up channel is determined from out of band in case a PU appears on the rendezvous channel. In hybrid protocols, medium access is achieved by utilizing random access and time-slotted schemes. For example, in opportunistic spectrum MAC (OS-MAC) [77], there are predetermined intervals for communication coordination. CCC is used to exchange control packets, and each node is a member of a cluster.

From a multimedia communication perspective, MAC protocols face challenging difficulties. Existing MAC layer approaches do not support real-time, seamless communication as a result of PU and high-throughput requirements, jitter, and delay bound. An important MAC protocol has been proposed to support multimedia communication in CRNs [78]. It is a distributed QoS-aware MAC protocol for multichannel CRNs. Based on channel usage statistics, the channels to be sensed and the data channels are determined to satisfy certain QoS requirements. For various traffic types, spectrum-sensing duration is changed to enhance QoS provisioning. Cai et al. [78] offer a priority-based spectrum access scheme for heterogeneous traffic to further improve QoS. MAC protocols for multimedia applications must consider QoS requirements such as traffic, PU activities, real-time communication, and delay bound. Furthermore, cognitive cycle operations must be considered for medium access such that spectrum-sensing results and spectrum decision are fundamental operations that affect the performance of the communication.

3.6.3 Open Research Issues for the MAC Layer

There are many approaches for the MAC layer in WSNs that satisfy the requirements of multimedia communication. In contrast, the protocols proposed for CRNs are mainly concerned with decreasing interference with PUs and increasing channel utilization. These protocols generally do not consider multimedia communication. Hence, there is a need to design a MAC protocol to realize multimedia communication in CR multimedia ad hoc and sensor networks.

The proposed MAC protocol must minimize the delay caused by spectrum handoff, as well as contention. Furthermore, it must offer a high throughput against changing the operating channel and its condition. Hence, designing a MAC protocol to satisfy the requirements of multimedia communication is a challenging task.

3.7 Conclusions

In this chapter, we surveyed the existing literature on multimedia communication in WSNs, CRNs, CRSNs, and WMSNs. We also investigated the protocols proposed for wireless networks and pointed out their advantages and disadvantages for realizing multimedia communication in CR ad hoc and sensor networks. Existing approaches were scrutinized from the perspective of network layers. The challenges posed by multimedia communication and the CR ad hoc and sensor network paradigm were clearly indicated for each network layer. Open research avenues for realizing multimedia communication over CR ad hoc and sensor networks were presented.

Acknowledgment

This work was supported by The Scientific and Technological Research Council of Turkey (TUBITAK) under grant 110E249.

References

1. Akyildiz, I.F., Su, W., Sankarasubramaniam, Y., Cayirci, E. Wireless sensor networks: A survey. *Computer Networks* 38(4), 393–422, 2002.
2. Misra, S., Reisslein, M., Xue, G. A survey of multimedia streaming in wireless sensor networks. *Communications Surveys & Tutorials, IEEE* 10(4), 18–39, 2008.
3. Gürses, E., Akan, O.B. Multimedia communication in wireless sensor networks. In: *Annales des Télécommunications*, volume 60, pp. 872–900. Springer, 2005.
4. Akyildiz, I.F., Lee, W.Y., Vuran, M.C., Mohanty, S. Next generation/dynamic spectrum access/cognitive radio wireless networks: A survey. *Computer Networks* 50(13), 2127–2159, 2006.
5. Akan, O.B., Karli, O., Ergul, O. Cognitive radio sensor networks. *Network, IEEE* 23(4), 34–40, 2009.
6. Haykin, S. Cognitive radio: Brain-empowered wireless communications. *IEEE Journal on Selected Areas in Communications* 23(2), 201–220, 2005.
7. Akyildiz, I.F., Melodia, T., Chowdhury, K.R. A survey on wireless multimedia sensor networks. *Computer Networks* 51(4), 921–960, 2007.
8. Vuran, M.C., Akan, O.B., Akyildiz, I.F. Spatio-temporal correlation: Theory and applications for wireless sensor networks. *Computer Networks* 45(3), 245–259, 2004.
9. Wiegand, T., Sullivan, G.J. The H.264/AVC video coding standard. *IEEE Signal Processing Magazine* 24(2), 148–153, 2007.
10. Ohm, J., Sullivan, G.J. High efficiency video coding: The next frontier in video compression [standards in a nutshell]. *Signal Processing Magazine, IEEE* 30(1), 152–158, 2013.
11. Slepian, D., Wolf, J.K. Noiseless coding of correlated information sources. *IEEE Transactions on Information Theory* 19(4), 471–480, 1973.

12. Girod, B., Aaron, A.M., Rane, S., Rebollo-Monedero, D. Distributed video coding. *Proceedings of the IEEE* 93(1), 71–83, 2005.
13. Aaron, A., Rane, S., Zhang, R., Girod, B. Wyner–Ziv coding for video: Applications to compression and error resilience. In: *Proceedings of Data Compression Conference*, pp. 93–102. IEEE, Snowbird, UT, 2003.
14. Aaron, A., Setton, E., Girod, B. Towards practical Wyner–Ziv coding of video. In: *Proceedings of International Conference on Image Processing, ICIP*, volume 3, pp. III–869. IEEE, Barcelona, Spain, 2003.
15. Brites, C., Pereira, F. Correlation noise modeling for efficient pixel and transform domain Wyner–Ziv video coding. *IEEE Transactions on Circuits and Systems for Video Technology* 18(9), 1177–1190, 2008.
16. Brites, C., Pereira, F. An efficient encoder rate control solution for transform domain Wyner–Ziv video coding. *IEEE Transactions on Circuits and Systems for Video Technology* 21(9), 1278–1292, 2011.
17. Yu, F.R., Sun, B., Krishnamurthy, V., Ali, S. Application layer QoS optimization for multimedia transmission over cognitive radio networks. *Wireless Networks* 17(2), 371–383, 2011.
18. Dastpak, A., Liu, J., Hefeeda, M. Video streaming over cognitive radio networks. In: *Proceedings of the 4th Workshop on Mobile Video*, pp. 31–36. ACM, Chapel Hill, NC, 2012.
19. Zhang, H., Zhang, Z., Chen, X., Yin, R. Energy efficient joint source and channel sensing in cognitive radio sensor networks. In: *IEEE International Conference on Communications (ICC)*, pp. 1–6. IEEE, Kyoto, Japan, 2011.
20. Wang, C., Sohraby, K., Li, B., Daneshmand, M., Hu, Y. A survey of transport protocols for wireless sensor networks. *IEEE Network* 20(3), 34–40, 2006.
21. Lee, W.Y., Akyildiz, I.F. Optimal spectrum sensing framework for cognitive radio networks. *IEEE Transactions on Wireless Communication* 7(10), 3845–3857, 2008.
22. Hull, B., Jamieson, K., Balakrishnan, H. Mitigating congestion in wireless sensor networks. In: *Proceedings of the 2nd International Conference on Embedded Networked Sensor Systems*, pp. 134–147. ACM, Baltimore, MD, 2004.
23. Wan, C.Y., Eisenman, S.B., Campbell, A.T. CODA: Congestion detection and avoidance in sensor networks. In: *Proceedings of the 1st International Conference on Embedded Networked Sensor Systems*, pp. 266–279. ACM, Los Angeles, CA, 2003.
24. Ee, C.T., Bajcsy, R. Congestion control and fairness for many-to-one routing in sensor networks. In: *Proceedings of the 2nd International Conference on Embedded Networked Sensor Systems*, pp. 148–161. ACM, Baltimore, MD, 2004.
25. Stann, F., Heidemann, J. RMST: Reliable data transport in sensor networks. In: *Proceedings of the 1st IEEE International Workshop on Sensor Network Protocols and Applications*, pp. 102–112. IEEE, Anchorage, Alaska, 2003.

26. Felemban, E., Lee, C.G., Ekici, E. MMSPEED: Multipath multi-SPEED protocol for QoS guarantee of reliability and. timeliness in wireless sensor networks. *IEEE Transactions on Mobile Computing* 5(6), 738–754, 2006.

27. Wan, C.Y., Campbell, A.T., Krishnamurthy, L. PSFQ: A reliable transport protocol for wireless sensor networks. In: *Proceedings of the 1st ACM International Workshop on Wireless Sensor Networks and Applications*, pp. 1–11. ACM, Atlanta, GA, 2002.

28. Sankarasubramaniam, Y., Akan, O.B., Akyildiz, I.F. ESRT: Event-to-sink reliable transport in wireless sensor networks. In: *Proceedings of the 4th ACM International Symposium on Mobile Ad Hoc Networking & Computing*, pp. 177–188. ACM, Annapolis, Maryland, 2003.

29. Paek, J., Govindan, R. RCRT: Rate-controlled reliable transport for wireless sensor networks. In: *Proceedings of the 5th International Conference on Embedded Networked Sensor Systems*, pp. 305–319. ACM, Sydney, Australia, 2007.

30. Gungor, V.C., Akan, O.B., Akyildiz, I.F. A real-time and reliable transport (RT)² protocol for wireless sensor and actor networks. *IEEE/ACM Transactions on Networking* 16(2), 359–370, 2008.

31. Chowdhury, K.R., Di Felice, M., Akyildiz, I.F. TCP-CRAHN: A transport control protocol for cognitive radio ad hoc networks. *IEEE Transactions on Mobile Computing* 12(4), 790–803, 2013.

32. Slingerland, A.M.R., Pawelczak, P., Venkatesha Prasad, R., Lo, A., Hekmat, R. Performance of transport control protocol over dynamic spectrum access links. In: *2nd IEEE International Symposium on New Frontiers in Dynamic Spectrum Access Networks, DySPAN 2007*, pp. 486–495. IEEE, Dublin, Ireland, 2007.

33. Chowdhury, K.R., Di Felice, M., Akyildiz, I.F. TP-CRAHN: A transport protocol for cognitive radio ad-hoc networks. In: *IEEE INFOCOM 2009*, pp. 2482–2490. IEEE, Rio de Janerio, Brazil, 2009.

34. Luo, C., Yu, F.R., Ji, H., Leung, V.C.M. Cross-layer design for TCP performance improvement in cognitive radio networks. *IEEE Transactions on Vehicular Technology* 59(5), 2485–2495, 2010.

35. Bicen, A.O., Akan, O.B. Reliability and congestion control in cognitive radio sensor networks. *Ad Hoc Networks* 9(7), 1154–1164, 2011.

36. Yaghmaee, M.H., Adjeroh, D. A new priority based congestion control protocol for wireless multimedia sensor networks. In: *IEEE WoWMoM 2008*, pp. 1–8. IEEE, Newport Beach, CA, 2008.

37. Al-Karaki, J.N., Kamal, A.E. Routing techniques in wireless sensor networks: A survey. *IEEE Wireless Communications* 11(6), 6–28, 2004.

38. Kulik, J., Heinzelman, W., Balakrishnan, H. Negotiation-based protocols for disseminating information in wireless sensor networks. *Wireless Networks* 8(2/3), 169–185, 2002.

39. Intanagonwiwat, C., Govindan, R., Estrin, D., Heidemann, J., Silva, F. Directed diffusion for wireless sensor networking. *IEEE/ACM Transactions on Networking* 11(1), 2–16, 2003.

40. Braginsky, D., Estrin, D. Rumor routing algorithm for sensor networks. In: *Proceedings of the 1st ACM International Workshop on Wireless Sensor Networks and Applications*, pp. 22–31. ACM, Atlanta, GA, 2002.
41. Heinzelman, W.R., Chandrakasan, A., Balakrishnan, H. Energy-efficient communication protocol for wireless microsensor networks. In: *Proceedings of the 33rd Annual Hawaii International Conference on System Sciences*, pp. 1–10. IEEE, Hawaii, USA, 2000.
42. Bereketli, A., Akan, O.B. Event-to-sink directed clustering in wireless sensor networks. In: *Wireless Communications and Networking Conference, 2009, WCNC 2009*. IEEE, pp. 1–6. IEEE, Budapest, Hungary, 2009.
43. Ye, F., Chen, A., Lu, S., Zhang, L. A scalable solution to minimum cost forwarding in large sensor networks. In: *Proceedings of 10th International Conference on Computer Communications and Networks*, pp. 304–309. IEEE, Scottsdale, AZ, 2001.
44. Yu, Y., Govindan, R., Estrin, D. Geographical and energy aware routing: A recursive data dissemination protocol for wireless sensor networks. Technical report, *Technical Report UCLA/CSD-TR-01-0023*, UCLA Computer Science Department, Los Angeles, CA, 2001.
45. Rodoplu, V., Meng, T.H. Minimum energy mobile wireless networks. *IEEE Journal on Selected Areas in Communications* 17(8), 1333–1344, 1999.
46. Akkaya, K., Younis, M. An energy-aware QoS routing protocol for wireless sensor networks. In: *Proceedings of 23rd International Conference on Distributed Computing Systems Workshops*, pp. 710–715. IEEE, Providence, RI, 2003.
47. Chipara, O., He, Z., Xing, G., Chen, Q., Wang, X., Lu, C., Stankovic, J. et al. Real-time power-aware routing in sensor networks. In: *14th IEEE International Workshop on Quality of Service*, pp. 83–92. IEEE, New Haven, CT, 2006.
48. Cesana, M., Cuomo, F., Ekici, E. Routing in cognitive radio networks: Challenges and solutions. *Ad Hoc Networks* 9(3), 228–248, 2011.
49. Ma, M., Tsang, D.H.K. Joint spectrum sharing and fair routing in cognitive radio networks. In: *5th IEEE Consumer Communications and Networking Conference, CCNC 2008*, pp. 978–982. IEEE, Las Vegas, Nevada, 2008.
50. Lin, S.C., Chen, K.C. Spectrum aware opportunistic routing in cognitive radio networks. In: *IEEE Global Telecommunications Conference (GLOBECOM 2010)*, pp. 1–6. IEEE, Miami, FL, 2010.
51. Liu, Y., Cai, L.X., Shen, X. Spectrum-aware opportunistic routing in multi-hop cognitive radio networks. *IEEE Journal on Selected Areas in Communications* 30(10), 1958–1968, 2012.
52. Pan, M., Zhang, C., Li, P., Fang, Y. Joint routing and link scheduling for cognitive radio networks under uncertain spectrum supply. In: *INFOCOM, 2011 Proceedings IEEE*, pp. 2237–2245. IEEE, Shanghai, China, 2011.
53. Cheng, G., Liu, W., Li, Y., Cheng, W. Spectrum aware on-demand routing in cognitive radio networks. In: *2nd IEEE International Symposium on New Frontiers in Dynamic Spectrum Access Networks*, pp. 571–574. IEEE, Dublin, Ireland, 2007.

54. Ma, H., Zheng, L., Ma, X., Luo, Y. Spectrum aware routing for multi-hop cognitive radio networks with a single transceiver. In: *3rd International Conference on Cognitive Radio Oriented Wireless Networks and Communications, 2008. CrownCom 2008.*, pp. 1–6. IEEE, Singapore, 2008.

55. Shah, G.A., Alagoz, F., Fadel, E., Akan, O.B. A spectrum-aware clustering for efficient multimedia routing in cognitive radio sensor networks. *IEEE Transactions On Vehicular Technology* 63(7), 3369–3380, 2013.

56. Abazeed, M., Faisal, N., Zubair, S., Ali, A. Routing protocols for wireless multimedia sensor network: A survey. *Journal of Sensors* 1–11, 2013.

57. Li, S., Neelisetti, R., Liu, C., Lim, A. Delay-constrained high throughput protocol for multi-path transmission over wireless multimedia sensor networks. In: *International Symposium on a World of Wireless, Mobile and Multimedia Networks, WoWMoM 2008*, pp. 1–8. IEEE, Newport Beach, CA, 2008.

58. Hamid, Md.A., Alam, M.M., Hong, C.S. Design of a QoS-aware routing mechanism for wireless multimedia sensor networks. In: *IEEE Global Telecommunications Conference, 2008, IEEE GLOBECOM 2008*, pp. 1–6. IEEE, New Orleans, LA, 2008.

59. Maimour, M. Maximally radio-disjoint multipath routing for wireless multimedia sensor networks. In: *Proceedings of the 4th ACM Workshop on Wireless Multimedia Networking and Performance Modeling*, pp. 26–31. ACM, Vancouver, Canada, 2008.

60. Medjiah, S., Ahmed, T., Asgari, A.H. Streaming multimedia over WMSNs: An online multipath routing protocol. *International Journal of Sensor Networks* 11(1), 10–21, 2012.

61. Stankovic, J.A., Abdelzaher, T.F., Lu, C., Sha, L., Hou, J.C. Real-time communication and coordination in embedded sensor networks. *Proceedings of the IEEE* 91(7), 1002–1022, 2003.

62. Demirkol, I., Ersoy, C., Alagoz, F. MAC protocols for wireless sensor networks: A survey. *IEEE Communications Magazine* 44(4), 115–121, 2006.

63. Cormio, C., Chowdhury, K.R. A survey on MAC protocols for cognitive radio networks. *Ad Hoc Networks* 7(7), 1315–1329, 2009.

64. De Domenico, A., Strinati, E.C., Di Benedetto, M. A survey on MAC strategies for cognitive radio networks. *IEEE Communications Surveys & Tutorials* 14(1), 21–44, 2012.

65. Ye, W., Heidemann, J. Medium access control in wireless sensor networks. *Wireless Sensor Networks*, Springer, pp. 73–91, 2004.

66. Pei, G., Chien, C. Low power TDMA in large wireless sensor networks. In: *IEEE MILCOM 2001*, volume 1, pp. 347–351. IEEE, Washington, DC, 2001.

67. Sohrabi, K., Pottie, G.J. Performance of a novel self-organization protocol for wireless ad-hoc sensor networks. In: *Vehicular Technology Conference, 1999. VTC 1999-Fall. IEEE VTS 50th*, volume 2, pp. 1222–1226. IEEE, Amsterdam, Holland, 1999.

68. Karn, P. MACA—A new channel access method for packet radio. In: *ARRL/CRRL Amateur Radio 9th Computer Networking Conference*, volume 140, pp. 134–140, 1990.
69. Bharghavan, V., Demers, A., Shenker, S., Zhang, L. MACAW: A media access protocol for wireless LAN's. In: *ACM SIGCOMM Computer Communication Review*, volume 24, pp. 212–225. ACM, London, UK, 1994.
70. Lin, C.R., Gerla, M. Real-time support in multihop wireless networks. *Wireless Networks* 5(2), 125–135, 1999.
71. IEEE 802 LAN/MAN Standards Committee et al. Wireless LAN medium access control (MAC) and physical layer (PHY) specifications. *IEEE Standard*, 802(11), 1999.
72. Rhee, I., Warrier, A., Aia, M., Min, J., Sichitiu, M.L. Z-MAC: A hybrid MAC for wireless sensor networks. *IEEE/ACM Transactions on Networking (TON)* 16(3), 511–524, 2008.
73. Ma, L., Han, X., Shen, C.C. Dynamic open spectrum sharing MAC protocol for wireless ad hoc networks. In: *1st IEEE International Symposium on New Frontiers in Dynamic Spectrum Access Networks, DySPAN 2005*, pp. 203–213. IEEE, Baltimore, MD, 2005.
74. Timmers, M., Pollin, S., Dejonghe, A., Van der Perre, L., Catthoor, F. A distributed multichannel MAC protocol for multihop cognitive radio networks. *IEEE Transactions on Vehicular Technology* 59(1), 446–459, 2010.
75. Hu, W., Willkomm, D., Abusubaih, M., Gross, J., Vlantis, G., Gerla, M., Wolisz, A. Cognitive radios for dynamic spectrum access—Dynamic frequency hopping communities for efficient IEEE 802.22 operation. *IEEE Communications Magazine* 45(5), 80–87, 2007.
76. Cordeiro, C., Challapali, K. C-MAC: A cognitive MAC protocol for multi-channel wireless networks. In: *2nd IEEE International Symposium on New Frontiers in Dynamic Spectrum Access Networks*, pp. 147–157. IEEE, Dublin, Ireland, 2007.
77. Hamdaoui, B., Shin, K.G. OS-MAC: An efficient MAC protocol for spectrum-agile wireless networks. *IEEE Transactions on Mobile Computing* 7(8), 915–930, 2008.
78. Cai, L.X., Liu, Y., Shen, X., Mark, J.W., Zhao, D. Distributed QoS-aware MAC for multimedia over cognitive radio networks. In: *IEEE Global Telecommunications Conference (GLOBECOM 2010)*, pp. 1–5. IEEE, Miami, FL, 2010.

4

Multimedia Streaming in Wireless Multimedia Sensor Networks

AHMED HUSSEIN ABBAS SALEM AND RANIA AHMED ABUL-SEOUD

Contents

4.1 Introduction

Multimedia streaming is the process of sending and delivering multimedia content to an end user or to the base station, where it will pass through further processing or be stored for further research. The choice of delivery method is driven by the content that is being distributed. In the case of telecommunications networks, the system uses streaming technology to deliver multimedia content, which might be a video, picture, or audio. Wireless multimedia sensor networks (WMSNs) are a special case where power is critical, as the nodes are mostly battery-operated; advances in the protocols and methods of streaming are crucial in this case. For video, there is a recommended broadband speed; if this recommendation is satisfied, the video content will be meaningful and useful. The minimum recommended broadband for video is 2.5 MB/s, which consumes a great deal of power, particularly if the network is used for real-time monitoring and surveillance. For high definition video, the minimum recommended broadband is 10 MB/s. As a result, compressing the multimedia content is crucial; audio and video codecs are used to compress the data as much as possible without harming it or causing it to be meaningless. Compression conserves power and increases efficiency in many applications, such as monitoring nearby areas. However, high resolution with raw, unmodified content can be useful, especially if the field of view is broad; the user can then magnify an area of the picture without distortion. This functionality is advantageous if the area being monitored is very large, such as a whole town; although in this case a very expensive camera would be required.

Particular interest has been shown in developing an advanced multimedia streaming method to prevent the occurrence of dead nodes, which is especially important if the nodes cooperatively send content to the base station using routing protocols. However, such situations can be solved by choosing the best-fitting MAC protocols, routing protocols, network topology, and method of power supply. Nodes can be powered using solar cells, although this method has drawbacks because the cells need to be directed toward the sun; solar power is not always guaranteed, especially in harsh environments like forests. Developing streaming techniques differs from computer networks. A computer network works toward a primary issue, to prevent delays, but WMSNs work toward a different primary issue—to prevent high power consumption, which may lead to dead nodes in the network. These problems will be solved by using the smart advanced multimedia streaming techniques that will be shown in this chapter.

4.2 Differences between Wireless Sensor Network and WMSN Requirements in Multimedia Streaming

WSNs measure scalar data such as temperature, humidity, and other data that can be represented as a measured value. These data are measured by a sensor and is then sampled, calibrated, packetized, and sent to the base station. This process and its requirements are very different from those in WMSNs, which primarily send multimedia content. The hardware differences are very clear; scalar data require only a sensor and an integrated circuit (IC) that has an analog to digital channel (ADC) channel. By contrast, multimedia requires a camera, microphone, and hardware that can provide the required and needed processing for such data. The differences between a WSN and a WMSN are as follows:

- Quality-of-service requirements: Multimedia applications need different requirements to supply different functionalities, such as snapshots, playback, and storage. Different functionalities will require specific limits on the delays encountered and the jitter.
- Bandwidth: WMSNs require several times more bandwidth than was needed to support ordinary scalar sensor networks.
- Power: Power consumption is higher for WMSNs, because it is consumed by data storage activities, high transmission rates, and the aggressive processing applied to multimedia content.
- In-network processing support: WMSNs have the availability and the support to extract targeted data from the content stored, which could be used in object identification applications, and the usage of image fusion capabilities will enhance the capabilities of such application.
- In-node processing support: Such support is needed to compress the raw files stored and supplied from the cameras and the microphones in WMSNs.
- Cross-layer design: Complete implementation and optimization is necessary in WMSNs from the application layer to the physical layer for the node to work and cooperate in the network without encountering any incompatibility or lack of support issues.
- Better hardware design: WMSN design has been concerned with managing power consumption in a better way to conserve energy, which has accelerated the need to investigate energy-harvesting methods.

4.3 Multimedia Streaming Optimization Techniques

Optimization techniques are a necessity in WMSNs to increase the efficiency of data transfer. Some of these techniques are as follows:

- Deduplication: Redundancy data will be eliminated by using references instead of the actual data by working on the bytes of the data. The benefits of such a technique will be obvious in IP applications.

- Compression: Compression in WMSNs is similar to ordinary compression programs as it relies on data patterns that can be represented in an efficient manner. It is very important to observe the difference between compression technique and compressive sensing. Compressive sensing is also known as compressive sampling and sparse sampling. It is an efficient way to acquire the signal and reconstruct it by finding solutions to some underdetermined linear systems that use the sparseness and the compressibility of the signal, which will extract the entire desired signal with few measurements.
- Latency optimization: Latency optimization is accomplished by giving the authority of answering and replying to different requests from the nodes in a local manner instead of sending such requests to remote administrative nodes to reply.
- Forward error correction: Its main goal is to reduce retransmissions, which occur especially in harsh environments or bad weather, by adding a loss recovery packet for every specific number of packets being sent.
- Connection limits: Connection limits represent a security method to ensure the avoidance of denial of service in WMSNs.
- Simple rate limits: Congestion can be avoided by limiting the rate at which packets are sent to any user.
- Multimedia in-network processing: Multimedia processing was mostly dealt with as a separate problem from network design. Studies have primarily taken an interest in the cross-layer interactions among the lower layers of the protocol stack. However, the processing and streaming of multimedia content are not separate or independent from each other, and their function has a great impact on the quality of service delivered to the user and required by the application, as well. Processing is crucial in the case of WMSNs and, in point of fact, in any video streaming application. Video is first recorded as a raw file, which is a digital or analog record that has been digitized without any occurrence of compression or distortion to the file itself. Using this type of file will consume a great deal of storage and processing as well as considerable power, which is a big disadvantage

for WMSNs. Thus, files must be compressed to be ready for streaming. Compression may decrease the quality of the files and make low-quality videos worse; audio files will be hard to hear or understand. Therefore, methods for reducing file size are similar to taking smaller pictures or reducing the frame rate. Reducing the frame rate would be useful in many applications, such as monitoring melting polar ice. For this application, it would suffice to record video at specific predefined intervals for short periods, or just to take a picture. There are many advances necessary to make such an application possible. Problems include the power, the supports for the camera, and how to keep the camera lens and microphone clean.

4.4 Key Video Parameters

The key video parameters must be known and identified to determine the quality of the received multimedia content through the wireless channels. The parameters are as follows:

- Sample quantization rate: This parameter is the number of bits being used to quantize each sample, measured in bits/sample unit. The lower the number of bits used, the lower the amount of information sent for each sample. This will allow a greater number of samples to be sent, which is advantageous. However, a greater quantization error will be encountered in each sample. The benefit of sending more samples is to outweigh the distortion encountered in the samples; a minimum rate would be 5 bits/sample. Moreover, image corruption is acceptable, as a corrupted image might appear once in every 103 sent images.
- Samples per frame: This parameter is the required number of samples that must be supplied to reconstruct an image with a predefined level of quality. Clearly, the quality of the image will increase with an increase in the number of samples sent. All this will depend on the required quality of the video.
- Channel encoding rate: This could be identified by determining the channel coding strategy that is best suited for transmitting packets over a multihop wireless network.

4.5 Operations on Multimedia Content

This section will illustrate the operations that must be performed on multimedia content to prepare it for packetizing and sending. Raw files cannot be sent in their original form; some operations must be performed on them to make them ready and to conserve the power, processing, storage, and bandwidth usage. There are many operations that could be done; we will illustrate some of the most popular methods in the WMSN and multimedia arenas. Much of the recent research discusses compression, which is found in almost every multimedia application. The JPEG is a common image compression algorithm that is found in most CMOS camera sensor chips, as JPEG can achieve a compression ratio from 10:1 to 20:1 without a noticeable loss in color images. A compression ratio from 30:1 to 50:1 is also possible with small or moderate distortion in the image. Compression of JPEG images is mostly lossy, and lossy compression means that some of the image content will be reduced. In color images, the raw file is divided into two components: luminance and color components. The difference here is only in the representation of the data; no loss or reduction have been achieved. The human observer is much more observant of the intensity information than the color information itself. Therefore, the color information can be subsampled without any noticeable defect in the image, although the amount of data will be highly reduced. The image is then divided into 8 × 8 pixel blocks and the algorithm is performed on these blocks. The blocks will be transformed by using the discrete cosines transformation method. The next step is the quantization step, which is crucial for the quality that the user needs. As the quality increases, the size of the image will increase, which might require more storage, power, processing, and bandwidth. The JPEG is a block-based compression method. The compressed sensing (CS) method is also common and is heavily used, especially in WMSNs; the CS method is more flexible than JPEG and consumes less power. The CS method has several advantages—for example, an inherent resilience to channel errors, which are caused by unstructured image representation; this will lead to a zero loss in image quality. In the CS method, the transmitted samples constitute a random and incoherent combination of the original data itself. No single sample is given priority over any other sample, and only the number of completely received samples that have not encountered any errors are used to construct the image. Thus, the complete samples are the main parameters for achieving a certain quality to the image; clearly, the image quality will increase when the corrupted samples are dropped. The corrupted samples are dropped in adaptive parity-based channel coding, which was an advance introduced to the CS method. In adaptive parity-based channel coding, the quality of the video stream can be improved by dropping the samples that are corrupted or have encountered some errors that might impair image reconstruction by introducing incorrect information. Adaptive parity-based channel coding can be achieved by using even parity on a definable number of samples that will be dropped at the receiver or at an intermediate node in a multihop scenario if the parity check has failed. Adaptive parity was tested against rate compatible punctured convolutional (RCPC) codes; it outperformed it at all levels of the RCPC codes. The adaptive parity method has performed better in all the bit error rate (BER) levels. BER is the number of bits received by a receiver through a wireless channel that has encountered noise, interference, and distortion errors. Adaptive parity performs better. Although forward error correction (FEC) schemes have more powerful error correction methods, FEC has no additional overhead. This additional overhead is needed to increase video quality, but instead FEC drops the samples that have encountered errors. There are several error correction schemes, codes, and methods, but the parameters that were targeted while designing them were the capability to correct any kind of error, the time needed to correct such errors, and sufficient memory to power the algorithms. These systems were created for computers, where power was not a large problem because the processor, RAM, and storage cooperated with the interfaces and peripherals of the system. However, in WMSNs, power is a great concern, so data must be sent in a lossy manner. In WMSNs, the algorithms depend on dropping the error rather than retransmitting the packet to extract the correct information. Future development in WMSNs should target reliable, fast, and energy-efficient methods.

4.6 Conclusion

It was shown that, although JPEG encoded images are used extensively, they are not best suited for WMSNs. The CS method will perform much better because of its inherent resiliency to channel errors.

It was also shown that FEC methods and schemes are not best suited or beneficial for WMSN applications. The adaptive parity method will perform much better because it is able to drop samples that have encountered errors, thus improving the quality of the multimedia content that was received, while maintaining low complexity.

5

Coverage Problems for Wireless Multimedia Sensor Networks

XIAOLAN LIU, GUILIN CHEN, AND BIN YANG

Contents

Recently, the rapid development and progress of low complexity, high flexibility sensor facilities (visual sensor nodes, digital signal processing devices, etc.) has encouraged the emergence of wireless multimedia sensor networks (WMSNs). Multimedia sensor nodes are capable of gathering richer multimedia information (besides scalar physical phenomena) from a monitored region. Hence, WMSNs have been widely applied to various scenarios, such as smart homes, medical applications, and so on. Recently, coverage as a measure of the quality of service (QoS) has drawn much attention in WMSNs. Compared to traditional sensor networks, multimedia sensor networks have exclusive properties, such as sensor viewing direction and angle, as well as object facing direction and location. Based on the above considerations, the coverage problems in WMSNs require specific algorithms and solutions. In this chapter, we mainly survey the existing research in the field of multimedia device coverage. First, we list and classify off-the-shelf sensor hardware, as well as available coverage models. Furthermore, we describe the state of the art in influencing factors, deployment mechanisms, sensor selections, and performance metrics for WMSN node coverage. The coverage problem in WMSNs can be divided into three categories: barrier coverage, area coverage, and target coverage. We discuss the three types of coverage and note representative solution algorithms. Finally, we discuss the existing problems and new research trends in key areas. We conclude that WMSN coverage research is still an open issue that has not been fully addressed.

5.1 Introduction

The recent development of low complexity, high flexibility sensor devices, such as audio and visual sensors, has motivated the emergence of WMSNs, that is, a system of interconnected multimedia sensor motes that consists of a sensing unit, processing unit, communication unit, memory units, power unit, coordination unit, and so on. WMSNs can obtain richer multimedia information, as well as scalar physical phenomena, from a monitored site. In addition, they are also capable of storing, processing, transferring, and fusing multimedia content originating from heterogeneous sensor devices [1]. Hence, WMSNs promise a number of prospective applications. Most of the key applications are divided into surveillance, management, monitoring, detection, object tracking, and virtual reality.

Coverage, which evaluates how well a target area is monitored, is a fundamental performance metric to measure QoS [2]. It has drawn researchers' attention recently, leading to several papers about coverage. For the most part, research has focused on traditional sensor coverage [3–6]. However, the coverage problem in WMSNs has drawn a great deal of attention from the research community in recent years. Ma and Liu [7] present the concept of WMSNs and discuss multimedia sensor coverage problems. Compared to traditional sensor nodes, multimedia sensor nodes have exclusive properties, such as sensor viewing direction and angle, as well as object facing direction and location [8]. A comprehensive discussion of the traditional coverage problems in WMSNs is provided in Ref. [9].

Because most of the existing coverage algorithms are confined to the field of traditional sensor networks, they are not a good fit for multimedia sensor networks. The coverage problem requires specific solutions and techniques in WMSNs. In this chapter, we mainly survey the existing research in the field of multimedia node coverage, including hardware devices, coverage models, affecting factors, deployment mechanisms, sensor management, performance metrics, and typical coverage, and discuss future research problems in detail.

In this chapter, we further divide the coverage content into four stages: design stage, deployment stage, management stage, and coverage metrics. For the design stage, we list some relevant factors to determine how many multimedia nodes are needed to provide complete field coverage in the monitored environment. For the deployment stage, we divide the deployment type into two groups: random placement and deterministic placement. Random placement, where multimedia nodes may be scattered via a plane or launched by artillery, is mainly adapted to inhospitable or remote regions. Multimedia nodes may also be placed in a predetermined position in a deterministic way. In order to satisfy the specified application requirements, sensor management mainly applies to select nodes and schedule the activity of different nodes, while maintaining multimedia node coverage. Finally, the coverage metric which includes network connectivity, sensor lifetime, and node energy is an indicator of the quality of coverage.

In this chapter, the reader may gain better understanding of current coverage research in the field of WMSNs. Simultaneously, it may also promote discussion and encourage new research topics within the research community.

The reminder of the chapter is organized as follows. In Section 5.2, we list real-world multimedia node devices and present their off-the-shelf hardware platforms as well as architecture. In Section 5.3, we list and classify available coverage models, such as mathematical model, physical model, etc. In Section 5.4, we introduce the key factors affecting multimedia sensor coverage. In Section 5.5, we discuss multimedia sensor deployment and possible scheduling plans. In Section 5.6, we investigate the existing research in sensor management. Section 5.7 presents several coverage performance metrics. The coverage type in WMSNs can be classified into three categories: barrier coverage, target coverage, and area coverage. In Section 5.8, we describe several different types of coverage and review representative solution algorithms in the chapter. Open research issues are discussed briefly in Section 5.9. Section 5.10 concludes the chapter.

5.2 WMSN Hardware

In this section, we first introduce and classify existing sensor nodes that can satisfy the special applications in WMSNs. Additionally, we describe multimedia node structure with a particular emphasis on multimedia node sensing motes. Moreover, we show existing hardware platforms and test beds. Eventually, we review existing wireless multimedia network architecture which contains homogeneous and heterogeneous.

5.2.1 Multimedia Sensors

In addition to traditional sensor nodes such as temperature sensors, pressure sensors, and humidity sensors, WMSN sensors also include some other multimedia sensors. Figure 5.1 shows several real-world multimedia sensors, including video sensors, infrared (IR) sensors, and ultrasound sensors. In the following subsection, we introduce several multimedia sensor nodes and describe their unique performance.

5.2.1.1 Video Sensors   Video sensors, in the form of numerous low-cost complementary metal–oxide-semiconductor (CMOS) camera nodes, have brought new opportunity for applications within the scope of visual surveillance and traffic security monitoring. In these applications, video sensors retrieve information-rich visual data from a monitored physical environment.

With the development of high-resolution visual technology, the large-scale products of video sensor nodes have been used in WMSNs, which contain robots, toys, computers, cell phones, etc.

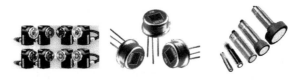

Figure 5.1   Multimedia sensors, from left to right: video sensors, infrared sensors, and ultrasound sensors.

Some related research is found in Ref. [10], where Akyildiz et al. present an overview of WMSNs, including networking architectures, communication protocol, and multimedia sensor hardware. To discuss video sensor nodes robustly, Ref. [11] consider future research directions in the field, including sensor hardware processing, communication, and sensor management.

To illustrate the physical properties of video sensors, we first introduce some camera terminology [12]: depth of field (DoF), focal length (f), focus distance (s), hyperfocal distance (H), the angle of view (AoV) [13], and so on. In the following introduction, we focus on AoV. As the maximum visible volume, AoV can be measured vertically, horizontally, and diagonally. In some literature, the term field of view (FoV) denotes AoV [13]. But the FoV differs slightly from AoV, as is proven by Ref. [14], which describes the sensing radius as equal to the AoV of a 1/3" lens for a video sensor.

Recently, with the improvement of image capturing devices, charge-coupled device webcam, and the CMOS imaging device [15], video sensors have been produced extensively. Most video sensors are manufactured by Agilent [16] and Omnivision [17]; Table 5.1 provides a description of the features of several video sensor products (e.g., ADCM-1700, 2650, 2700 vs. OV6620, 7620, 9630).

5.2.1.2 IR Sensors   IR sensors are used to monitor specific properties of the physical environment according to emit and detect IR radiation. They also have the ability to detect a target's heat and motion [18]. We classify IR sensors into several types. One type is passive IR (PIR) sensors, which are mainly used to detect IR rays, rather than emit them [13].

Table 5.1   Comparison of Several Video Sensors

VIDEO SENSOR	COMPANY	PLATFORM	IMAGE TECHNOLOGY	LENS SIZE	f-NUMBER	DEFAULT RESOLUTION
ADCM-1700	Agilent	MeshEye	CMOS	N/A	2.8	352×288
ADCM-2650	Agilent	N/A	CMOS	N/A	2.8	480×640
ADCM-2700	Agilent	MeshEye	CMOS	N/A	N/A	640×480
OV6620	Omnivision	CMUCam3	CMOS	1/4	N/A	352×288
OV7620	Omnivision	CMUCam3	CMOS	1/3	N/A	640×480
OV9630	Omnivision	N/A	CMOS	1/3	N/A	1280×1024

Source: Amac Guvensan, M., and Gokhan Yavuz, A., *Ad Hoc Networks*, 9, 1238–1255, 2011.
Note: N/A, not available.

This ray is not visible to the human eye, but it is extremely vulnerable to be interpreted by other IR radiation [18].

A special IR sensor such as a motion sensor can use optics or acoustics to detect an object's behavior. Such behavior might be either active or passive. Active IR sensors detect objects' behavior by measuring the feedback of optics or sound waves. In addition, PIR sensors are typically used to monitor indoor environments and linked to IR burglary protection systems [19]. There exist many other IR sensors (e.g., reflective IR sensors and interrupter IR sensors); it is impossible to introduce all IR sensors individually.

The working principle for IR sensors is as follows. First, the IR sensor detects IR rays. The next step is to transform IR rays into electric current. Finally, we detect motion using an amperage or voltage detector [20]. Compared to other radiation, the wavelengths of IR radiation are longer than visible ray wavelengths in the electromagnetic spectrum and shorter than microwaves [21]. We often find IR radiation in daily life. For instance, there is an IR detector in every television, which can analyze the signal from a remote base station. All in all, IR sensors have been used in a wide range of applications because of their unique features—low power, portability, and simplicity [21].

5.2.1.3 Ultrasound Sensors   An ultrasonic sensor is a device that uses high-frequency sound to measure distance [22]. The basic operating principle for ultrasonic sensors is as follows. The ultrasonic sensor launches a sonic pulse, and then the pulse bounces off an object. The transducer converts among electrical, sonic, and mechanical energies [23].

In addition, ultrasonic sensors have many applications. For example, medical facilities often use ultrasonic sensors to visualize areas within the human body. Industrial machines often use these sensors to detect the presence of a living being in an automated factory. Security installations also use sonic sensors to detect the presence of an unauthorized person [22]. However, the drawbacks of ultrasonic sensors are that we cannot tell the difference between large bodies and small bodies. The reason is that the emitted sonic pulse is cone-shaped. Ref. [23] proposes to use multiple sensors or rotating sensors to solve this problem.

5.2.2 Node Structure

The structure of a WSMN node is designed to be simple, small, and low cost. The typical hardware components of a multimedia sensor device include a sensing unit, central processing unit (CPU), memory unit, communication unit, and power supply unit, and so on, as shown in Figure 5.2. We will illustrate the major component motes of WMSN nodes.

- The sensing unit contains several different multimedia sensors and analog-to-digital converters (ADCs). In the sensing stage, the multimedia sensors collect the analog signals from a monitored environment. Then the analog signals are converted into digital signals through the ADC. Finally, the digital signals are delivered into the processing unit.
- The processing unit is often designed for a specific application such as digital signal processors, because of better performance and lower power consumption. In addition to regulate of communication, coordination, network synchronization of the unit, and so on, the most important assignment of the

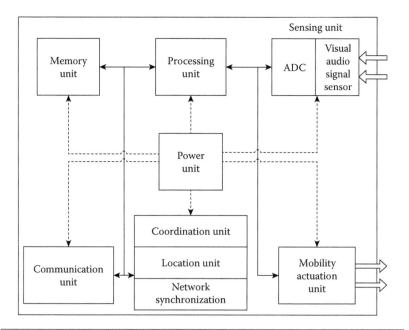

Figure 5.2 Basic components of the multimedia node.

processing unit is to process the data from the sensing unit. Afterwards, the processed data are conveyed to the base station or the memory unit.

- Generally speaking, the memory unit is used for storing the sensed data or procedure code. Once in a while, it functions as a multimedia data buffer. Hence, there is a high storage requirement for WMSNs, as WMSNs handle a large amount of multimedia data, such as images, audio, video, as well as scalar sensor information. In total, the storage requirements for WMSNs are at least ten times higher than scalar networks.

- Currently, the communication protocols are mainly based on the Institute of Electrical and Electronic Engineers (IEEE) 802.14.3 or ZigBee standard [10]. The coordination unit is responsible for regulating location and network synchronization. The mobility/actuation unit can move or manipulate targets.

Most multimedia devices are powered by portable batteries that cannot be recharged or replaced without delay. Therefore, energy efficiency has become an important research topic for WMSNs. However, all research on battery energy efficiency has been for scalar sensors. The content for multimedia sensors has yet to be explored.

5.2.3 Hardware Platforms and Test Beds

To handle more multimedia node applications and to test and examine the above-mentioned algorithms and protocols for WMSNs, we survey some existing hardware platforms and test beds. We examine multimedia data transmission efficiency in terms of bandwidth, storage, data rate, power consumption, and so on [24]. In this subsection, we introduce available hardware prototypes and categorize the existing platforms and test beds based on their capabilities and functionalities. Figure 5.3 shows the classification for most off-the-shelf platforms and test beds.

5.2.3.1 Hardware Platforms Existing multimedia platforms and research prototypes are shown in Table 5.2, which displays the different capabilities and features of hardware platforms. In terms of node structures such as the processing unit, memory unit, power unit, sensing unit, and radio, we classify these hardware platforms

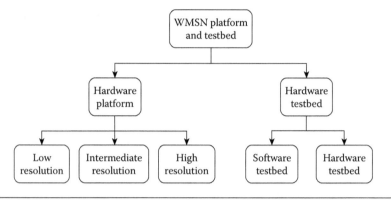

Figure 5.3   Wireless multimedia sensor network platforms and test beds.

Table 5.2   Comparisons of Hardware Platforms for Wireless Multimedia Sensor Networks

PLATFORM	IMAGE SENSOR	PROCESSING UNIT	MEMORY	RADIO	ENERGY (mW)
Cyclops [25]	CMOS	8-bit ATMEL ATmega128L MCU + CPLD	512 KB flash 64 KB SRAM	ZigBee	110–0.76
CMUcam3 [26]	CMOS	ARM7TDMI (32-bit) 60 MHz	64 KB RAM 128 KB flash	ZigBee	572.3–0.29
Stargate [27]	Webcam	PXA255 XScale 400 MHz	32 MB flash 64 MB SDRAM	IEEE 802.11 Bluetooth	N/A
Imote2 [28]	Webcam	32-bit PXA271 XScale	256 KB SRAM, 32 MB flash 32 MB SDRAM	ZigBee	322–1.8
Panoptes [30]	Webcam	400 MHz 32-bit PXA255 XScale CPU (Stargate)	32 MB flash 64 MB SDRAM	IEEE 802.11	5300–58
MeshEye [31]	CMOS	55 Hz 32-bit ARM7 TDMI ATMEL AT91SAM7S	64 KB SRAM, 256 KB flash	ZigBee	175.9–1.8

Note: N/A, not available.

into three groups: low-resolution hardware platforms, intermediate-resolution hardware platforms, and high-resolution hardware platforms.

- Low-resolution hardware platforms are the low-power processing devices platforms; they were specifically designed for simple object detection task from multiple disparate viewpoints. Cyclops, Cyclops Electronics Company, Glasgow [25] and CMUCam3, Carnegie Mell University, Pennsylvania [26] are examples of low-resolution hardware platforms.

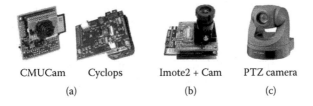

CMUCam   Cyclops   Imote2 + Cam   PTZ camera

(a)   (b)   (c)

Figure 5.4 Examples of wireless multimedia sensor network hardware platforms. (a) low-resolution camera; (b) intermediate-resolution camera; and (c) high-resolution camera. (From Almalkawi, I.T. et al., *Sensors*, 10, 6662–6717, 2010.)

- Intermediate and high-resolution hardware platforms are designed for sophisticated high-quality applications, such as network management, target detection, and monitoring. These two kinds of hardware platforms can consume a great deal of energy. As the examples of intermediate resolution hardware platform, the Stargate board [27] and the Imote2 [28] platforms (Intel company, California) and beyond that PTZ camera [29] (Sony Corporation, Tokyo, Japan), Panoptes camera [30] (Logitech company, California), and MeshEye camera [31] (Agilent Technologies incorporated Corporation, California) are considered as high-resolution cameras. Figure 5.4 shows several commercial products of hardware platforms used in WMSNs.

5.2.3.2 Test Beds To evaluate different processing algorithms and communication protocols or test various applications in WMSNs, researchers obtain experiment results and theoretical analysis according to conduct simulations, because the experimental formula in WMSNs is inefficient and complex, and it is difficult to be repeatedly used by other researchers. As a result, simulation reduction is considered the best measurement methodology in WMSNs. However, current simulators cannot model the major characteristics of real-time multimedia systems. Obviously, simulation reduction is somewhat dubious and has limited credibility [32]. In order to remedy the gap between theoretical and actual approaches, researchers have evaluated proposed protocols and algorithms in a test bed.

According to whether they can test and evaluate application, protocols, research prototypes, or network performance metrics in real environments, test beds can be divided into two categories: hardware test beds and software test beds [24]. Software test beds are designed on application program interfaces, which provide testing and evaluation of application conditions via abstraction layers that hide the low-level hardware devices. WiSNAP [28,33] is an example of a software test bed. Hardware test beds consist of some hardware devices, such as multiple sensor nodes, wireless communication hardware, base stations, supporting tools for user interface and information monitoring.

According to the hierarchal organization in WMSN, we further divided hardware test beds into single-tier and multitier test beds. A single-tier hardware test bed, Meerkats [34] is used for detecting and monitoring wide surroundings. IrisNet [35], a multitier hardware test bed, builds large-scale distributed networks for heterogeneous WMSN applications. Table 5.3 gives a summary of the features for existing software and hardware test beds.

5.2.4 Network Architecture

Similar to traditional sensor networks, the network architecture of WMSNs is also a flat, homogeneous architecture, where each multimedia node device has a similar or identical processing capability. However, homogeneous architecture is not suited for processing multimedia applications. We introduce various heterogeneous architectures for WMSNs in Figure 5.5, where the network architecture of WMSNs can be divided into three categories in accordance with different network application characteristics.

- Single-tier flat architecture consists of homogeneous multimedia nodes. They have the same processing capabilities in the network architecture, where all the nodes have the ability to accomplish any function to the sink by means of multihop route, as shown in Figure 5.5a.
- Figure 5.5b shows a single-tier clustered deployment architecture, which contains heterogeneous multimedia nodes, such as visual, image, scalar sensors, and so on. They pass on the sensed information to the cluster head, which has a more complex ability to process data. The cluster head is joined with the gateway or the sink either directly or through other cluster heads through a multihop route [24].

Table 5.3 WMSN Test Beds

	TEST BED NAME	CAMERA AND RESOLUTION	WIRELESS MOTE	ADDITIONAL FEATURES
Software Test Beds	WiSNAP	Includes device library Agilent ADCM-1670	Includes device library of Chipcon CC2420DB IEEE 802.15.4	-MATLAB®-based test bed -Open source APIs -Multimedia processing Primitives
	AER Emulator	OmniVision OV7649 640 × 480 @ 30fps 320 × 240 @ 60fps	XYZ, Imote2 IEEE 802.15.4	-Visual C++ based test bed -AE recognition
Hardware Test Beds	Meetkat	Logitech QuickCam Pro 4000 640 × 480	Stargate IEEE 802.11b	-Energy efficient -Event detection
	SenseEye	Cyclops, CMUcam3, PTZ Sony SNC-RZ30N Different resolutions	MICA2 IEEE 802.15.4 Stargate IEEE 802.11	-Multilevel resolution -Surveillance application
	IrisNet	Logitech QuickCam Pro 4000 640 × 480	Stargate	-Internet-like queries -Scalable
	Explorebots	X10 Cam2 320 × 240	MICA2 IEEE 802.15.4	-Mobile robot -Electronic compass Ranging devices for navigation
	Mobile Emulab	Overhead Hitachi KP-D20A 768 × 494	MICA2 IEEE 802.15.4 Stargate IEEE 802.11b	-Mobile robot -Evaluate mobility-related network protocols
	WMSN test bed	Logitech QuickCam Pro 4000 640 × 480 176 × 144 @15fpx	MICAz IEEE 802.15.4 Stargate IEEE 802.11b	-Mobile robot -Multilevel resolution

Source: Almalkawi, I.T. et al., *Sensors*, 10, 6662–6717, 2010.

- The middle section presents a multitiered network, with heterogeneous multimedia sensors. In the architecture, the low section is composed of tradition sensors, which executes simple tasks like object sensing. The middle section deployed with visual nodes may execute more complicated tasks such as target capturing. The upper section, with high-resolution multimedia nodes, has the ability to execute more complex tasks, like target tracking. Any tier has a central hub for processing data and exchanging information with the upper tier. The final tier is used for linking the gateway or the sink [24], as illustrated in Figure 5.5c.

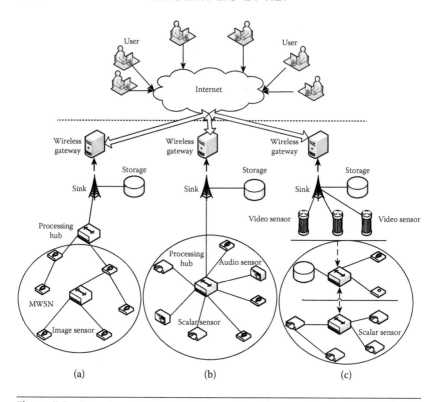

Figure 5.5   Network architecture of wireless multimedia sensor networks: (a) single-tier flat architecture; (b) single-tier clustered architecture; and (c) multitier architecture.

Table 5.4   Hardware Platforms, Typical Tasks for Each Tier in a Multitiered Hierarchical Architecture

HIERARCHY	TYPICAL TASK	HARDWARE PLATFORMS
Low tier	Object sensing	Cylops/XYZ-ALOHA/ MeshEye
Medium tier	Object capturing	MeshEye/Firefly Mosaic/CITRIC
High tier	Object tracking	Panoptes/Meerkats

Source: Tavli, B. et al., *Multimed. Tools Appl.* 60, 689–726, 2012.

Several network architectures have many applications, especially for multitiered heterogeneous network architecture, where each tier sensor is in charge of different functionalities and with different hardware platforms. Table 5.4 presents hardware platforms for each tier in a multitiered hierarchical architecture [36].

5.3 Coverage Models

The coverage problem estimates the capturing capability of multimedia nodes and QoS by obtaining the geometric relation among the target and sensor nodes. Generally speaking, coverage models might be formulated as the function of the angles or the Euclidean distances between the target and the sensor node [37]. There are several attributes for categorizing available coverage models, as shown in Figure 5.6.

In this section, we mainly discuss two coverage models: the mathematical coverage model [38] and physical coverage model. In addition, we review the other off-the-shelf coverage models such as the two-dimensional (2D)/three-dimensional (3D) coverage model and full-coverage model, as well as the full-view coverage model and non-overlapping and overlapping coverage models. In the following, we will provide a detailed introduction to the above-mentioned coverage models.

5.3.1 Mathematical and Physical Coverage Models

Mathematical coverage models depict the geometric relationship of coverage by a multimedia node or node system. To deal with the coverage relation, we divided coverage model into the Boolean (binary) coverage model and the probabilistic coverage model.

In the Boolean coverage model, the coverage measurement is either 0 or 1 to express a target. If an object is located through sensor's capturing scope, the coverage measure is considered as 1. Otherwise, it is 0 and the object will not be perceived due to interference factors, even if the target is located within the sensing area in practical applications.

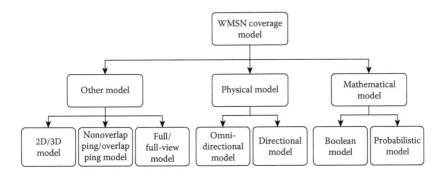

Figure 5.6 Comparisons of coverage models.

As a result, the Boolean coverage model is an ideal model for multimedia sensor coverage.

The probabilistic coverage model [39] describes sensed objects within the scope of the multimedia node via the probability function, which function is described by either the distance or angle between the multimedia nodes and the target, and the value of the probability function decreases as the distance/angle descends.

Physical coverage models can provide sensing direction information for multimedia sensors. We classify physical coverage models into the omnidirectional (isotropic) coverage model and directional coverage model.

The sensing range of the omnidirectional model is often abstracted as a circular area and a target is considered to be captured or covered by a multimedia node if it is in the field of the sensing range for the multimedia node [40]. At present, most of researches mainly use the circular sensing model to solve coverage issues [41–44].

Unlike omni-directional model, directional model can record different views of the target or different direction targets [40]. Directional nodes have a finite AoV and cannot sense the entire circular scope. Consequently, the coverage range of directional sensors is a fan-shaped area in a 2D plane.

According to a simple geometrical abstraction, the sector coverage model of directional nodes is expressed by fourfold $<S_i, r, \varphi, f>$, where S_i expresses the location of the directional node, r is the maximum sensing radius, φ is a FoV angle, and f represents the working orientation of the object. The sensing area of the directional sensor for a 2D plane is shown in Figure 5.7a. A point P is covered by a node S_i if P is within the sensing scope of S_i, as shown in Figure 5.7b.

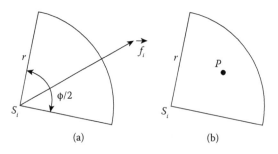

(a)   (b)

Figure 5.7   (a) The directional sensor S_i sensing sector and (b) an object point covered by node S_j.

5.3.2 Other Coverage Models

In addition to the above-mentioned coverage models, there are some other coverage models according to different classifications. For example, coverage models might be divided based on their description of a spatial region into 2D and 3D coverage models. Based on the directional relationship between target and multimedia sensor, coverage model can be divided into full-coverage model and full-view coverage model. We divide coverage models into overlapping and nonoverlapping coverage models according to the relationship between multimedia sensors. In the following subsection, we will introduce several different coverage models in detail.

5.3.2.1 2D/3D Coverage Model To simplify the experimental estimation of the proposed algorithms in the existing publications, most coverage models regard the monitored area as 2D coverage model. However, the 2D coverage model does not meet real-world application requirements. Compared to the 2D model, the 3D model can deliver more accuracy. The establishment of the 3D model mainly focuses on two distinct features for pan–tilt–zoom (PTZ) directional sensors; one is a multimedia sensor with a fixed 3D point. The other is the coverage area as a projecting quadrilateral field in a 2D surface.

The 3D coverage model is represented by five elements (P, W_d, A, α, and β), where P expresses the sensor position (x,y,z), W_d indicates the working direction for the directional node, A is the maximum value of the FoV angle, and α versus β represent the horizontal and vertical offset angles in sight around W_d. $W_d = (dx(t),dy(t),dz(t))$ denotes a unit length, where $dx(t)$, $dy(t)$, and $dz(t)$ are elements along the x, y, and z axes, respectively [13]. Figure 5.8 shows the 3D coverage model [45]. If an object P is covered by a sensor S_i, the following condition must be satisfied: the object P must be fixed in the projecting quadrilateral area in a 2D surface.

5.3.2.2 Full/Full-View Coverage Model The full-coverage model has nothing to do with target direction, if only the object is within the node's sensing range. As to some special applications, multimedia sensors not only record an object image, but they must also obtain a frontal view of the object to identify the target clearly. As a result,

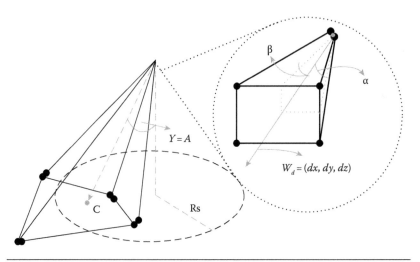

Figure 5.8 A 3D coverage model. (From Ma, H. et al., *Proceedings of the IEEE International Conference on Computer Communications*, 2009.)

in addition to the target location, the working orientation of the target has vital impact on the quality of coverage.

However, the nonexistence of commercially available coverage models was used to solve the problems of the target working orientation in the past few years, until Wang and Guohong [40] put forward the full-view coverage model. In this model, a target is recognized as full-view coverage if no matter which direction the target faces, the target is within the sensing range of at least one sensor and the target's orientation is sufficiently close to that sensor's orientation. The angle θ between the front direction of object and the sensor's orientation is a predefined parameter, we call it the effective angle. Figure 5.9 shows full-view coverage models for omnidirectional sensors and directional sensors.

5.3.2.3 Nonoverlapping/Overlapping Coverage Model In this subsection, we further divide coverage types into the overlapping model and nonoverlapping model [46], as shown in Figure 5.10. Directional sensors with the nonoverlapping coverage model only take a limited series of directions and mutually disjoint coverage sectors (see Figure 5.10a).

Compared to the nonoverlapping model [47], directional sensors with the overlapping coverage model (see Figure 5.10b) have a

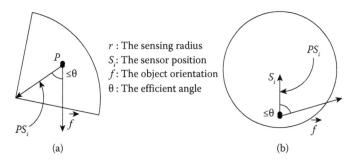

Figure 5.9 The full-view coverage models for (a) directional sensors and (b) omnidirectional sensors.

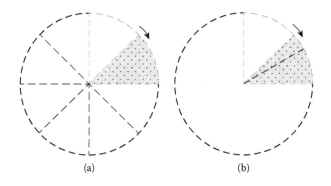

Figure 5.10 Two typical directional sensing models. (a) Nonoverlapping model and (b) Overlapping model.

limitless number of available coverage sectors based on different orientations. However, each directional node can only choose one active coverage direction at any moment. Generally speaking, the overlapping coverage model is developed to sweep all directions continuously along its center. The aim is to combine a finite set of coverage sectors to generate a whole circular viewpoint.

5.4 Factors Influencing Coverage

There are several problems (e.g., sensor deployment, movement, characteristics, location, organization) to be solved in WMSNs, because these problems generate a significant effect on coverage optimization. In this section, we mainly introduce sensor characteristics and sensor behaviors, which are the most affecting factors

Table 5.5 Research Publications on Affecting Factors in Wireless Multimedia Sensor Network Coverage

PUBLICATION	COVERAGE MODEL	SENSOR BEHAVIOR	DEPLOYMENT	COVERAGE TYPE
Wang and Cao [8]	Directional model	Static sensor	Random deployment	Barrier coverage
Yang and Qiao [39]	Omnidirectional model	Active Static sensor	Random deployment	Barrier coverage
Wang and Guohong [40]	Directional model	Static sensor	Random deployment	Area coverage
Zhang et al. [47]	Directional model	Static sensor	Deterministic deployment	Barrier coverage
Liu et al. [63]	Directional model	Static sensor	Random deployment	Target coverage
Chang et al. [64]	Directional model	Static sensor	Random deployment	Area coverage

for coverage problems. Moreover, deployment strategy, location information, and application requirements have some influence on coverage schemes. To simplify comparison, Table 5.5 lists some notable and leading publications for several different factors affecting WMSN coverage.

5.4.1 Sensor Characteristics

Compared to traditional sensors, multimedia sensors possess some unique characteristics, such as sensing radius, communication ranges, line of sight, AoV, and working direction, which bring new challenges for coverage optimization. In the following, we will introduce some of these characteristics. We have already noted these properties in the Section 5.3 except for line of sight and communication ranges; we will focus on these two characteristics in the following.

5.4.1.1 Line of Sight Unlike traditional omnidirectional sensors, each multimedia node has its own working orientation. When multimedia nodes are arranged, some issues associated with the direction need to be considered. For example, some obstacles (e.g., buildings or mountains) which are reflected in the deployment environment will affect node coverage [48]. This condition is known as the *occlusion effect*, and it directly affects the line of sight and area size for sensor coverage. The line of sight of multimedia sensors is undoubtedly decided by the size and distance between obstacles. If the intersection angle between the node and the object is 0°, we can obtain useful information from the coverage area [10]. However, the above theory is impracticable. As a result, traditional coverage models are insufficient for multimedia sensor networks.

5.4.1.2 Communication Ranges Communication range defines the farthest distance which data between nodes can be exchanged. To maximize coverage area, the basic principal is to avoid overlapping coverage where two or more multimedia sensors intersect. Existing solutions for WMSNs guarantee that communication range between nodes is at least twice that of the sensing scope [49].

5.4.2 Sensor Behaviors

In WMSNs, some sensor behaviors can often be used for achieving high coverage rates. In Subsections 5.4.2.1 through 5.4.2.3, we will introduce several characteristics of multimedia sensors: node organization, motility, and mobility.

5.4.2.1 Node Organization Generally speaking, node organization is either homogeneous or heterogeneous. A homogeneous architecture expresses that every multimedia sensor has the same processing capability. Heterogeneity is another kind of node organization that has been proposed [50]. A heterogeneous architecture expresses that some multimedia sensors are more powerful than the others. Usually, the powerful nodes are regarded as cluster heads, which can obtain information from the less powerful nodes [51]. In heterogeneous architecture, there exist multimedia sensors with different functions to meet application requirements. As a result, low-level and high-level sensors are deployed at different times or places [52].

5.4.2.2 Motility Motility—as one of the sensor behaviors—consists of actuation, pan, tilt, and zoom. Actuation yields a significant improvement in the field of sensor coverage, which is determined to actuate by cooperative relationship between neighboring multimedia sensor nodes. In Ref. [53], an intelligent sensor actuation mechanism is presented to reduce the redundancy of node information through actuating a certain number of multimedia nodes while still providing the necessary target coverage.

Pan, tilt, and zoom (PTZ), defined as motions for multimedia sensor nodes, can move and rotate the multimedia sensor along the x, y, or z axis. A PTZ multimedia sensor can randomly deploy fewer sensors at the initial phase. Meanwhile, we move and adjust multimedia sensors to meet coverage requirements. Owning to its low-cost overhead, there are a larger numbers of studies on the motility problem [54].

5.4.2.3 Mobility Motility can improve coverage performance, within reasonable delay constraints on behavior [54]. To remedy motility hole in the coverage issue, some deployment mechanisms take full advantage of mobility to redeploy nodes to sparsely covered fields after an initial random deployment [55]. Hence, mobility is feasible for improving coverage and prolonging lifetime.

In the above subchapter, we introduce the two behaviors of multimedia nodes: motility and mobility. They can improve network coverage to minimize the overlapped areas and the occlusion effect. Nevertheless, motile and mobile multimedia nodes are expensive. Consequently, Ref. [13] proposes balancing the coverage ratio and cost with hybrid multimedia sensors.

5.4.3 Other Factors

5.4.3.1 Deployment Strategy Deployment strategy plays a vital role in constructing WMSNs. Generally speaking, we construct WMSNs via two styles, deterministic deployment and random deployment. In deterministic deployment, the location and orientation of each multimedia sensor node is placed in advance. Usually, deterministic deployment can be used for a small to medium WMSN. In military applications, inhospitable surroundings, disaster sites, and remote locations, the positions and direction of sensor nodes cannot be placed in advance. In these conditions, random placement might be a good choice. Recently, a popular form of random deployment is to scatter sensors from an aircraft or to launch sensors via artillery. There has been some research in the field of random deployment [7]. Concrete deployment strategy will be explained in Section 5.5.

5.4.3.2 Location Information   In WMSNs, many coverage applications including object surveillance and monitoring are dependent on location information. Hence, it is crucial to obtain location information in terms of objects and sensors. Earlier location information can be obtained through GPS (global positioning system). If it lacks the information of sensor orientation, cost, and energy, we can not obtain location data [56].

Currently, it is common to use localization algorithms to decide object and sensor location information. Sayed et al. [57] proposed a centralized algorithm. The work in Ref. [58] is an extension of Ref. [56]. Lee and Aghajan [59] presented distributed localization methods. The study in Ref. [60] obtained the position of the cameras by moving target. A localization algorithm for WMSNs was investigated in Ref. [61], which proposed an algorithm to estimate node locations to identify the areas where cameras overlap. The work presented in Ref. [62] uses 3D node localization to obtain node location information. Liu et al. [63] present a novel localization-oriented sensing model for randomly deployed nodes.

5.4.3.3 Application Requirements   Application requirements for the coverage problem mainly refers to factors including coverage type, degree, ratio, and so on. Coverage type refers to the subject to be covered by nodes; coverage types can be divided into area coverage, point (target) coverage, and barrier coverage. Coverage degree describes how a target is covered. Chang et al. [64] propose *k*-barrier coverage. Coverage ratio measures how many nodes are needed to finish coverage in an area or how many targets satisfy the application requirement for coverage degree. Wang and Guohong [40] estimate node density for achieving full-view coverage with any given probability (e.g., 0.99). Other available studies on application requirements will be discussed in detail in Sections 5.7 and 5.8.

5.5 Sensor Deployment and Scheduling

As described in Section 5.4.3.1, sensor deployment in WMSNs can be divided into two categories, deterministic (for short deterministic deployment) and random (for short random deployment), as shown in Figure 5.11. In this section, we discuss algorithms for

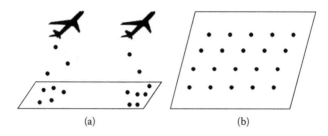

(a)   (b)

Figure 5.11 Comparison of sensor deployment. (a) Random deployment and (b) Deterministic deployment.

deterministic deployment (see Figure 5.11a), which convey that optimal node placement brings about coverage problems. Further, we present algorithms for node management and node localization in random deployment (see Figure 5.11b). Finally, we introduce several special sensor scheduling algorithms, especially for the art gallery problem.

5.5.1 Deterministic Deployment

As shown in Figure 5.11b, with deterministic deployment, MWSN nodes are deployed in an orderly fashion in predetermined locations. Through this method, we can use a minimal number of nodes to achieve maximum coverage and further reduce the cost of WMSNs [65]. However, deterministic deployment can only apply to indoor environments without any obstacles. In military applications, inhospitable or remote locations, or disaster sites, this deployment strategy is not feasible because of some overlapping and occlusion problems.

We may divide deterministic deployment into two groups: static and dynamic deployment. In static deployment, multimedia nodes can stay in the same place and cannot change their position once they are deployed [66]. The algorithm for static deployment is executed only once. If multimedia sensors can change their working directions or position after initial deployment, it is known as dynamic deployment. The algorithm in Ref. [67] provides maximal coverage through node movement with location information. In dynamic deployment, coverage can be recalculated over time, and multimedia sensors allow a new configuration to overcome the problem of coverage holes. For some scenarios, multimedia sensors can dynamically configure themselves. Ref. [68] proposes the concept of self-calibration for traditional networks. In general, a dynamic multimedia node is much more complicated than a static sensor node. Fortunately, dynamic sensors can prolong the lifetime and increase the connectivity of nodes, while maintaining or improving coverage [69].

In the past few years, research on deterministic deployment has mainly underscored working direction. A multimedia node may be deployed in N different directions. We may determine the best working direction for this node, in which overlapped and occlusion regions are minimized. In Ref. [70], optimal node deployment with 360° rotation is investigated. Other works that have investigated deterministic deployment have focused on camera placement (such as the art gallery problem) [71], the floodlight illumination problem [72], and the next-best view problem [73]. Recently, many studies have further discussed deterministic deployment based on more realistic assumptions. Clearly, occlusion and overlapping have significant influence on deployment problems. Mittal and Davis [74] present deterministic deployment of cameras with unchangeable orientation in a dynamic and occluded scene, which aims to cover a field of interest with minimal nodes. Similarly, Refs. [75,76] take into account the impact of the obstacle and occlusion.

The above-mentioned research has made contributions to solutions for the real-time deployment problems in covering an area of interest. In addition to deterministic deployment, there exist some additional influencing factors such as deployment structure and model. As the example of deployment model, Horster and Lienhart [77] modeled the monitored field as a grid. Zhao et al. [78] proposed a visibility model to solve the deployment problem through a binary integer programming approach. Ram et al. [79] proposed a realist node model in 3D environments. Adriaens et al. [80] found the worst-case coverage problem with camera networks. For deployment structure, the authors of Ref. [81] considered two-level deployment. Schwager et al. [82] proposed a decentralized control strategy with heterogeneous degrees of mobility. Its purpose is to use a flying robot to rotate the cameras in order to cover the monitored regions with minimal sensors.

5.5.2 *Random Deployment*

In military applications, inhospitable or remote locations, and disaster sites, random deployment may be the best option. Sensor nodes could be massively scattered from an aircraft or launched via artillery (see Figure 5.11b). Compared to deterministic placement, random deployment is more suitable for WMSNs. Therefore, random deployment can generate numerous redundant nodes and cause overlapped and occluded areas, while compensating for a hole in node coverage and improving fault tolerance. An interesting approach is to solve the problem using strategies such as redeployment and mobile nodes [83].

During random deployment, sensor nodes are deployed anywhere. To obtain their current location and direction, the traditional positioning system depends on GPS. The current method for node localization requires specific algorithms. There are two kinds of common localization algorithms, centralized algorithms and distributed algorithms. In centralized algorithms, the sink or a central server is used for processing data, while the other sensing node is used for capturing information. It is a useful method for saving energy. In distributed algorithms, each node needs to run all functions independently [84].

In addition, to maximize area coverage and reduce their overlap, sensor nodes adjust their current positions after initial deployment. Cai et al. [85] discuss the random deployment of nodes with changeable directions. Tezcan and Wang [86] present a distributed algorithm to adjust node direction for minimizing the effects of occlusion. Kandoth and Chellappan [87] investigate mobile multimedia sensors, where these nodes can avoid undesired overlapping and blanket spaces.

5.5.3 *Sensor Scheduling*

Scheduling problems have a strong correlation with coverage optimization in WMSNs. Recently, there have been several examples of sensor scheduling issues, such as the art gallery problem, robotic systems coverage, the circle covering problem, the floodlight illumination problem, the next-best view problem, and so on. In this subsection, we focus on describing the art gallery problem.

The art gallery problem is related to the concept of coverage [51]. O'Rourke [88] first gave a more formal definition for the art gallery problem. In the art gallery problem, the manager places sensors in a gallery such that the whole gallery is covered. The specific operation is to model the gallery into a polygon, such as nonoverlapping triangles [55]. This method is not feasible for a 3D space [51]; it is only suitable for a 2D space. In this model, we suppose the view angle of the node deployed in the art gallery is 360° and the sensing range is unlimited. However, this scenario is not feasible for the real world.

5.6 Sensor Management

In WMSNs, sensor nodes can obtain continuous information from the covered area with a desired quality. However, these sensor nodes can be changed as time goes by. In this scenario, the instructions and duration for sensor nodes' activity rely on the strategy of sensor management, including sensor selection and scheduling. Coverage metrics are used for evaluating the strategy of sensor management, for example, network connectivity, energy efficiency, coverage degree, coverage ratio, and so on.

A similar application on coverage metrics for selecting sensors is investigated in Ref. [89]. Similarly, Dagher et al. [90] discuss the application for complete real-time coverage of an area and provide a strategy for assigning each node's coverage area to keep minimizing energy consumption. However, this strategy is only suitable for 2D spaces without occlusions, which cannot be extended to a 3D space. Ercan et al. [91] further consider the occlusion problem.

There is currently some relevant research on sensor selection. Ref. [92] considers sensor selection with the constraints of energy costs. Considering the next-best view problem, Park et al. [93] propose a realistic 3D coverage model for sensor selection. In addition, Shen et al. [94] assign a general coverage metric to coverage space and allow task-specific weighting of the individual factors. Akyildiz and Vuran [95] present sensor selection problems. Kulkarni et al. [96] define the topological coverage overlap model with purely empirical.

The purpose of sensor scheduling is to decide the status and duration of sensor nodes, so we can guarantee the coverage requirement and prolong the network lifetime. If an area is covered by multiple sensors simultaneously, the other sensors can be considered redundant, except for a few sensors with satisfying coverage conditions. The redundant sensors should be temporarily transitioned into their energy-saving sleep state [2]. There are two node scheduling algorithms that are proposed in the literature, distributed algorithms and centralized algorithms. Because these two algorithms have been mentioned in the Section 5.5, we will not discuss them again.

5.7 Coverage Metrics

After deployment, multimedia nodes are distributed in the monitored area, with unpredicted overlapping and occlusions. Some corresponding algorithms can be used to improve the coverage of deployed nodes, but coverage benchmarks are subject to multiple factors, such as network connectivity, energy efficiency, and network lifetime. In addition, there are some other influencing factors which contain coverage performance, coverage degree, coverage ratio, and so on. In the following, we will mainly introduce several remarkable and leading coverage metrics. The related literature for coverage metrics of multimedia sensor nodes are listed in Table 5.6 to simplify comparison.

5.7.1 Network Connectivity

The coverage area of only one sensor is limited, so wireless collaboration between sensors is vital for covering larger areas [84]. Hence, network connectivity is closely related to coverage problems. It can ensure that there is at least one communication path between any two nodes. Recently, connected coverage problems have drawn much attention. Ref. [97] introduces how to determine optimal deployment to accomplish connectivity and full coverage.

The sensing model and communication radius of a node directly affects network connectivity. In WMSNs, the communication mode between nodes is omnidirectional, and most existing research assumes that the communication radius of a node is at least twice the sensing radius of this node. Under connectivity constraints, we reconsider coverage problems while assuring network connectivity. Han et al. [98] first surveyed the connected coverage problem in MWSNs; they used minimum number of directional sensors to maximize the entire target area. In addition, Ma and Liu [99] presented a deployment mechanism that maintains node coverage and network connectivity. Further, the latest research [100] solves the relationship between coverage and network connectivity in deterministic deployment.

Table 5.6 Research Publications on Coverage Metrics in Wireless Multimedia Sensor Networks

	COVERAGE METRICS				
PUBLICATION	NETWORK CONNECTIVITY	ENERGY EFFICIENCY	NETWORK LIFETIME	COVERAGE RATIO	COVERAGE DEGREE (k)
Kranakis et al. [97]	√	×	×	×	×
Han et al. [98]	√	×	×	√	×
Bai et al. [100]	√	×	×	×	×
Margi et al. [101]	×	√	×	√	×
Cardei and Wu [102]	√	√	√	√	√
Ai and Abouzeid [49]	×	√	√	√	√
Osais et al. [103]	√	√	×	√	×
Pescaru et al. [104]	×	√	√	√	×
Istin et al. [105]	×	√	×	√	×
Istin et al. [106]	×	√	√	√	×
Cai et al. [85]	×	√	√	×	×
Fusco and Gupta [109]	×	√	×	√	√
Kumar et al. [110]	√	×	×	√	√
Wan and Yi [111]	×	×	×	×	√
Wang et al. [112]	√	√	×	√	√
Liu et al. [113]	√	×	×	√	√
Zhao and Zheng [114]	×	×	×	√	×
Bay et al. [115]	×	×	×	√	√
Tezcan and Wang [116]	√	×	×	√	×
Chang et al. [64]	×	×	×	×	√

Note: √ indicates that coverage metrics are satisfied; × indicates that coverage metrics are not satisfied.

5.7.2 Network Lifetime

Most sensor nodes with limited battery capacity have a large influence on network lifetime. It is not feasible to replace a sensor node or recharge a battery after sensors are deployed. To prolong the network lifetime, the primary method is avoiding unnecessary energy consumption, which reflects on hardware, local processing, communication and sensing functions, and so on.

An energy-aware strategy for minimizing the energy consumption has been proposed. One pattern is to schedule redundant sensors into sleep mode. The other pattern is to adjust the transmission distance between nodes. In addition, Ref. [51] conserves energy by enhancing the efficiency of information gathering and routing. In WMSNs, scheduling redundant sensors into sleep mode or reducing the amount of active nodes is a relatively better way which can prolong network lifetime. Conversion between them may require considerable energy and time [101].

In deployment networks, especially for random deployment networks, there are a large number of redundant nodes. On one hand, redundant nodes can be used for remedying holes to improve area coverage. On the other hand, we turn off redundant nodes to save energy. The authors of Ref. [102] propose four fundamental questions for node redundancy. The first question is which sensor to put into sleep mode. The next problem is when this node should enter sleep mode; another issue is how long the node can last in this status. The last problem should consider mode feature. In addition, Ai and Abouzeid [49] present centralized and distributed algorithms to solve redundant nodes. Osais et al. [103] present an ILP model to reduce the number of sensors.

To balance coverage and network lifetime, Ref. [104] proposes the "Sensing Neighborhood Cooperative Sleeping" protocol, where the less significant nodes are shut down. Ref. [105] considers nodes with rechargeable batteries. Similar research [106] considers coverage and network lifetime with moving obstacles. Ref. [107] considers an energy-efficiency strategy based on sleeping sensor network. In Ref. [108], power management policies are defined to reduce energy consumption in MWSNs.

5.7.3 Other Coverage Metrics

5.7.3.1 Coverage Degree Depending on the application requirements, coverage degree describes how many sensors can cover an object area. The related literature proposed k-coverage, which indicates that an area is covered by at least k different nodes. For example, if a deployment field is 5-coverage, each area is covered by at least five sensor nodes, and it can accept four failed nodes while maintaining region coverage. The purpose of k-coverage is to improve coverage robustness and reliability.

There are some research papers on k-coverage problems. Ref. [109] uses a minimal number of sensors to finish k-coverage. Ref. [110]

uses *k*-barrier coverage to detect the target. The authors of Ref. [111] survey a *k*-covered region. Wang et al. [112] discuss a *k*-connected network problem. Liu et al. [113] use *k*-coverage to measure coverage performance.

5.7.3.2 Coverage Ratio   As one of the coverage performance metrics, the coverage ratio measures how much area or how many targets satisfy the coverage requirement [2]. The study in Ref. [114] increased the coverage ratio by 3%. The paper [115] achieved 90% coverage. In Ref. [116], the authors studied self-orientation of multimedia nodes for maximizing coverage with occlusions. Simulations showed that the coverage ratio with occlusion-free viewpoints was significantly increased by 41%. In addition, quality of coverage, scalability, robustness, latency, jitter, adaptively, distortion, and energy consumption are also coverage metrics in WMSNs. We will not explain the coverage metrics one by one.

5.8 Typical Coverage

Cardei et al. [4] categorized available coverage problems in WMSNs into three main categories: point (target) coverage, area coverage, and barrier coverage. Point (target) coverage refers to some assigned point (the target) with a known location (see Figure 5.12). Area coverage refers to covering (monitoring) a region of interest (see Figure 5.13). Barrier coverage constructs a barrier for intrusion detection, to avoid undetected penetration, or searches for a penetration path across the monitored area (see Figure 5.14).

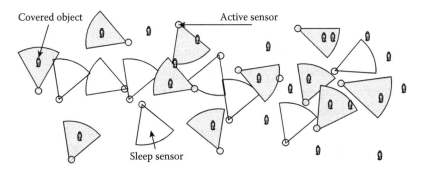

Figure 5.12   Point (target) coverage.

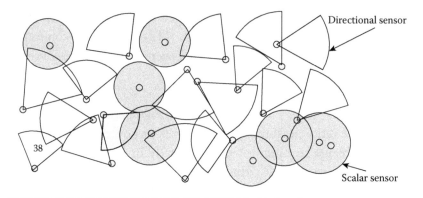

Figure 5.13   Area coverage.

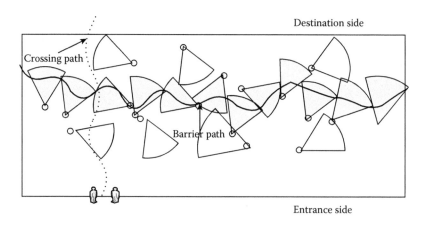

Figure 5.14   Barrier coverage.

5.8.1 Target Coverage

To cover an assigned target, researchers have defined target coverage. As shown in Figure 5.12, target coverage mainly studies how to deploy and schedule sensor nodes to satisfy maximum coverage for objects. In target coverage, each target within the monitored area is covered continuously by at least one node. Because the target within a sensor's sensing region is a discrete distribution, target coverage is also called point coverage.

There are several typical target coverage algorithms. The investigators in Ref. [117] have done extensive research to detect, classify, and track objects. The authors of Refs. [118–122] considered whether energy has an influence on target coverage. In the pioneer study of directional network coverage, Ai and Abouzeid [49] presented the problem of maximum coverage with minimum sensors problem. Considering that some deployed nodes fail and some new objects may be added as the mission requirement changes, Ref. [123] suggests reconfiguring the network by letting existing sensors steer and serve the targets periodically and solve service delay problems. To our knowledge, it is the first research on the minimum service delay problem in WMSNs.

5.8.2 Area Coverage

As shown in Figure 5.13, area coverage requires that the whole monitored area be covered by more than one node. To provide high coverage quality in WMSNs, Ref. [124] introduces the approach of utilizing a mixture of static and mobile sensors, where mobile sensors can move to make up coverage holes. To maximize multimedia sensor coverage with less time, movement distance, and message complexity, the authors of Ref. [125] use Voronoi diagrams to detect coverage holes and obtain movement trajectory. Meanwhile, Wang et al. [126] present a framework for redeployed mobile sensors in a balanced, efficient, and timely manner.

Considering directional nodes from different viewpoints can catch different views of the same objects. Ref. [40] proposes a novel concept called full-view coverage. A target point is considered to have full-view coverage if, no matter which orientation the object faces, the target is within the sensor's range and the target's facing orientation is sufficiently close to that sensor's viewing orientation. Based on the concept of full-view coverage, Ref. [52] discusses two random deployment schemes.

5.8.3 Barrier Coverage

As shown in Figure 5.14, the purpose of barrier coverage is to detect intruders that attempt to pass the monitored area. Currently, it has a large range of applications, for example: monitoring coastal waters, country borders, and boundaries of battlefields. Unlike area coverage, barrier coverage is concerned with the detectability of intruders traversing the region of interest. Unlike full coverage, barrier coverage needs a much lower number of sensors. Hence, barrier coverage in MWSNs has gained considerable attention in practice.

There have been some studies on barrier coverage, while the majority focus on traditional networks which coverage range is a circular. In recent years, there have been some requirements in WMSNs [127–129]. Compared to WSNs, the barrier coverage range for WMSNs is fan-shaped. Hence, it can capture different viewpoints for the same target point.

Barrier coverage in WSNs was first proposed in Ref. [129]. In barrier coverage, any intruding object can be identified once it passes the barrier path, regardless of the direction the object is facing. In addition, Ref. [130] proposes the maximum breach and minimum exposure path problem. In this article, the authors quantify coverage improvement when other nodes are added to the network.

Barrier coverage can be further divided into weak and strong coverage [131]. The concepts are as follows. If intruders choose the shortest path to pass through the monitored area, they can be detected. This is a weak barrier coverage. If intruders take any path from one side to the other, they can be detected; no objects can pass the undetected area. This is a strong barrier coverage.

To handle the special application requirements, Ref. [132] introduces the novel concept of full-view coverage, which we mentioned in Section 5.8.2. Based on this concept, Wang and Cao [133] construct a full-view barrier, where the monitored area is first separated into small subparts. Next, every subpart is marked up to form a graph. Further, each subpart is verified to be full-view covered. Finally, full-view covered subparts are chosen as the construct barriers.

The above distribution is not rigorous. To further reduce the number of sensors, Ma et al. [134] improved on the algorithm in Ref. [133] and proposed the minimum camera barrier coverage problem in WMSNs.

5.9 Other Research Issues

In the above-mentioned content, we have introduced some aspects of coverage problems in WMSNs. However, other currently relevant research issues are still uninvestigated. In the following content, we suggest some open research topics, such as realistic environments, 3D networking, privacy and security, node state transformation, and so on.

- Most studies of coverage problems make unrealistic assumptions (e.g., sensor model). In random deployment, the conditions in inhospitable or remote regions are not considered. Additionally, most simulation and analysis results are obtained in a fairly idealistic environment, which causes some unrealistic analysis of coverage problems. Hence, it is unreasonable for investigators to ignore these issues. Some real-world research should be considered in the future.

- To simplify coverage models, most existing research concentrates on a 2D plane. However, such network models are miles away from realistic environments. Under present conditions, research on 3D network models is still a new topic, due to high complexity in the design and analysis. These network models are largely unexplored, and the 3D network model is an extremely complex problem. As a result, the road leading to a 3D network model in WMSNs is still far away.

- WMSNs cause many challenges, while bringing gains such as people's private information. With network coverage enlarging, more and more multimedia sensors are being deployed into people's everyday lives. This circumstance causes many privacy and security issues. Certainly, there are several ways to solve this issue, such as excluding camera coverage from the network or sacrificing a bit of privacy. Nonetheless, it is still a marginal topic and is not treated seriously.

- In the area being monitored, the states of sensor nodes need to be adjusted for some application requirements. As states transformation of sensor nodes need to last for a long time, other coverage properties may be changed during this period. For example, when a multimedia sensor is switched from on to off, some routings will be broken. Coverage under such conditions is very vulnerable, and some complex and robust solutions are required to solve this issue.

5.10 Conclusions

In this article, we gave a broad survey of the ongoing research that has been solving coverage issues in WMSNs. Coverage problems can be classified into different research fields. First, we introduced and classified existing available WMSN hardware. Moreover, we presented several coverage models, which can measure sensing capability and quality through the geometric relation between objects and sensor nodes.

Second, we further divided coverage problems into four stages: the design stage, deployment stage, management stage, and coverage metrics. In the design stage, we noted some factors that can significantly influence coverage optimization. In the deployment stage, we mainly considered deterministic and random deployment. In the management stage, we discussed scheduling different sensor nodes to work alternatively to prolong network lifetime while preserving network coverage. In addition, we also related benchmarks for measuring coverage performance, such as network connectivity, energy consumption, and so on.

Finally, we touched on several typical coverage classifications including area coverage, target coverage, and barrier coverage. We reviewed representative solution algorithms in each category. In addition, coverage problems are still a recent, open research topic. We surveyed and classified existing recent studies on topics such as realistic environments, 3D networks, privacy and security, and node state transformation for WMSNs. We hope our work is useful for other researchers.

References

1. Akyildiz, I.F., Melodia, T., Chowdhury, K.R. Wireless multimedia sensor networks: Applications and testbeds. *Proceedings of the IEEE* 96(10), 1588–1605, 2008.
2. Wang, B. Coverage problems in sensor networks: A survey. *ACM Computing Surveys* 43(4), 32, 2011.
3. Liu, H., Wan, P., Yi, C.W., Jia, X., Makki, S., Pissinou, N. Maximal lifetime scheduling in sensor surveillance networks. *The 24th Annual Joint Conference of the IEEE Computer and Communications Societies*, pp. 2482–2491, 2005. DOI: 10.1109/INFCOM.2005.1498533.
4. Cardei, M., Thai, M., Li, Y., Wu, W. Energy-efficient target coverage in wireless sensor networks. *The 24th Annual Joint Conference of the IEEE Computer and Communications Societies*, pp. 1976–1984, 2005. DOI:10.1109/INFCOM.2005.1498475.

5. Huang, C.F., Tseng, Y.C. A survey of solutions to the coverage problems in wireless sensor networks. *Journal of Internet Technology* 6, 1–8, 2005.

6. Megerian, S., Koushanfar, F., Potkonjak, M., Srivastava, M. Worst and best-case coverage in sensor networks. *IEEE Transactions on Mobile Computing* 4, 1, 84–92, 2005. DOI: 10.1109/TMC.2005.1(410).

7. Ma, H., Liu, Y. On coverage problems of directional sensor networks. In: Lecture Notes in Computer Science. *Mobile Ad-Hoc and Sensor Networks* 3794, 721–731, 2005.

8. Wang, Y., Cao, G. Achieving full-view coverage in camera sensor networks. *ACM Transactions on Sensor Networks*, 2013.

9. Soro, S., Heinzelman, W. On the coverage problem in video-based wireless sensor networks. In: *Proceedings of the 2nd International Conference on Broadband Networks*, pp. 932–939, IEEE: Boston, MA, USA, October 3–7, 2005.

10. Akyildiz, I.F., Melodia, T., Chowdhury, K.R. A survey on wireless multimedia sensor networks. *Computer Networks* 51, 4, 921–960, 2007.

11. Soro, S., Heinzelman, W. A survey of visual sensor networks. *Hindawi Advances in Multimedia* 2009. DOI: 10.1155/2009/640386.

12. Greenleaf, A., Photographic Optics, Macmillan, London, England, 1950.

13. Amac Guvensan, M., Gokhan Yavuz, A. On coverage issues in directional sensor networks: A survey. *Ad Hoc Networks* 9, 1238–1255, 2011.

14. Carnegie Mellon University, CMUcam3 Datasheet Version 1.02, Pennsylvania, September 2007.

15. Yap, F.G.H., Yen, H.H. A survey on sensor coverage and visual data capturing/processing/transmission in wireless visual sensor networks. *Sensors* 14, 3506–3527, 2014. DOI: 10.3390/s140203506.

16. Omnivision Technologies. http://www.ovt.com

17. Agilent Technologies. http://www.home.agilent.com

18. Wise GEEK. http://www.wisegeek.org/what-is-an-infrared-sensor.htm

19. Wise GEEK. http://www.wisegeek.com/what-is-a-motion-detector.htm

20. eHow. http://www.ehow.com/how-does_5561845_do-ir-sensors-work.html

21. azosensors. http://www.azosensors.com/Article.aspx?ArticleID=339

22. Wise GEEK. http://www.wisegeek.com/what-is-an-ultrasonic-sensor.htm

23. eHow. http://www.ehow.com/how-does_4947693_ultrasonic-sensors-work.html

24. Almalkawi, I.T., Guerrero Zapata, M., Al-Karaki, J.N., Morillo-Pozo, J. Wireless multimedia sensor networks: current trends and future directions. *Sensors* 10, 6662–6717, 2010. DOI: 10.3390/s100706662.

25. Rahimi, M., Baer, R., Iroezi, O., Garcia, J., Warrior, J., Estrin, D., Srivastava, M. Cyclops: In situ image sensing and interpretation in wireless sensor networks. In: *Proceedings of the 3rd ACM Conference Embedded Network Sensor Systems (SenSys)*, ACM Press, San Diego, CA, USA, Nov. 2005.

26. Carnegie Mellon University. CMUcam3 datasheet, version 1.02. Pittsburgh, PA, USA, Sep. 2007.

27. The Stargate Platform. http://www.xbow.com/Products/Xscale.htm
28. Teixeira, T., Culurciello, E., Park, J., Lymberopoulos, D., Barton-Sweeney, A., Savvides, A. Address-event imagers for sensor networks: Evaluation and modeling. In: *Proceedings of the 5th International Conference on Information Processing in Sensor Networks, IPSN 2006*, pp. 458–466, IEEE: Nashville, TN, USA, April, 2006.
29. Kulkarni, P., Ganesan, D., Shenoy, P., Lu, Q. SensEye: A multi-tier camera sensor network. In: *Proceedings of the 13th Annual ACM International Conference on Multimedia, MULTIMEDIA'05*. pp. 229–238, ACM: New York, NY, USA, 2005.
30. Feng, W.C., Kaiser, E., Feng, W.C., Baillif, M.L. Panoptes: Scalable low-power video sensor networking technologies. *ACM Transactions on Multimedia Computing, Communications, and Applications* 1, 151–167, 2005.
31. Hengstler, S., Prashanth, D., Fong, S., Aghajan, H. MeshEye: A hybrid-resolution smart camera mote for applications in distributed intelligent surveillance. In: *Proceedings of the International Conference on Information Processing in Sensor Networks (IPSN)*, pp. 360–369, IEEE: Cambridge, MA, USA, 2007.
32. Kurkowski, S., Camp, T., Colagrosso, M., MANET simulation studies: The incredibles. *ACM SIGMOBILE Mobile Computing and Communications Review* 9(4), 50–61, 2005.
33. Hengstler, S., Aghajan, H. WiSNAP: A wireless image sensor network application platform. In: *Proceedings of 2nd International Conference on Testbeds and Research Infrastructures for the Development of Networks and Communities, TRIDENTCOM 2006*, pp. 6–12, Barcelona, Spain, 1–3 March 2006.
34. Boice, J., Lu, X., Margi, C., Stanek, G., Zhang, G., Obraczka, K. Meerkats: A power-aware, self-managing wireless camera network for wide area monitoring. In: *Distributed Smart Cameras Workshop - SenSys06*, Boulder, CA, USA, 2006.
35. Campbell, J., Gibbons, P.B., Nath, S., Pillai, P., Seshan, S., Sukthankar, R. IrisNet: An Internet-scale architecture for multimedia sensors. In: *Proceedings of the 13th annual ACM International Conference on Multimedia, MULTIMEDIA'05*, pp. 81–88, ACM: New York, NY, USA, 2005.
36. Tavli, B., Bicakci, K., Zilan, R., Barcelo-Ordinas, J.M. A survey of visual sensor network platforms. *Multimedia Tools and Applications* 60, 689–726, 2012.
37. Wang, Y. Coverage Problems in Camera Sensor Networks. *The Pennsylvania State University*, Pennsylvania, 2013.
38. Onur, E., Ersoy, C., Delic, H., Akarun, L. Surveillance wireless sensor networks: Deployment quality analysis. *Network, IEEE* 21, 6, 48–53. DOI: 10.1109/MNET.2007.4395110, 2007.
39. Yang, G., Qiao, D. Barrier information coverage with wireless sensors. In: *Proceedings of the IEEE Infocom Conference on Computer Communications*, IEEE: Rio de Janeiro, Brazil, 918–926, 2009.

40. Wang, Y., Guohong, C. On full-view coverage in camera sensor networks. *IEEE International Conference on Computer Communications* 1781–1789, 2011.
41. Huang, C.F., Tseng, Y.C. The coverage problem in a wireless sensor network. *Mobile Network and Applications* 519–528, 2005.
42. Shen, C., Cheng, W., Liao, X., Peng, S. Barrier coverage with mobile sensors. In: *International Symposium on Parallel Architectures, Algorithms, and Networks*, pp. 99–104, 2008.
43. Kloder, S., Hutchinson, S. Barrier coverage for variable bounded-range line-of-sight guards, in Robotics and Automation. *IEEE International Conference* 391–396, 2007.
44. Kloder, S., Hutchinson, S. Partial barrier coverage: Using game theory to optimize probability of undetected intrusion in polygonal environments, *2008 IEEE International Conference on Robotics and Automation, Pasadena, CA, USA*, May 19–23, 2671–2676, 2008.
45. Ma, H., Zhang, X., Ming, A. A coverage-enhancing method for 3d directional sensor networks. In: *Proceedings of the 28th IEEE International Conference on Computer Communications (INFOCOM'09)*, pp. 2791–2795, IEEE: Rio de Janerio, Brazil, 2009. DOI: 10.1109/INFCOM.2009.5062233.
46. Tao, D., Ma, H. Coverage control algorithms for directional sensor networks. *Journal of Software* 22(10), 2315–2332, 2011.
47. Zhang, L., Tang, J., Zhang, W. Strong barrier coverage with directional sensors. In: *Proceedings of IEEE Global Telecommunications Conference (Globecom)*, 1–6, IEEE: Honolulu, HI, USA, 2009. DOI: 10.1109/GLOCOM.2009.5425893.
48. Tezcan, N., Wang, W. Self-orienting wireless multimedia sensor networks for occlusion-free viewpoints. *Computer Networks: International Journal of Computer and Telecommunications Networking* 52(13), 2558–2567, 2008. DOI: http://dx.doi.org/10.1016/j.comnet.2008.05.014.
49. Ai, J., Abouzeid, A.A. Coverage by directional sensors in randomly deployed wireless sensor networks. *Journal of Combinatorial Optimization* 11(1), 21–41, 2006. DOI: 10.1007/s10878-006-5975-x.
50. Wang, X., Wang, X., Zhao, J. Impact of mobility and heterogeneity on coverage and energy consumption in wireless sensor networks. In: *Proceedings of IEEE ICDCS 2011*, pp. 477–487, Minneapolis, MN, USA, June 21–24, 2011.
51. Mulligan, R., Ammari, H.M. Coverage in wireless sensor networks: A survey. *Network Protocols and Algorithms*. ISSN 1943-3581. 2(2), 2010.
52. Wu, Y., Wang, X. Achieving full view coverage with randomly-deployed heterogeneous camera sensors. *The 32nd IEEE International Conference on Distributed Computing Systems*, pp. 556–565, 2012. DOI: 10.1109/ICDCS.2012.9.
53. Devarajan, D., Radke, R. Calibrating distributed camera networks using belief propagation. *EURASIP J. Appl. Signal Process.* 2007.

54. Kansal, A., Kaiser, W.J., Pottie, G.J., Srivastava, M.B. Actuation techniques for sensing uncertainty reduction, Technical Reports, pp. 1–16, 2005.

55. Fan, G.J., Jin, S.Y. Coverage problem in wireless sensor network: A survey. *Journal of Networks* 5(9), 2010. DOI: 10.4304/jnw.5.9.1033-1040.

56. Fuiorea, D., Guia, V., Pescaru, D., Toma, C. Using registration algorithms for wireless sensor network node localization. In: *Proceedings of 4th IEEE International Symposium on Applied Computational Intelligence and Informatics*, pp. 209–214, IEEE: Timisoara, Romania, May 17–18, 2007.

57. Sayed, A.H., Tarighat, A., Khajehnouri, N. Network-based wireless location: Challenges faced in developing techniques for accurate wireless location information. Signal Processing Magazine, IEEE 22, 24–40, 2005.

58. Fuiorea, D., Gui, V., Pescaru, D., Paraschiv, P., Codruta, I., Curiac, D., Volosencu, C. Video-based wireless sensor networks localization technique based on image registration and SIFT algorithm. *WSEAS Transactions on Computers*, pp. 990–999, 2008.

59. Lee, H., Aghajan, H. Vision-enabled node localization in wireless sensor networks. In: *Proceedings of Cognitive Systems with Interactive Sensors*, pp. 1–8. ACM Press, Paris, France, March 15–17, 2006.

60. Funiak, S., Paskin, M., Guestrin, C., Sukthankar, R. Distributed localization of networked cameras. In: *Proceedings of the 5th International Conference on Information Processing in Sensor Networks*, pp. 34–42, IEEE: Nashville, TN, USA, April 19–21, 2006.

61. Shafique, K., Hakeem, A., Javed, O., Haering, N. Self calibrating visual sensor networks. In: *Proceedings of IEEE Workshop on Applications of Computer Vision*, pp. 1–6, Copper Mountain, CO, USA, January 7–9, 2008.

62. Barton-Sweeney, A., Lymberopoulos, D., Savvides, A. Sensor localization and camera calibration in distributed camera sensor networks. In: *Proceedings of the 3rd International Conference on Broadband Communications, Networks and Systems*, pp. 1–10, IEEE: San Jose, CA, USA, October 1–5, 2006.

63. Liu, L., Zhang, X., Ma, H. Localization-oriented coverage in wireless camera sensor networks. *IEEE Transactions on Wireless Communications* 10(2), pp. 484–494, 2011.

64. Chang, C.Y., Hsiao, C.Y., Chang, C.T. The k-barrier coverage mechanism in wireless visual sensor networks. *IEEE Wireless Communications and Networking Conference: Mobile and Wireless Networks*, pp. 2318–2322, 2012.

65. Osais, Y.E., St-Hilaire, M., Riu, F.R. Directional sensor placement with optimal sensing ranging, field of view and orientation. *Mobile Networks and Applications* 15, 216–225, 2010.

66. Younis, M., Akkaya, K. Strategies and techniques for node placement in wireless sensor. networks: A survey. *Ad Hoc Networks*, pp. 621–655, 2008.

67. Howard, A., Mataric, M.J., Sukhatme, G.S. An incremental self deployment algorithm for mobile sensor networks. *Autonomous Robots* 13(2), 113–126, 2002.
68. Zhou, Z., Das, S., Gupta, H. Variable radii connected sensor cover in sensor networks. *ACM Transactions on Sensor Networks*, pp. 1–36, 2009.
69. Gasparri, A., Krishnamachari, B., Sukhatme, G.S. A framework for multi-robot node coverage in sensor networks. *Annals of Mathematics and Artificial Intelligence* 52(2–4), 281–305, 2008.
70. Couto, M., Souza, C., Rezende, P. Strategies for optimal placement of surveillance cameras in art galleries. In: *Proceedings of 18th International Conference on Computer Graphics and Vision*, pp. 1–4, Moscow, Russia, June 23–27, 2008.
71. Marengoni, M., Draper, B., Handson, A., Sitaraman, R. A system to place observers on a polyhedral terrain in a polynomial time. *Image and Vision Computing* 773–780, 1996.
72. Bose, P., Guibas, L., Lubiw, A., Overmars, M., Souvaine, D., Urrutia, J. The floodlight problem. *International Journal of Computational Geometry & Applications* 153–163, 1997.
73. Pito, R. A solution to the next best view problem for automated surface acquisition. *IEEE Transactions on Pattern Analysis and Machine Intelligence* 21, 1016–1030, 1999.
74. Mittal, A., Davis, L. Visibility analysis and sensor planning in dynamic environments. In: *Proceedings of 8th European Conference on Computer Vision*, pp. 175–189, Prague, Czech Republic, May 11–14, 2004.
75. Lin, Y.T., Saluja, K.K., Megerian, S. Adaptive cost efficient deployment strategy for homogeneous wireless camera sensors. *Ad Hoc Networks* 9, 713–726, 2011.
76. Karakaya, M., Qi, H. Coverage estimation for crowded targets in visual sensor networks. *ACM Transactions on Sensor Networks*, pp. 41–49, 2012.
77. Horster, E., Lienhart, R. Approximating optimal visual sensor placement. In: *Proceedings of IEEE International Conference on Multimedia and Expo*, pp. 1257–1260, Toronto, ON, Canada, July 9–12, 2006.
78. Zhao, J., Cheung, S., Nguyen, T. Optimal camera network configurations for visual tagging. *IEEE Journal of Selected Topics in Signal Processing* 464–479, 2008.
79. Ram, S., Ramakrishnan, K., Atrey, P., Singh, V., Kankanhalli, M. A design methodology for selection and placement of sensors in multimedia surveillance systems. In: *Proceedings of the 4th ACM International Workshop on Video Surveillance and Sensor Networks*, pp. 121–130, Santa Barbara, CA, USA, October 27, 2006.
80. Adriaens, J., Megerian, S., Pontkonjak, M. Optimal worst-case coverage of directional field-of-view sensor networks. In: *Proceedings of 3rd Annual IEEE Communications Society Conference on Sensor, Mesh and Ad Hoc Communications and Networks*, pp. 336–345, Reston, VA, USA, September 25–28, 2006.

81. Li, H., Pandit, V., Agrawal, D.P. Deployment optimization strategy for a two-tier wireless visual sensor network. *Wireless Sensor Network* 91–106, 2012.

82. Schwager, M., Julian, B., Angermann, M., Rus, D. Eyes in the sky: Decentralized control for the deployment of robotic camera networks. *Proceedings of the IEEE* 1541–1561, 2011.

83. Pescaru, D., Gui, V., Toma, C., Fuiorea, D. Analysis of post-deployment sensing coverage for video wireless sensor networks. In: *Proceedings of 6th International Conference RoEduNet*, Craiova, Romania, November 23–24, 2007.

84. Costa, D.G., Guedes, L.A. The coverage problem in video-based wireless sensor networks: A survey. *Sensors 2010*, 10, 8215–8247, 2010. DOI: 10.3390/s100908215.

85. Cai, Y., Lou, W., Li, M., Li, X.Y. Target-oriented scheduling in directional sensor networks. In: *Proceedings of IEEE Infocom*, pp. 1550–1558, Anchorage, AK, USA, May 6–12, 2007.

86. Tezcan, N., Wang, W. Self-orienting wireless sensor networks for occlusion-free viewpoints. *Computer Networks* 52, 2558–2567, 2008.

87. Kandoth, C., Chellappan, S. Angular mobility assisted coverage in directional sensor networks. In: *Proceedings of International Conference on Network-Based Information Systems*, pp. 376–379, Indianapolis, IN, USA, August 19–21, 2009.

88. O'Rourke, J. *Computational Geometry in C.* Cambridge University Press, Cambridge, Britain, March 25, 1994.

89. Soro, S., Heinzelman, W. Camera selection in visual sensor networks. In: *Proceedings of the IEEE Conference on Advanced Video and Signal Based Surveillance (AVSS '07)*, pp. 81–86, 2007.

90. Dagher, J.C., Marcellin, M.W., Neifeld, M.A. A method for coordinating the distributed transmission of imagery. *IEEE Transactions on Image Processing* 15(7), 1705–1717, 2006.

91. Ercan, A., Gamal, A.E., Guibas, L. Camera network node selection for target localization in the presence of occlusions. In: *Proceedings of the ACM SenSys Workshop on Distributed Smart Cameras*, 2006.

92. Mavrinac, A., Chen, X. Modeling coverage in camera networks: A survey. *Springer Science Business Media New York* 2012. DOI: 10.1007/s11263-012-0587-7.

93. Park, J., Bhat, P.C., Kak, A.C. A look-up table based approach for solving the camera selection problem in large camera networks. In: *Proceedings of International Workshop on Distributed Smart Cameras*, 2006.

94. Shen, C., Zhang, C., Fels, S. A multi-camera surveillance system that estimates quality-of-view measurement. In: *Proceedings of IEEE International Conference on Image Processing*, pp. 193–96, 2007.

95. Akyildiz, I.F., Vuran, M.C. *Wireless Sensor Networks.* John Wiley and Sons, 2010.

96. Kulkarni, P., Shenoy, P., Ganesan, D. Approximate initialization of camera sensor networks. In: *Proceedings of 4th European Conference on Wireless Sensor Networks*, pp. 67–82, 2007.

97. Kranakis, E., Krizanc, D., Urrutia, J. Coverage and connectivity in networks with directional sensors. In: *Euro-Par 2004 Parallel Processing, Lecture Notes in Computer Science*, vol. 3149, pp. 917–924, Springer: Berlin, Heidelberg, 2004.

98. Han, X., Cao, X., Lloyd, E., Shen, C.C. Deploying directional sensor networks with guaranteed connectivity and coverage. In: *Proceedings of 5th Annual IEEE Communications Society Conference on Sensor, Mesh and Ad Hoc Communications and Networks (SECON'08)*, pp. 153–160, San Francisco, CA, USA, 2008. DOI: 10.1109/SAHCN.2008.28.

99. Ma, H., Liu, Y. Some problems of directional sensor networks. *International Journal of Sensor Networks* 2(1/2), 44–52, 2007.

100. Bai, X., Yun, Z., Xuan, D., Lai, T.H., Jia, W. Optimal patterns for four-connectivity and full coverage in wireless sensor networks. *IEEE Transactions on Mobile Computing* 9(3), 435–448, 2010.

101. Margi, C.B., Manduchi, R., Obraczka, K. Energy consumption tradeoffs in visual sensor networks. In: *Proceedings of 24th Brazilian Symposium on Computer Networks*, Curitiba, Brazil, May 2006.

102. Cardei, M., Wu, J. Energy-efficient coverage problems in wireless ad hoc sensor networks. *Computer Communications* 413–420, 2006.

103. Osais, Y., St-Hilaire, M., Yu, F. Directional sensor placement with optimal sensing range, field of view and orientation. In: *Proceedings of IEEE International Conference on Wireless and Mobile Computing (WIMOB'08)*, pp. 19–24, Avignon, France, 2008. DOI: 10.1109/WiMob.2008.88.

104. Pescaru, D., Istin, C., Curiac, D., Doboli, A. Energy saving strategy for video-based wireless sensor networks under field coverage preservation. In: *Proceedings of IEEE International Conference on Automation, Quality and Testing, Robotics*, pp. 289–294, Cluj-Napoca, Romania, May 22–25, 2008.

105. Istin, C., Pescaru, D., Ciocarlie, H., Curiac, D., Doboli, A. Reliable field of view coverage in video-camera based wireless networks for traffic management applications. In: *Proceedings of IEEE International Symposium on Signal Processing and Information Technology*, pp. 63–68, Sarajevo, Bosnia and Herzegovina, December 16–19, 2008.

106. Istin, C., Pescaru, D., Doboli, A., Ciocarlie, H. Impact of coverage preservation techniques on prolonging the network lifetime in traffic surveillance applications. In: *Proceedings of 4th International Conference on Intelligent Computer Communication and Processing*, pp. 201–206, Cluj-Napoca, Romania, August 28–30, 2008.

107. Kumar, S., Lai, T.H., Balogh, J. On k-coverage in a mostly sleeping sensor network. *MobiCom'04*, Sept. 26–Oct. 1, 2004.

108. Misra, S., Reisslein, M., Xue, G. A survey of multimedia streaming in wireless sensor networks. *IEEE Communications Surveys & Tutorials* 10(4), 18–39, 2008.

109. Fusco, G., Gupta, H. Selection and orientation of directional sensors for coverage maximization. In: *Proc. of IEEE Intl. Conf. on Sensor, Mesh and Ad Hoc Communications and Networks (SECON'09)*, Rome, Italy, pp. 1–9, 2009. DOI: 10.1109/SAHCN.2009.5168968.

110. Kumar, S., Lai, T.H., Arora, A. Barrier coverage with wireless sensors. In: *Proc. of ACM Intl. Conf. on Mobile computing and networking (MobiCom'05)*, pp. 284–298, 2005. DOI: http://doi.acm.org/10.1145/1080829.1080859.

111. Wan, P., Yi, C. Coverage by randomly deployed wireless sensors networks. *IEEE Transactions on Information Theory* 52, 2658–2669, 2006.

112. Wang, X., Xing, G., Zhang, Y., Lu, C., Pless, R., Gill, C. Integrated coverage and connectivity configuration in wireless sensor networks. In: *Proceedings of 1st ACM Conference on Embedded Networked Sensor Systems*, pp. 28–39, Los Angeles, CA, USA, November, 2003.

113. Liu, L., Ma, H., Zhang, X. On directional k-coverage analysis of randomly deployed camera sensor networks. In: *Proceedings of IEEE International Conference on Communications*, pp. 2707–2711, Beijing, China, May 19–23, 2008.

114. Zhao, J., Zeng, J.C. An electrostatic field-based coverage-enhancing algorithm for wireless multimedia sensor networks. In: *Proc. of IEEE Intl. Conf. on Wireless Communications, Networking and Mobile Computing (WiCom'09)*, pp. 1–5, Beijing, China, 2009. DOI: 10.1109/WICOM.2009.5302443

115. Bay, H., Ess, A., Tuytelaars, T., Van Gool, L. Speeded-up robust features (surf). *Computer Vision and Image Understanding* 110(3), 2010.

116. Tezcan, N., Wang, W. Self-orienting wireless multimedia sensor networks for maximizing multimedia coverage. *IEEE Communications Society ICC*, 2206–2210, 2008.

117. Arora, A., Dutta, P. et. al. A line in the sand: A wireless sensor network for target detection, classification, and tracking, *Computer Networks. Computer and Telecommunications Networking*, pp. 605–634, 2004.

118. Cardei, M., Thai, M., Yingshu, L., Weili, W. Energy-efficient target coverage in wireless sensor networks. *INFOCOM 2005*, 1976–1984, 2005.

119. Cardei, M., Du, D. Improving wireless sensor network lifetime through power aware organization. *Wireless Networks*, pp. 330–333, 2005.

120. Cardei, M., Wu, J., Lu, M., Pervaiz, M. Maximum network lifetime in wireless sensor networks with adjustable sensing ranges. *Wireless and Mobile Computing, Networking And Communications*, pp. 438–445, 2005.

121. Zhang, H., Wang, H., Feng, H. A distributed optimum algorithm for target coverage in wireless sensor networks. *Asia-Pacific Conference on Information Processing*, pp. 144–147, 2009.

122. Zhang, H. Energy-balance heuristic distributed algorithm for target coverage in wireless sensor networks with adjustable sensing ranges. *Asia-Pacific Conference on Information Processing*, pp. 452–455, 2009.

123. Wang, Y., Cao, G. Minimizing service delay in directional sensor networks. *Computer Communications. Piscataway* 2011, 1790–1798, 2011.

124. Wang, G., Cao, G., LaPorta, T. A bidding protocol for deploying mobile sensors. *ICNP'03*, pp. 315–324, 2003.

125. Wang, G., Cao, G., LaPorta, T. Movement-assisted sensor deployment. *IEEE INFOCOM*, 2004.

126. Wang, G., Cao, G., LaPorta, T., Zhang, W. Sensor relocation in mobile sensor networks. *IEEE INFOCOM*, 2005.
127. Devarajan, D., Ranke, R.J., Chung, H. Distributed metric calibration of ad-hoc camera networks. *ACM Transactions on Sensor Networks*, pp. 33–44, 2006.
128. Johnson, M.P., Bar-Noy, A. Pan and scan: Configuring cameras for coverage. *INFOCOM*, pp. 1071–1079, 2011.
129. Shih, K.P., Chou, C.M., Liu, I.H., Li, C.C. On barrier coverage in wireless camera sensor networks. *IEEE AINA*, pp. 873–879, 2010.
130. Meguerdichian, S., Koushanfar, F., Potkonjak, M., Srivastava, M. Coverage problems in wireless ad-hoc sensor networks. *IEEE Infocom 2001*, 1380–1387, 2001.
131. Chen, A., Kumar, S., Lai, T.H. Designing localized algorithms for barrier coverage. In: *MOBICOM*, 2007.
132. Balasubramaniam, S., Kangasharju, J. Realizing the Internet of nano things: Challenges, solutions, and applications. *IEEE Computer Society* 62–68, 2013.
133. Wang, Y., Cao, G. Barrier coverage in camera sensor networks. *ACM International Symposium on Mobile Ad Hoc Networking and Computing*, May 16–19, 2011.
134. Ma, H., Yang, M., Li, D. Minimum camera barrier coverage in wireless camera sensor networks. *IEEE INFOCOM 2012*, 217–225, 2012.

6

A SECURITY SCHEME FOR VIDEO STREAMING IN WIRELESS MULTIMEDIA SENSOR NETWORKS

NOUR EL-DEEN MAHMOUD KHALIFA

Contents

Wireless sensor networks (WSNs) have become an important component of our daily life. In the near future, they will dominate the technology industry around the world. WSNs have gained importance
due to the variety of vital applications they can participate in, such
as applications for the military, health care, agriculture, surveillance,
and monitoring natural phenomena.

Wireless multimedia sensor networks (WMSNs) are a special
type of WSN. WMSNs typically consist of wirelessly interconnected devices that are able to ubiquitously retrieve multimedia
content such as video and audio streams, still images, and scalar sensor data from the environment. These wireless devices, called sensor nodes, are limited in energy and storage capabilities. The sensor
nodes collect data from physical or environmental phenomena.
They cooperatively pass the sensed data through the network to a
certain location or sink node where the data can be collected and
analyzed.

The unprotected nature of wireless communication channels and
untrustworthy transmission medium of WMSNs are vulnerable to
many types of security attacks. Attackers ultimately seek to eavesdrop,

steal confidential data, inject false data, or even jam the whole network, so securing these networks has become essential.

This chapter will propose a security scheme for WMSNs. The proposed security scheme is appropriate for the nature of real-time video streaming. It constructs its security features within the application and transport layers, because the information that attackers ultimately seek exists within these layers. The proposed security scheme consists of two security levels. The first level is encryption of the packet data by means of applying the Advanced Encryption Standard (AES); http://csrc.nist.gov/publications/fips/fips197/fips-197.pdf, while the second level consists of generating a Message Authentication Code (MAC) using Cipher-based Message Authentication Code (CMAC). The rationale for using both these security techniques will be justified in detail in this chapter. Both levels achieve the principles of security—authentication, confidentiality, data integrity, and availability.

Performance comparisons between the proposed security scheme and other security frameworks will be presented. All the work presented in this chapter was developed and implemented using Network Simulator version 2 (NS2). According to our literature review, this study is one of the first attempts to use NS2 as a security simulator; NS2 has not supported security features before.

Finally, it is hoped that the research presented in this chapter will help other researchers to simulate their security ideas and mechanisms based on the suggested development and integration of security libraries into NS2.

6.1 Wireless Multimedia Sensor Networks

A WMSN is composed of low cost, low power, multifunctional sensor nodes (Figure 6.1), which are small in size and communicate wirelessly over short distances. WMSNs can also be introduced as self-configured wireless networks used to collect data (video, image, audio, and scalar sensor data) from physical or environmental phenomena and deliver the multimedia content through sensors [1]. The networks cooperatively pass their sensed data through the network to a main location or sink where the data can be monitored and analyzed. A sink node or base station performs like a gate between users and the network [1] (Figure 6.2).

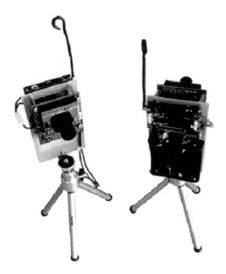

Figure 6.1   An example of a wireless multimedia sensor node. (From Akyildiz, I.F., and Vuran, M.C.: *Wireless sensor networks*. 2010. Copyright Wiley-VCH Verlag GmbH & Co. KGaA.)

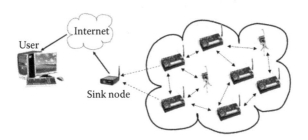

Figure 6.2   A generic wireless multimedia sensor network architecture. (From Akyildiz, I.F., and Vuran, M.C.: *Wireless sensor networks*. 2010. Copyright Wiley-VCH Verlag GmbH & Co. KGaA.)

In general, a WMSN may contain hundreds or thousands of sensor nodes. The sensor nodes can communicate among themselves using radio signals as illustrated in Figure 6.2. After the sensor nodes are deployed in the area to be monitored, they are accountable for self-organizing an acceptable network infrastructure, often using multihop communication with each other. They then start gathering information of interest [1].

There is greater flexibility in deployment options for WMSNs compared to other networks. Once WMSN nodes are distributed randomly in an environment, they organize themselves into a coherent information-sharing network. WMSN nodes may also be deployed in an organized way by creating a network topology before deploying them in the actual environment. Wireless sensor devices also respond to orders sent from an "administration site" to do specific instructions or provide sensing data samples. The working style of the sensor nodes may be either continuous or event driven [1].

6.1.1 WMSN Node Structure

A WMSN node consists of five main components: a processing unit, memory, a transceiver, sensors (video camera), and a power supply, as shown in Figure 6.3. Every unit in the WMSN node has specific tasks to be done. The following points will illustrate those tasks [2]:

- The *transceiver unit* allows the node to communicate with neighboring nodes.
- The *sensor unit* consists of two parts. First, there is an analog sensing component such as a video camera, which physically measures environmental characteristics. Second, there is an analog-to-digital converter, which transforms analog environmental readings into a digital representation that can be handled by the node processor.
- The *power source unit* provides the node with life and is normally limited, so that once the node's power supply is exhausted the node can no longer operate.

A node may contain other elements, such as power-generating components (e.g., solar panels and thermocouples) to recharge the

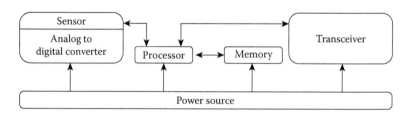

Figure 6.3 The structure of a wireless multimedia sensor network node. (From Sohraby, K.: *Wireless sensor networks: technology, protocols, and applications.* 2007. Copyright Wiley-VCH Verlag GmbH & Co. KGaA.)

node's power supply. However, the five components discussed are crucial for a node to be considered a WMSN node, whereas the other components are optional [2].

6.1.2 WMSN Protocol Stack

The sensor nodes are often scattered in a sensor field. Each sensor node has the functionality to collect and send data to the sink node and end users. Sensed data are sent to the end user by a multihop architecture through the sink node as shown in Figure 6.4. The sink node may communicate with the end user via Internet or satellite [4].

The protocol stack applied by the sink and the sensor nodes is given in Figure 6.4. The protocol stack of WSNs or WMSNs consists of the application layer, transport layer, network layer, data link layer, and physical layer. A brief account of every layer will be listed in the following sections.

The protocol layers can be viewed as a set of management planes across each layer. Each layer includes power, connection, and task management planes [3].

- The *power management plane* is responsible for managing the power level of a sensor node for processing, sensing, transmission, and reception, which can be applied by employing efficient power management schemes at different protocol layers.

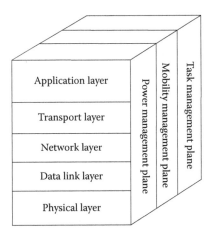

Figure 6.4   The protocol stack for a wireless multimedia sensor network. (From Akyildiz, I.F. et al., *IEEE Communications Magazine*, 40(8), 102–114, © 2002 IEEE.)

- The *connection management plane* handles the configuration and reconfiguration of sensor nodes to establish and maintain the connectivity of a network in the case of node deployment and topology change due to node addition, node failure, or node movement.
- The *task management plane* is in charge of assigning tasks among sensor nodes in a sensing area to improve energy efficiency and extend network lifetime.

6.1.2.1 Application Layer   The application layer is a program or a group of programs that is prepared for the end user [2]. There are two types of services: global and local. Global services make direct contributions to the mission objective for a program. For example, a node's decision to track a vehicle would be a global service. Local services are the services that the node provides to itself. For instance, determining the quality of service, performing authentication, and determining communication partners are all examples of local services. Generally, for WMSNs, the application layer determines the system level behavior of a node [2,3].

6.1.2.2 Transport Layer   The transport layer is responsible for passing data to the application layer in such a manner as to relieve the application layer of responsibility for cost-effective transmission and connection reliability [2]. The transport layer manages connections, provides congestion and flow control, and maintains connection reliability. Examples of reliable transport protocols used for wireless communications include the User Datagram Protocol (UDP) and Transmission Control Protocol (TCP). It should be noted that in some WSNs a formal transport layer may not exist [2].

6.1.2.3 Network Layer   The network layer establishes, maintains, and terminates network connections [2]. The protocol in the network layer is assigned to route, address, and possibly task the node roles if nodes can perform multiple roles, for example, as sensors or sinks. Examples of routing protocols for ad hoc multihop WSNs include the Destination-Sequenced Distance Vector, Ad Hoc On-Demand Distance Vector Routing Protocol, and Temporally Ordered Routing Algorithm [4].

6.1.2.4 Data Link Layer   The data link layer is divided into two sub-layers: the logical link control (LLC) layer and the media access control (MAC) layer. The LLC layer is assigned to provide a reliable, error-free link between the MAC and network layers. The MAC layer is primarily assigned to minimize collisions in the medium [3].

The MAC layer minimizes packet collisions using techniques such as carrier sensing multiple access and by multiplexing wireless data from different sensor nodes using time division multiple access, frequency division multiple access, or code division multiple access. In addition to minimizing collisions, the MAC layer may also provide some link reliability services, such as cyclical redundancy checking and unique addressing [3].

6.1.2.5 Physical Layer   The physical layer is accountable for the transmission and reception of data across wireless and possibly wired channels [1]. For sensor nodes, the physical layer is essentially the Radio Frequency (RF) section of the node. However, a sink node might be connected to more than one medium. For example, the sink node may be connected to the Internet, as well as wirelessly to sensor nodes. In this instance, the sink's physical layer would need to include an RF section as well as a wired modem section.

An effective sensor network is the one that achieves or exceeds the specific performance requirements for its particular application. To achieve specific performance requirements, any proposed scheme design may need to be optimized within and across the node architecture layers.

6.1.3 WMSN Applications

There are several applications for wireless multimedia sensors, in many areas, from military and homeland security, to medical, to increasing efficiency of businesses. The generation of sensors provides tremendous flexibility to applications developers.

Sensors can run while unconnected to the Internet; they can continue to sense, filter, and process local information. Smart sensors can join context to sensed data; for instance, depending on what the item is, sensors can determine if it is broken or spoiled.

There is a range of diverse applications that lend themselves to WMSNs. We will categorize them here into five areas: military, environment, industrial, health, and home and commercial areas [5].

6.1.3.1 Military Applications WMSNs are suitable for use in many military applications, including command and control applications, surveillance and reconnaissance of enemy targets, monitoring for deployment of biological and chemical weapons, and ordinance tracking. The ability of WMSN nodes to be quickly deployed and organize themselves autonomously into functional, fault-tolerant networks makes WMSN technology ideal for these and many other military applications. Some examples of such military applications are listed below [5]:

- Monitoring friendly forces, equipment, and ammunition
- Battlefield surveillance
- Reconnaissance of opposing forces and terrain
- Targeting guidance
- Battle damage assessment
- Nuclear, biological, and chemical attack detection and reconnaissance

6.1.3.2 Environmental Applications Environmental applications for WMSNs include monitoring the movement of wildlife, such as animals and birds, monitoring factors that affect the expansion of crops, exploring inhospitable parts of the earth that remain unexplored, detecting and tracking forest fires, detecting and monitoring the headways of floods, and measuring levels of pollution across distributed locations [2].

6.1.3.3 Industrial Applications In industry, WMSNs can be applied for observing manufacturing processes or the condition of manufacturing equipment; wireless sensors can be attached to production and assembly lines to monitor and control production processes [1].

6.1.3.4 Medical Applications One of the most important applications for WMSNs is in the health-care field. WMSNs provide the potential to offer vulnerable populations a greater level of independence in their lives. Potential applications comprise integrated control of household devices from a single controller, remote patient monitoring, better real-time monitoring of patients in hospitals, and tracking staff and equipment in hospitals [2]. Other examples of WMSN medical applications are as follows:

- Providing interfaces for the disabled
- Integrated patient monitoring
- Administration in hospitals
- Video monitoring of human physiological data
- Tracking and monitoring doctors and patients inside a hospital

6.1.3.5 WMSN Home and Commercial Automation Applications   Home and commercial automation technology has been a subject of research for many years. The potential applications for home automation technology are diverse, including multimedia entertainment, automatic houseplant watering, domestic robots, home security, and energy saving [5].

6.1.4 WMSN Research Areas

WMSNs are currently receiving significant attention due to their unlimited potential. Practically, WMSNs encounter numerous problems. The following section will present some areas of research for WMSNs.

6.1.4.1 Real Time in WMSNs   WMSNs transact with real-world environments. In many cases, sensed data must be delivered within time constraints so that actions can be taken. There are a few current solutions for meeting real-time requirements in WMSNs [6]. The majority of protocols either ignore real-time processes or simply attempt to process as fast as possible and presume that this speed is enough to meet deadlines.

Researchers have performed several trials in this field to suggest new ideas to solve this problem, namely Real-Time Communication Architecture for Large-Scale Wireless Sensor Networks (RAP) [7] and a Real-Time Routing Protocol for Sensor Networks (SPEED) [8].

Working with real-time protocols usually requires differentiated services. For example, routing solutions need to uphold different classes of traffic: guarantees for the important traffic and less support for unimportant traffic [6]. It is important to design not only real-time protocols for WMSNs but also analysis techniques associated with these protocols.

6.1.4.2 Power Management in WMSNs

Limited processor bandwidth and small memory are two arguable constraints in sensor networks, which will gradually disappear with the development of fabrication techniques by manufacturers [9]. However, energy constraints are unlikely to be solved in the near future, due to slow progress in improving battery capacity. Furthermore, the untended nature of sensor nodes and dangerous sensing environments prohibit battery replacement as a logical solution.

By contrast, the monitoring functions of many sensor network applications demand a longer lifetime; therefore, providing a form of energy-efficient monitoring for a surveillance area is a notable research issue [9].

6.1.4.3 Programming Abstractions in WMSNs

A key growth area for WMSNs is promoting the level of abstraction for programmers. Currently, developers deal with too many low-level details regarding sensing and node-to-node communication [10]. As an example, they typically deal with sensing data, fusing data, and moving data. If the level of abstraction were raised to consider aggregate behaviors, application functionality, and direct support for scaling issues, then productivity would increase. There have been a few attempts at this type of research; one of these trials was the environment-based abstraction EnviroTrack [11].

Programming abstractions for WMSNs will likely remain rare. Rather, a number of solutions will emerge, each more suited to a certain domain. Research in this area is important in order to expand the development and deployment of WMSNs by general programmers, not by WMSN engineering specialists [11].

6.1.4.4 Security and Privacy in WMSNs

WMSNs are limited in their energy, computation, and communication capabilities. In contrast to traditional networks, sensor nodes may be deployed in easily accessible areas, presenting a risk of vandalism. Sensor networks react closely with their physical environment and with people, arguing additional security problems [12].

Because of the above-mentioned problems, the current security mechanisms are inadequate for WMSNs. The new constraints create new research challenges in the areas of key establishment, secrecy and authentication, robustness, stand against denial-of-service (Dos) attacks, secure routing, and node capture [12].

To establish a secure scheme, security should be integrated into every component, since components designed without security in mind can become a point of attack. Eventually, security is a difficult challenge for any system. The strict resource constraints of WMSNs make any computer security for these systems even more challenging [12].

6.1.5 Scope

The work presented in this chapter can be classified under the umbrella of the following areas:

- Real time
- Power management (energy consumption)
- Security and privacy

6.2 Security in WMSNs

Since computers were invented, there has been a need for a strategy to keep data on these computers secured; scientists termed this strategy computer security. With the advent of distributed systems connected by networks across the Internet, there arose a need to keep data safe between these networks; this was called Internet security. With the appearance of WSNs and WMSNs in the research and practical fields, security in these networks has become a necessity. Security here is concerned with how to protect sensed data against unauthorized access and modification and to ensure the availability of network communication and services despite malignant activities.

6.2.1 Security Properties

To consider any scheme secured, there are general security properties that must be satisfied; these properties include authentication, confidentiality, data integrity, and availability [13]. The following sub-sections will discuss these categories in more detail.

6.2.1.1 Authentication   The authentication process is concerned with verifying the identity of an entity (peer authentication) or verifying the source of a message (data authentication) [13].

- In *peer authentication*, the identity of an entity is confirmed to grant physical access to a building or electronic access to a service [13].
- In *data authentication*, the data received are validated to ensure that the data were sent from the entity claimed. The objective of data authentication is to prevent third parties from insert-ing data into preexisting communications with authenticated entities [13].

The most common approach to peer authentication is provid-ing username and password combinations, smart cards, or biomet-ric data to authenticate users, before providing them with physical access to a building or services. In data authentication, a secret key is used, only known by the sender and the receiver, to encrypt and decrypt data [13].

6.2.1.2 Confidentiality   Confidentiality is concerned with keeping data secret from third parties not authorized to view the contents of communications. A system that implements confidentiality must protect data from direct and indirect interpretation by unauthorized entities [13].

Direct interpretation involves unauthorized entities intercepting and viewing data. Indirect interpretation involves unauthorized enti-ties viewing communication traffic patterns and deriving the contents of the communications, through traffic analysis [13].

The primary approach for providing confidentiality is encryp-tion. There are two categories of encryption used to provide con-fidentiality: symmetric key cryptography [14] and public key cryptography [15].

6.2.1.3 Integrity   Data integrity is concerned with preventing the unau-thorized modification of data, without detection by a legitimate user.

There are three established approaches for verifying that a message has not been tampered with, namely, message encryption, MACs [16], and hash functions [17].

6.2.1.4 Availability The availability of an item is its state of readiness to execute a required function at a given instant of time or at any instant of time within a given time interval, assuming that the exterior resources, if required, are provided [13].

In the security domain, service availability research focuses on the protection of service-providing systems from attackers that attempt to overwhelm the resources of these systems in an attempt to either permanently remove the service from availability or to sufficiently degrade a service to intermittently remove it from availability. Threats to the availability of services are collectively termed denial-of-service attacks [18].

6.2.2 Security Constraints for WMSNs

Section 6.2.1 discussed general security properties. As already stated, for any system to be considered secure, it must give consideration to the properties of security (i.e., authentication, confidentiality, data integrity, and availability). However, due to the extremely resource-constrained nature of sensor nodes, their security properties may be slightly different compared to those of conventional networks. Revisiting the security properties from a WMSN perspective yields the following [19]:

- *Authentication*: As a WMSN communicates, critical data participates in a number of decision-making procedures. The sink node needs to ensure that the data used in any decision-making process are produced from the correct source node. Similarly, authentication is substantial during the exchange of controlled information in the network.
- *Integrity*: During its journey across the network, data can be changed by adversaries. Data loss or deterioration can also occur without the presence of a malicious node, due to the severe communication environment. Data integrity assures that information is not changed during conveyance, either due to malicious intent or by coincidence.

- *Confidentiality*: Applications such as monitoring of information, industrial secrets, and key distribution depend on confidentiality. The standard approach for keeping confidentiality is through the use of encryption techniques.
- *Availability*: Sensor nodes may use up their battery power due to extreme computation or communication and become unavailable. Security requirements not only influence the operation of the network but are also highly important in maintaining the availability of the network.

Because of the resource-constrained nature of WMSNs, other properties and limitations should be taken into consideration while designing security scheme such as the following [19]:

- *Freshness*: Even if confidentiality and data integrity are indisputable, we also need to ensure the freshness of each message. Freshness of sensed data confirms that the data are recent, and it ensures that no old messages have been replayed. To ensure that no old messages are replayed, a time stamp can be added to the packet.
- *Scalability*: Scalability is required in most WMSN applications, as the number of sensor nodes to be deployed is in the order of hundreds, thousands, or more. The protocols must be sufficiently scalable to reply and operate with such a large number of sensor nodes.
- *Unattended operation*: In many applications, there is no human interference after sensor nodes are deployed. Thus, the nodes are responsible for reconfiguration in case of any modifications. This constrains any security scheme to be as energy sufficient as possible.
- *Untethered*: The sensor nodes are not attached to any energy source. They have only a limited source of energy, which should be optimally used for data processing and communication. To attain optimal energy use, communication must be reduced as much as possible.
- *Limited memory and storage space*: A sensor is a tiny device with only a small amount of memory and storage space for the code. To build an effective security scheme, it is necessary to limit the code size of the security algorithm.

6.2.3 Attacks on WMSNs

Security in any network system does not involve only one or two layers, but rather needs to be viewed across all layers as a whole. The security issues for a conventional network differ greatly from the security issues in WMSNs because of the extremely limited resources available in sensor nodes. Attacks in a WMSN can be categorized into two types, passive and active attacks [15].

- In a passive attack, the attacker can get information from the WMSN by eavesdropping on wireless communications and trying to steal confidential data.
- In an active attack, the attacker can get information from the WMSN by spoofing or altering packets to breach authenticity of communication or by injecting false data to impasse the network.

The prime objective of this research is to stand against eavesdropping, stealing confidential data, and injecting false packets into the network; for example, in terms of military applications, an attacker may cause the following:

- Jamming and/or confusing the network protocols by injecting false packets, which leads to DoS in the whole WMSN network (i.e., violating WMSN availability and integrity)
- Eavesdropping on classified information (i.e., violating WMSN confidentiality)
- Supplying misleading information, for example, enemy movements in the east, when in fact they are in the west (in technical terms, violating WMSN authenticity)

Additionally, in health applications, attacks can lead to fatal errors in the health-care system by providing incorrect physiological measurements to the nurse or doctor on behalf of a patient; an offender may cause a potentially fatal diagnosis and treatment to be performed on the patient (i.e., a violation of WMSN integrity and authenticity).

The following subsections will explain the attacks on the WMSN from the perspective of the WMSN layer stack and how to defend against them. Particular emphasis will be placed on attacks on the upper layers (application and transport layer), which are the main focus of this chapter.

6.2.4 Attacks on WMSN Layers

Attacks can also happen on different layers of the WMSN stack layers. The standard layered architecture of the communication protocol for WSNs was introduced in Section 6.1.2 in detail. Attacks and their security solution approaches in different layers with respect to the WMSN layer stack are summarized [20] in Table 6.1. This table provides a classification of the various security attacks on each layer of a WMSN.

6.2.4.1 Transport Layer Attacks
The focus of transport layer attacks is to exploit communication protocols that use connection-oriented communications and maintain connection information. The main transport layer attacks against WMSNs include desynchronization attacks and flooding attacks.

Table 6.1   Wireless Multimedia Sensor Network Layer Attacks and Security Approaches

LAYER	POSSIBLE ATTACKS	SECURITY APPROACHES
Application layer	Path-based denial-of-service attack [21] Node reprogramming attacks [19]	Cryptographic approach Authentication
Transport layer	Desynchronization attack [22] Flooding attack [22]	Authentication Complex puzzles [22]
Network layer	Sybil attack [23] Sinkhole attack [23] Wormhole attack [23] Hello flooding attack [23]	Three-way handshake [24] Authentication Cryptographic approach
Data link layer	Collision attack [12] Interrogation attack [12] Denial-of-sleep attacks [25]	Spread spectrum techniques [26] Error correcting codes [27] Rate control mechanisms [27]

Physical layer	Node-tampering attack [19]
	Jamming and interception attack [19]
		Spread spectrum techniques
		MAC layer admission [28]
		Tamper proofing (camouflaging
		  nodes) [19]
		Directional antenna for access
		  restriction [29]

- *Desynchronization attack*: An attacker objects active communications and modifies or fakes the parameters of captured messages, such as control flags and sequence numbers. The modified or faked messages are sent back into an active communication stream between two nodes [22]. Consequently, when modified or faked messages arrive at their respective destinations, they are rejected as out of sequence or as corrupted, leading the sender to resend messages and wasting energy and network bandwidth. The encryption of message headers or the whole message with authentication can ban attackers from modifying existing messages and creating fake packets. Moreover, anti-replay mechanisms [22] can prevent false messages from being inserted into false communication streams undetected.
- *Flooding attack*: The target of the attacker in a flooding attack is a network employing connection-oriented communication protocols. The attacker requests a connection from a node in the WSN; the node detains space in its open connection buffer and sends a synchronization acknowledgment. After a period of time has elapsed, a time-out counter expires, causing the victim to clear its open connection buffer. However, an attacker may repeatedly order a number of connections and leave them half open, thereby exhausting the victim's connection buffer and preventing false connection requests for the duration of the attack [22].

One approach for protecting against flooding attacks in WMSNs demands connecting nodes to complete a complex puzzle [22] before a node reserves connection space. Nevertheless, the use of complex puzzles requires all nodes in the WMSN to have additional hardware to solve complex puzzles. Moreover, each connection attempt will incur false hosts, additional energy, and processing costs.

There are two major protocols in the transport layer, TCP and UDP [3]. In TCP, the attacker creates a large number of half-opened TCP connections with a receiver node, but never finishes the handshake to fully open up the connection, leading to a drain in energy.

Another type of attack in TCP is session hijack. Here, the attacker mimics the victim's Internet Protocol (IP) address, determines the correct sequence number that is expected by the target, and then executes a DoS attack on the victim node [14]. To hijack a session over UDP, the attacker takes the same action as in TCP, except that UDP attackers do not need to concern themselves with the overhead of treating sequence numbers and other TCP control fields. Because UDP is connectionless, phasing into a session without being detected is much easier than in TCP [3].

In this chapter, we concentrate on UDP and how to secure it using authentication mechanisms and encryption techniques, which both stand against the above-mentioned attacks; however, flood attacks will not be included as they require special hardware.

6.2.4.2 Application Layer Attacks   Attacks targeting the application layer of WSNs focus either on a weakness in application software specific to a particular WSN or on more general inherent weaknesses in the application layer of WSNs. The most popular forms of application layer attacks include path-based DoS attacks and node reprogramming attacks.

- A *path-based DoS attack* is an attack on the reliability of the WMSN network. An attacker floods counterfeit or replayed packets along a multihop, end-to-end routing path. There are a number of methods proposed for defending against path-based DoS attacks; the primary response of most defense approaches is to detect and remove spurious packets along a communication path. There are three generic defense approaches against such attacks [21]:
    - Each node along a communication path shares a secret key with the sender. The sender generates authentication and integrity material for each key/node and appends it to each packet.
    - A modified approach to that discussed in (1) involves a node storing a path key for every potential path in a WMSN; if any node in the network is subverted, an attacker can flood a whole communication path.
    - Rate control mechanisms can also be applied to each node, limiting the amount of replayed packets accepted from any one node. However, due to the nature of WMSNs, certain nodes—such as nodes directly around a coordinator or router nodes—have different packet rates.

- *Node reprogramming attack*: Due to the nature of many WMSN applications, where nodes are located in inaccessible and remote locations, it is desirable to remotely and wirelessly update node software. The process of updating node software is referred to as code dissemination. There are numerous approaches and protocols for disseminating software, such as the approach adopted by TinyOS, which is called Deluge [30]. In the Deluge approach, nodes periodically send advertisements containing their software version. Secure methods for reprogramming nodes have emerged; one such scheme is called Seluge [31]—a secure extension of the Deluge approach.

From the protocol perspective, the application layer contained user data, and it supported many protocols such as HTTP, SMTP, RTP, and FTP [32], which have vulnerabilities and provide access points for attackers. As mentioned earlier, preprogramming node attacks (malicious code attacks), such as viruses, worms, spyware, and Trojan horses [32], can attack both operating systems and user applications. These malicious programs can usually spread themselves through the network and cause the WSN node and networks to slow down or even become damaged.

In the current research, the focus is on the first solution presented in path-based DoS attack, thereby using the cryptographic approach and adding the MAC authentication mechanism. This research will further focus on Real-Time Transfer Protocol (RTP) as it is commonly used in data streaming.

6.2.5 Attacks and Scope of Work for the Proposed Security Scheme

The preceding sections have illustrated attacks that might occur in every layer in the WMSN layer stack. The focus of this study is to defend against attacks in the application and transport layers, as long as the attackers ultimately seek the information that exists within these layers. However, security in any network system does not involve only one or two layers, but rather needs to be viewed across all layers as a whole.

The scope of the work has widened to improve the performance of the proposed security scheme in terms of energy consumption and other metrics. Section 6.3 will describe the structure of the proposed security scheme in detail. We kept providing security features in the application and transport layers to stand against attacks within these layers, but some attacks were hard to defend against as they required hardware or a sensor operating system that was beyond the research objective.

The research objective is to propose a security scheme for multimedia streaming using RTP and UDP within the application and transport layers of the WSN protocol stack. The scope of the proposed security scheme and the attacks that the scheme will stand against are set forth in Table 6.2.

6.2.6 Existing Security Frameworks

Few security solutions exist for WSNs. Most current security solutions have been developed to be quite general to fit various platforms and scenarios. The existing security solutions deliver security features

Table 6.2   Scope of Protection Offered by the Proposed Security Scheme against Wireless Multimedia Sensor Network Attacks

	ATTACKS THAT THE PROPOSED SECURITY SCHEME WILL STAND AGAINST		ATTACKS THAT THE PROPOSED SECURITY SCHEME WILL NOT STAND AGAINST	
LAYER	ATTACK NAME	DEFENSIVE MECHANISM	ATTACK NAME	REASON
Application layer	Path-based DoS	Authentication mechanism		
	Node reprogramming attack (viruses, worms, spywares, and Trojan horses)	Authentication mechanism and encryption technique	Node reprogramming attack (node operating system software update)	Requires nodes with running operating system (TinyOS)
Transport layer	Desynchronization attack	Authentication mechanism	Flooding attack	Require special hardware
Network layer	Hello flooding attack	Authentication mechanism and encryption technique	Sybil attack Sinkhole attack Wormhole attack	Beyond research scope
Data link layer			Collision, interrogation Packet replay Denial-of-sleep attacks	Beyond research scope
Physical layer	Node jamming	DSDV routing	Node tampering	Beyond research scope

at the link and network layers using the TinyOS or Contiki (http://www.contiki-os.org/) operating systems. They did not cover security in the application and transport layers together.

A common problem with all existing security solutions is that they failed to reduce energy consumption and to fit real-time multimedia streaming.

6.2.6.1 TinySec TinySec (http://tinyos.stanford.edu/tinyos-wiki/index.php/TinySec) is a security architecture currently integrated into TinyOS. TinySec was introduced in 2004 and exists in the data link layer. It provides two different modes of operation [33], authenticated encryption or authentication only.

TinySec uses the SkipJack block cipher [33] with the cipher block chaining (CBC) mode of operation. To assure that the ciphertext length is the same as the plaintext, it uses CBC in conjunction with ciphertext stealing (CS). This is usually written as CBC-CS.

6.2.6.2 MiniSec MiniSec (https://sparrow.ece.cmu.edu/group/minisec.html), released in 2007, claims to address and resolve several obstacles with other security architectures proposed for TinyOS. It has two modes of operation, one for unicast and the other for multicast [34]. Both modes suggest using replay protection with synchronized counters or a bloom filter [34], respectively. Like TinySec, MiniSec uses the Skipjack cipher but with offset code book (OCB) as the mode of operation. OCB provides both authenticity and data secrecy while avoiding ciphertext expansion.

6.2.6.3 TinyECC TinyECC (http://discovery.csc.ncsu.edu/software/TinyECC/) was one of the first successful trials to provide public key cryptography in WSNs [35]. It utilizes elliptic curve cryptography, which has a shorter key length than traditional public key cryptology schemes. The shorter key length results in faster computations and less energy consumption and saves on both memory and bandwidth.

6.2.6.4 ContikiSec The first, and currently only, security solution aimed at the Contiki operating system, ContikiSec (http://www.cse.chalmers.se/research/group/dcs/masters/contikisec/) was implemented in 2009 and provides two modes of operation, like TinySec [36]. The first mode provides authenticity and data secrecy, whereas the second provides authenticity only. ContikiSec employs a 128-bit AES as cipher, with OCB for the first mode and CBC-MAC for the second [37].

6.3 Proposed Security Scheme Design

The proposed security scheme in this research built two levels of security. The first level was the encryption of payload data using AES encryption technique [38], while the second level was the generation of the MAC authentication code by using CMAC authentication mechanism [39]. Both levels achieved the security principles (authentication, confidentiality, data integrity, and availability), which were previously introduced in Section 6.2.1.

This section will introduce the design of the proposed security scheme for multimedia streaming in more detail. It will be divided into three sections. The first section will explain the proposed secured packet structure. A diagram of the sending and receiving process for will be outlined in the next section. A proposed scheduling algorithm will then be presented.

The proposed scheduling algorithm led to a significant decrease in the energy consumed by the network for multimedia streaming. At the end of this section, a brief explanation will be given to justify the selection of NS2 for the development of the proposed security scheme.

The significant contribution of this research is the proposed security scheme for multimedia streaming; in addition, an attempt has been made to implement security features with NS2, since NS2 did not support any security features before. The proposed implementation will help other researchers to begin to use NS2 as a security simulator.

6.3.1 Security Scheme Design

The first element in the proposed security scheme design is the packet structure. The packet structure design should take into consideration the two levels of security (in the application and transport layer). It should also maintain the normal functions of the usual structure of the WMSN packet format, presented in Figure 6.5.

The research concentrated on RTP [40] in the application layer with UDP in the transport layer, due to the nature of the applications,

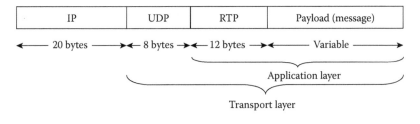

Figure 6.5 Packet format for wireless multimedia sensor networks using RTP and UDP.

such as military and monitoring applications. For example, in military applications, there are two kinds of data transmission. The first type is message transmission, for example, "tank moved in location *X*, *Y*," and the second type is streamed video from sensor cameras, such as video frames.

RTP packets could not be transferred as it was over the WMSN. RTP used UDP to be transferred across the WMSN. To transfer a UDP packet over the WMSN, UDP packets were encapsulated with IP packets [40].

- An IP header contained the information required to route data on the WMSN; it contained the address, the source and destination, and the UDP header.
- The UDP header consisted of four fields, each of which was 2 bytes. The use of the fields "Checksum" and "Source port" was optional. UDP did not guarantee the delivery of payload, which fits the nature of RTP.
- The RTP header had a size of 12 bytes. The RTP was followed by the RTP payload.
- Timestamp and sequence number are the most important fields in the proposed security scheme because they assure the data freshness of the WMSN.

6.3.1.1 Secured Packet Structure   Figure 6.6 illustrates the proposed secured packet format for the WMSN. The generated CMAC code depends on UDP, RTP, and the encrypted payload message. The IP header was not included in CMAC calculation, as the research focus was on providing security for the application and transport layers. The generated code would be stored in the MAC header field (4 bytes).

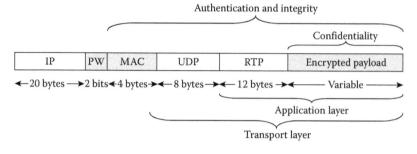

Figure 6.6   Proposed secured packet format for wireless multimedia sensor networks.

The research decision was to select a CMAC authentication mechanism as long as it was developed to fit variable payload data with different sizes. The payload of RTP would carry video frames.

Data freshness was achieved by applying the sequence number and timestamp in the RTP header. A new password (PW) field was added to the proposed secured scheme. The PW field holds 2 bits, and it would contain the values {00, 01, 10, and 11}. The PW values would notify the secured scheme which key password would be used to encrypt and decrypt the payload.

The PW field allowed the proposed security scheme to be more computationally secured against known attacks than any other security solution. The generated MAC field and PW field data in the proposed security scheme were counted as an overhead and will be studied in Section 6.4.9 with the other WMSN security properties.

6.3.2 Proposed Idea for Multimedia Streaming

Multimedia streaming is quite different from message transmission across WMSNs. The difference can be itemized as follows:

- Large data size (frame size varying from 1000 to 3000 bytes).
- Real-time characteristics (frames should be sent and received in a bounded delay).
- Video should be sent at a certain frame rate (standard 24 frames per second).
- The energy consumed by sensors should be taken into consideration while sending and receiving frames.

The above issues made any proposed security mechanism very hard to implement. It encountered some problems in multimedia streaming, because the time between each frame was very small (between 35 and 45 ms), and frame size was more than 1000 bytes to be encrypted, decrypted, and authenticated. The problems can be summarized in three points:

1. *Large frame size*: The size of frames varied from 1000 to 3000 bytes, which would affect encryption, decryption time, and energy. This problem was solved by using a video encoder, which fits the video in the standard frame size for RTP multimedia streaming. The standard frame size will be 1536 bytes, and frame height and width will be 352 × 288 pixels.

    The standard frame size and dimension [41] values were used to calculate the needed time and energy to encrypt, decrypt, and authenticate video frames. This calculation led to a significant savings in the energy consumed by the network for multimedia streaming, while applying the proposed security scheme.

2. *Real-time property* means that the video frames should be sent and received in a bounded delay. Adding security features to real-time video was challenging. We investigated the time needed to encrypt, decrypt, and authenticate a frame size of 1536 bytes in milliseconds. We found that the proposed scheme can be used in real time.

3. *High energy consumption* refers to the energy consumed to send and receive packets, plus the packet processing function. The proposed security features were studied in terms of the amount of consumed energy. Moreover, the research conducted the process of encryption, decryption, and authentication, but it did not consume a lot of energy compared to the sending and receiving function in WMSNs.

Figure 6.7 clarifies the sent function of the proposed security scheme for multimedia streaming. The scenario is as follows:

1. A frame (F) is going to be transmitted by a video camera sensor node.
2. Before sending the frame, a decision must be made by the proposed scheduler whether to send the frame or not.

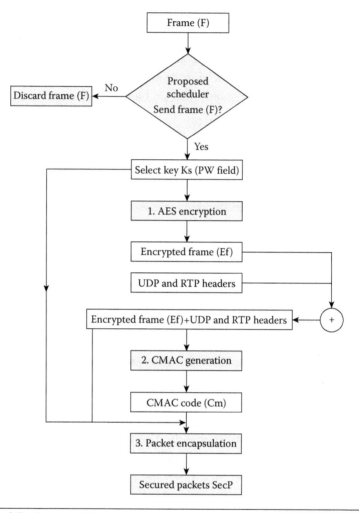

Figure 6.7 Flow chart of the sent function to secure a video frame in wireless multimedia sensor networks.

3. If the scheduler decides to send the frame, then a key will be selected from four different keys that exist in the sent function. If the scheduler decides not to send the frame, no action is taken.

4. The frame will be encrypted with the selected key (Ks), producing an encrypted frame (Ef).

5. The encrypted frame with UDP and RTP headers will be used to generate a CMAC code (Cm).

6. The selected key value, encrypted frame, UDP and RTP headers, and generated CMAC code will be encapsulated together to produce a secured packets (SecP).
7. The secured packet will be sent through the wireless transmission medium.

A frame could be lost for three reasons in the proposed security scheme for multimedia transmission:

1. Due to the encryption process by the sender node, a new frame needs to be sent while the current frame is being encrypted
2. Due to the decryption process in the receiver node, a new frame needs to be displayed while the current frame is being decrypted
3. Due to network traffic congestion

The scheduler proposed by the author led to a significant savings in the network energy consumption for multimedia streaming. The process is introduced below (see also Figure 6.8):

1. Initialize the time of encryption, decryption, and authentication as T_{ENC}, T_{DEC}, and T_{AUTH}.
2. Calculate the time needed to secure a frame $\{T_{SEC} = T_{ENC} + T_{DEC} + T_{AUTH}\}$.
3. Buffer two frames, frame A and frame B, and calculate the time between them as T_{AB}.
4. If $T_{AB} > T_{SEC}$, then pass frame A to the proposed security scheme, or else discard frame A and continue until the end of all video frames.

For instance, if T_{SEC} is equal to 40 ms, and the time between frames A and B is 42 ms, then T_{AB} is greater than T_{SEC}, so frame A will be secured and sent across the network to the receiver node. Otherwise, the frame will be discarded by the sender (the video camera sensor).

The proposed scheduler would decrease network energy consumption, because some frames were going to be dropped by the receiver node due to the decryption and authentication processes.

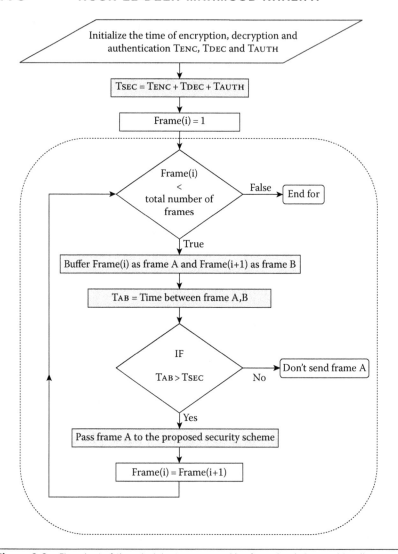

Figure 6.8 Flow chart of the scheduler to secure a video frame in wireless multimedia sensor networks.

Figure 6.9 illustrates the receiving process of the proposed security scheme for multimedia streaming:

1. A secured packets (SecP) is received by the receiver node.
2. The receiver node decapsulates the packet into fields.
3. The receiving process calculates the CMAC code (CCm) by using the encrypted frame (EF) and the UDP and RTP headers.

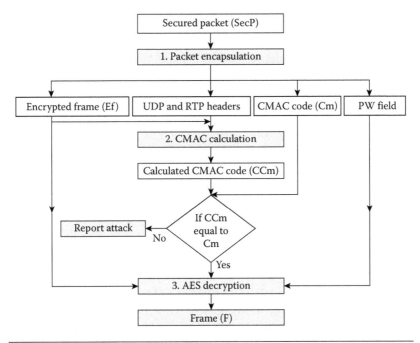

Figure 6.9 Flow chart of the proposed received function to secure a video frame in wireless multimedia sensor networks.

4. If the calculated CMAC code is equal to the sent CMAC code (Cm), then the proposed security scheme sends the encrypted frame to the decryption process; otherwise it reports an attack and shuts down all sensor nodes.
5. The decryption process decrypts the encrypted frame using the AES decryption process and produces frame (F) if the calculated CMAC is equal to the sent CMAC code.

6.3.3 Security Scheme Implementation

There were two possible methods of evaluating the proposed security scheme. The first possibility was to implement the scheme on real sensor nodes in the TinyOS [42] operating system. It was very difficult to choose this method as it required between 80 and 100 sensor motes, which exceeded the research budget. The second method was to implement the proposed security scheme in WMSN simulators; this solution was satisfactory, since it met the research budget and schedule.

A simulator is software that imitates selected parts of the real world and is normally used as a tool for research and development [43]; there are more than 60 simulators for WSNs and WMSNs. Table 6.3 outlines some of the most well-known WSN simulators.

The NS2 simulator was selected from the list of WSN and WMSN simulators. It was decided to implement the proposed security scheme within NS2 for the following reasons:

- It is open-source software.
- It has a large number of protocols available.
- It is used by many researchers around the world.
- It has not supported any security features so far.

Although NS2 has a complicated design, the purpose for using it was to make a valuable contribution to the research community. Appendix 6A will deal with the installation of NS2 and will explain the main components of the simulator. In addition, a detailed structure of the proposed security scheme and its implementation in NS2 will be given.

Appendix 6A will provide further details on how to implement the proposed security scheme for multimedia streaming in NS2.

6.4 Evaluation of the Proposed Security Scheme

Section 6.3 introduced the design of the proposed security scheme for multimedia streaming. In this section, the simulation assumptions, parameters, scenarios, metrics, and results of the proposed security scheme will be presented. It is important to note that all the simulation trials are based on NS2.

6.4.1 Simulation Assumptions

There is a set of assumptions that should first be listed before running the simulations, and they are as follows:

- There is no mobility feature on the nodes. Once nodes are deployed, they cannot be moved or replaced.
- Traffic flow follows a pattern determined by the application. Most of the traffic is assumed to be directed from the nodes to the sink node.

Table 6.3 Comparison of Well-Known Wireless Sensor Network Simulators

SIMULATOR	PROGRAMMING LANGUAGE	GUI	OPEN SOURCE	MAIN FEATURES	LIMITATIONS
QualNet [44]	C/C++	Yes	Commercial	Comprehensive set of advanced wireless modules and user-friendly tools	High-cost annual license
OPNET [44]	C/C++	Yes	Commercial	Uses a hierarchical model to define each characteristic of the system Capable of recording a large set of user-defined results	Scalability problems Expensive tool
J-Sim [45]	Java	Yes	Yes	Ability to simulate the use of sensors for phenomena detection Support for using the simulation code for real hardware sensors	Comparatively complicated to use Unnecessary overhead in the intercommunication model
SENS [44]	C++	No	Yes	Provides very basic network and physical layer support Source codes can be compiled for TinyOS	Simulators do not seem to be developed any further
NS2 [46]	C++	No	Yes	A large number of protocols available publicly Ability to support multiple radio interfaces and multiple channels	Complex configuration Does not run real hardware code

Sources: Eriksson, J., Detailed simulation of heterogeneous wireless sensor networks, Uppsala University, Uppsala, Sweden, 2009.
Kellner, K. et al., Simulation environments for wireless sensor networks, Georg-August University, Gottingen, Germany, 2010.

- All the sensors use integrated circuits that are tamper-resistant. Thus, if a node is captured, the attacker is unable to extract data from the sensor, especially the network keys.
- Traffic generation is based on a fired triggered event in the simulation environment.
- All nodes always have a way to the sink node through other nodes or a direct connection to the sink node.
- Multimedia sensors are more powerful than normal sensors in terms of initial energy and memory.
- The standard frame size for multimedia streaming is 1536 bytes, and screen width and height is 352 × 288 pixels.

6.4.2 Simulation Parameters

To simulate the proposed scheme, the following general NS2 parameters should be set up first:

1. The appearance of the network, which indicates the full view of the topology of the sensor network; this includes the position of nodes with (x, y, and z) coordinates.
2. The internal configuration: Because the simulation is conducted on network traffic, it is important to configure the following:
   a. Which nodes will be the sources?
   b. What is the status of the connections?
   c. What kind of secure connection will be used?
3. The configuration of the layered structure of each node in the network, including the following:
   a. The detailed configuration of network components on a sensor node.
   b. Where to produce the simulation results (the trace file).
   c. Organizing the simulation process.

6.4.2.1 Appearance of the Network for Multimedia Streaming   In the multimedia streaming scenario, node positions were generated according to uniform distribution. The monitored area was 1000 × 1000 m. There were 25 nodes deployed. The simulation included from one to four sensor cameras with different x and y coordinates.

The location of x and y coordinates of sensor cameras can be away from the sink node by one to four hops. Figure 6.10 shows an example

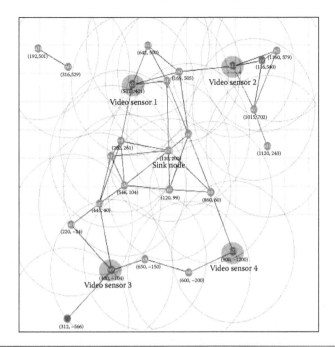

Figure 6.10 Example of one of the network appearance for nodes in 1 km² area for multimedia streaming.

of the network appearance of the nodes in a 1 km² area with sensor cameras.

6.4.2.2 Internal Configuration Because the simulation is conducted on network traffic, the traffic sources are all deployed nodes except for the sink node. Most of the traffic is assumed to be directed from the nodes to the sink node. The reason for that assumption is that the ultimate goal of the WMSN is to get information from the network. Every node in the simulation scenario is connected to a set of neighboring sensor nodes. There is always a path to the sink node.

6.4.2.3 Layered Structure Configuration of Nodes The layer structure of multimedia streaming is quite different from any other transmission type. Table 6.4 lists the NS2 parameters for a multimedia streaming scheme. WMSNs not only have high traffic flow but also a large frame size for a bounded time. In WMSNs, the unsuccessful reception of large packets is due to the number of hops packets must make to reach the sink; every packet with large multimedia data

Table 6.4   NS2 Simulation Parameters for Multimedia Streaming

SIMULATION PARAMETER	VALUE
MAC layer protocol	IEEE 802.11
Transmission radius	250 M
Data packet size	64 bytes
Data rate	24 frame/s
Traffic type	Multimedia frame
Simulation area	1 km^2
Number of sensor nodes	25
Node initial energy	1000 J
Transmission energy	0.007 J
Reception energy	0.007 J
Simulation times	120 s, 360 s
Routing protocols	AODV

passes from 1 to 20 nodes to reach the sink. The authors suggested using a minimum number of nodes to be deployed in an area 1 km^2. The proposed number of nodes is 25.

The WMSNs had initial energy larger than the WSNs. The initial energy was 1000 J. The times for simulation were 120 and 360 seconds.

The above simulation times were chosen because the simulations had two multimedia streamed videos. The duration of the first video was 20 seconds, and the duration of the second video was 120 seconds. The simulation experiments (Appendix 6A) will give more details about the videos used in such simulations.

6.4.3 Simulation Scenarios

The multimedia streaming scenario was quite different and more complicated than any transmission. Scenarios for multimedia streaming were divided into two scenarios: short multimedia streaming and long multimedia streaming.

The short multimedia streaming duration was approximately 20 seconds. The long multimedia streaming duration was approximately 120 seconds. For both types, simulation experiments should be conducted when there are between one and four videos to be streamed in the network.

The positions of video cameras sensor nodes should be away from the sink node by one hop, two hops, three hops, and four hops;

moreover, some experiments will be executed when video cameras are deployed in random places in the network. The simulation scenarios are quite numerous so as to study the proposed security scheme for multimedia streaming in different conditions and environments.

6.4.4 Simulation Hardware

All simulation scenarios were performed in Windows Server 2003 Enterprise Edition Service Pack 2 (Kansas) using the compiler GCC 2.9.6. All experiments were run on a Dell PowerEdge 2800 tower server (Texas) with an Intel Xeon CPU, 3.40 GHz, and 4 GB of RAM.

The execution of simulation scenarios consumed a large amount of time. The specifications of the machine had no relation to the simulation performance and results. NS2 simulates the specifications of the wireless sensor node hardware. The machine used helped in processing the resulting trace files and videos before and after simulations.

6.4.5 Performance Metrics

In a multimedia streaming scenario, the metrics are the total network energy consumption, network packet delivery ratio, video frames lost due to network congestion or due to the proposed security scheme, and peak signal-to-noise ratio (PSNR).

The main challenges for the proposed security scheme are the energy consumption and the strength of the security to stand against all known attacks without missing the network delivery ratio.

6.4.5.1 Network Delivery Ratio   The network delivery ratio is defined as the number of successful received packets during a specific time. Equation 6.1 is used to calculate the network delivery ratio.

$$\text{Network delivery ratio} = \frac{\sum_{i=1}^{n} RP_i}{\text{All Transmitted Packets}} \qquad (6.1)$$

where n represents the total number of nodes, RP_i represents the received packets by node i.

6.4.5.2 Average Energy Consumption per Received Packets The average energy consumption per received packet is defined as the total energy consumed by the whole network to deliver control and data packets to the destination during a specific time. Equation 6.2 is employed to calculate that metric.

$$\text{Average energy consumption per received packets} = \frac{\sum_{i=1}^{n} E_i}{\sum_{i=1}^{n} RP_i} \tag{6.2}$$

where n represents the total number of nodes, E_i represents the consumed energy by node i, RP_i represents the received packets by node i.

6.4.5.3 Frame Loss Frame loss is defined as one or more frames of data traveling across the network that fail to reach their destination during a specific time or due to node calculations. Equation 6.3 is drawn upon to calculate the frame loss.

$$\text{Frame Loss} = \text{Dropped frames due to network congestion} \\ + \text{dropped frames due to node calculations} \tag{6.3}$$

6.4.5.4 PSNR PSNR is defined as the normalized average difference between each pixel in the transmitted video and the received video through the network. This is the most commonly used method to measure video quality. Equations 6.4 and 6.5 are used to calculate PSNR.

This measurement has a nonlinear relationship with the subjective video quality. Excellent values for video encoding range from 30 to 50 dB, whereas the acceptable range in wireless transmission settles from 20 to 25 dB.

$$PSNR = 10 \log_{10} \frac{L^2}{MSE} \tag{6.4}$$

$$MSE = \frac{1}{N * M} \sum_{i=0}^{N-1} \sum_{j=0}^{M-1} \left[X(i,j) - Y(i,j) \right]^2 \tag{6.5}$$

where L represents the maximum value a pixel can take in a video frame, MSE represents the mean square error, X represents the transmitted video frame, Y represents the received video frame, and i,j represents the location of the pixel in a video frame.

6.4.6 Simulation Results

The simulation results of the proposed security scheme for multimedia streaming are included in two sections. The first section will represent the results for short multimedia streaming, while the second one will show the results for the long multimedia streaming. The short and long multimedia streaming have been selected to test the behavior of the proposed security scheme in terms of light and heavy network traffic load.

The metrics to be measured for both sections are the total network energy consumption, network packet delivery ratio, lost video frames due to network congestion or due to the proposed security scheme, and PSNR. The above metrics are commonly used to measure the performance of any proposed work for multimedia streaming [47,48].

6.4.6.1 Simulation Results for Short Multimedia Streaming Streaming short duration video files is very important in many applications such as monitoring and military applications. To classify a movie as short, the standard movie data set classification was used in the proposed work. This classification considers a movie short when its duration is less than 20 seconds and long when its duration is more than 1 minute long, when the wireless transmission medium is used.

All the following simulations result in short multimedia streaming using a movie entitled "Container" with a duration of 20 seconds to be sent through the network (Appendix 6A explains how to prepare a movie for simulation). There were four scenarios in short multimedia streaming with one, two, three, and four video cameras, respectively, placed in the network topology in different positions. The metrics to be measured were the total network energy consumption, network packet delivery ratio, and video frame loss due to network congestion or due to the proposed security scheme.

6.4.6.1.1 The Total Network Energy Consumption The first metric to be measured in the current work was the total network energy consumption. Figures 6.11 through 6.14 represent the energy consumed by the network when there are one, two, three, and four videos streamed through the network, respectively. The x axis represents the location of the video cameras, while the y axis indicates the network energy consumption in joules.

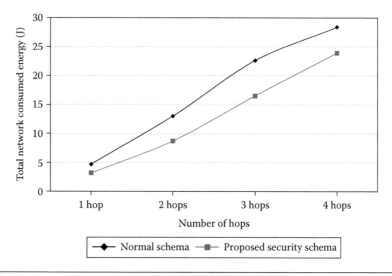

Figure 6.11   The total network energy consumption for one streamed video with different locations.

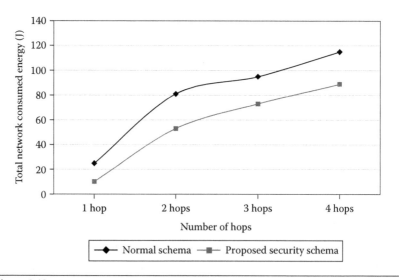

Figure 6.12   The total network energy consumption for two streamed videos with different locations.

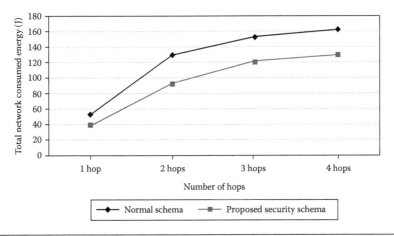

Figure 6.13   The total network energy consumption for three streamed videos with different locations.

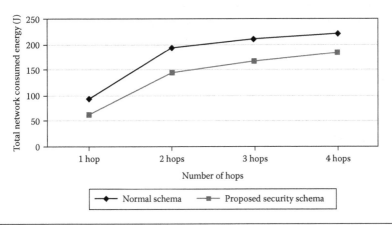

Figure 6.14   The total network energy consumption for four streamed videos with different locations.

Figures 6.11 through 6.14 illustrate that the proposed security scheme achieved less energy consumption than the normal scheme. The proposed scheduler that was presented in Section 6.3.2 achieved this improvement in network energy consumption. The video camera sensor would discard any frame that would not burden the process of encryption, decryption, and authentication before sending it to their destination. This idea conserved a lot of consumed energy, as there were frames that were going to consume a lot of energy during their journey to the sink node. When they reached the sink node, they would be dropped, as it could not burden the process of decryption. The energy consumed during its journey was proportional to the video camera location: the farther away the video camera was located, the more energy the frame consumed to reach the sink node.

The question that might arise here is what the times were when two, three, and four videos were streamed through the network. If the two, three, and four videos were streamed, and there was a pause time between them, then there would not be a problem; the network would handle this situation because there was one video at a time.

Random start times were generated for the videos with a uniform distribution. The uniform distribution would generate two numbers between 0 and 40 for two videos streamed through the network. The value 40 was the result of multiplying the duration of the movie by the number of videos to be streamed. For three videos, the random times to start streaming would be between 0 and 60, and so forth.

The simulations were executed 10 times for every scenario, and the average was calculated from these values to conclude network energy consumption and the other metric.

Note that the behavior of the energy consumption curve for the proposed security scheme was the same in all cases. The proposed security scheme always achieved lower energy consumption than the normal scheme because of the proposed scheduler. The proposed security scheme achieved from 15% to 20% lower energy consumption than the normal scheme.

6.4.6.1.2 The Network Delivery Ratio   The second metric to be measured through the proposed work is the total network delivery ratio. Figures 6.15 through 6.18 illustrate the network delivery ratio when there are one, two, three, and four videos streamed through the network, respectively. The x axis indicates the location of the video cameras, whereas the y axis refers to the achieved network delivery ratio as a percentage.

Figure 6.15 shows that the delivery ratio for the proposed security scheme is 81%. The 81% delivery ratio was achieved due to the discarded frames by the proposed scheduler. When the video camera was four hops away from the sink, the delivery ratio of the normal scheme was below 81%, while the proposed secured scheme is

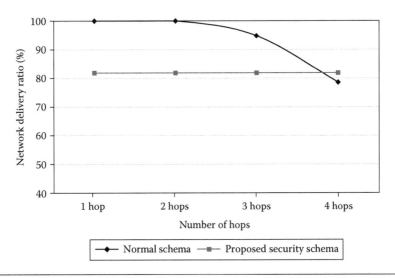

Figure 6.15   The network delivery ratio for one streamed video with different locations.

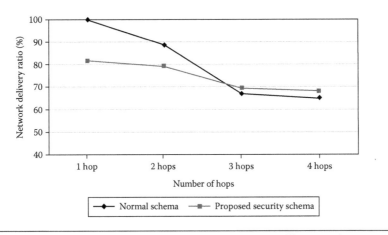

Figure 6.16   The network delivery ratio for two streamed videos with different locations.

constant at 81%. The delivery ratio for the normal scheme was below 81% because of the network traffic congestion.

From Figures 6.16 through 6.18, it is clear that the delivery ratio of the proposed secured scheme was not constant at 81% as when there was one video streamed through the network. The delivery ratio of the proposed security scheme was below 81%. The reason for that phenomenon was due to network traffic congestion as there were two, three, and four video cameras, and their locations were two, three, and four hops away from the sink, respectively.

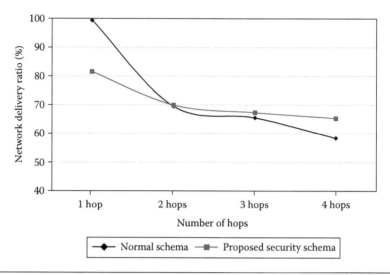

Figure 6.17   The network delivery ratio for three streamed videos with different locations.

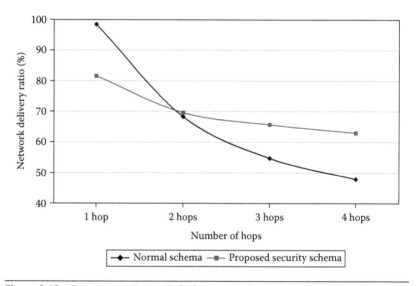

Figure 6.18   The network delivery ratio for four streamed videos with different locations.

For multimedia streaming, the video was considered to be at a good quality for watching when no more 1/3 of frames were being lost. The proposed security scheme and the normal scheme achieved more than 65% delivery ratio as shown in Figures 6.16 and 6.17, which was a good indicator for movie quality. The PSNR will strengthen our indication at the end of the multimedia results section.

Note that, in Figure 6.18 at four hops away from the sink node, the delivery ratio of the normal scheme and the proposed secured scheme was below 65%. This value was not acceptable for video quality. However, this was the worst-case scenario for the whole simulation. Random deployment of video cameras was thus required to draw the final conclusion of the proposed security scheme performance. The PSNR will also have the final decision concerning the quality of the streamed videos.

6.4.6.1.3 Frame Loss The frame loss metric was one of the most important metrics to be measured in the proposed security scheme. This metric presents the reasons for the frames that were being lost. A frame could be lost for two reasons. The first reason for loss was due to network congestion, which occurred with both the proposed security scheme and the normal one, whereas the second reason for loss was the security calculations performed by the proposed security scheme.

Figures 6.19 through 6.22 represent the frame loss when there are one, two, three, and four videos streamed through the network, respectively. The x axis indicates the location of the video cameras, whereas the y axis represents the number of lost frames.

Figure 6.19 reveals that all the lost frames in the proposed security scheme were due to security process calculations; it did not lose any frames due to network traffic congestion, as it had already dropped

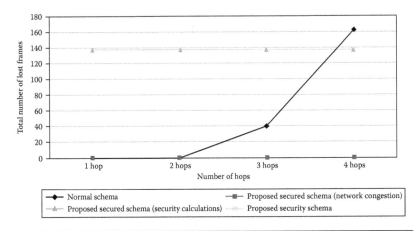

Figure 6.19 The total number of lost frames for one streamed video with different locations.

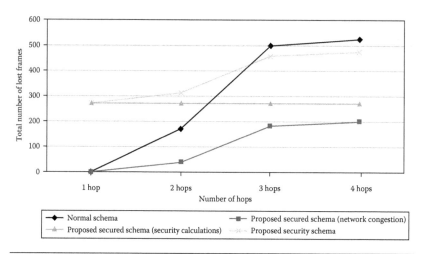

Figure 6.20   The total number of lost frames for two streamed videos with different locations.

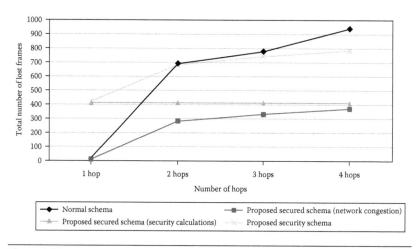

Figure 6.21   The total number of lost frames for three streamed videos with different locations.

the frames that could not burden the security process by the video camera. Hence, it had a lower number of lost frames than the normal scheme; even if the video camera was four hops away from the sink node, all frames were successfully delivered to the sink under the proposed security scheme. In general, the normal scheme had fewer lost frames when the video camera was close to the sink and more lost frames when the video camera was farther away from the sink.

From Figures 6.20 and 6.21, it is apparent that the lost frames of the proposed secured scheme were due to network traffic congestion and the security calculations. Generally, there were two proportional

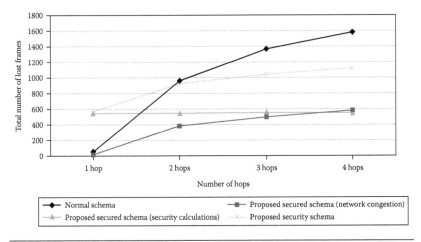

Figure 6.22   The total number of lost frames for four streamed videos with different locations.

relationships; the first one was that the more video cameras existed in the network topology, the more lost frames the network had. The second relationship was that increasing distance from the sink also increased the number of lost frames.

The proposed security scheme was biased to achieve fewer lost frames than the normal scheme when there were more cameras deployed and when they were located farther away from the sink, since the number of sent frames was less than the normal scheme. According to the WMSN application, the video cameras were always deployed far from the sink to monitor the whole region. The choice of deploying video cameras will constitute a design variable controlled by the network engineer in our proposed scheme.

Note that the worst-case scenario happened when four video cameras were deployed away from the sink node by four hops. The network delivery ratio was 62%, and the number of lost frames due to network traffic congestion was equal to the lost frames due to the security calculations. This result poses the question of what the behavior of the proposed security scheme was when the four video cameras were deployed in random locations.

6.4.6.2 Performance Evaluations for Short Multimedia Streaming When the Four Video Cameras Were Deployed in Random Locations   Table 6.5 exhibits the random locations for four video cameras when they were deployed in a random fashion. For every combination, the simulations

Table 6.5   Random Locations for Four Video Cameras in Short Multimedia Streaming

	LOCATION OF VIDEO CAMERAS (NUMBER OF HOPS FROM SINK)			
COMBINATION NAME	VIDEO CAMERA 1	VIDEO CAMERA 2	VIDEO CAMERA 3	VIDEO CAMERA 4
Combination 1	1	1	2	2
Combination 2	1	1	3	2
Combination 3	1	1	2	4
Combination 4	1	2	3	4
Combination 5	2	3	3	3
Combination 6	3	3	3	4
Combination 7	3	3	4	4

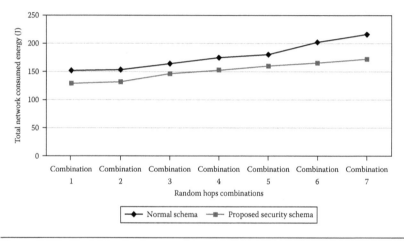

Figure 6.23   The total network energy consumption for four streamed videos with random locations.

were executed 10 times, and the average was calculated from these runs. The metrics to be measured were network energy consumption, network delivery ratio, and total number of lost frames. The random location deployment was a strategy to draw a final conclusion about the performance of the proposed security scheme to figure out its behavior under random deployment.

The first metric to be measured was network energy consumption. Figure 6.23 represents the energy consumed by the network when four videos were streamed from random locations in the network topology. The time to start streaming the four videos was a random time between 0 and 80.

Figure 6.23 illustrates that the proposed security scheme was sufficiently stable with random locations for video cameras according to the energy consumption metric. The proposed security scheme's energy consumption curve always achieved lower energy consumption. There was no doubt that, although the proposed security scheme added security features to the network, the network nonetheless achieved less energy consumption.

It is notable that the proposed security scheme achieved better results when the video cameras were away from the sink by three or four hops. Figure 6.23 illustrates that, in Combinations 6 and 7, the proposed security scheme curve margin was 40 J less than the normal one. It seems that the proposed security scheme had a strong tendency to achieve better results when video cameras were away from sink by more than two hops.

Figure 6.24 demonstrates the network delivery ratio for both the security scheme and the normal scheme when four videos were streamed through the network from random locations. The proposed security scheme achieved a lower delivery ratio when Combinations 1, 2, and 3 were executed, but it achieved a better delivery ratio when Combinations 4, 5, 6, and 7 were executed. The reason for this result was the locations of video cameras; the farther away the video cameras were placed, the better delivery ratio the network had. That is why the number of frames delivered in the proposed scheme was less than the normal one.

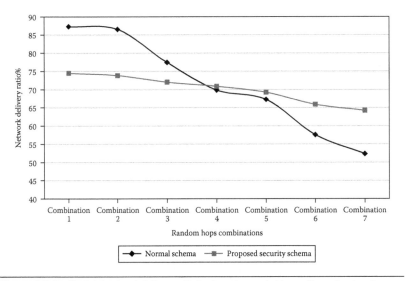

Figure 6.24   The total network delivery ratio for four streamed videos with random locations.

With Combinations 6 and 7, the network delivery ratio of the proposed security scheme was approximately 65%. This ratio was good enough to strengthen our analysis for the case of four video cameras deployed four hops away from the sink; that was the worst-case scenario in the network.

Figure 6.25 shows the network total number of lost frames. It was clear that the proposed security scheme achieved fewer lost frames than the normal one. The frames lost due to the security calculations were always constant, at 18%–20% of the original video. The frames lost due to network congestion in the proposed security scheme were proportional to the locations of video cameras. The farther the video cameras were located from the sink, the more network congestion there would be.

The results of the short multimedia streaming simulation, as presented in Sections 6.4.6.1 and 6.4.6.2, can be summarized as follows:

1. The proposed security scheme achieved lower energy consumption than the normal scheme in all simulation scenarios.
2. The lower energy consumption of the proposed security scheme was achieved because of the proposed scheduler, as already discussed in Section 6.3.2.

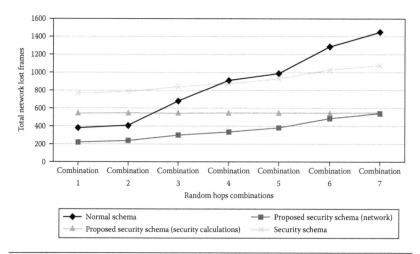

Figure 6.25 The total number of frames lost by the network for four streamed videos with random locations.

3. The network delivery ratio for the proposed security scheme was better when the video camera was deployed farther away from the sink node. The farther the video cameras were deployed from the sink node, the better the delivery ratio.

4. The delivery ratio for the proposed security scheme was always above 65%, which was acceptable for video streaming unless the worst-case scenario occurred.

5. The proposed security scheme fits the light traffic on WMSNs, whether one, two, three, or four video cameras were used.

6. Deciding how many sensor cameras to deploy and where to deploy them would be a network engineer design parameter.

6.4.6.3 Simulation Results for Long Multimedia Streaming   The proposed security scheme proved its effectiveness versus the normal scheme for short multimedia streaming. This section will describe the behavior of the proposed security scheme in the simulation when long multimedia content was streamed through the network. The duration of the streamed video here was 120 s, longer than the short video by 100 s.

6.4.6.4 Long Multimedia Streaming with Four Video Cameras Deployed in Different Locations   In this scenario, there were four video cameras at different locations in the topology of the network; the video cameras were at a distance of one hop, two hops, three hops, and four hops from the sink. Figure 6.26 represents the energy consumption.

The time at which streaming of the four videos was begun was a random time between 0 and 480. Figure 6.26 shows that the behavior of the energy consumption metric for the proposed security scheme when streaming long multimedia content was the same as when streaming short multimedia content.

Note that, when four videos were streamed, the margin between the proposed security scheme and the normal one became larger. This was a good indicator that the proposed scheme performed well in heavy traffic streaming according to the energy metric.

The good performance of the energy metric of the proposed scheme was because of the proposed scheduler introduced in this work. Figure 6.27 displays the network delivery ratio for four streamed videos with different locations.

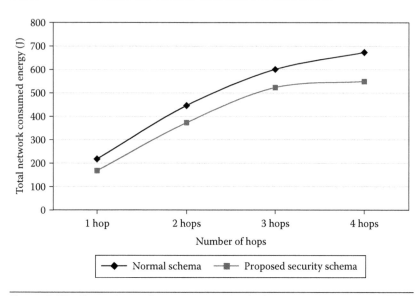

Figure 6.26 The total network energy consumption for four streamed videos with different locations in long multimedia streaming.

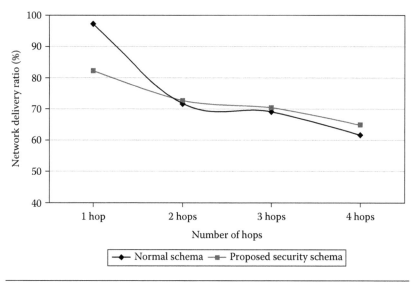

Figure 6.27 The total network delivery ratio for four streamed videos with different locations in long multimedia streaming.

As seen in Figure 6.27, when four video cameras were located one hop away from the sink, the proposed security scheme achieved a delivery ratio of 81%, whereas the normal one achieved 98%. The lower delivery ratio was caused by the security calculations and the proposed scheduler. When the four video cameras were away from the sink by two, three, and four hops, the proposed security scheme achieved a better delivery ratio than the normal one. This better ratio was due to the proposed scheduler.

It was surprising that the proposed security scheme achieved a better delivery ratio when streaming long multimedia content than short content. An investigation of this phenomenon revealed that the reason was the random start time of the video. The random start time range was between 0 and 480 for the long videos. In short multimedia streaming, when the random value for the start time was between 0 and 80, at least three videos would margin with each other, while in long multimedia streaming at least two videos would margin together. This factor made the network more relaxed and enabled a higher delivery ratio. Figure 6.28 shows the total number of lost frames for both the normal scheme and proposed security scheme.

Figure 6.28 demonstrates that the proposed security scheme's lost frames were due to network congestion and the security calculations. The frames lost due to the security calculations were always between 18% and 20% of the original video to be streamed. If the network had more resources, the proposed security scheme would only have lost frames due to the security calculations.

Note that the above scenario was the worst case for the entire simulation done for this study. There was no need to simulate random locations of video cameras, as the worst case achieved 65% delivery ratio.

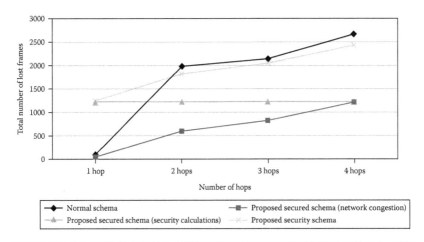

Figure 6.28 The total network of lost frames for four streamed videos with different locations in long multimedia streaming.

6.4.7 PSNR Results for Multimedia Streaming

The PSNR metric had a nonlinear relationship with the subjective video quality. Therefore, it was important to use a utility function that describes subjective video quality as a function of the PSNR. The excellent range of values for optimal video quality is from 30 to 50 dB, while an acceptable range in wireless transmission settled between 20 and 25 dB.

The PSNR metric had to be calculated for every video streamed through the network with every simulation scenario. More than 110 PSNR graph could have been constructed, but the author decided to calculate the PSNR when the worst delivery ratio occurred in the network. The worst delivery ratio was 62% and occurred when four videos were streamed, each four hops away from the sink.

To calculate the PSNR value, both the original video and the resulting streamed video needed to be in YUV format. The researchers of this work used the FFmpeg tool [59] to convert both videos. Figure 6.29 illustrates the PSNR values of the streamed video when the worst-case scenario happened in the network.

The PSNR mean value was 20.43 dB. This value was quite low but acceptable, because the acceptable region for the PSNR value was between 20 and 25 dB for wireless transmission. The PSNR value indicated that the proposed security scheme for multimedia streaming

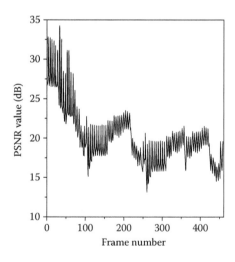

Figure 6.29 The peak signal-to-noise ratio between the original video file and the received video file in the worst-case scenario.

achieved not only lower energy consumption but also an acceptable delivery and PSNR value while proposing a strong security scheme—in other words, four times stronger than any proposed security scheme.

6.4.8 Results Discussion

We have demonstrated that the proposed security scheme for multimedia streaming was more effective than the normal scheme. The effectiveness of the proposed security scheme was measured and tested against the normal scheme according to four metrics—energy consumption, network delivery ratio, frame loss, and PSNR.

The proposed security scheme for multimedia streaming has advantages and disadvantages. The forthcoming points will tackle the advantages of the proposed security scheme for multimedia streaming:

- The proposed security scheme added security features to WMSNs and was four times stronger than any other proposed security scheme.
- Although the proposed security scheme added security features to WMSNs, it achieved lower energy consumption due to the proposed scheduler.
- It achieved an acceptable delivery ratio when video cameras were deployed farther away from the sink node.
- In the worst-case scenario, although the proposed security achieved a delivery ratio of 62%, the PSNR illustrated that the subjective quality of the video was acceptable at 20.43 dB.
- The proposed security scheme was biased to better performance when streaming long content rather than short and achieved better results in delivery ratio.
- The farther the video cameras were deployed, the better the delivery ratio that the proposed security scheme achieved.
- Deciding how many sensor cameras to deploy and where to deploy them should be a network engineer design parameter.

The proposed security scheme for multimedia streaming also had the following disadvantages:

- The proposed security scheme achieved a lower delivery ratio than the normal scheme when the network had only one video camera deployed in the network at all times.

- Moreover, it had a lower delivery ratio than the normal scheme when video cameras were deployed only one hop away from the sink node.

6.4.9 Evaluation of the Proposed Security Operations

Any proposed security scheme will have some trade-off to offer security features. We have already discussed the cost paid by the network in terms of energy consumption, delivery ratio, frame loss, and PSNR.

This section will detail the cost of the security processes. Although NS2 included many features and modules, it did not include any modules for node process calculations in terms of time or energy.

The proposed security scheme based its security features on two processes: the process of encryption and decryption using the AES encryption technique and the process of authentication and deauthentication by the CMAC mechanism.

Refs. [49–51] maintain that both the AES encryption technique and CMAC mechanism are applicable to WSN and WMSN motes. The authors measured the energy consumption and RAM and ROM size for both algorithms; the results are as shown in Tables 6.6 and 6.7.

Table 6.6   Energy Consumed by AES and CMAC Algorithms

ALGORITHM	ENERGY (mJ/byte)
AES encryption	1.62
AES decryption	2.49
CMAC process	1.4

Source: Wang, Y. et al., *IEEE Communications Surveys and Tutorials*, 8, 2–23, © 2006 IEEE.

Table 6.7   Size of Reserved RAM and ROM by AES and CMAC Algorithms

ALGORITHM	RAM (KB)	ROM (KB)
AES	2	10
CMAC	1	6

Source: Wang, Y. et al., *IEEE Communications Surveys and Tutorials*, 8, 2–23, © 2006, IEEE.

The energy consumed by encryption, decryption, and authentication was low compared to that consumed by the transmission and reception functions; data transmission accounts for 70% of the total energy consumption of a WSN [51].

6.4.10 *Performance Comparison with Other Related Works*

Security in WMSNs is a new field of study in the research community. To date, there have only been a few security frameworks presented for WSNs. The most well-known frameworks for WSN security are TinySec, SenSec (http://ieeexplore.ieee.org/xpl/login.jsp?tp=&arnumber=5961521), MiniSec, TinyECC, and ContikiSec. An overview of these frameworks was given in Section 6.2.6.

Table 6.8 provides references for these frameworks and compares them with the proposed security scheme for multimedia streaming.

6.5 Conclusions

At the beginning of this study, an initial study was carried out to determine the key challenges facing WMSN security. The research objectives became obvious after the initial study, and the main objective was to propose a security scheme that would fit the nature of streaming multimedia in WMSNs. There are a number of frameworks that have been implemented for WSNs that may fit WMSNs, but due to time and budget limitations, the current research was restricted to working on WSN simulators.

The selection criterion for a WSN simulator was provision of security features. Various simulation tools were matched including OPNET, QualNet, GloMoSim, and NS2, none of which supported security features. NS2 was determined to be the most appropriate simulation tool based on its flexibility, in addition to the fact that it was publically available free software. It is still regarded by the research community as the most credible network simulator.

After NS2 was selected as the main simulator for this research, several trials were executed and numerous modifications were made to the NS2 infrastructure to adapt it to the security features of the

Table 6.8 Comparison between the Proposed Security Scheme and Other Security Frameworks

FRAMEWORK NAME	YEAR	IMPLEMENTED/ SIMULATED	SECURITY PROPERTIES	ALGORITHMS	LAYER	OVERHEAD	KEY LENGTH	SUPPORT MULTIMEDIA
TinySec [33]	2004	Implemented (NesC)	Access control, integrity, confidentiality, replay protection	Skipjack CBC-CS mode	Link layer	8 bytes/packet	80	—
SenSec [52]	2005	Implemented (NesC)	Access control, integrity, confidentiality, key management	Skipjack-X CBC-CS mode	Link layer	5 bytes/packet	80	—
MiniSec [34]	2007	Implemented (NesC)	Predeployed symmetric keys, confidentiality, replay protection, authentication	Skipjack OCB mode	Network layer	3 bytes/packet	80	—
TinyECC [35]	2007	Implemented (NesC)	Key Exchange, Public key encryption, Digital signature	ECC SECG-160	Link Layer	Keys overheads	256	—
ContikiSec [36]	2009	Implemented (C)	Authentication, Integrity & Confidentiality	AES CBC-CS mode	Network Layer	4 bytes/packet	128	—
Proposed Security Scheme	2013	Simulated (NS2 – C)	Authentication, Integrity, Confidentiality & freshness	AES CMAC Authentication	Transport and Application layer	4 bytes/packet + 2 bits/ packet	256 – 4 times stronger than TinyECC	Yes

proposed security scheme. More than 200 hours of development and simulation were put into implementing the security features in NS2 for multimedia streaming.

At the end of the development and implementation phase, comparisons between the proposed security scheme and the normal one were drawn according to the network delivery ratio and energy consumption, which were the main interests of this study. Moreover, a comparison was made between other frameworks for security in WSNs and the proposed security scheme.

The most significant contributions of this study are as follows:

- It managed to add security libraries to NS2, which did not support security features before. Appendix 6A illustrates the steps that were taken to integrate security features into NS2.
- It attempted to propose a security scheme for WMSNs for multimedia streaming.
- The proposed secured scheme for multimedia streaming achieved a significant savings in network energy consumption, consuming 15%–20% less energy consumption than the normal scheme despite the addition of security features. This significant savings was due to the proposed scheduler for WMSNs, which predicts video frames that cannot handle the process of encryption, decryption, and authentication and discards them before sending them through the network.
- The suggested security scheme for multimedia streaming outperforms the normal scheme in delivery ratio when the sensor cameras are farther away from the sink node. The farther away the video cameras are deployed, the better the delivery ratio provided by the proposed security scheme. Moreover, the proposed security scheme achieved acceptable subjective video quality (PSNR value), even though the main goal of the research was energy consumption.
- The proposed security scheme was four times stronger than other security frameworks: every packet contains a PW field with four values, which makes the proposed security scheme computationally secure, but is considered as overhead by 2 bits/packet.

6.6 Implications for Future Works

There are still several research challenges that need to be addressed before use of the proposed security scheme in real WMSN deployment. The following list will offer some implications for future research related to the study presented in this chapter:

- Simulating the proposed security scheme with other application and transport layer protocols, for example, TCP, FTP, and HTTP
- Building a computational processing model for NS2 to calculate the consumed energy for the code executed inside WMSN nodes
- Concerning the proposed work in multimedia streaming, extending the video codec used in this research to such video codecs as MPEG-4, H.261, H.264, and so on
- Comparing the AES encryption algorithm with video encryption algorithms by means of using NS2
- Implementing the proposed security scheme in WMSN operating systems, such as TinyOS or Contiki, and comparing it with the current security frameworks implemented on these operating systems

Finally, it is hoped that the research presented in this chapter will help other researchers to simulate their security ideas and mechanisms based on the suggested development and the integration of security libraries into NS2.

Appendix 6A: Proposed Security Scheme Implementation

This appendix will provide a detailed description of the implementation of the proposed secured scheme using NS2. It will describe how to install NS2 and how to implement multimedia streaming into it within the proposed secured scheme.

6A.1 NS2

NS2 is a simulation tool primarily targeted for networking research and educational use. The simulator was derived from the old network simulator Real and Large (REAL) in 1989, which was developed with the goal of studying flow and congestion-control schemes in packet-switched data networks [44].

In 1995, the first generation of NS was completed through the VINT project with the hope of becoming a common simulator with advanced features to change the then-prominent protocol engineering practices [44]. The simulator continued to evolve and the second generation, NS2, was first released in 1996 based on NS1.

NS2 is extensively used by the networking research community. It provides substantial support for simulation of TCP, UDP, routing, multicast protocols over wired and wireless (local, satellite, sensor) networks, and so forth. [44]. The simulator is event-driven. It consists of C++ core methods and uses Tool Command Language (Tcl) and Object Tcl shell as interface allowing the input file (simulation script) to describe the model to simulate. Users can define arbitrary network topologies composed of nodes, routers, links, and shared media [44].

6A.1.1 NS2-Supported Platforms

NS2 is supported by many platforms; it runs over the Linux, FreeBSD, and Solaris operating systems. It is also supported in Windows 98/2003/XP/Vista/7 operating systems, but it requires the Cygwin platform [53]. The Cygwin platform is a collection of tools that provide an environment with a Linux look and feel for the Windows operating system. Windows 2003 with the Cygwin platform was the preferred choice for the present study, due to the researchers' experience with Windows 2003.

The first step in the implementation phase was the installation of the Cygwin platform. This step was achieved by following the tutorials in Ref. [54]. This reference gives excellent instructions for how to install the Cygwin platform on a Windows operating system.

6A.1.2 NS2 Installation

The second step is installing the NS2 simulator over the Cygwin platform, which was installed on a Windows 2003 operating system. The researchers installed NS version 2.29. It was the latest version of NS2 at the time. Ref. [55] describes how to install NS2 over the Cygwin platform.

6A.1.3 NS2 Layered Structure Modifications

The implementation of the proposed security scheme in this research for both message transmission and multimedia streaming is developed across the layers of NS2. Figure 6A.1 represents the implementation modifications that have been made to adapt the proposed secured scheme.

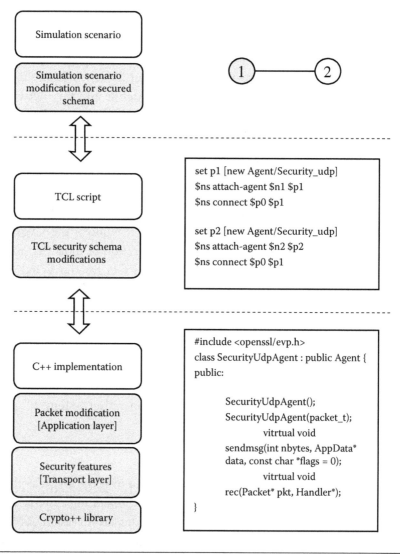

Figure 6A.1   Modification of the layered structure of NS2.

Implementing the modifications of the proposed security scheme detailed in Section 6.3.2 can be summarized by the following steps:

1. Add the Crypto++ library [56] to NS2 libraries and structure (C++ implementation layer).
2. Modify the packet format to add MAC-generated code (C++ implementation layer).
3. Modify the UDP to adapt the security features mentioned in the proposed security scheme, namely, CMAC generation, AES encryption, and C++ implementation layer.
4. Add the proposed security scheme to the Tcl script layer to deal with it in the simulation scenario layer (Tcl layer).
5. Call the proposed security scheme from the simulation scenario layer and initialize simulation parameters.

6A.1.3.1 C++ Implementation Layer Modification The modification of the C++ implementation layer consists of two steps. The first step is adding the Crypto++ library to the NS2 C++ implementation layer, whereas the second step involves adding CMAC code to the WSN packet format and encrypting the payload data with the AES encryption technique.

Crypto++ is a free open-source C++ class library of general purpose cryptographic algorithms and schemes. It provides a C++ application programming interface (API) for cryptographic functionality, such as encryption and decryption, hashing, key agreement schemes, random number generation, and others [56]. Adding the Crypto++ library to the NS2 C++ implementation layer was achieved after several trials and took more than 50 hours of research time. This length of time was a result of the fact that NS2 will not accept a new library unless it is integrated into its structure without any errors. The following points were applied to implement this step:

1. Download the Crypto++ library from Ref. [56]
2. Set the downloaded library in the Cygwin library directory
3. Select Install File in the NS2 simulator and add the Crypto++ library to the NS2 library
4. Install NS2 again with the modified NS2 install file
5. Select Make File in NS2 and add the line {-lm -lm -lcrypto} to the library code line
6. Build the whole NS2 simulator and run the make file

The second step, adding CMAC code to the WSN packet format and encrypting payload data, required numerous attempts. The author investigated NS2 books to study its structures. The work done in the present study concentrated on Ref. [54], which provides a detailed account of how to add new protocols into the structure of NS2 without facing errors. The following points describe how to implement this second step:

1. For WMSN packet modification, create a duplicate copy of the files rtp.h and rtp.cc in the Apps folder in the NS2 directory.
2. Name these copies "secured_rtp.h" and "secured_rtp.cc", respectively.
3. Open secured_rtp.h and rename all named RTP names to "secured_rtp".
4. Open secured_rtp.cc and rename all named RTP names to "secured_rtp".
5. Add a char variable of 4 bytes of cmac_code in the hdr_secured_rtp structure.
6. Add a 2-bit variable of PW in the hdr_secured_rtp structure.
7. The CMAC code generation will be added to the received and sent functions of the proposed secured scheme.
8. For the proposed secured scheme, create a duplicate copy of udp.h and udp.cc in the Apps folder in the NS2 directory.
9. Name these copies "secured_udp.h" and "secured_udp.cc", respectively.
10. Open secured_udp.h and make the following changes:
    a. Include the security library by the following line: {#include <openssl/evp.h>}.
    b. Define the block of AES by the following line: {#define AES_BLOCK_SIZE 256}.
    c. Add the following functions of AES encryption and decryption to the class of secured_upd.

```
int aes_initiation(unsigned char *key_d, int key_d_len,
  unsigned char *salt, E_C_CT*e_ct, E_C_CT*d_ct);

unsigned char *aes_encryption(E_C_CT *e, unsigned char
  *pt, int *len);

unsigned char *aes_decryption(E_C_CT *e, unsigned char
  *ct, int *len);
```

11. Open secured_udp.cc and make the following changes:
   a. Initiate AES using the aes_initiation function in the constructor of secured_upd class.
   b. Modify the send function of secured_udp by calling the aes_encryption function, then call the function CMAC and pass the encrypted payload and WSN fields to it. The generated code will be appended the secured_rtp.
   c. Modify the receive function of secured_udp by calling the function CMAC and pass the encrypted payload and WSN fields to it. If the generated code is equal to the CMAC code in the header, then call the aes_decryption function or report attack.

6A.1.3.2 Tcl Layer Modification The modification in the second layer (the Tcl layer) is related to the first layer (the C++ implementation layer). The modifications to the second layer may be implemented as follows:

1. Modify the file {tcl/lib/ns-default.tcl} inside the NS2 directory and add the following lines:

```
Agent/Security_udp instproc done {} { }
Agent/Security_udp instproc process_data {from } { }
```

2. Modify the file {tcl/lib/ns-packet.tcl} inside the NS2 directory and add the line in bold:

```
foreach prot {
AODV
# others:
Security_udp # Proposed Security Schema
}
```

3. Modify the file located in {Makefile} inside the NS2 directory and add the following line:

```
apps/Security_udp.o \
```

The modification in the file {tcl/lib/ns-default.tcl} is considered a mirror of the modification made in the first layer (the C++

implementation layer). The other lines are added to define the packet size and process data in the proposed security scheme in the form of text messages. The modification in the file {tcl/lib/ns-packet.tcl} is made to define the new secured packet format in the file, which contains all packet formats on NS2 protocols.

The modification in the file {Makefile} is the link between the first layer (the C++ implementation layer) and the second layer (the Tcl layer), which notifies the C++ implementation layer that a new protocol has been added to NS2 protocols.

After the above modifications are carried out, NS2 must be recompiled. The recompile of NS2 is needed to execute the changes that have been developed in the NS2 structure.

6A.1.3.3 Simulation Scenario Layer Modification   After applying the modification to the first layer (the C++ implementation layer) and the second layer (the Tcl layer), the implementation of the proposed security scheme is complete. The last step is building a simulation scenario of the proposed security scheme in the Simulation Scenario layer. In order to call the new proposed security scheme, you can add the following lines to any simulation scenario. The following lines describe the calling of the proposed security scheme; for example, in this case WMSN node n1 is attached to WMSN node n0 {sink node}.

```
#Create two secured agents of the proposed secured
  schema and attach them to the nodes n0 and n1
set p0 [new Agent/Security_udp]
$ns attach-agent $n0 $p0
#------------------------------------------------------------
set p1 [new Agent/Security_udp]
$ns attach-agent $n1 $p1
$ns connect $p0 $p1
```

6A.2 Multimedia Streaming Modification

To study the problems mentioned above in greater detail and propose a solution for them, the author implemented the steps proposed by Chih-Heng Ke [57]. Chih-Heng Ke proposed a tool, called "EvalVid," that can be integrated with NS2 to stream multimedia in real time over a WMSN. Figure 6A.2 represents the EvalVid tool components.

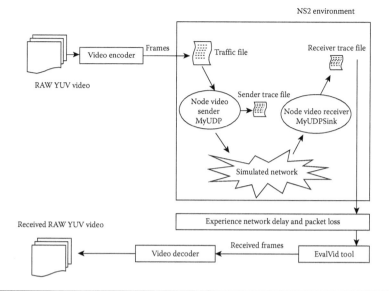

Figure 6A.2 Design diagram of the EvalVid tool. (From Ke, Chih-Heng et al. *J. Inf. Sci. Eng.* 24.2 (2008): 425–440.)

MyUDP is an extension of the UDP agent for the node video sender. This new agent allows users to specify the output file name of the sender trace file, and it records the timestamp of each transmitted packet, the packet ID, and the packet payload size. The task of the MyUDP agent corresponds to the task that tools such as RTP-dump do in a real network environment [57].

MyUDPSink is the receiving agent of the receiver node for the fragmented video frame packets sent by MyUDP. This agent also records the timestamp, packet ID, and payload size of each received packet in the user-specified file [57].

After installing the EvalVid tool in NS2 and making sure that it was working without errors, the author began to investigate the code and to modify it to add security features as mentioned in the proposed security scheme in Section 6.3.2.

6A.2.1 Secured Version for EvalVid Tool

The secured design of the EvalVid tool is presented in Figure 6A.3. The main changes are 1) the proposed mechanism was added to the NS2 scheduler and 2) the security feature of the proposed security scheme was added to both the video sender and receiver.

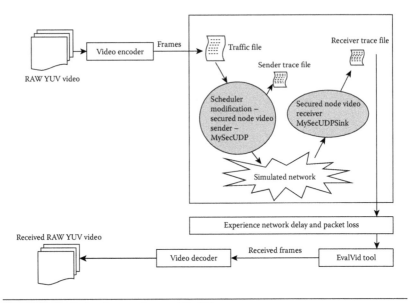

Figure 6A.3 Design diagram of secured EvalVid.

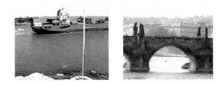

Figure 6A.4 Screenshot of both videos used in simulations. (From National Science Foundation, Arizona State University, 2000.)

6A.3 Experiment Data Preparations

The researchers of this work used standard video sequences that are commonly used for multimedia experiments. The video sequences can be found at the following website: http://trace.eas.asu.edu/yuv/index. html [58].

The standard video used in short multimedia streaming can be found at the above-mentioned site with the name "Container." The standard video used in long multimedia streaming can also be reached on the same website with the name "Bridge (Close)." A screenshot for both videos is displayed in Figure 6A.4.

Both videos are presented in raw YUV sequence format. The size of the short multimedia streaming video (Container) is 45 mega-bytes, whereas the long multimedia streaming video (Bridge [Close])

1364566535.613739 RTP len=1328 from=193.227.14.69:1728 v=2 p=0 x=0 cc=0 m=0 pt=33 (MP2T,0,90000) seq=17574 ts=764884950

ssrc=0x6062

data=4700441830087810a0009804c3d84267041160010703e9049fd900d8a0244f862eeb003f01593a0007a50c01288ae0411600b80250d049f4cdc

01a006408bf64d008fc005881d005ee9c031cc01381c81402770369041140100022fe10c2d31c00f085ba920549f303081d309800000107113e521042

2804a3cc48fab01400134824814a6ee003d040b1006201a00c434988210064a4f3c0a61f5a0835000ac114180300490 7d2d17e6f13099c113e90149204

b80401890044fac01124814700441974a5041aa005608a0a01802484620cc9040ac0056904404000038990a1f17e601046807430349a58150c28a2b3a

52941794 1f7ad040d7040d42804f8004c00f1001600645125949018960 04cb01e0ed6e006e081a400cc01993124202a02748184a5c0c2158408badeae

f4e50eba48403be4c21861358668182d09183dbdf37e0816808007690074031417c06e42e05c0744d412908ecce064e55f4e1b177a9242259b3e5fbf

98940819800c099c04c3001b809834033010ac4700441a9a03b4b801f00e8ac480c267602e330042bbaa0056081880186007008228006121a1a4b70

0ac04e9412897d20391802b235ee33dc7040330 05c9004a00ac040030f80503496 58e1852e829899944 0b6e0302596352bbf0c0805600a0004800c0

04c3402726c01b96028dcf38fb9a4a1860250222c65f4108219995907 2b5a8b00cc07485a58127f711a961a6d992156e91a4dc089f48015 2a24c00b4

306e042fa2dc09e7fa2083c80191c84164d141986ca5006a0310d01c4700441b006059587 9696f0103f43fba09a4221931018 90094c199c3eb096430

09034124015562 1a4602182963620169340090c81904bf6ee05470856a380c4090693aac9658fab2b00f644a9 12eef03203b024980d01df3 13509260

0f665231a1704a9819bb988639337 01b8e485d512f80484fa604704c17006209776821 7b8e0b4ca4a013869e4eaa74a4908d40321b80fcc95036e200

749412406fc412a549089981 17f0023605958796 96f0103f43fba09a4221931018900 94c199605958796 96f0103f43fba0605958

Figure 6A.5   An example of a frame to be sent by a node in multimedia streaming simulations.

is 297 megabytes. The YUV format cannot be used in WMSNs because the size of frames is very large. To overcome this problem, the researchers applied a multimedia encoder to encode the video files into the standard encoding format used in RTP protocol. The standard RTP encoding is moving picture experts group (MPEG). In the current work, the FFmpeg [59] encoder was used to convert video files to MPEG format. The FFmpeg encoder is a cross-platform solution for recording, converting, and streaming audio and video files. The following commands are used to convert both videos using the FFmpeg encoder.

```
ffmpeg -s cif -i container_cif.yuv -qscale 7 -r 40 container.mpeg
ffmpeg -s cif -i bridge-far_cif.yuv -qscale 7 -r 40 bridge-far.mpeg
```

The –qscale was equal to 7 to reduce the quality of the video from 10 to 7. The –r was set equal to 40, as 40 is the number of frames per second. The previous command was achieved after several trials, as FFmpeg has about 70 parameters to be used while converting video files.

The newly produced sizes for both videos were 1.4 megabytes for the file Container and 5.9 megabytes for the file Bridge (Close). After converting files into MPEG format, these files were used in the NS2 simulation. One of the frames is shown in Figure 6A.5.

References

1. Akyildiz, I.F., Vuran, M.C. *Wireless sensor networks*, First Edition, John Wiley and Sons, New Jersey, USA, 2010.
2. Sohraby, K., Minoli, D., Znati, T. *Wireless sensor networks: Technology, protocols, and applications*, First Edition, John Wiley and Sons, New Jersey, USA, 2007.
3. Akyildiz, I.F., Su, W., Sankarasubramaniam, Y., Cayirci, E. A survey on sensor networks, *IEEE Communications Magazine*, 40(8), 102–114, 2002.
4. Gupta, A.K., Sadawart, H., Verma, A.K. Performance analysis of AODV, DSR & TORA routing protocols, *International Journal of Engineering and Technology*, 2(2), 226–231, 2010.
5. Prasanna, S., Rao, S. An overview of wireless sensor networks applications and security, *International Journal of Soft Computing and Engineering*, 2(2), 2231–2307, 2012.
6. Prabh, K.S. Real-time wireless sensor networks, *PhD Thesis*, Faculty of the School of Engineering and Applied Science, University of Virginia, May 2007.

7. Lu, C., Blum, B.M., Abdelzaher, T.F., Stankovic, J.A., He, T. RAP: A real-time communication architecture for large-scale wireless sensor networks. In: *IEEE Real-Time and Embedded Technology and Application Symposium*, IEEE, San Jose, CA, USA, pp. 55–67, September 2002.

8. He, T., Stankovic, J.A., Lu, C., Abdelzaher, T.F. SPEED: A real-time routing protocol for sensor networks, *Technical Report CS-2002-09*, Virginia Polytechnic Institute and State University, Virginia, USA, March 2002.

9. Sinha, A., Chandrakasan, A. Dynamic power management in wireless sensor networks, *IEEE Design and Test of Computers*, 18(2), 62–74, 2001.

10. Mottola, L., Picco, G. Programming wireless sensor networks: fundamental concepts and state of the art, *ACM Computing Surveys*, 43(3), 1–51, 2011.

11. Abdelzaher, T., Blum, B., Cao, Q., Chen, Y., Evans, D., George, J., George, S. et al. EnviroTrack: Towards an environmental computing paradigm for distributed sensor networks. In: *24th International Conference on Distributed Computing Systems*, Department of Computer science and Engineering, Ohio State University, Tokyo, Japan, pp. 582–589, 2004.

12. Mohammadi, S.H., Jadidoleslamy, H. A comparison of link layer attacks on wireless sensor networks, *International Journal on Applications of Graph Theory in Wireless Ad Hoc Networks and Sensor Networks*, 3(1), 69–84, 2011.

13. Stallings, W. *Cryptography and network security*, Fourth Edition, Prentice Hall, New Jersey, USA, 2006.

14. Agrawal, M. A comparative survey on symmetric key encryption techniques, *International Journal on Computer Science and Engineering*, 4(5), 877–882, 2012.

15. Koblitz, N., Menezes, A.J. A survey of public-key cryptosystems, *SIAM Review*, 46(4), 599–634, 2004.

16. Black, J.R. Message authentication codes, *PhD Thesis*, Computer Science Department, University Of California, California, USA, 2000.

17. Bakhtiari, S., Safavi-Naini, R., Pieprzyk, J. Cryptographic hash functions: A survey, *Technical Report TR 95-09*, Computer Science Department, University of Wollongong, New South Wales, USA, 1995.

18. Sandström, H. A survey of the denial of service problem, *Master Thesis*, Computer Science and Electrical Engineering Department, Lulea University of Technology, Kiruna, Sweden, 2001.

19. Cayirci, E., Rong, C. *Security in wireless ad hoc and sensor networks*, First Edition, John Wiley and Sons, New Jersey, USA, 2009.

20. Kavitha, T., Sridharan, D. Security vulnerabilities in wireless sensor networks: A survey, *Journal of Information Assurance and Security*, 5(1), 31–44, 2009.

21. Deng, J., Han, R., Mishra, S. Defending against path-based DoS attacks in wireless sensor networks. In: *3rd ACM Conference on Security of Ad Hoc and Sensor Networks*, Association for Computing Machinery, New York, NY, USA, pp. 89–96, November 2005.

22. Singh, V.P., Jain, S., Singhai, J. Hello flood attack and its countermeasures in wireless sensor networks, *International Journal of Computer Science Issues*, 7(11), 23–27, 2010.

23. Karlof, C., Wagner, D. Secure routing in wireless sensor networks: Attacks and countermeasures, *Ad Hoc Networks*, 1(3), 293–315, 2003.

24. Huang, J.H., Buckingham, J., Han, R. A level key infrastructure for secure and efficient group communication in wireless sensor network. In: *1st International Conference on Security and Privacy for Emerging Areas in Communications Networks*, IEEE, Athens, Greece, pp. 249–260, September 2005.

25. Brownfield, M., Yatharth, G., Nathaniel D. Wireless sensor network denial of sleep attack. In: *6th Annual IEEE Systems, Man and Cybernetics (SMC) Information Assurance Workshop*, IEEE, New York, NY, USA, pp. 356–364, June 2005.

26. Rgheff, A., Ali, M. Fundamentals of spread-spectrum techniques, 2007. Last accessed May 2013. http://v5.books.elsevier.com/bookscat/samples/9780750652520/9780750652520.pdf

27. Islam, M.R. Error correction codes in wireless sensor network: An energy aware approach, *International Journal of Computer and Information Engineering*, 4(1), 59–64, 2010.

28. Li, M., Prabhakaran, B. MAC layer admission control and priority re-allocation for handling QoS guarantees in non-cooperative wireless LANs, *Mobile Networks and Applications*, 10(6), 947–959, 2005.

29. Cho, J., Lee, J., Kwon, T., Choi, Y. Directional antenna at sink (DAAS) to prolong network lifetime in wireless sensor networks. In: *12th European Wireless Conference for Enabling Technologies on Wireless Multimedia Communications*, IEEE, Athens, Greece, pp. 1–5, April 2006.

30. Hue, J. Deluge 2.0 - TinyOS network programming, 2005. Last accessed May 2013. http://www.cs.berkeley.edu/~jwhui/deluge/deluge-manual.pdf.

31. Hyun, S., Ning, P., Liu, A., Du, W. Seluge: Secure and DoS-resistant code dissemination in wireless sensor networks. In: *7th International Conference on Information Processing in Sensor Networks*, New York, NY, USA, pp. 445–456, April 2008.

32. Pathan, A.K. *Security of self-organizing networks: MANET, WSN, WMN, VANET.* First Edition, Auerbach Publications, 2010.

33. Karlof, C., Sastry, N., Wagner, D. TinySec: A link layer security architecture for wireless sensor networks. In: *2nd International Conference on Embedded Networked Sensor Systems*, Association for Computing Machinery, New York, NY, USA, pp. 162–175, November 2004.

34. Luk, M., Mezzour, G., Perrig, A., Gligor, V. MiniSec: A secure sensor network communication architecture. In: *6th International Conference on Information Processing in Sensor Networks*, Association for Computing Machinery, New York, MA, USA, pp. 479–488, April 2007.

35. Liu, A., Ning, P. TinyECC: A configurable library for elliptic curve cryptography in wireless sensor networks. *Technical Report TR-2007-36*, Department of Computer Science, North Carolina State University, North Carolina, USA, November 2007.

36. Casado, L., Tsigas, P. ContikiSec: A secure network layer for wireless sensor networks under the Contiki operating system. In: *14th Nordic Conference on Secure IT Systems*, Springer - International Publisher Science, Oslo, Norway, pp. 133–147, October 2009.

37. Black, J., Rogaway, P. CBC MACs for arbitrary-length messages: The three-key constructions, *Journal of Cryptology*, 18(2), pp. 111–132, 2005.

38. Mahmoud, N. Securing real-time video over IP transmission, *Master Thesis*, Department of Information Technology, Cairo University, Giza, Egypt, May 2009.

39. Yasmin, R. An efficient authentication framework for wireless sensor networks, *PhD Thesis*, College of Engineering and Physical Sciences, The University of Birmingham, Birmingham, UK, November 2012.

40. Schulzrinne, H., Casner, S., Frederick, R., Jacobson, V. RFC 1889 – RTP: A transport protocol for real-time applications, *Internet Engineering Task Force*, IETF RFC 1889, January 1996.

41. Fitzek, F., Reisslein, M. A prefetching protocol for continuous media streaming in wireless environments, *IEEE Journal on Selected Areas in Communications*, 19(6), pp. 2015–2028, 2001.

42. Levis, P., Madden, S., Gay, D., Polastre, J., Szewczyk, R., Whitehouse, K., Woo, A. et al. TinyOS: An operating system for sensor networks. In: *Ambient Intelligence*, Springer-Verlag, New York, NY, USA, pp. 115–148, 2004.

43. Eriksson, J. Detailed simulation of heterogeneous wireless sensor networks, Department of Information Technology, Uppsala University, PhD Thesis, Thunbergsvägen, Sweden, April 2009.

44. Kellner, A., Behrends, K., Hogrefe, D. Simulation environments for wireless sensor networks, *Technical Report TR IFI-TB-2010-04*, Institute of Computer Science, Georg-August University, Göttingen, Germany, June 2010.

45. Sobeih, A., Chen, W., Hou, J.C., Kung, L., Li, N., Lim, H., Tyan, H. et al. J-Sim: A simulation and emulation environment for wireless sensor networks. *IEEE Wireless Communications Magazine*, 13(4), 104–19, 2006.

46. Xue, Y., Lee, H.S., Yang, M., Kumarawadu, P., Ghenniwa, H., Shen, W. Performance evaluation of ns-2 simulator for wireless sensor networks. In: *Canadian Conference on Electrical and Computer Engineering*, IEEE, Vancouver, BC, Canada, pp. 1372–1375, April 2007.

47. Khater, J. NS-2 simulation based study of E2E video streaming over ultra-wideband (UWB) wireless mesh networks, *Master Thesis*, Athens Information Technology, Peania, Athens, 2006.

48. Khan, A., Lingfeng, S., Ifeachor, E. Impact of video content on video quality for video over wireless networks. In: *5th International Conference on Autonomic and Autonomous Systems*, Valencia, Spain, pp. 277–282, May 2009.

49. Lee, J., Kapitanova, K., Son, S.H. The price of security in wireless sensor networks, *Computer Networks*, 54(17), pp. 2967–2978, 2010.

50. Wang, Y., Attebur, G., Ramamurthy, B. A survey of security issues in wireless sensor networks, *IEEE Communications Surveys and Tutorials*, 8(2), pp. 2–23, 2006.
51. Bala, S., Secure routing in wireless sensor networks, *Master Thesis*, Computer and Engineering department, Thapar University, Punjab, India, May 2009.
52. Tieyan, L., Hongjun, W., Xinkai, W., Feng, B. SenSec design, sensor network flagship project, *Technical Report TR v1.0*, InfoComm Security Department, Institute for Infocomm Research in Singapore, February 2005.
53. Faylor, C. Cygwin, 1995. Last accessed May 2013. http://www.cygwin.com/
54. Yan, S.F. How to implement protocol in NS2. Last accessed May 2013. http://netlab.cse.yzu.edu.tw/ns2/html/chu-workshop/session2-2.pdf
55. The Vint Project. Network Simulator - ns-2, 1989. Last accessed May 2013. http://www.isi.edu/nsnam/ns/
56. Bider, D. Crypto ++ library, 2007. Last accessed May 2013. http://www.cryptopp.com/
57. Chih-Heng, K., Shieh, C., Hwang, W., Ziviani, A. An Evaluation Framework for More Realistic Simulations of MPEG Video Transmission, *Journal of Information Science and Engineering*, 24(2), pp. 425–440, 2008.
58. National Science Foundation, Arizona State University. YUV Video Sequences Datasets, 2000. Last accessed May 2013. http://trace.eas.asu.edu/yuv/
59. Bellard, F. FFmpeg: Software to record, convert and stream audio and video, 2004. Last accessed May 2013. http://www.ffmpeg.org/

7

POWER MANAGEMENT FOR WIRELESS MULTIMEDIA SENSOR NETWORKS

RAGHIED MOHAMMED ATTA

Contents

Wireless multimedia sensor networks (WMSNs) cover several branches of communication, computation with signal processing, and control with embedded computing. This cross-disciplinary research field enables distributed systems of heterogeneous embedded devices that sense, interact, and control the physical environment. There are several factors that mainly influence the design of WMSNs, such as high bandwidth demand, integration with other wireless technologies, and power consumption.

Batteries have been the source of energy for most mobile, embedded, and remote system applications. To prolong the lifetime of batteries, hardware power optimizations have been the focus of a vast amount of research in WMSNs. This research includes dynamic optimization of voltage and clock rate, wake-up procedures to keep power-consuming electronics inactive most of the time, and energy-optimized protocol development for sensor communications.

It is clear that alternative sources of energy to power up WMSNs are required. There is a need to supply energy to prolong the lifetime of a system with self-powered devices that use energy-harvesting techniques. Such energy supply might be achieved by extracting energy from the environment where the sensor itself lies, which offers another important means to prolong the lifetime of sensor devices. There are various forms of energy that can be harvested, such as thermal, mechanical, magnetic, solar, acoustic, wind, and water.

Collecting energy from the background environment might provide an additional source of energy to help prolong the lifetime of the sensor devices. However, it will yield power that is several orders of magnitude lower compared to the power consumption of state-of-the-art multimedia devices.

In this chapter, we will look into various ways of optimizing the power consumption of existing WMSNs. We will also identify various unconventional sources of energy that can be harvested based on the available techniques and compare their advantages.

7.1 Introduction

A WMSN is defined as a network of wireless embedded devices that allow retrieval of audio and video streams, images, and scalar sensor data from the physical environment. More recently, there have been rapid improvements in miniaturization of inexpensive hardware such as CMOS cameras and microphones that are able to universally capture multimedia content from the environment; a single sensor device module has enhanced the development of WMSNs [1,2].

A critical issue for most of the applications for which WMSNs are installed is battery replacement; therefore, battery lifetime would ideally be unlimited [3]. The energy capacity of batteries has doubled roughly every 35 years [4]. To a large extent, this development has accelerated in recent years, due to the needs of portable electronic devices; however, the rate of improvement is still fairly slow compared to Moore's law.

Therefore, power consumption is a fundamental concern in WMSNs, even more than in traditional wireless sensor networks (WSNs). In traditional sensor nodes, energy consumption is dominated by communication functions, while multimedia applications produce large amounts of data, which require high transmission rates with large bandwidth and extensive processing. Thus, both power and bandwidth are even more constrained than for other types of WSNs. In the meantime, the faster processors used in WMSNs tend to require more power to operate. It is necessary to come up with techniques to reduce and manage power consumption in high-speed networks.

Sensing power varies with the nature of applications. In applications such as environmental and habitat monitoring, WMSNs are positioned in remote and inaccessible regions such as mountains, forests, deserts, and rural areas to collect multimedia information for an extended duration. Such applications typically consume more energy than in the case of traditional WSNs. Irregular sensing might consume less power than constant event monitoring; however, the complexity of event detection also plays a crucial role in determining power consumption. For example, for the visual processing component, which focuses on detecting and characterizing events within a node camera's field of view, the more images acquired, the more accurate its decision of whether or not an event worth reporting is needed. However, the more images are taken, the more power will be consumed. Higher ambient noise levels might also cause significant corruption and increase detection complexity.

The collapse of a few nodes in the network because of power loss can cause significant topological changes and might require rerouting of packets and reorganization of the network. Therefore, the following issues are critical: a proper management strategy for residual energy; an optimal choice of energy-aware routing protocols, algorithms, and architectures; adequate topological placement of the sensors to maximize the network lifetime; and an efficient energy-harvesting mechanism from the deployment environment [5]. Consequently, there have been investigations into lowering the energy consumption of wireless networks. Researchers have concentrated on developing low-power techniques at all levels, from designing energy-efficient circuits [6] to adapting central processing unit (CPU) frequencies [7] and enhancing network protocols [8].

Another important aspect addressed in WMSNs is whether it is more efficient to send the full video stream or to perform the processing on board, hence saving bandwidth by transmitting only a higher level representation of the data. To make such decisions, it is necessary to know all the information about the power budget of the nodes involved, the power consumed by different operations involved, and the application performance requirements.

7.2 Energy Characterization

WMSN nodes have four major components:

- A microcontroller (MCU), consisting of the processor itself, memory (RAM and flash), and associated hardware
- A radio system, consisting of wireless communication circuitry and an antenna
- A sensor system, consisting of multimedia sensing devices
- A power supply subsystem, consisting of the battery, a DC–DC converter, and an energy harvester

These different components can be in different states. A set of basic operations can be considered representative of tasks performed by a sensor node. These operations consist of five main task categories, namely idle, processing intensive, storage intensive, communication intensive, and visual sensing [9].

1. Idle: Idle state behavior consumes energy when the node runs basic operating system tasks. In addition to characterizing energy consumption when the system is idle, this task also serves as a reference for all other tasks.
2. Processing intensive: Fast Fourier transform, an industry-standardized CPU-intensive efficient algorithm, is used to characterize processing-intensive tasks.
3. Storage intensive: The storage media is a memory that can store and recall files as input parameters.
4. Communication intensive: Energy consumed by communication-related tasks can be characterized by transmitting a certain amount of random bytes to the server.
5. Visual sensing: To characterize power consumed by the webcam, a sequence of frames is acquired.

Analysis of the energy consumption profile helps with the selection of hardware components for multimedia applications.

7.2.1 Microcontroller

Most WMSN computing subsystems are implemented as fully static CMOS MCU devices, which operate at frequencies ranging from very low (1 kHz) to a maximum speed of 1 MHz at 1.8 V, to 100 MHz at 5 V depending on the technology. The current drawn at 32 kHz is about 100 μA, when the MCU is running continuously, which is not sufficient to achieve multiyear battery life. In this case, it is necessary that the MCU be put into a power-savings mode, such as idle, sleep, or stop mode.

When the MCU is built entirely of clocked CMOS logic circuitry, the current consumption is a linear function of clock speed, with zero offset current. However, in modern mixed-mode MCUs, the flash-based type is packed with analog circuitry. Therefore, the total current consumed when the MCU is active is composed of two elemental components: static and dynamic current. The dynamic current consumption is the current change when clock frequency changes. The static current is the current that has different components that are independent of operating frequency; they are analog-block current, flash-module current, and leakage current.

Independent of the MCU clock frequency, most analog blocks have a significant current drain when they are powered. The flash memory typically draws current to power the array and read from the flash cell, which in some cases draws more current than the CPU itself, especially at low clock speed. The leakage current depends very much on the fabrication process technology.

In active mode, static current can reach 10 times as high as that in the power-savings mode. To minimize the active static current, the WMSN must operate at a low duty cycle, which means that faster speed results in more power savings. In addition, as lithography advances for low-voltage submicron technology, the dynamic current goes down, while the static leakage current tends to increases. Thus, for more advanced fabrication technologies, low duty-cycle operation is more beneficial. Table 7.1 shows the power consumption of the most popular CPU installed in standard sensor nodes [10].

7.2.2 Radio Communication System

Radio frequency (RF) communication requires modulation, band pass filtering, and multiplexing circuitry, which makes it more complex and power hungry. The path loss of the transmitted signal between two sensor nodes can be as high as the fourth-order exponent of the distance between them. Nevertheless, RF communication is preferred in most of the ongoing sensor network research projects, because the packets conveyed in sensor networks are small, data rates are low, and the frequency reuse is high due to short communication distances [11].

Several factors affect the power consumption characteristics of the communication system. These include the type of modulation scheme, data transfer rate, transmit power, and the operational duty cycle. Additionally, as device sizes shrink, wireless power consumption is becoming a dominant part of device power budget [12]. Communication energy consumption in both the transmitter and the receiver can be modeled as [13]

$$E_{tx} = (\alpha_t + \alpha_{amp} d^2)^* r \qquad (7.1)$$

and

$$E_{rx} = (\alpha_r {}^* r) \qquad (7.2)$$

Table 7.1 Power Consumption for Some Common CPUs

CPU	POWER SUPPLY (V)	POWER ACTIVE (mW)	POWER DOWN (μW)	SENSOR NODE
4-BIT CPU				
EM6603	1.2–3.6	0.0054	0.3	
EM6605	1.8–5.5	0.012	0.9	
8-BIT CPU				
ATtiny261V/461V/861V	1.8–5.5	*0.38 mA @ 1.8 V 1 MHz	*0.1	
PIC16F877	2.0–5.5	1.8		CIT
MC68HC05PV8A	3.3–5.0	4.4	485	
AT90LS8535	4.0–6.0	15	45	WeC Rene
ATmega163L	2.7–5.5	15		Rene2 Dot
ATMega103L	2.7–3.6	15.5	60	Mica IBadse
C8051F311	2.7–3.6	21	0.3	Parasitic
ATmega128L	2.7–5.5	26.7	83.15	Mica Mica2 Dot Mica2 BTnode
PIC18F452	2.0–5.5	40.2	24	EnOcean TCM
80C51RD+	2.7–5.5	48	150	RFRAIN
16-BIT CPU				
MSP430F149	1.8–6.0	3	15	Eyes.BSN
MSP430F1611	1.8–3.6	3	15	Telos
		1.5	6	SNoW[5]
MC68EZ326	3.3	60	60	SpotON
32-BIT CPU				
Atmel AT91 ARM Thumb	2.7–3.6	114	480	
Intel PXA271	2.6–3.8	193	1800	iMote2
Intel StrongArm SA-1100	3.0–3.6	230	25	WINS μAMPS

where E_{tx} is the energy to send r bits and E_{rx} is the energy consumed to receive r bits, α_t is the energy/bit consumed by the transmitter circuit, α_{amp} is the energy dissipated in the transmitter amplifier, α_r is the energy/bit consumed by the receiver circuit, and d is the distance that the message traverses, assuming a $1/d^2$ path loss. Table 7.2 shows power consumption of the most popular transceiver radio modules used by sensor nodes [14].

Table 7.2   Power Consumption for Some Common Radio Modules

TYPE	CLOCK (MHz)	Rx POWER (mA)	Tx POWER (mA/dBm)	POWER DOWN (µA)
LOW-POWER RADIO MODULES				
MPR300CB	916	1.8	12	1.0
SX1211	868–960		25/10	
TR1000	916	3.8	12.0/1.5	0.7
CC1000	315–915	9.6	16.5/10	1.0
MEDIUM-POWER RADIO MODULES				
nRF401	433–434	12	26/0	
CC2500	2400	12.8	21.6	
XE1205	433–915	14	33/5	0.2
CC1101	300–928	14.7	15	0.2
CC1010	315–915	16	34/0	0.2
CC2520	2400	18.5	17.4/0	<1.0
CC2420	2400	19.7	17.4/0	1.0
CC1020	402–915	19.9	19.9	0.2
CC2430	2400	19.9	19.9	
PH2401	2400	20	20	
nRF2401	2400	22	10/0	0.4
CC2400	2400	24	19/0	1.5
CC2530F32	2400	24	29/1	
RC1180	868	24	37/0	
LMX3162	2450	27	50	
STD302N-R	869	28	46.0	
MCl13191/92	2400	37	34/0	1
HIGH-POWER RADIO MODULES				
ZV4002	2400	65	65/0	140

Source: Stojcev, M.K. et al., *9th International Conference on Telecommunication in Modern Satellite, Cable, and Broadcasting Services*, © 2009 IEEE.

7.2.3 Sensing System

Sensor transducers convert physical quantities into electrical signals. According to the type of output they produce, sensors can be classified as analog or digital circuits. There exists a diversity of sensors that measure environmental parameters such as light intensity, temperature, humidity, proximity, magnetic fields, acoustic, etc. In general, passive sensors such as temperature sensors consume negligible power relative to other components of the sensor node. By comparison to passive sensors, active sensors such as imagers and proximity, pressure, flow control, and level sensors usually have an acquisition time that is longer than the transmission time, especially in the case of multimedia sensors such as CCDs and CMOS image sensors; accordingly, they consume more energy than communication [15,16].

Power consumption in WMSN sensors is mainly a result of signal sampling and conversion of physical signals, signal conditioning, and analog-to-digital conversion. Sensors such as acoustic and image sensors generally require high-rate and high-resolution power-hungry analog-to-digital converters. The power consumption of the converters can account for the most significant power consumption of the sensing system [17].

Direct power consumption is not the only factor affecting the selection of sensor for use in WMSNs; several other factors need to be considered. These factors include volume, suitability for power cycling, fabrication and assembly, compatibility with other components of the system, and packaging needs. Table 7.3 lists the power consumption of some common sensors.

Sensors can be divided into five groups, as shown in Table 7.3. The on/off sensors belong to the micropower group, with power consumption less than 1 mW. The second group, referred to as "low power," is characterized by power consumption less than 10 mW and a small amount of linear signal processing. Sensors from the medium-power group have a power consumption within the range of 10 to 50 mW and are realized with mixed circuits (analog and digital electronics). The sensors in the high-power group are enabled with some kind of dedicated signal processor, making the sensors of this group smart devices. The power consumption of this group is from 50 mW to 1 W. The last group, the ultra-high-power group, is characterized by consumption that is greater than 1 W. Due to higher power consumption in the last two groups, harvesting electronics are usually essential [18].

Table 7.4 provides an overview of the power consumption of multimedia sensors by comparing the power consumed by four classes of cameras, from very low-power, low-resolution cameras, to web cameras, to advanced, high-resolution cameras are available commercially. At the lowest end of the spectrum is the tiny Cyclops [19], which consumes a mere 46 mW and can capture low-resolution video. CMUcams [20] are cell-phone-class cameras with onboard processing for motion detection, histogram computation, and so on.

Table 7.3 Power Consumption for Some Common Sensors

SENSOR TYPE	SENSING	POWER CONSUMPTION (mW)
MICRO POWER		
SFH 5711	Light sensor	0.09
DSW98A	Smoke alarm	0.108
SFH 7741	Proximity	0.21
SFH 7740	Optical switch	0.21
ISL29011	Light sensor	0.27
STCN75	Temperature	0.4
LOW POWER		
TSL2550	Light sensor	1.155
ADXL202JE	Accelerometer	2.4
SHT 11	Humidity/ temperature	2.75
MS55ER	Barometric pressure	3
QST108KT6	Touch	7
SG-LINK(IOOOΩ)	Strain gauge	9
MEDIUM-POWER		
SG-LINK(350Q)	Strain gauge	24
iMEMS	Accelerometer	30
OV7649	CCD	44
2200/2600 series	Pressure	50
HIGH POWER		
TI50	Humidity	90
DDT-651	Motion detector	150
EM-005	Proximity	180
BES 516-371-S49	Proximity	180
EZ/EV-18M	Proximity	195
GPS-9546	GPS	198
LUC-M10	Level sensor	300
CP18.VL18.GM60	Proximity	350
TDA0161	Proximity	420
ULTRA HIGH POWER		
FCS-GL1/2A4- AP8X-H1141	Flow control	1250
FCBEX11D	CCD	1900/2800
XC56BB	CCD	2200

Source: Stojcev, M.K. et al., *9th International Conference on Telecommunication in Modern Satellite, Cable, and Broadcasting Services*, © 2009 IEEE.

Table 7.4 Power Consumption and Capabilities of Four Classes of Camera Sensors

MULTIMEDIA SENSOR	POWER USED FOR IMAGE CAPTURING	IMAGE CAPTURING CAPABILITY
Cyclops	42 mW	Fixed-angle lens, 352 × 288 at 10 fps
CMUcam	200 mW	Fixed-angle lens, 352 × 288 up to 60 fps
Webcam	200 mW	Auto-focus lens, 640 × 480 at 30 fps
High-end PTZ camera	1 W	PTZ lens, 1024 × 768 up to 30 fps

Source: Margi, C.B. et al., *Proceedings of 24th Brazilian Symposium on Computer Networks*, 2006.

Table 7.5 Average Power Requirements in Watts

SYSTEM STATE	POWER
Idle	1.473
CPU loop	2.287
Camera with CPU	3.049
Camera in sleep mode with CPU	1.617
Networking on with CPU	2.557
Camera, networking, CPU	4.280
Capture running	5.268
Sleep	0.058

Source: Soro, S., Heinzelman, W., *Advances in Multimedia*, pp. 1–22, 2009.

At the high end, webcams can capture high-resolution video at a full frame rate while consuming 200 mW, whereas pan–tilt–zoom cameras are retargetable sensors that produce high-quality video while consuming 1 W. An interesting example of power consumption for different tasks performed by a camera node is shown in Table 7.5 [21,22]. Each task has an associated cost and execution time.

7.2.4 Batteries System

From the system's point of view, a good microbattery should have the following features [23]:

- High energy density
- Rechargeable, in case the system has an energy harvester
- Small cell potential (0.5–1.0 V), such that digital circuits might take advantage of the quadratic reduction in power consumption with supply voltage

- Efficiently divided into series batteries to provide a variety of cell potentials for various components of the system without requiring voltage converters
- Large active volume-to-packaging ratio

Three small cell chemistries are currently dominating the application market for WMSNs: lithium–ion (Li-ion), nickel–metal hydride (NiMH), and lithium polymer (Li-polymer) [24]. Each of these battery types has its advantages and disadvantages for use in a node. The first step in selecting a cell for a node is to study the specific characteristics of each cell in terms of voltage, charging time, discharging rates, cycles, load current, and energy density. Following is a brief overview of the characteristics, advantages, and disadvantages of each of the three cell chemistries. The crucial battery parameters are given in Tables 7.6 and 7.7 [25].

Lithium–ion (Li-ion): The Li-ion battery has a nominal voltage of 3.6 V, 1000 duty cycles per lifetime, less than 1 C optimal load current,

Table 7.6 Battery Parameters

VOLTAGE	NOMINAL CELL VOLTAGE
Capacity	The amount of electrical charge that can be stored
Specific energy	The volume-related content, measured in energy/weight
Energy density	The volume-related content, measured in energy/volume
Internal resistance	Characterizes the ability to handle a specific load
Self-discharge	The internal leakage and aging effects
Recharge cycles	The number of charge cycles before performance degrades
Charging procedure	Type of charge circuit required

Source: Stojcev, M.K. et al., *9th International Conference on Telecommunication in Modern Satellite, Cable, and Broadcasting Services*, © 2009 IEEE.

Table 7.7 Battery Types

BATTERY TYPE	VOLTAGE (V)	ENERGY DENSITY (Wh/dm^3)	SPECIFIC ENERGY (Wh/kg)	SELF-DISCHARGE PER MONTH (%)
Lead–acid	2.0	60–75	30–40	3–20
Nickel–cadmium	1.2	50–150	40–60	10
Nickel–metal hydride	1.2	140–300	30–80	30
Lithium-ion	3.6	270	160	5
Lithium polymer	3.7	300	130–200	1–2

Source: Stojcev, M.K. et al., *9th International Conference on Telecommunication in Modern Satellite, Cable, and Broadcasting Services*, © 2009 IEEE.

an average energy density of 160 Wh/kg, a charging time of less than 4 hours, a typical discharge rate of approximately 10% per month when stored, and a rigid form factor. These characteristics make the Li-ion battery a good option when requirements include lower weight, higher energy density or aggregate voltage, and a greater number of duty cycles and when the price is not critical. To increase the voltage, Li-ion battery systems can be connected with up to seven series cells, resulting in a maximum aggregate voltage of 25.2 V [26].

Nickel–metal hydride (NiMH): The NiMH battery has a nominal voltage of 1.25 V, 500 duty cycles per lifetime, less than 0.5 C optimal load current, an average energy density of 100 Wh/kg, less than 4-hour charge time, a typical discharge rate of approximately 30% per month when in storage, and a rigid form factor. NiMH battery systems excel when lower voltage requirements or price sensitivities are primary considerations in cell selection. To increase the voltage, NiMH systems can be connected with up to ten series cells, resulting in a maximum aggregate voltage of 12.5 V [26].

Lithium polymer (Li-polymer): The Li-polymer battery has a nominal voltage of 3.6 V, 500 duty cycles per lifetime, less than 1 C optimal load current, an average energy density of 160 Wh/kg, less than a 4-hour charge time, a typical discharge rate of less than 10% per month when in storage, and a semi-rigid form factor. To increase the voltage, Li-ion cells can be connected with up to seven series cells, resulting in a maximum aggregate voltage of 25.2 V [26]. Li-polymer cells have a similar performance to Li-ion cells, but have the advantage of being packaged in a slightly flexible form as long as it remains flat when installed in a device.

7.3 Power Management Techniques

Various power management techniques are used to reduce the power consumption in different types of networks. Many of these techniques are used in common practice to reduce the power of devices in WMSNs. Doing so requires the use of a structured, interconnect-oriented design methodology at all layers, starting from the application layer all the way down to the physical layer of a networking protocol stack.

7.3.1 Application Layer

At the application layer, different techniques can be used to reduce the power consumption in a wireless device. In a load-partitioning technique, the application has the option to perform all of its power-intensive computations at the base station rather than locally. The wireless device sends a request for the computation to be performed and then waits for the result to be received. Another technique uses proxies to inform an application about battery power changes. Applications use this information to limit their functionality to provide only their most essential features and eliminate some unnecessary visual effects that accompany a process [27].

These techniques can be adapted to work with most applications that wish to support them. A number of other techniques also exist for specific classes of applications. Two such common applications are database operations and video processing. For database systems, techniques are able to reduce power consumed during data retrieval, indexing, and querying operations. In these cases, energy is conserved by reducing the number of transmissions needed to perform such operations.

For video-processing applications, energy is conserved by reducing the number of bits transmitted over the wireless channels using compression techniques. However, performing the compression itself may consume more power than that saved in transmission. Other techniques that slightly degrade video quality have been explored to reduce the power even further [28].

7.3.2 Transport Layer

All the various techniques used to conserve energy at the transport layer work by reducing the number of retransmissions necessary due to packet losses because of a faulty wireless link. In a wired network, packet losses indicate congestion, requiring back-off mechanisms to account for it. In wireless networks, however, packet losses can occur sporadically, which does not necessarily indicate the onset of congestion. With this knowledge in mind, TCP-Probing [29] and Wave and Wait protocols [30] have been developed as replacements for traditional TCP. They guarantee end-to-end data delivery with high throughput and low power consumption.

Congestion control is another important issue that should be considered in transport protocols. Congestion is an essential problem in WSNs. It not only wastes scarce energy due to a large number of retransmissions and packet drops, but also hampers the event detection reliability. Congestion in WMSNs has a direct impact on energy efficiency and application quality of service. Two types of congestion can occur in sensor networks [31]. The first type is node-level congestion that is caused by buffer overflow in the node, which can result in packet loss and increased queuing delay. Not only can packet loss degrade reliability and application quality of service, but it can also waste the limited node energy and degrade link utilization. In each sensor node, when the packet arrival rate exceeds the packet service rate, buffer overflow may occur. It is more likely to occur at sensor nodes close to the sink, as they usually carry more combined upstream traffic. The second type of congestion is link-level congestion related to the wireless channels, which are shared by several nodes using protocols such as CSMA/CD (Carrier Sense, Multiple Access with Collision Detection). In this case, collisions can occur when multiple active sensor nodes try to seize the channel at the same time. To avoid the negative aspects of congestion in WMSNs, congestion must be effectively controlled. Each congestion control solution consists of three important parts: congestion detection, congestion notification, and rate adjustment [32].

In traditional TCP protocol, congestion is detected at the end nodes based on a time-out or redundant acknowledgments. In general, link-by-link congestion detection in sensor networks has better performance than traditional end-to-end congestion detection using time-out or duplicate acknowledgment. Thus, in sensor networks, proactive methods are used, based on some form of congestion indicator. Different congestion indicators have been proposed, such as queue length [33], packet service time, or the ratio of packet service time to packet interarrival time at the intermediate nodes [34]. After detecting congestion, to prevent the negative aspects of congestion in the networks, the transport protocol needs to propagate congestion information from the congested node to the upstream sensor nodes or the source nodes that contribute to congestion. This can be done explicitly by sending a special control message to the other sensors, or implicitly by using a piggybacking technique in data packets.

When a node receives a congestion notification message, it will adjust its transmission rate using a rate control technique such as additive increase multiplicative decrease.

7.3.3 Network Layer

Power management techniques at the network layer level are responsible for performing power-efficient routing through a multihop network [35,36]. Despite the large volume of research activities and the significant progress made in recent years, routing in WMSNs still harbors many open issues that need to be resolved [37]. Because an idle receive circuit can consume almost as much power as an active transmitter, a good power-saving technique should permit as many nodes as possible to turn their radio receivers off most of the time. At the same time, it should forward packets between source and destination with almost the same delay as if all nodes were awake. This expectation implies that enough nodes should be awake to form a connected network.

The protocols used for the network layer are typically backbone-based, topology-control-based, or a hybrid of the two. In a backbone-based protocol, some nodes must remain active all the time to form a backbone, while others might sleep periodically. The backbone nodes will establish a path between all source and destination nodes in the network. This design means that paths that could operate without interference in the original network should be represented in the backbone. Therefore, any node in the network, including backbone nodes themselves, must be within one hop of at least one backbone node. The power savings is achieved by permitting nonbackbone nodes to sleep periodically, as well as by periodically choosing which nodes in fact make up the backbone. The algorithm for picking this backbone should be distributed, requiring each node to make a local decision. Furthermore, the backbone nodes should provide about as much total capacity as the original network, otherwise congestion may increase.

Each node in the network periodically makes local decisions on whether to sleep or stay awake as a coordinator to participate in the forwarding backbone structure. A node volunteers to become a coordinator if it discovers, using information gathered from local broadcast messages, that two of its neighbors are not communicating with each other directly or through existing coordinators. This provision will preserve the capacity of the network. To keep the number of redundant coordinators low, each node delays announcing its willingness to become a coordinator by a random time interval. The length of this time interval considers two factors: the amount of remaining battery charge and the number of pairs of neighbors that can connect together. This role will rotate among all nodes, ensuring, with high probability, a capacity-preserving connected backbone at any point in time, where nodes lean to consume power at about the same rate.

Backbone-based protocols, such as ASCENT [38] and SPAN [39], utilize local information to assess the connectivity of a node with its neighbors and then decide whether or not the node should stay active to join a communication backbone. These protocols concentrate on maintaining continuous connectivity of the network and are best suited for high data rate ad hoc multihop networks.

Topology-based routing protocols can achieve power savings differently. Their goal is to reduce the transmission power by making all nodes operate with their lowest possible transmission power, such that the network just remains connected. In a homogeneous network, this design would mean that the all nodes adjust their transmission powers so that they are just within the range of their nearest one-hop neighbor. In heterogeneous networks, the transmission powers will be adjusted based on the needs of that network. A summary of the different types of existing topology-based protocols is shown in Figure 7.1.

Certain location-based topology control protocols try to use the topology of the network to provide the most power-efficient communication path possible. These protocols produce a localized power-aware routing mechanism for the network. In some cases, providing

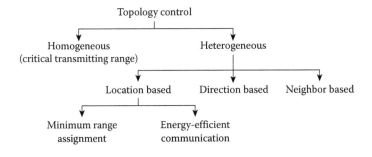

Figure 7.1   Topology-based routing protocols.

such a path means taking a larger number of hops through the network than that taken by direct transmission from one node to another. It is more energy efficient to transmit over several short distances than it is to transmit over a few long distances [40]. Short distances require less energy to transmit across and enable better signals, resulting in fewer retransmissions due to packet loss. Other power-aware routing protocols using connected dominating sets elect fewer coordinators because they actively prevent redundant coordinators using randomized slotting and damping [41].

Introducing new sensor nodes and allowing the network to self-organize and learn often offer better solutions. Such a plan allows the network to perform better in a dynamic environment according to its acquired knowledge [42]. For such dynamic networks, nodes cannot know *a priori* the optimal route to other nodes, because the paths keep changing as nodes move, enter, or leave the network. Therefore, the network protocol coordinates the discovery and tracking of routes in the network. This discovery and tracking, however, consumes energy because it requires communication between nodes. With the low data rates and fast dynamics of some nodes, the network discovery and maintenance overhead may dominate the power consumed for data transmission itself [43]. Because environmental conditions and user constraints can vary over time, the use of static algorithms and protocols can result in less than optimal energy consumption. Thus, wireless sensors must allow adaptation of underlying hardware by higher level algorithms. By giving upper layers the opportunity to adapt the hardware in response to changes in the state of the system, the user's quality constraints and the energy consumption of the node can be better controlled [44].

Finally, transmission power control schemes might be combined with backbone-based ones to produce a hybrid of both, as the benefits of these protocols can be achieved simultaneously.

7.3.4 Data Link Layer

Automatic Repeat Request (ARQ) and Forward Error Correction (FEC) schemes are the most common techniques used to conserve energy at the data link layer to reduce the transmission overhead. These schemes aim to reduce the number of packet errors at a receiving node.

By enabling ARQ, a router can directly request a retransmission of a packet from its source without first having to require the receiver node to detect if a packet error has occurred. Power-saving results have shown that occasionally it is more efficient to transmit at a lower transmission power while sending multiple ARQs than to transmit at a high transmission power and achieve better throughput. Adding FEC to ARQ codes will result in a reduction of the number of retransmissions necessary at a lower transmission power, which increases energy efficiency [27].

Another power management technique applied at the data link layer based on a packet-scheduling protocol [45] allows multiple packet transmissions to occur back to back. It might be possible to reduce the power associated with sending each packet individually. To announce the presence of sent packets on the radio channel, preamble bytes need to be sent for the first packet only, while all subsequent packets will follow this announcement. A packet-scheduling algorithm might also reduce the number of retransmissions necessary only if the packet is sent during a scheduled time when its destination is able to receive packets. By reducing the number of retransmissions necessary, the overall power consumption will consequently be reduced.

7.3.5 MAC Layer

Idle listening—the time spent listening while waiting to receive packets—is a significant cost. The energy cost for a node in idle mode is approximately the same as in receive mode. Even when no communication is taking place, a considerable amount of energy is spent searching for the next packet. In many application scenarios, the energy spent while waiting for a transmission can represent more than 90% of a node's total energy budget. It has become clear that to reduce power consumption in radios, the radio must be *turned off* during idle times (sleep) [46–47].

Power-saving techniques at the MAC layer are primarily concerned with sleep-scheduling protocols. Such protocols switch a radio's power on and off to reduce the effects of this idle listening. They are used to wake up the radio whenever it is required to transmit or receive packets; otherwise, it will sleep.

Battery-Aware MAC (BAMAC) protocol [48] decides which node should send next based on the battery level of all surrounding nodes in the network. Battery level information is attached with each transmitted packet, and decisions about sending packets from individual nodes will be based on this information.

To complete the above procedure, several challenges must be overcome. First, efficient mechanisms are needed to selectively activate sleeping nodes with the most remaining energy according to the appropriate positions around the target. Second, the activated nodes need to cooperate to distribute the required signal processing tasks with a certain quality of service, aggregate the results, and route the final decision to the base station. Third, network management can be complicated when different nodes have varying energy levels, processing capabilities, and sensing modalities [49].

Sleep-scheduling protocols are divided into two categories: synchronous and asynchronous [50,51]. Synchronous sleep-scheduling policies rely on a synchronized clock between all nodes in a network. Senders and receivers each know when the other should be on and only send packets to one another during these slotted time intervals; otherwise, they go to sleep. Slotted time division has a natural structure that leaves traffic uncorrelated and provides end-to-end fairness with high power efficiency. Global schedules can be generated with reserved bandwidth from source to sink and make it clear when to turn the radio on and off locally. Slotted time-division schemes have static global schedules that require centralized control and very precise time synchronization [52].

PAMAS (Power Aware Multi-Access Signaling) [53,54] is a synchronous solution that has proven to be very effective in reducing the power consumed by nodes by detecting when a packet on the channel is sent for someone else and putting themselves to sleep. This approach is suitable for radios in which processing a received packet is expensive compared to listening to an idle radio channel. PAMAS can be combined with some of the other sleep-scheduling protocols to produce even more power savings.

In the AFECA protocol [55], each node listens to the transmissions on the channel and maintains a count of the number of nodes within radio range. A node then switches between listening and sleeping, with randomized sleep times proportional to the number of nearby nodes with a net effect of maintaining the number of listening nodes roughly constant, regardless of node density. As the node density increases, more power can be saved. To be conservative, AFECA tends to make nodes listen even when they could be asleep if a node does not know whether it is required to listen to maintain connectivity. Setting the on/off periods based on application hints reduces both power and delay [56].

Asynchronous sleep scheduling, on the other hand, does not rely on any node clock synchronization at all. According to the MAC protocol in use, nodes can send and receive packets whenever they like. Nodes wake up and go to sleep periodically in the same way they do for synchronous sleep scheduling.

However, it has been shown that in some situations poor interaction between high-level power-saving techniques and low-level communication protocols might lead to an increase in power consumption when using these mechanisms [56]. Therefore, there must be a way to ensure that receiving nodes are awake to hear other nodes' transmissions. Precise control over the power state of the radio allows the protocol to turn off the radio between each sample. To synchronize the starting point of an incoming data stream between the transmitter and receiver, preamble bytes are sent by a packet. Once detected, the preamble will cause the receiver to search for the pending start symbol. The duty cycle of the receiver becomes proportional to the length of this preamble.

A sufficient number of extra preamble bytes are sent per packet to assure that a receiver has the chance to synchronize with it at some point. In the worst case, a packet will be transmitted just as its receiver goes to sleep, and preamble bytes will have to be sent for a time equal to the receiver's sleep interval. However, the frequency with which a receiver checks for a wake-up signal controls the amount of time that it takes for the network to wake up. Once the receiver wakes up, it will synchronize to these preamble bytes and stay on until it completely receives the packet. This protocol optimization trades power consumption by the sender for power consumption by the receiver, because the sender must transmit longer but the receiver can sample the radio channel less frequently. The optimal ratio is dependent on the communication patterns of the application.

The receiver overhead can be reduced arbitrarily at the expense of bandwidth, latency, and transmission overhead depending on application-specific goals. Moreover, based on network activity with flexible communication protocols, an application can change the protocol at runtime by exploiting the ability to tailor protocols to application-specific criteria [52].

The Low Power Listening (LPL) [57] asynchronous sleep-scheduling protocol is quickly becoming the effective standard for sleep-scheduling policies. LPL operates in a similar fashion to any other asynchronous sleep-scheduling protocol, but with one key difference. LPL turns the radio on to check for an incoming packet through the channel very quickly and reliably so that it can go back to sleep immediately afterward. The time between each of these checks is known as a check interval. LPL only achieves significant power savings if many check intervals are allowed to pass before a packet is actually detected on the channel, which makes LPL ideal for the low data rate environment in WSNs.

Another asynchronous technique known as remote access switch is used to wake up a receiver only when data are being sent for it. A low-power radio circuit is always running to detect a certain type of activity on the channel. The circuit wakes up the rest of the system for reception of a packet only when this activity is detected. However, a transmitter has to know what type of activity needs to be sent on the channel to wake each of its receivers up [35].

An event starts when a sensor node picks up a signal above a predetermined threshold power. Every node is assumed to have a uniform radius of visibility r, while in real applications the terrain might influence the visible radius. An event, such as a localized change in parameters in an environment-monitoring application, can be static or can propagate, such as signals generated by a moving object.

In general, events have a characterized distribution in space and time. There are three distinct classes of events:

- The event occurs as a stationary point.
- The event propagates at a fixed velocity.
- The event propagates at a fixed speed but in a random direction.

The processor must watch for preprogrammed wake-up signals. Prior to entering the sleep state, the CPU programs these signal conditions. The node must be able to predict the arrival of the next event to wake up on its own.

A pessimistic strategy results in some events being missed, while an optimistic prediction might result in the node waking up unnecessarily. There are two possible approaches:

1. Disallow the state completely, which will result in events being missed because the node was not alerted. If the sensing task is critical and events cannot be missed, this state must be disabled.
2. Disallow the state selectively, resulting in events being missed because the node was not alerted. This technique can be used if the events are spatially distributed and not all critical.

Both random and deterministic approaches can be used. In the clustering protocol, the cluster heads can have a disallowed state, whereas normal nodes can transit to this state, which makes the scheme more homogeneous. Every node that satisfies the sleep-threshold condition for the selectively disallowed node can enter sleep with a system defined by a probability for a certain time duration.

The advantage of this algorithm is that an energy-efficiency compromise can be made with event detection probability. By increasing this probability, the probability of missed events will increase, while the system energy consumption will be reduced, and vice versa. Hence, the overall shutdown policy is controlled by two implementation-specific probability parameters.

The protocols described here explain only some of the main sleep-scheduling protocols that have been developed to date. They do provide a good indication of the different domains to which variable sleep-scheduling protocols are most applicable.

Unlike for the energy-efficient routing protocols, it does not make sense to have a hybrid sleep-scheduling protocol based on these two techniques. The energy savings achieved using each of these techniques varies from system to system and application to application. Efforts are being made to define exactly when each technique should be used, as one technique is not better than the other in this sense.

7.3.6 Physical Layer

Techniques can be implemented at the physical layer not only to preserve energy but also to generate it. Proper hardware design techniques can decrease the level of leak currents in an electronic device due to parasitic capacitance to almost nothing [58], resulting in a longer lifetime for these devices, because they consume less power while idle. Variable clock CPUs, CPU voltage scaling, flash memory, and disk spin-down techniques can also be used to further reduce the power consumed at the physical layer [35].

Energy-harvesting techniques allow a device to actually gather energy from its surrounding environment. Ambient energy is all around in the form of vibration, strain, inertial forces, heat, light, wind, magnetic forces, and so on [59]. Energy-harvesting techniques allow this energy to be harnessed and either converted directly into usable electric current or stored for later use within an electrical system.

In the next sections, the latest technological advances in both low-power design and energy-harvesting techniques will be introduced.

7.4 Dynamic Power Management of Very Large Scale Integrated Circuit (VLSI) Systems

Power awareness can be enhanced by applying systematic techniques to VLSI systems at several levels of the system hierarchy: multipliers, register files, digital filters, dynamic voltage scaled processing, and data-gathering wireless networks. The power awareness of these systems can be significantly enhanced, leading to increases in battery lifetimes.

A related motivation for power awareness is that a well-designed system must gracefully decline in quality and performance as the available energy resources are depleted. In this context, making a scalable system refers to enabling the user to compromise the performance of the system parameters by hard-wiring them. Scalability allows the end user to implement operational policy, which often varies significantly over the lifetime of the system.

While the above argues for power awareness from a user-centric and user-visible perspective, one can also motivate this paradigm in more fundamental, system-oriented terms. With burgeoning system complexity and the accompanying increase in integration, there is more diversity in operating scenarios than ever before. Even if there is little explicit user intervention, there is an imperative to track operational diversity and scale power consumption accordingly. This necessity naturally leads to the concept of power awareness. For instance, the embedded processor that decodes the video stream in a portable multimedia terminal can display tremendous workload diversity depending on the temporal correlation of the incoming video bit stream. Hence, even if the user does not change the quality criteria, the processor must exploit this operational diversity by scaling its power as the workload changes.

Architecture and VLSI technology trends point in the direction of increasing energy budgets for register files. The key to enhancing the power awareness of register files is the observation that over a typical window of operation, a microprocessor accesses a small group of registers repeatedly, rather than the entire register file. More than 75% of the time, no more than 16 registers are accessed by the processor in a 60-instruction window. Equally importantly, there is strong locality from window to window. More than 85% of the time, fewer than five registers change from window to window.

The number of registers the processor typically needs over a certain instruction window is considered a scenario. The smaller files have lower costs of access because the switched bit-line capacitance is lower. Hence, from a power awareness perspective, over any instruction window, as small as possible a file is used.

There are significant motivations for investigating power-aware filters. As an example, consider the adaptive equalization filters that are ubiquitous in communications application-specific integrated circuits. The filtering quality requirements depend strongly on the channel conditions (line lengths, noise, and interference), the state of the system (training, continuous adaptation, freeze, etc.), the standard dictated specifications, and the quality of service desired.

All these considerations lead to tremendous scenario diversity, which a power-aware filtering system can exploit. This is because using all available time allows the frequency of the processor to be lowered, which in turn allows scaling down of the voltage, leading to significant energy savings. In terms of the power awareness framework, a scenario would be characterized by the workload. The point systems would be processors designed to manage a specific workload. As the workload changes, we would ideally want the processor designed for the instantaneous workload to execute it. It is clear that implementing such an ensemble spatially is meaningless and must be done temporally using a dynamic voltage scaling (DVS) system.

Increased levels of integration and advanced low-power techniques are enabling dedicated wireless networks of sensor nodes. Replacing high-quality sensors with such networks has several advantages, including robustness, fault tolerance, and autonomous operation for years [60].

Traditionally, energy-efficient VLSI design has been focused on low-power techniques. As the issue of energy efficiency becomes more pervasive, the policy of using the bare minimum of energy will face different challenges: semiconductor technology, circuit design, design automation tools, system architecture, operating system, and application design [61].

7.4.1 On-Chip Power Management

Interconnect wires account for a significant fraction of the power consumption in an integrated circuit that can reach up to 50% [62], which is expected to grow in future, making on-chip interconnects crucial. As the technology scales to the nanometer regime, the delay and energy consumption of global interconnect structures will be a major bottleneck for the system-on-chip (SOC) design [63,64].

A suggested approach is to use an on-chip router-based interconnect architecture, as shown in Figure 7.2 [65], similar to that adopted at the board level for interconnecting components in a wireless multimedia node [66]. In theory, the router could be a fully connected crossbar. However, every component on the chip will not need to talk

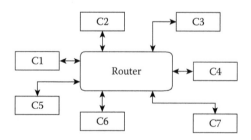

Figure 7.2 A router-based communication architecture.

to all other components; hence, it might be optimized for reduced complexity. Furthermore, optimizations can be used to reduce latency and improve crossbar utilization [67]. Other advantages of the router-based architecture are [65] as follows:

Components being isolated from each other leads to reduced capacitive loading during data transfers, which results in lower power consumption.

The increased parallelism enabled by the router results in a higher throughput, which can be further improved through the use of frequency/supply voltage scaling or other power-performance-improving techniques.

As the number of components present in the system increases, the power benefits of router-based communication architecture also increase [66]. Adopting router-based communication architecture will help future SOCs, which are expected to have a large number of components [68], which will potentially lead to significant power savings.

Researchers have just begun to investigate the merits and demerits of such an approach by analyzing and modeling the power consumption of routers and switches [69,70]. Efforts are also underway to develop modeling and simulation frameworks for on-chip communication architectures [71]. Such frameworks will enable SOC designers to quickly and efficiently explore the communication architecture design space.

7.4.2 Sensing Power Management

To reduce power consumption for the WMSNs containing power-consuming sensors, two approaches are considered: duty cycling and adaptive sensing. Duty cycling consists of powering the sensing system on only for the time needed to obtain a new set of samples, while switching it off immediately afterwards, provided that the dynamics of the sensed phenomenon are time invariant and known in advance. For fixed sampling, the rate should be computed *a priori*, which might have oversampling, inducing, in turn, waste of power. A better approach would require adopting a dynamically adaptive sensing strategy that tracks the real dynamics of the process. By reducing the number of samples, an efficient sensing strategy will also reduce the amount of data to be processed and transmitted to other network nodes. To provide effective handling of the duty-cycle issue, some aspects of the sensor drivers for the operating system must be considered. Failing to consider these aspects might result in invalid acquired data and power consumption larger than that associated with the traditional continuous powering mode. Those aspects that impact the power-managed sensor are defined by a set of functional characteristics, mainly wake-up latency and break-even cycle. The wake-up latency is defined as the time required by the sensor to produce a correct value once activated. It is clear that the active time of the sensor (t_{on}) needs to be long enough for the sensor to wake up (t_{wakeup}) and to obtain the measured information ($t_{acquire}$) [72]:

$$t_{on} \geq t_{wakeup} + t_{acquire} \tag{7.3}$$

The break-even cycle is defined as the rate at which the power consumption of a power-managed node equals that of non-power-managed node. This value is in inverse proportion to the overhead power consumption introduced by the nonideal on/off sensor transition, which represents the highest sampling rate for which applying power management is worth.

Adaptive sensing can be implemented by developing three main different approaches: hierarchical sensing, adaptive sampling sensing, and model-based active sensing, as indicated in Figure 7.3.

1. Hierarchical sensing techniques assume that multiple sensors are installed on the sensor nodes to measure the same physical quantity, each characterized by its own accuracy and

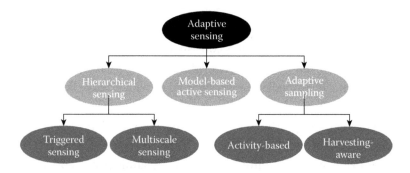

Figure 7.3   Classification of adaptive sensing strategies. (From Jeličić, V., Qualifying doctoral examination, University of Zagreb, Croatia, 2011.)

power consumption. Simple sensors are usually energy-efficient, but provide very limited resolution, whereas complex sensors can give a more accurate characterization of the sensed phenomenon at the expense of higher power consumption. At first, low-power sensors are activated to provide a coarse-grained characterization of the sensing field or to trigger an event, then accurate but power-hungry sensors can be turned on to provide measurements to improve the original coarse description. Two main approaches are used for hierarchical sensing: triggered sensing and multiscale sensing.

a. Triggered sensing [73]: Activation of the more accurate and power-consuming sensors after the low-resolution ones detect some activity within the sensed area is referred to as "triggered sensing." A central node, which supervises all the activities of the WMSN, is endowed with a triggering system.

b. Multiscale sensing [74]: A different use of hierarchical sensing consists of identifying areas within the monitoring field that need a higher resolution observation. Such areas can be identified by relying on a coarse-grained description of the field from lower accuracy sensors and activating additional high-resolution ones only in areas where it is requested to have accurate acquisitions.

2. Adaptive sampling techniques are aimed at dynamically adapting the sensor sampling rate by exploiting spatial and temporal correlations among acquired data and the available energy whenever the sensor node is able to harvest energy from the environment as follows:

a. Activity-driven adaptive sampling: Activity-driven adaptive sampling exploits both temporal and spatial correlation among the acquired data.

b. Harvesting-aware adaptive sampling: Harvesting-aware adaptive sampling techniques develop knowledge about the residual and predicted energy coming from the harvester module at the unit level to optimize its power consumption. The approach requires developing models able to characterize the progress of energy availability over time and the energy consumption of sensor units.

3. Model-based active sampling [75] consists of building a model of the sensed phenomenon on top of an initial set of sampled data. Once the model is available, instead of sampling the quantity of interest, the next data can be predicted by the model, hence saving the data-sensing power consumption. The model needs to be updated or reestimated whenever the requested accuracy is no longer satisfied to adopt the new dynamics of the physical phenomenon under observation. Correlation-based sampler selection is performed at each cluster head in order to determine the nodes that capture the best spatial and temporal correlations among the other sensor readings [76].

7.4.3 Low-Power System Design

Currently, most WMSN components are fabricated using CMOS technology. Intelligent, wireless microsensor node technology, based on commercial, low-cost CMOS fabrication and bulk micromachining, has demonstrated the capability to have multiple sensors, electronic interfaces, control, and communication in a single device. However, they face challenges in the form of the requirements for power consumption and the complete integration of a CMOS RF transceiver [77].

The main reason for the bias toward CMOS is that this technology is cost-efficient and inherently consumes less power than other technologies. The dominant factor of power consumption in CMOS is *dynamic*. A first-order approximation of the dynamic power consumption P_d of CMOS circuitry is given by the following formula [61]:

$$P_d = C_{eff} V^2 f \qquad (7.4)$$

where C_{eff} is the effective switch capacitance, V is the supply voltage, and f is the frequency of operations. The power dissipation arises from the charging and discharging of the circuit node capacitance found on the output of internal circuit capacitances. C_{eff} combines two factors: C, the capacitance being charged and discharged, and the *activity weighting* α, which is the probability that a transition will occur.

$$C_{eff} = \alpha C \qquad (7.5)$$

Therefore, lower level power consumption can be decreased by reducing the supply voltage, the capacitive load, or the switching frequency. Good system design attempts to make a system optimal for a certain application and environment, which takes into consideration various parameters such as supply voltage and clock frequency. However, energy efficiency in WMSNs is not a one-time design problem, to be solved during the design phase. Rather, it requires frequent adaptations to the system so that it can fulfill requirements in terms of a general quality of service model. This multidimensional design space offers a wide range of possible optimization.

7.4.4 Dynamic Voltage Scaling

It is well known that processor workloads can vary significantly, and it is highly desirable for the processor to scale its energy with the workload. The dynamic computing slowdown factor procedure is to alter the supply voltage and operating frequency of the system dynamically during task scheduling in accordance with recent tasks and execution history.

Although shutdown techniques can yield substantial energy savings in idle system states, additional energy savings are possible by optimizing the sensor node performance in the active state. DVS is an effective technique for reducing CPU energy. Simply reducing the operating frequency during periods of reduced activity results in linear decreases in power consumption, but does not affect the total energy consumed per task. Reducing the operating voltage implies greater critical path delays, which in turn compromise peak performance.

DVS is the active adjustment of the supply voltage in conjunction with the clock frequency in response to fluctuations in a processor's utilization. Peak performance is not always required and, therefore, the processor's operating voltage and frequency can be dynamically adapted according to the instantaneous processing requirement, which results in a nearly quadratic savings in energy and reduces leakage current. A voltage scheduler, running in tandem with an operating system's task scheduler, can adjust voltage and frequency in response to a priori knowledge or predictions of the system's workload. DVS has been successfully applied to custom chip sets.

DVS can be implemented using a DC–DC converter circuit with a dynamically digitally adjustable voltage that delivers power to a microprocessor core and is controlled by a multithreaded, power-aware operating system, as shown in Figures 7.4 and 7.5. A buck regulator composed of discrete components is driven by a commercial step-down switching regulator controller [78]. This controller is programmed with a 5-bit digital value to regulate 1 of 32 voltages between 0.9 and 2.0 V. The operating system running on the microprocessor commands the core voltage as a 5-bit digital value that is passed to the regulator controller. External programmable logic between microprocessor and the regulator controller prevents the regulator from delivering a voltage beyond the microprocessor core's rated maximum.

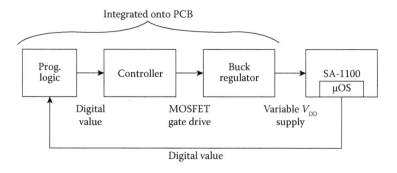

Figure 7.4 Overview of the adjustable DC–DC converter. (From Hac, A.: *Wireless sensor network designs*, 2003. Copyright Wiley-VCH Verlag GmbH & Co. KGaA.)

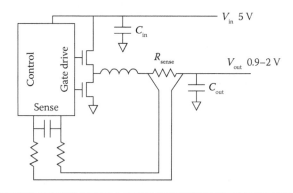

Figure 7.5 Simplified schematic for the buck regulator. (From Hac, A.: *Wireless sensor network designs*, 2003. Copyright Wiley-VCH Verlag GmbH & Co. KGaA.)

In the implementation, the microprocessor operation system monitors load on the processor and adjusts the clock frequency and supply voltage together to meet throughput requirements imposed by the tasks. Though the majority of throughput requirements and real-time deadlines on a sensor network are known *a priori*, more sophisticated load prediction algorithms may be needed for more optimal voltage scheduling for nondeterministic workload.

The rate at which DVS is carried out also has a significant bearing on performance and energy. A low update rate implies greater workload averaging, which results in lower energy use. The update energy and performance cost is also amortized over a longer time frame. Conversely, a low update rate also implies a greater performance hit, because the system will not respond to a sudden increase in workload.

7.4.5 Lifetime Prolongation Evaluation

To evaluate the scheduling scheme in terms of power conservation, we compare the cooperative scheduling scheme with a single-tier network or one tier of a multitier architecture consisting of N nodes monitoring without coordination among them, in which, nodes are awakened at a time period of T [79,80]. We note that the evaluation is over the sensing subsystem and that the radio subsystem (i.e., transmission and reception of packets) is not taken into account.

The energy (E) consumed in the network for object detection by N nodes during a duty-cycle interval of T in the noncollaborative scheduling is

$$E = N \cdot (T_{\text{sleep}} \cdot P_{\text{sleep}} + E_{\text{w\_up}} + E_{\text{cap}} + E_{\text{detect}}) \qquad (7.6)$$

where T_{sleep} and P_{sleep} are the period and power consumption for a node in sleep mode. $E_{\text{w\_up}}$, E_{cap}, and E_{detect} are the energies consumed in waking up a node, capturing a picture, and performing object detection, respectively.

Consider the cooperative scheduling algorithm in a clustered tier/network; both the interval between waking up consecutive nodes in the same cluster and the period during which a given node is awakened, are functions of the size of the cluster that the nodes belong to.

Note that, in large clusters, T_{interval} is small and thus cluster duty-cycle frequency is increased. Moreover, a larger number of nodes in the cluster takes a longer period T_p to awaken a given node of the cluster and thus enhances the power conservation in the cluster members. Assuming an average cluster size for all clusters in the tier/network, T_p will be

$$T_P = \frac{T \cdot \mu C_{\text{size}}}{\mu C_{\text{size}} - \gamma \cdot (\mu C_{\text{size}} - 1)} \tag{7.7}$$

where T is the base period for waking nodes in the base uncoordinated tier, C_{size} is the size of the cluster, μC_{size} is the average cluster size, and γ is the clustering scale.

Figure 7.6 shows the evolution of T_p normalized by T (i.e., $\mu C_{\text{size}}/\beta$) for several node densities and γ [18]. The factor β represents the increment of area that the cluster senses with respect to an individual sensor.

Consequently, the total average energy consumption by nodes for object detection in the coordinated tier during T_p will be

$$E_P = E + N \cdot P_{\text{sleep}} \cdot (T_P - T) \tag{7.8}$$

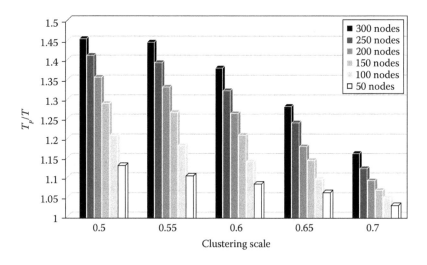

Figure 7.6 T_P/T for several node densities and clustering scales. (From Alaei, M., and Barceló, J., *Wireless communications and networks: Recent advances*, Rijeka, Croatia, InTech, 2012.)

7.5 Energy Harvesting

Energy-harvesting techniques, also referred to as "energy scavenging," extract energy from the environment where the sensor itself exists, offering another important means to prolong the lifetime of sensor devices. Traditionally, energy has been harvested through solar light, background radio signals, thermoelectric conversion, vibrational excitation, and the human body [81]. Solar panels are made up of *photovoltaic* cells that convert sunlight directly into electrical current, coupled with super capacitors and rechargeable batteries [82]. However, the primary disadvantage of solar panels is that they are large and require continuous sunlight to work. In most wireless networking situations, it is not practical to be limited by such constraints. Solar panels achieve only about 16–18% efficiency [66].

Super capacitors can also be used in these systems to effectively lower the impedance of a battery of the energy-harvesting system to allow larger peak currents or to store charge from the energy harvester to compensate for lulls, such as nighttime for a solar cell. Super capacitors can store up to 10 mJ/mm^3, which is less than 1% of the energy density of lithium cells [24].

Most recently, technology using piezoelectric materials has been used for power generation. Piezoelectricity is an electric current created by subjecting certain types of crystal to mechanical stress. The primary advantage of piezoelectric materials over solar panels is that they are small, do not require access to direct sunlight, and operate with about a 70% mechanical-to-electrical transduction efficiency.

For collecting energy from background radio signals, an electric field of 1 V/m yields only 0.26 1 W/cm^2, in contrast to 100 1 W/cm^2 produced by a crystalline silicon solar cell exposed to bright sunlight [3]. Electric fields of intensity of a few V/m are only encountered when it is close to strong transmitters. Another practice of broadcasting RF energy deliberately to power electronic devices is severely constrained by legal limits set for health and safety concerns.

Unlike thermoelectric conversion, which may not be suitable for wireless devices, harvesting energy from vibrations in the surrounding environment can provide another useful power source. Vibration-based magnetic power generators derived by moving magnets or coils may yield power that ranges from tens of microwatts when

Table 7.8 Power Output from Various Energy-Scavenging Technologies

HARVESTING TECHNOLOGY	POWER DENSITY
Solar cells—direct sun	15 mW/cm²
Solar cells—cloudy day	0.15 mW/cm²
Solar cells—indoors	0.006 mW/cm²
Solar cells—desk lamp <60 W	0.57 mW/cm²
Piezoelectric—shoe inserts	330 µW/cm²
Vibration—microwave oven	0.01–0.1 mW/cm²
Thermoelectric—10°C gradient	40 µW/cm²
Acoustic noise—100 dB	9.6–4 mW/cm²
Passive human-powered system	1.8 mW²
Nuclear reaction	80 mW/cm³ 1E6 mWh/cm³

Source: Stojcev, M.K. et al., *9th International Conference on Telecommunication in Modern Satellite, Cable, and Broadcasting Services,* © 2009 IEEE.

generated by microelectromechanical system technologies to over a milliwatt for larger devices. Other vibration-based microgenerators are relying on charged capacitors with moving plates and, depending on their excitation and power conditioning, yield power in the order of 10 1 W [3]. However, recent microgenerators [83] have yielded up to 800 µW/cm³ from machine-induced stimuli, which is orders of magnitude greater than the power provided by currently available microgenerators [81]. Hence, this seems to be a promising technology for small battery-powered devices. Table 7.8 shows power outputs for typical energy-scavenging devices.

Although these techniques may provide an additional source of energy and help prolong the lifetime of sensor devices, they yield power that is several orders of magnitude lower compared to the power consumption of state-of-the-art multimedia devices. Hence, they may currently be suitable only for very low duty-cycle devices.

7.5.1 Energetic Sustainability

A workload can be called energetically sustainable if, at each node, the power required for processing data packets and routing them to base stations is sustained completely by the power harvested from the environment.

The maximum energetically sustainable workload (MESW) is defined as a workload that can be energetically sustained by each node involved in packet processing and routing and that cannot be incremented without violating the energetic sustainability at some nodes. In the case of continuous uniform monitoring applications, the MESW is defined as the maximum rate at which data packets are produced by all sensors and delivered to base stations. Both the MESW of the routing algorithm under study and the theoretical optimal MESW, that is, the MESW of the best routing algorithm applicable to the network, need to be determined to evaluate the optimality of a routing algorithm.

To determine to what extent packet energy P_e spent by a node n can be sustained by the power it harvests from the environment, a recovery time (T_e) is defined as the amount of time required by the energy scavenger to provide packet energy P_e to a node n. The recovery time is the ratio between P_e and the environmental power P_n available at the node n:

$$T_e = P_e/P_n \tag{7.9}$$

The workload can be considered energetically sustainable and the lifetime of the network is theoretically unlimited if the average inter-arrival time of packets on each edge is longer than the corresponding recovery time.

Recovery time directly correlates packet processing rate with available power. Channel capacity (C_e) of the maximum packet rate across an edge (e) is usually limited by the channel bandwidth, which represents energetic sustainability constraints. Hence, the channel capacity of edge e corresponds to its inverted recovery time:

$$C_e = 1/T_e \tag{7.10}$$

The flow F_e across the edge e is limited by its energetically sustainable channel capacity, which is expressed by

$$Fe \le C_e = 1/T_e = P_n/P_e \tag{7.11}$$

Effective algorithms exist for determining the maximum flow between any pair of nodes in flow networks (networks with annotated channel capacities) by solving the so-called max flow problem [84]. It has been suggested that energy-harvesting WSNs can be viewed as flow networks and MESW problems cast into instances of max flow [85]. However, if Equation 7.11 is used to compute edge capacities, the overall maximum flow might end up being over-estimated, due to the fact that all edges with the same source share the same power budget available at the common source node.

Therefore, a more general class of flow networks, called "node-constrained flow networks" [86], is needed to properly model the flow *Fe* across any edge *e* exiting from node *n*, which is limited not only by its maximum capacity, given by Equation 7.11, but also by the overall power budget of node *n*. This is expressed by

$$\sum_{e \text{ exiting from } n} F_e P_e \leq Pn \qquad (7.12)$$

For only one outgoing edge node, Equation 7.12 is equivalent to Equation 7.11.

7.6 Summary

WMSNs have several factors that mainly influence their design, such as high bandwidth demand, integration with other wireless technologies, and power consumption. Prolonging the lifetime of operating battery and hardware power optimizations have been the focus of a vast amount of research in WMSNs. This research includes dynamic optimization of voltage and clock rate, wake-up procedures to keep high power-consuming electronics inactive most of the time, and energy-optimized protocol development for sensor communications.

Extracting energy from the environment is another important field. There are various forms of energy that can be harvested, such as thermal, mechanical, magnetic, solar, acoustic, wind, and wave. Additional sources of energy can help prolong the lifetime of sensor devices.

In this chapter, we looked into various ways of optimizing the power consumption of existing WMSNs. We also identified various unconventional sources of energy-harvesting based on available techniques and compared their advantages.

References

1. Gürses, E., Akan, O.B. Multimedia communication in wireless sensor networks. In: *Annales des Télécommunications* 60(7–8), pp. 872–900. Springer-Verlag, 2005.

2. Misra, S., Reisslein, M., Xue, G. A survey of multimedia streaming in wireless sensor networks. *Communications Surveys & Tutorials, IEEE* 10(4), 18–39, 2008.

3. Akyildiz, I.F., Melodia, T., Chowdhury, K.R. A survey on wireless multimedia sensor networks. *Computer Networks* 51(4), 921–960, 2007.

4. Aaron, A., Rane, S.D., Setton, E., Girod, B. Transform-domain Wyner-Ziv codec for video. In: *Electronic Imaging 2004*, pp. 520–528. International Society for Optics and Photonics, 2004.

5. Yang, Z., Liao, S., Cheng, W. Joint power control and rate adaptation in wireless sensor networks. *Ad Hoc Networks* 7(2), 401–410, 2009.

6. Chandrakasan, A.P., Brodersen, R.W. Minimizing power consumption in digital CMOS circuits. *Proceedings of the IEEE* 83(4), 498–523, 1995.

7. Gonzalez, R., Horowitz, M. Energy dissipation in general purpose microprocessors. *IEEE Journal of Solid-State Circuits* 31(9), 1277–1284, 1996.

8. Chang, J.H., Tassiulas, L. Energy conserving routing in wireless ad-hoc networks. In: *INFOCOM 2000. 19th Annual Joint Conference of the IEEE Computer and Communications Societies. Proceedings. IEEE*, vol. 1, pp. 22–31. IEEE, 2000.

9. Boice, J., Lu, X., Margi, C., Stanek, G., Zhang, G., Manduchi, R., Obraczka, K. Meerkats: A power-aware, self-managing wireless camera network for wide area monitoring. In: *Proc. Workshop on Distributed Smart Cameras*. 2006.

10. Atmel Corporation Datasheets. www.atmel.com/products/15.03.2009

11. Akyildiz, I.F., Su, W., Sankarasubramaniam, Y., Cayirci, E. Wireless sensor networks: A survey. *Computer Networks* 38(4), 393–422, 2002.

12. Miao, G., Himayat, N., Li, Y.G., Swami, A. Cross-layer optimization for energy-efficient wireless communications: A survey. *Wireless Communications and Mobile Computing* 9(4), 529–542, 2009.

13. Gupta, G., Younis, M. Load-balanced clustering of wireless sensor networks. In: *IEEE International Conference on Communications, 2003. ICC'03*, vol. 3, pp. 1848–1852. IEEE, 2003.

14. Polastre, J., Szewczyk, R., Culler, D. Telos: Enabling ultra-low power wireless research. In: *4th International Symposium on Information Processing in Sensor Networks, 2005. IPSN 2005.*, pp. 364–369. IEEE, 2005.

15. Alippi, C., Anastasi, G., Galperti, C., Mancini, F., Roveri, M. Adaptive sampling for energy conservation in wireless sensor networks for snow monitoring applications. In: *IEEE International Conference on Mobile Ad-Hoc and Sensor Systems, 2007. MASS 2007*, pp. 1–6. IEEE, 2007.

16. Raghunathan, V., Spanos, P., Srivastava, M.B. Adaptive power-fidelity in energy-aware wireless embedded systems. In: *Real-Time Systems Symposium, 2001.(RTSS 2001). Proceedings of 22nd IEEE*, pp. 106–115. IEEE, 2001.

17. Schott, B., Bajura, M., Czarnaski, J., Flidr, J., Tho, T., Wang, L. A modular power-aware microsensor with >1000x dynamic power range. In: *Proceedings of the 4th International Symposium on Information Processing in Sensor Networks*, p. 66. IEEE Press, 2005.

18. Alaei, M., Barceló, J. Power management in sensing subsystem of wireless multimedia sensor networks. In: *Wireless communications and networks: Recent advances*. Rijeka, Croatia: InTech—Open Access Company, 2012, pp. 549–570.

19. Rahimi, M., Baer, R., Iroezi, O.I., Garcia, J.C., Warrior, J., Estrin, D., Srivastava, M. Cyclops: In situ image sensing and interpretation in wireless sensor networks. In: *Proceedings of the 3rd International Conference on Embedded Networked Sensor Systems*, pp. 192–204. ACM, 2005.

20. Rowe, A., Rosenberg, C., Nourbakhsh, I. A low cost embedded color vision system. In: *IEEE/RSJ International Conference on Intelligent Robots and Systems, 2002*, vol. 1, pp. 208–213. IEEE, 2002.

21. Margi, C.B., Manduchi, R., Obraczka, K. Energy consumption tradeoffs in visual sensor networks. In: *Proceedings of 24th Brazilian Symposium on Computer Networks*. 2006.

22. Soro, S., Heinzelman, W. A survey of visual sensor networks. *Advances in Multimedia*, pp. 1–22, 2009.

23. Pistoia, G. *Battery operated devices and systems: From portable electronics to industrial products*. Elsevier, 2008.

24. Stojcev, M.K., Kosanovic, M.R., Golubovic, L.R. Power management and energy harvesting techniques for wireless sensor nodes. In: *9th International Conference on Telecommunication in Modern Satellite, Cable, and Broadcasting Services, 2009. TELSIKS'09*, pp. 65–72. IEEE, 2009.

25. Eliasson, J. Low-power design methodologies for embedded Internet systems. *PhD Thesis*, Department of Computer Science and Electrical Engineering, Luleå University of Technology, Luleå, Sweden, 2008.

26. Crompton, Thomas, PJ. *Battery reference book*. Newnes, 2000.

27. Jones, C.E., Sivalingam, K.M., Agrawal, P., Chen, J.C. A survey of energy efficient network protocols for wireless networks. *Wireless Networks* 7(4), 343–358, 2001.

28. Negri, L., Barretta, D., Fornaciari, W. Application-level power management in pervasive computing systems: A case study. In: *Proceedings of the 1st Conference on Computing Frontiers*, pp. 78–88. ACM, 2004.

29. Tsaoussidis, V., Badr, H. TCP-probing: Towards an error control schema with energy and throughput performance gains. In: *Proceedings of 2000 International Conference on Network Protocols, 2000*, pp. 12–21. IEEE, 2000.

30. Zhang, C., Tsaoussidis, V. TCP-real: Improving real-time capabilities of TCP over heterogeneous networks. In: *Proceedings of the 11th International Workshop on Network and Operating Systems Support for Digital Audio and Video*, pp. 189–198. ACM, 2001.

31. Ee, C.T., Bajcsy, R. Congestion control and fairness for many-to-one routing in sensor networks. In: *Proceedings of the 2nd International Conference on Embedded Networked Sensor Systems*, pp. 148–161. ACM, 2004.

32. Yaghmaee, M.H., Adjeroh, D. A new priority based congestion control protocol for wireless multimedia sensor networks. In: *2008 International Symposium on a World of Wireless, Mobile and Multimedia Networks, 2008. WoWMoM 2008*, pp. 1–8. IEEE, 2008.

33. Hull, B., Jamieson, K., Balakrishnan, H. Mitigating congestion in wireless sensor networks. In: *Proceedings of the 2nd International Conference on Embedded Networked Sensor Systems*, pp. 134–147. ACM, 2004.

34. Wang, C., Li, B., Sohraby, K., Daneshmand, M., Hu, Y. Upstream congestion control in wireless sensor networks through cross-layer optimization. *IEEE Journal on Selected Areas in Communications* 25(4), 786–795, 2007.

35. Murthy, C.S.R., Manoj, B.S. *Ad hoc wireless networks: Architecture and protocols*. Prentice Hall Publishers, May 2004, ISBN 013147023X.

36. Karl, H. An overview of energy-efficiency techniques for mobile communication systems. Telecommunication Networks Group, Technical University Berlin, Berlin, Germany, Tech. Rep. TKN-03-017 (2003).

37. Ehsan, S., Hamdaoui, B. A survey on energy-efficient routing techniques with QoS assurances for wireless multimedia sensor networks. *Communications Surveys & Tutorials, IEEE* 14(2), 265–278, 2012.

38. Cerpa, A., Estrin, D. ASCENT: Adaptive self-configuring sensor networks topologies. *IEEE Transactions on Mobile Computing* 3(3), 272–285, 2004.

39. Chen, B., Jamieson, K., Balakrishnan, H., Morris, R. Span: An energy-efficient coordination algorithm for topology maintenance in ad hoc wireless networks. *Wireless Networks* 8(5), 481–494, 2002.

40. Pottie, G.J., Kaiser, W.J. Wireless integrated network sensors. *Communications of the ACM* 43(5), 51–58, 2000.

41. Wu, J., Dai, F., Gao, M., Stojmenovic, I. On calculating power-aware connected dominating sets for efficient routing in ad hoc wireless networks. *Journal of Communications and Networks* 4(1), 59–70, 2002.

42. Doumit, S.S., Agrawal, D.P. Self-organizing and energy-efficient network of sensors. In: *MILCOM 2002. Proceedings*, vol. 2, pp. 1245–1250. IEEE, 2002.

43. Rabaey, J.M., Ammer, M.J., da Silva Jr, J.L., Patel, D., Roundy, S. PicoRadio supports ad hoc ultra-low power wireless networking. *Computer* 33(7), 42–48, 2000.

44. Shih, E., Cho, S.H., Ickes, N., Min, R., Sinha, A., Wang, A., Chandrakasan, A. Physical layer driven protocol and algorithm design for energy-efficient wireless sensor networks. In: *Proceedings of the 7th Annual International Conference on Mobile Computing and Networking*, pp. 272–287. ACM, 2001.

45. Alghamdi, M.I. PARM: A power-aware message scheduling algorithm for real-time wireless networks. In: *11th IEEE International Conference on Computational Science and Engineering Workshops, 2008. CSEWORKSHOPS'08*, pp. 299–306. IEEE, 2008.

46. Mangione-Smith, W., Ghang, P.S. A low power medium access control protocol for portable multi-media systems. *3rd International Workshop on Mobile Multi Media Communications*, September 25–27, 1996.

47. Stemm, M. Measuring and reducing energy consumption of network interfaces in hand-held devices. *IEICE Transactions on Communications* 80(8), 1125–1131, 1997.

48. Jayashree, S., Manoj, B.S., Murthy, C. On using battery state for medium access control in ad hoc wireless networks. In: *Proceedings of the 10th Annual International Conference on Mobile Computing and Networking,* pp. 360–373. ACM, 2004.

49. Yu, Y., Krishnamachari, B., Prasanna, V.K. Issues in designing middleware for wireless sensor networks. *Network, IEEE* 18(1), 15–21, 2004.

50. Zheng, R., Hou, J.C., Sha, L. Asynchronous wakeup for ad hoc networks. In: *Proceedings of the 4th ACM International Symposium on Mobile Ad Hoc Networking & Computing,* pp. 35–45. ACM, 2003.

51. Van Dam, T., Langendoen, K. An adaptive energy-efficient MAC protocol for wireless sensor networks. In: *Proceedings of the 1st International Conference on Embedded Networked Sensor Systems,* pp. 171–180. ACM, 2003.

52. Hohlt, B., Doherty, L., Brewer, E. Flexible power scheduling for sensor networks. In: *Proceedings of the 3rd International Symposium on Information Processing in Sensor Networks,* pp. 205–214. ACM, 2004.

53. Singh, S., Raghavendra, C.S. PAMAS—power aware multi-access protocol with signalling for ad hoc networks. *ACM SIGCOMM Computer Communication Review* 28(3), 5–26, 1998.

54. Singh, S., Woo, M., Raghavendra, C.S. Power-aware routing in mobile ad hoc networks. In: *Proceedings of the 4th Annual ACM/IEEE International Conference on Mobile Computing and Networking,* pp. 181–190. ACM, 1998.

55. Xu, Y., Heidemann, J., Estrin, D. Adaptive energy-conserving routing for multihop ad hoc networks. In: *Research report 527, USC/Information Sciences Institute.* 2000.

56. Stemm, M., Gauthier, P., Harada, D., and Katz, R. Reducing Power Consumption of Network Interfaces in Hand-Held Devices, In: *Proceedings 3rd Intl. Workshop on Mobile Multimedia Communications,* Princeton, NJ, 1996.

57. Polastre, J., Hui, J., Levis, P., Zhao, J., Culler, D., Shenker, S., Stoica, I. A unifying link abstraction for wireless sensor networks. In: *Proceedings of the 3rd International Conference on Embedded Networked Sensor Systems,* pp. 76–89. ACM, 2005.

58. Jacome, M., Catthoor, F. Special issue on power-aware embedded computing. *ACM Transactions on Embedded Computing Systems (TECS)* 2(3), 251–254, 2003. ISSN: 1539-9087.

59. Brown, C. Endless energy is harvesting's promise. EE Times. February 27, 2006. http://www.powermanagementdesignline.com/showArticle.jhtml?articleID=181400884

60. Hac, A. *Wireless sensor network designs.* West Sussex, UK: John Wiley & Sons, 2003.

61. Havinga, P.J.M., Smit, G.J.M. Energy-efficient wireless networking for multimedia applications. *Wireless Communications and Mobile Computing* 1(2), 165–184, 2001.

62. Liu, D., Svensson, C. Power consumption estimation in CMOS VLSI chips. *IEEE Journal of Solid-State Circuits* 29(6), 663–670, 1994.

63. Ho, R., Mai, K.W., Horowitz, M.A. The future of wires. *Proceedings of the IEEE* 89(4), 490–504, 2001.

64. Sylvester, D., Keutzer, K. A global wiring paradigm for deep submicron design. *IEEE Transactions on Computer-Aided Design of Integrated Circuits and Systems* 19(2), 242–252, 2000.

65. Raghunathan, V., Srivastava, M.B., Gupta, R.K. A survey of techniques for energy efficient on-chip communication. In: *Proceedings of the 40th annual Design Automation Conference*, pp. 900–905. ACM, 2003.

66. Lettieri, P., Srivastava, M.B. A QoS-aware, energy-efficient wireless node architecture. In: *1999 IEEE International Workshop on Mobile Multimedia Communications, 1999 (MoMuC'99)*, pp. 252–261. IEEE, 1999.

67. Chang, J., Ravi, S., Raghunathan, A. FLEXBAR: A crossbar switching fabric with improved performance and utilization. In: *Proceedings of the IEEE 2002 Custom Integrated Circuits Conference, 2002*, pp. 405–408. IEEE, 2002.

68. Chang, H., Cooke, L., Hunt, M., Martin, G., McNelly, A., Todd, L. Surviving the SoC revolution. *A Guide to Platform-Based Design*. Kluwer (1999).

69. Wang, H.S., Peh, L.S., Malik, S. A power model for routers: Modeling Alpha 21364 and InfiniBand routers. In: *Proceedings of the 10th Symposium on High Performance Interconnects, 2002*, pp. 21–27. IEEE, 2002.

70. Ye, T.T., De Micheli, G., Benini, L. Analysis of power consumption on switch fabrics in network routers. In: *Proceedings of the 39th Annual Design Automation Conference*, pp. 524–529. ACM, 2002.

71. Wang, H.S., Zhu, X., Peh, L.S., Malik, S. Orion: A power-performance simulator for interconnection networks. In: *Proceedings of the 35th Annual IEEE/ACM International Symposium on Microarchitecture, 2002. (MICRO-35)*, pp. 294–305. IEEE, 2002.

72. Dutta, P.K., Culler, D.E. System software techniques for low-power operation in wireless sensor networks. In: *Proceedings of the 2005 IEEE/ACM International Conference on Computer-Aided Design*, pp. 925–932. IEEE Computer Society, 2005.

73. Kijewski-Correa, T., Haenggi, M., Antsaklis, P. Wireless sensor networks for structural health monitoring: A multi-scale approach. In: *ASCE Structures 2006 Congress*. 2006.

74. Singh, A., Budzik, D., Chen, W., Batalin, M.A., Stealey, M., Borgstrom, H., Kaiser, W.J. Multiscale sensing: A new paradigm for actuated sensing of high frequency dynamic phenomena. In: *International Conference on Intelligent Robots and Systems, 2006 IEEE/RSJ*, pp. 328–335. IEEE, 2006.

75. Deshpande, A., Guestrin, C., Madden, S.R., Hellerstein, J.M., Hong, W. Model-driven data acquisition in sensor networks. In: *Proceedings of the 30th International Conference on Very Large Data Bases - Volume 30*, pp. 588–599. VLDB Endowment, 2004.

76. Jeličić, V. Power management in wireless sensor networks with high-consuming sensors. *Qualifying Doctoral Examination*, University of Zagreb, 2011.

77. Bult, K., Burstein, A., Chang, D., Dong, M., Fielding, M., Kruglick, E., Ho, J. et al. Low power systems for wireless microsensors. In: *International Symposium on Low Power Electronics and Design, 1996*, pp. 17–21. IEEE, 1996.

78. Hac, A. *Wireless sensor network designs*. West Sussex, UK: John Wiley & Sons, 2003.

79. Kulkarni, P., Ganesan, D., Shenoy, P., Lu, Q. SensEye: A multi-tier camera sensor network. In: *Proceedings of the 13th Annual ACM International Conference on Multimedia*, pp. 229–238. ACM, 2005.

80. Feng, W.C., Kaiser, E., Feng, W.C., Le Baillif, M. Panoptes: Scalable low-power video sensor networking technologies. *ACM Transactions on Multimedia Computing, Communications, and Applications (TOMCCAP)* 1(2), 151–167, 2005.

81. Paradiso, J.A., Starner, T. Energy scavenging for mobile and wireless electronics. *Pervasive Computing, IEEE* 4(1), 18–27, 2005.

82. Jiang, X., Polastre, J., Culler, D. Perpetual environmentally powered sensor networks. In: *4th International Symposium on Information Processing in Sensor Networks, 2005. IPSN 2005*, pp. 463–468. IEEE, 2005.

83. Mitcheson, P.D., Green, T.C., Yeatman, E.M., Holmes, A.S. Architectures for vibration-driven micropower generators. *Journal of Microelectromechanical Systems*, 13(3), 429–440, 2004.

84. Ford, L.R., Fulkerson, D.R. *Flows in Networks*, Princeton University Press, 1962.

85. Lattanzi, E., Regini, E., Acquaviva, A., Bogliolo, A. Energetic sustainability of routing algorithms for energy-harvesting wireless sensor networks. *Computer Communications* 30(14), 2976–2986, 2007.

86. Bogliolo, A., Lattanzi, E., Acquaviva, A. Energetic sustainability of environmentally powered wireless sensor networks. In: *Proceedings of the 3rd ACM International Workshop on Performance Evaluation of Wireless Ad Hoc, Sensor and Ubiquitous Networks*, pp. 149–152. ACM, 2006.

Index

Milton Keynes UK
Ingram Content Group UK Ltd.
UKHW040447071024
449327UK00020B/1063

9 780367 575366